Academic Pain Medicine

Yury Khelemsky • Anuj Malhotra
Karina Gritsenko
Editors

Academic Pain Medicine

A Practical Guide to Rotations, Fellowship, and Beyond

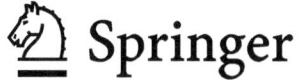 Springer

Editors
Yury Khelemsky
Pain Medicine Fellowship
Department of Anesthesiology, Perioperative and
Pain Medicine
Department of Neurology
Icahn School of Medicine at Mount Sinai
New York, NY
USA

Anuj Malhotra
Pain Medicine Fellowship
Department of Anesthesiology, Perioperative and
Pain Medicine
Icahn School of Medicine at Mount Sinai
New York, NY
USA

Karina Gritsenko
Regional Anesthesia and
Acute Pain Medicine Fellowship
Department of Anesthesiology
Albert Einstein College of Medicine
Montefiore Medical Center
Bronx, NY
USA

ISBN 978-3-030-18004-1   ISBN 978-3-030-18005-8   (eBook)
https://doi.org/10.1007/978-3-030-18005-8

This Springer imprint is published by the registered company Springer Nature Switzerland AG
The registered company address is: Gewerbestrasse 11, 6330 Cham, Switzerland

Preface

The specialty of Pain Medicine is relatively new, when compared to more established fields. Consequently, the base of required knowledge and skill is in a constant state of expansion and modification. The core requirements for the Accreditation Council for Graduate Medical Education (ACGME) accredited pain fellowships did not emerge until about 10 years ago and have since undergone multiple significant revisions.

There has been a clear, unmet need for a standardized text to be used by fellows in ACGME-accredited pain fellowship programs in order to provide a clinically relevant narrative to their training, as well as help prepare them for certification exams. This work was created to do just this. Additionally, it may serve as a valuable overview of the field for medical students, residents, non-physician providers, as well as physicians in other fields.

We believe that this text provides a blueprint for the emerging legitimate specialty of Pain Medicine and that it provides a common set of ideas for clinicians who have undergone the rigorous training and certification required in order to have the privilege of alleviating pain and suffering. And more than anything, we hope that the pages of future iterations of works like this are filled with new and ever-effective treatments of pain, developed by someone reading this preface.

New York, NY, USA   Yury Khelemsky
                                                                                                                    Anuj Malhotra
Bronx, NY, USA   Karina Gritsenko

Contents

Contributors

Rishi R. Agarwal, MD Department of Anesthesiology, Northwestern, Chicago, IL, USA

Rehan Ali, MD Icahn School of Medicine, Mount Sinai Department of Anesthesiology, Division of Pain Medicine, New York, NY, USA

Shawn Amin, DO Anesthesiology – Department of Pain Medicine, Rutgers University – New Jersey Medical School, Newark, NJ, USA

Michael Andreae, MD Department of Anesthesiology, Penn State Milton S. Hershey Medical Center, Hershey, PA, USA

Magdalena Anitescu, MD, PhD Department of Anesthesia and Critical Care, University of Chicago Medicine, Chicago, IL, USA

Christy Anthony, MD Department of Anesthesiology and Pain Management, University Hospital, Rutgers – NJMS, Newark, NJ, USA

Ingrid Fitz-James Antoine, MD Montefiore Medical Center, Albert Einstein College of Medicine, Bronx, NY, USA

Melinda Aquino, MD Montefiore Medical Center, Albert Einstein College of Medicine, Bronx, NY, USA

Sumeet Arora Metro Pain & Vein, Clifton, NJ, USA

Pavel Balduyeu, MD Department of Anesthesiology, College of Medicine, University of Florida, Gainesville, FL, USA

Jaime L. Baratta, MD Sidney Kimmel Medical College, Thomas Jefferson University, Philadelphia, PA, USA

Richard A. Barnhart, DO Department of Anesthesiology, Thomas Jefferson University Hospital, Philadelphia, PA, USA

Burton D. Beakley, MD Department of Anesthesiology, LSU School of Medicine, Shreveport, LA, USA

Ramsin M. Benyamin, MD, DABIPP Millennium Pain Center, Bloomington, IL, USA
College of Medicine, University of Illinois, Urbana-Champaign, IL, USA

Nicholas Bremer, MD Department of Anesthesiology and Pain Medicine, Columbia University Medical Center, New York, NY, USA

William Caldwell, DO Department of Anesthesiology, Pain Medicine, Stony Brook University Hospital, Stony Brook, NY, USA

Ellise Cappuccio, MD Montefiore Medical Center, Albert Einstein College of Medicine, Bronx, NY, USA

Veronica Carullo, MD Pediatric Pain Management, Pediatric Anesthesiology Fellowship Program, Montefiore Medical Center, The University Hospital for Albert Einstein College of Medicine, New York, NY, USA

Azem Chami, MD Department of Anesthesiology, LSU School of Medicine, Shreveport, LA, USA

Jianguo Cheng, MD, PhD Departments of Pain Management and Neurosciences, Cleveland Clinic, Cleveland, OH, USA

Paul K. Cheng, MD Departments of Pain Management and Neurosciences, Cleveland Clinic, Cleveland, OH, USA

Jeffrey Ciccone, MD Department of Anesthesiology, Perioperative and Pain Medicine, Icahn School of Medicine at Mount Sinai Health System, New York, NY, USA

Isaac Cohen, MD Frank H. Netter School of Medicine, Quinnipiac University, Hamden, CT, USA

Elyse M. Cornett, PhD Department of Anesthesiology, LSU School of Medicine, New Orleans, LA, USA

Chris J. Cullom, MD Department of Anesthesiology, LSU School of Medicine, Shreveport, LA, USA

Christopher Curatolo, MD, MEM Department of Anesthesiology, Perioperative and Pain Medicine, Icahn School of Medicine at Mount Sinai, New York, NY, USA

Pavan Dalal, MD Department of Anesthesiology, Perioperative and Pain Medicine, Mount Sinai Hospital, New York, NY, USA

Houman Danesh, MD Department of Anesthesiology, Perioperative and Pain Medicine, Mount Sinai Hospital, New York, NY, USA

Sukdeb Datta, MD, MBA Department of Anesthesiology, Mount Sinai Medical Center, New York, NY, USA

Miles Day, MD, DABA-PM, FIPP, DABIPP Department of Anesthesiology and Pain Medicine, Texas Tech University Health Sciences Center, Lubbock, TX, USA

Timothy R. Deer, MD, DABPM, FIPP The Spine and Nerve Centers of Virginia, Charleston, WV, USA

Guensley R. Delva, MD Dartmouth Hitchcock Medical Center, Theodore Geisel School of Medicine, Lebanon, NH, USA

Julia H. Ding, MD Department of Anesthesiology, Columbia University Medical Center, NewYork-Presbyterian Hospital, New York, NY, USA

Sudhir Diwan, MD Manhattan Spine and Pain Medicine, Lenox Hill Hospital, New York, NY, USA

Anis Dizdarević, MD Department of Anesthesiology and Pain Medicine, Columbia University Medical Center, New York, NY, USA

Theodore Eckman, MD Allegheny Health Network, Erie, PA, USA

Jason H. Epstein, MD Department of Anesthesiology, James J Peters Veterans Affairs Medical Center, Bronx, NY, USA

Lawrence Epstein, MD Department of Anesthesiology, Perioperative and Pain Medicine, Mount Sinai Hospital, New York, NY, USA

Samantha Erosa, MD Department of Physical Medicine and Rehabilitation, Montefiore Medical Center, Bronx, NY, USA

Alex Feoktistov, MD, PhD Clinical Research, Diamond Health Clinic, Glenview, IL, USA

Jacquelyn K. Francis, MD Hackensack University Medical Center, Hackensack, NJ, USA

Rishi Gaiha, MD Anesthesiology, Northwestern Hospital, Chicago, IL, USA

John S. Georgy Interventional Pain Medicine, The Spine and Spine and Pain Institute of New York, New York, NY, USA

Christopher Gharibo, MD Department of Anesthesiology, NYU Langone Medical Center, New York, NY, USA

Andrew Gitkind, MD Department of Rehabilitation Medicine, Montefiore Medical Center, Bronx, NY, USA

Kathryn Glynn, MD Department of Anesthesiology and Pain Management, Texas Tech University Health Sciences Center, Lubbock, TX, USA

Chaim Goldfeiz, MD Department of Anesthesiology, NYU Langone Medical Center, New York, NY, USA

Karina Gritsenko Department of Anesthesiology, Montefiore Medical Center and Albert Einstein College of Medicine, Bronx, NY, USA

Scott Grubb, MD Department of Anesthesia and Perioperative Care, University of California San Francisco, San Francisco, CA, USA

Amitabh Gulati, MD Department of Anesthesiology and Critical Care Medicine, Memorial Sloan Kettering Cancer Center, New York, NY, USA

Alexander Haroldson Medical College of Wisconsin, Wausau, WI, USA

Corey W. Hunter, MD, FIPP Ainsworth Institute of Pain Management, New York, NY, USA

Yuriy O. Ivanov, DO Physical Medicine and Rehabilitation, Montefiore Medical Center, Bronx, NY, USA

Erica B. John, MD, BS Department of Anesthesiology and Acute Pain Management, Thomas Jefferson University, Philadelphia, PA, USA

Mark R. Jones, MD Department of Anesthesiology, Critical Care and Pain Medicine, Beth Israel Deaconess Medical Center, Boston, MA, USA

Leonardo Kapural, MD, PhD Carolinas Pain Institute & Center for Clinical Research, Winston-Salem, NC, USA

Andrew G. Kaufman, MD Department of Anesthesiology, Rutgers, New Jersey Medical School, Newark, NJ, USA

Marc W. Kaufmann, DO Department of Anesthesiology, Thomas Jefferson University Hospital, Philadelphia, PA, USA

Alan David Kaye, MD, PhD, DABA, DABIPP, DABPM Department of Anesthesiology, Louisiana State University School of Medicine, Louisiana State University Interim Hospital and Ochsner Hospital at Kenner, New Orleans, LA, USA

Yury Khelemsky Department of Anesthesiology, Mount Sinai Medical Center, New York, NY, USA

Chong H. Kim, MD PM&R and Anesthesiology, Case Western Reserve University, Cleveland, OH, USA

Soo Y. Kim, MD Physical Medicine and Rehabilitation, Montefiore Medical Center, Bronx, NY, USA

Irena Kiliptch, MD Avalon University School of Medicine, Toronto, ON, Canada

Demetri Koutsospyros, MD Department of Anesthesiology, Montefiore Medical Center, Bronx, NY, USA

Nancy S. Lee, MD Department of Anesthesiology, Montefiore Medical Center, Bronx, NY, USA

Robert Levy, MD Institute for Neuromodulation, Boca Raton, FL, USA

James Lieber, BS University of Illinois College of Medicine, Urbana, IL, USA

Sean Li, MD Premier Pain Centers, Shrewsbury, NJ, USA

Scott Maddalo NYU Langone Medical Center, New York, NY, USA

Sylvia Malcore Department of Psychiatry and Behavorial Medicine, Spectrum Health, Grand Rapids, MI, USA

Anuj Malhotra, MD Department of Anesthesiology Perioperative and Pain Medicine, Icahn School of Medicine at Mount Sinai, New York, NY, USA

Mark N. Malinowski, DO Adena Regional Medical Center, Adena Spine Center, Chillicothe, OH, USA

Laxmaiah Manchikanti, MD Pain Management Center of Paducah, Paducah, KY, USA
University of Louisville, Louisville, KY, USA

Ricardo Maturana, MD Albert Einstein College of Medicine, Montefiore Medical Center, Bronx, NY, USA

Robert McCarron Department of Psychiatry and Human Behavior, University of California, Irvine School of Medicine, Orange, CA, USA

Ryan McKenna, MD, MBA Department of Anesthesiology and Pain Management, Texas Tech University Health Sciences Center, Lubbock, TX, USA

Michael Miller, DO Department of Neurology, SUNY Upstate Medical University, Syracuse, NY, USA

Patrick Milord, MD, MBA Department of Anesthesiology, NYU Langone Medical Center, New York, NY, USA

Susan M. Mothersele, MD Department of Anesthesiology, LSU School of Medicine, New Orleans, LA, USA

Bhargav Mudda, MD Department of Anesthesiology, Texas Tech University Health Sciences Center, Lubbock, TX, USA

Jeremy Naber, DO Carolinas Pain Institute & Center for Clinical Research, Winston-Salem, NC, USA

Sam Nia, MD Department of Anesthesiology, UMASS Memorial Healthcare, Worcester, MA, USA

Carl Noe, MD Department of Anesthesiology and Pain Management, University of Texas Southwestern Medical Center, Dallas, TX, USA

Matthew B. Novitch, MD Department of Anesthesiology and Critical Care Medicine, Froedtert Hospital, Milwaukee, WI, USA

Chukwuemeka Okafor, MD Forbes Hospital, Pittsburgh, Pennsylvania, USA

Robert Otterbeck, MD Department of Anesthesiology, NYU Langone Medical Center, New York, NY, USA

Kristoffer Padjen, MD Department of Anesthesiology, NYU Langone Medical Center, New York, NY, USA

Thomas Palaia, MD Department of Anesthesiology, Mount Sinai Medical Center, New York, NY, USA

Nisheeth Pandey, MD Pain Management, Fayette County Memorial Hospital, Washington Court House, OH, USA

Joseph Park Department of Anesthesiology, Icahn School of Medicine at Mount Sinai, New York, NY, USA

George W. Pasvankas, MD Department of Anesthesia and Perioperative Care, Pain Management Center, University of California San Francisco, San Francisco, CA, USA

Alopi Patel, MD Icahn School of Medicine at Mount Sinai, New York, NY, USA

Sunny Patel, MD Icahn School of Medicine at Mount Sinai, New York, NY, USA

Priya Pinto, MD Division of Palliative Medicine and Bioethics, NYU Winthrop Hospital, Mineola, NY, USA

Jason Pope, MD Evolve Restorative Center, Santa Rosa, CA, USA

Ravi Prasad, PhD Division of Pain Medicine, Stanford University, Redwood City, CA, USA

Rene Przkora, MD, PhD Department of Anesthesiology, College of Medicine, University of Florida, Gainesville, FL, USA

Gabor Racz, MD Texas Tech University Health Sciences Center, Lubbock, TX, USA

Amir Ramezani Physical Medicine & Rehabilitation, University of California, Davis, Sacramento, CA, USA

Yury Rapoport, MD Department of Anesthesiology, Tulane School of Medicine, New Orleans, LA, USA

Vibhav Reddy, MD Department of Anesthesiology, Tulane School of Medicine, New Orleans, LA, USA

Vincent Reformato, MD Department of Anesthesiology, Rutgers, New Jersey Medical School, Newark, NJ, USA

Rahul Sarna, MD Pain Specialists of Austin, Austin, TX, USA

Eric S. Schwenk, MD Sidney Kimmel Medical College, Thomas Jefferson University, Philadelphia, PA, USA

Stelian Serban, MD Department of Anesthesiology Perioperative and Pain Medicine, Icahn School of Medicine at Mount Sinai, New York, NY, USA

Sapan Shah, MD Department of Anesthesiology, Columbia University Medical Center, New York Presbyterian Hospital, New York, NY, USA

Naum Shaparin, MD, MBA Department of Anesthesiology, Montefiore Medical Center, Bronx, NY, USA

Lowell Shih, MD Department of Pain Management, Ochsner health Center, Covington, LA, USA

Jonathan Silverman, MD Department of Anesthesiology, Weill-Cornell Medical Center, New York, NY, USA

Adeepa Singh, MD Montefiore Medical Center, New York, NY, USA

William J. Smith, BS Millennium Pain Center, Bloomington, IL, USA

Jonathan Snitzer, MD Pain Management Specialist, Fairview Clinics, Blaine, MN, USA

Max Snyder, MD Department of Anesthesiology, Montefiore Medical Center, Bronx, NY, USA

Andrew So, MD Albert Einstein College of Medicine, Montefiore Medical Center, Bronx, NY, USA

Dmitri Souza, MD, PhD Western Reserve Hospital, Heritage College of Osteopathic Medicine, Ohio University, Cuyahoga Falls, OH, USA

Peter Staats, MD Premier Pain Centers, Shrewsbury, NJ, USA

Zakari A. Suleiman, MD, FIPP Department of Anaesthesia, University of Ilorin Teaching Hospital, Ilorin, Nigeria

Vinoo Thomas, MD Department of Anesthesiology, Mount Sinai Medical Center, New York, NY, USA

Andrea Trescot, MD Pain and Headache Center, Eagle River, AK, USA

Victor Tseng, MD Division of Regional Anesthesia & Acute Pain Management, Department of Anesthesiology, Westchester Medical Center, New York Medical College, Valhalla, NY, USA

Will Tyson, MD Icahn School of Medicine at Mount Sinai, New York, NY, USA

David Vahedi, MD Fellow in Pain Management, Mount Sinai Medical Center, New York, NY, USA

Cameran Vakassi, MD Department of Anesthesiology, Critical Care and Pain Medicine, Beth Israel Deaconess Medical Center, Boston, MA, USA

Ricardo Vallejo, MD Illinois Weslayan University, Bloomington, IL, USA

Katrina von-Kriegenbergh, MD Department of Anesthesiology, Pain Medicine, Texas Tech University Health Sciences Center, Lubbock, TX, USA

David R. Walega, MD, MSCI Division of Pain Medicine, Department of Anesthesiology, Northwestern University Feinberg School of Medicine, Chicago, IL, USA

Laura Wandner, PhD Walter Reed National Military Medical Center, Bethesda, MD, USA

Arjun Yerasi, MD Department of Anesthesiology, Perioperative and Pain Medicine, Icahn School of Medicine at Mount Sinai, New York, NY, USA

Xiao Zheng Icahn School of Medicine at Mount Sinai, New York, NY, USA

Awss Zidan, MD Department of Neurology, SUNY Upstate Medical University, Syracuse, NY, USA

Anatomy and Physiology: Mechanisms of Nociceptive Transmission

Scott Grubb and George W. Pasvankas

Introduction

Nociceptive pain is defined as sensation generated from actual or threatened damage to non-neural tissue and begins with the encoding of noxious stimuli in the nervous system [1]. Nociception itself is the initiation of a signal in peripheral nerves that is of sufficient intensity to trigger reflex withdrawal, autonomic responses, and/or the perception of pain by higher-order cortical structures [2]. The sensation of pain does not necessarily follow directly from nociceptive signaling, however, as pain perception is instead characterized as the unpleasant sensory or emotional experience which results from such signaling. Figure 1.1 depicts the fundamental process elements of the nociceptive pain pathway: transduction, transmission, perception, and modulation [3].

From peripheral nerves to the integrative network of the brain, the relay of pain signals is facilitated by a complex system of neural structures, each serving to modulate the experience that is the perception of pain. The key processes involved in nociception include transduction via specialized receptive elements and dorsal root ganglia (DRG), transmission via ascending relay tracts through the spinal cord and brainstem, and modulation in primary integrative sites in the thalamus and cortex. Each of these levels of neuronal signaling contributes to the totality of sensory input to the organism, and dysfunction at any level can contribute to the generation of chronic pain states [4].

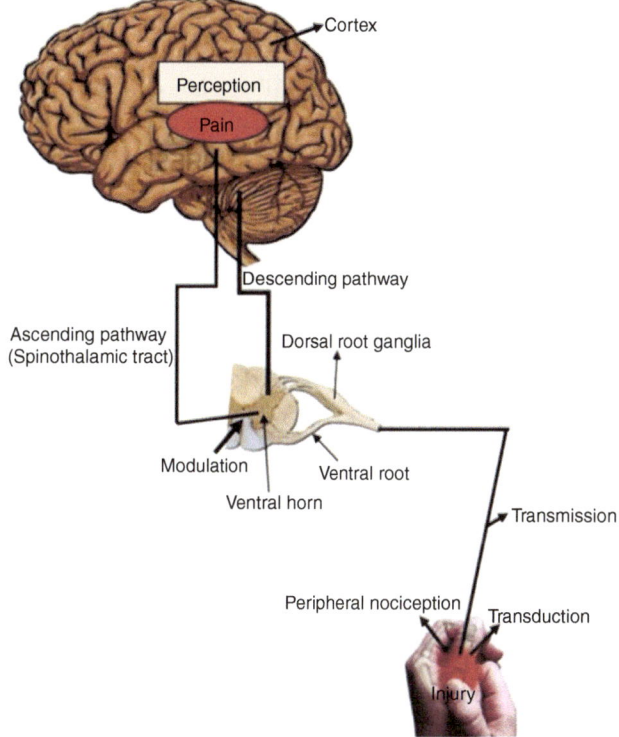

Fig. 1.1 The fundamental components of the nociceptive pain pathway. The system begins at the site of tissue injury which is transduced into a neuronal signal by peripheral nociceptive fibers. The nociceptive signal is then transmitted along the axon of the afferent nerve to synapse in the dorsal horn. Second-order projection neurons transmit the signal to higher order integrative centers in the CNS where pain perception occurs. Finally, pain sensation is modulated by specific integrative centers in the brain and via descending projection neurons which feedback to synapse in the spinal cord [3]

S. Grubb
Department of Anesthesia and Perioperative Care, University of California San Francisco, San Francisco, CA, USA

G. W. Pasvankas (✉)
Department of Anesthesia and Perioperative Care, Pain Management Center, University of California San Francisco, San Francisco, CA, USA
e-mail: george.pasvankas@ucsf.edu

Peripheral Mechanisms: Primary Peripheral Nociceptors, the Dorsal Root Ganglion (DRG), and Spinal Cord Projections

Noxious stimulation is generated through specialized peripheral structures located throughout tissue in skin, joints, muscle, dura, as well as the adventitia of blood vessels [5]. These

Y. Khelemsky et al. (eds.), *Academic Pain Medicine*, https://doi.org/10.1007/978-3-030-18005-8_1

nociceptors serve to detect mechanical, chemical, and thermal input which are potentially damaging to tissue and to relay those signals to central integrative centers which generate protective behaviors [6]. Nociceptors can be *polymodal* – meaning they may be activated by different forms of noxious input such as mechanical, chemical, or thermal stimuli – or may be specialized to one form of input [6]. A nociceptive peripheral nerve is comprised of the peripheral terminal in a target tissue, the axon which conducts an action potential to the CNS, the cell body located in the DRG or cranial nerve ganglion, and the central terminal where the cell synapses on second-order neurons in the CNS [2] (Fig. 1.2).

Primary afferent *C fibers* are small, unmyelinated nerves, which conduct nociceptive signals at velocities slower than 2.5 m/s. *Aδ fibers* are thinly-myelinated nerves and have conduction velocities of 4–30 m/s [5]. C fibers are more numerous in the dorsal roots than Aδ fibers; however, both C and Aδ fibers can travel with other somatic and autonomic motor axons. The cell bodies of these nociceptive nerves are invariably located in the DRG or trigeminal ganglia (CN V), enter the spinal cord on the dorsal surface, and synapse in the dorsal horn. Secondary neurons in the spinal cord project axons across the midline to ascend to the thalamus via the lateral and ventral *spinothalamic tracts (STT)*. STT cells located in the superficial dorsal horn ascend via the lateral STT, whereas cells projecting from the deep dorsal horn ascend in the ventral STT (see Fig. 1.3) [5]. Glial cells in the DRG serve to support the cell bodies and axonal projections of small and medium-sized nociceptive fibers, even playing a role in signal modulation and peripheral sensitization [7]. Discriminative touch, pressure, and proprioception are transmitted by large, myelinated *Aβ fibers*, whose cell bodies are also located in the DRG. These somatic mechanosensory fibers ascend in the dorsal column of the spinal cord to first synapse on the dorsal column nuclei of the medulla [5]. Motor neurons exit the spinal cord via the ventral horn and travel through large, richly myelinated, and rapidly conducting fibers contained within the ventral roots; however, autonomic motor afferents travel via small, slowly conducting fibers [5].

Fig. 1.2 Structure of a primary nociceptor. Information which reaches the central terminal is relayed to second-order neurons in the CNS, which are invariably located in the dorsal horn of the spinal cord [2]

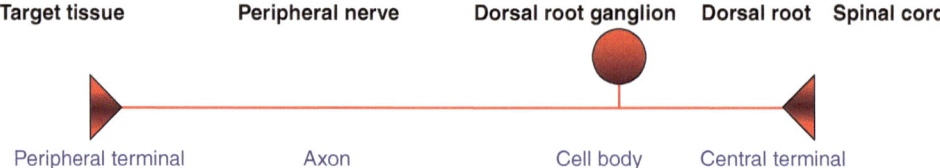

Fig. 1.3 Afferent nociceptor entry into the spinal cord. Somatic nociceptors enter the spinal cord on the dorsal surface via the dorsal root. The cell bodies of these neurons are located within the dorsal root ganglia. Primary somatic afferents undergo at least one synapse onto dorsal horn interneurons, which then project across the midline to ascend in the lateral and ventral white matter via the STT. Visceral nociceptive information, in contrast, is relayed through the dorsal horn and ascends via the ipsilateral dorsal column in the postsynaptic dorsal column pathway [5]

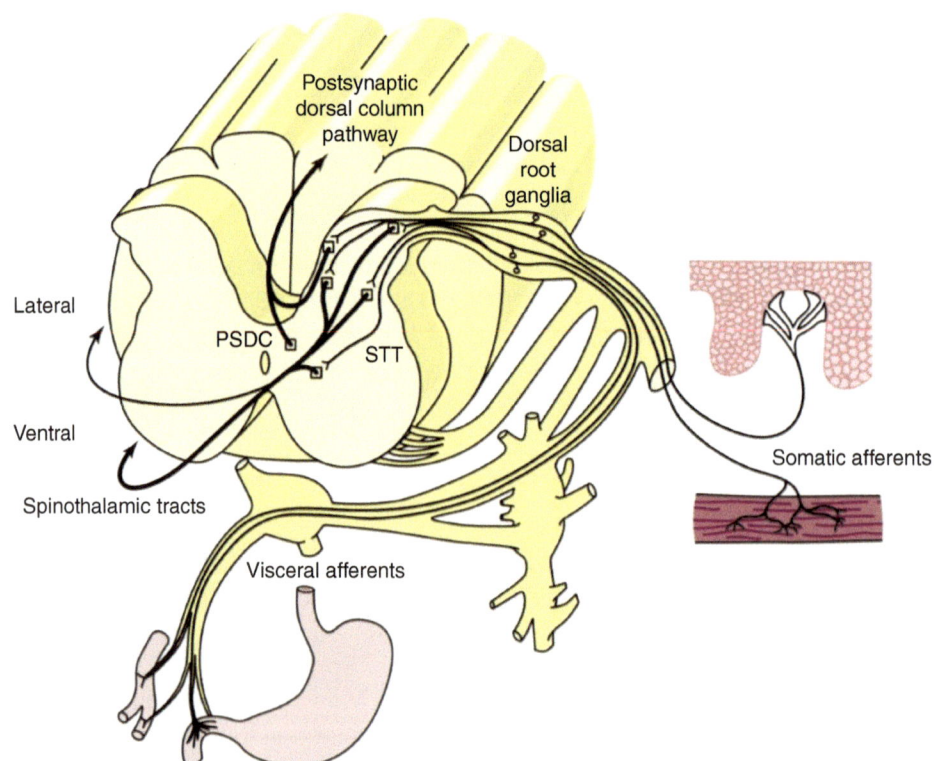

Nociceptive peripheral terminals are specialized, high-threshold endings which express ion channels that respond to mechanical, chemical, and thermal stimuli. Cool stimuli activate the TRPM8 channel, for instance, whereas noxious heat stimuli activate an array of TRP channels, including TRPV1-4 and the heat-sensitive potassium channel TREK-1 [8]. By contrast, non-nociceptive sensory neurons express ion channels which are activated at low-threshold by innocuous stimuli [2]. Genetic mutations in specific nociceptive receptor subtypes can produce an array of Hereditary Sensory and Autonomic Neuropathies (HSAN). HSAN Type IV, for example, results from a mutation in the TrkA receptor, thereby resulting in failure of nerve growth factor (NGF)-associated receptor differentiation and leading to pain hyposensitivity [2].

Glutamate is the primary excitatory neurotransmitter of nociceptive afferents and derangements in glutamate transport or the maintenance of glutamate homeostasis has been implicated in the development of chronic pain states [9]. An array of small molecules and neuropeptides have been found to reinforce and enhance glutamate signaling, including substance P (SP), neurokinin A, galanin, somatostatin, and calcitonin gene-related peptide (CGRP). Small, peptidergic nociceptors are the only source of CGRP in the spinal cord and, as such, CGRP is frequently used as a molecular marker for the study of nociceptive signaling in the spinal cord [10]. Inflammatory cytokines can activate nociceptors at their terminal endings, the DRG, or the spinal cord and include adenosine, NO, IL-1, IL-6, and TNFα [5]. In pathologic pain states, these inflammatory cytokines and signaling molecules can lead to further enhanced nociception, increased glutamate release, and increased dorsal horn activation, thereby bolstering the development of central sensitization [11].

Fine, discriminative sensory information from skin and joints enters the spinal cord as large, myelinated afferents in the dorsal root. The axons travel along the top of the dorsal horn and ascend in the ipsilateral dorsal column white matter to the medulla. These primary sensory neurons first synapse in the dorsal column nuclei of the medulla and then decussate in the *medial lemniscus* to synapse on the contralateral thalamic nuclei, most notably the *ventral posterolateral (VPL)* nucleus of the thalamus. Primary nociceptive and temperature information is carried within afferent myelinated and unmyelinated fibers which enter the dorsal surface of the spinal cord and traverse the top of the dorsal horn via Lissauer's Tract. They then enter the gray matter of the spinal cord and widely arborize onto dorsal horn interneurons [5]. Classically, axons traveling in Lissauer's Tract have been thought to either ascend or descend only 1–2 spinal segments before projecting into the dorsal horn; however, electrophysiologic studies have shown some Aδ-fibers to project as many as five spinal segments rostro-caudally in a rat model [12]. Visceral nociceptive afferents have been found to have more extensive terminal arborization in the dorsal horn than somatic nociceptors, which may account for the poor localization of symptoms and frequent incidence of "referred" pain in these cases [5].

Central Mechanisms: Spinal and Medullary Dorsal Horns, Segmental and Brainstem

The first site of nociceptive processing in the CNS is the gray matter of the spinal cord dorsal horn. Neurons entering the dorsal horn arborize to variable degrees and synapse at least once onto local interneurons. Second-order projection neurons then course to higher-order centers via the contralateral STT or ipsilateral postsynaptic dorsal column pathway (PSDC) (see Fig. 1.4). In contrast, discriminative touch and proprioception travel directly via the white matter of the dorsal columns to the dorsal column nuclei of the medulla.

The gray matter of the spinal cord is histologically and functionally divided into ten Rexed laminae, with the dorsal horns comprising laminae I–VI [13]. Visceral nociceptive C fibers are seen to project deeply into the dorsal horn, with wide branching synapses terminating in laminae I, II, V, and X ipsilaterally. Some visceral fibers even project across the midline and terminate in laminae V and X contralaterally. This wide degree of arborization explains the relatively poor localization of visceral pain, which is often referred to other areas of the body (see Fig. 1.5) [5]. The superficial dorsal horn (laminae I–III) is where most primary somatic afferent C fibers synapse, with laminae II and III comprising the *substantia gelatinosa* [14]. The reserved terminal arborization pattern of somatic C fibers in the substantia gelatinosa allows for geographic localization of painful stimuli, in contrast to the wide branching patterns of visceral C fibers.

Rexed lamina II contains a matrix of interneurons with large dense-core vesicles of excitatory (e.g., glutamate) and inhibitory (e.g., GABA) neurotransmitters [5]. In contrast to C fibers, Aδ fibers transmitting mechanical nociceptive information terminate in lamina I, as well as more deeply in the spinal cord gray matter of laminae V and X [15]. Distributive interneurons are located within laminae III, IV, and VI which project nociceptive information to the hypothalamus via the spinohypothalamic tract, and the brainstem via the spinoreticular and spinocervical tracts [5]. Areas deep to the dorsal horn extending into laminae VII–X are responsible for somatic and autonomic motor function. The central area of the spinal cord is comprised of laminae X and adjacent segments of the dorsal horn, and is responsible for the processing of purely visceral and autonomic nociception [5].

Spinal interneurons comprise a majority of the neurons in the dorsal horn and secrete a wide array of modulating neurotransmitters. GABA-ergic interneurons located in lamina II are thought to play an important role in the "*gate*

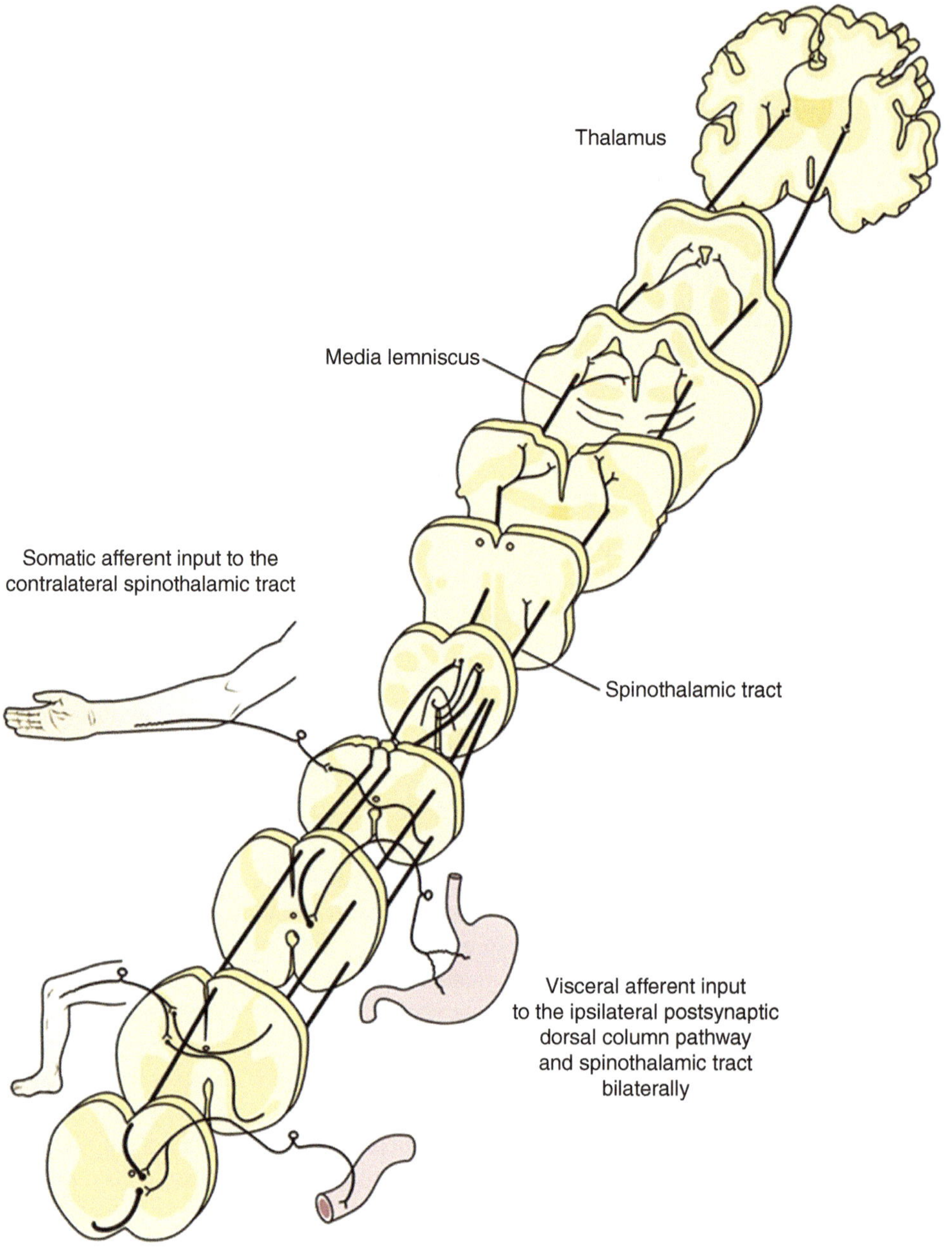

Fig. 1.4 Ascending nociceptive pathways in the spinal cord. Somatic nociceptors enter the spinal cord on the dorsal surface, travel in the Lissauer's Tract approximately 1–2 spinal segments along the cranio-caudal axis and synapse onto local interneurons in the gray matter of the dorsal horn. Second order projection neurons then decussate at the spinal cord level in the anterior white commissure ventral to the central canal and ascend to the thalamus via the STT. The lateral STT has its origins from the superficial dorsal horn, whereas the ventral STT projects from the deep dorsal horn. Visceral afferent nociception ascends via the ipsilateral PSDC pathway [5]

Thalamus

Media lemniscus

Somatic afferent input to the contralateral spinothalamic tract

Spinothalamic tract

Visceral afferent input to the ipsilateral postsynaptic dorsal column pathway and spinothalamic tract bilaterally

Fig. 1.5 Structure of the dorsal horn. Cutaneous nociceptors terminate in the substantia gelatinosa of Rexed laminae II and III, whereas visceral C fibers arborize extensively into laminae II, V, and X ipsilaterally, and X contralaterally [5]

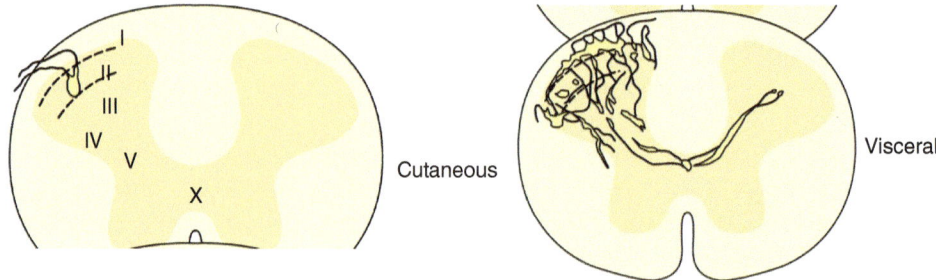

Cutaneous

Visceral

control theory" of nociceptive transmission, whereby noxious transmissions can be inhibited by somatic mechanical stimuli [16]. In this model, afferent nociceptive CRGP-ergic axons synapse onto inhibitory GABA-ergic interneurons in laminae II, inhibiting them through the secretion of the *glycine* and *dynorphin*. In this way, the signaling of downstream projection neurons is enhanced. It is when Aβ fibers carrying mechanical "touch" information are activated that the inhibitory activity of GABA-ergic interneurons is promoted and the downstream signal is quieted [16].

Nociceptive information arriving via the trigeminal nerve from the head, neck, and dura enter the CNS in the caudal medulla which serves as the functional equivalent to the spinal cord dorsal horn [17]. These afferent neurons synapse onto the *spinal trigeminal nucleus* which sends second-order projections via the trigeminal lemniscus to the contralateral *ventral posteromedial (VPM) nucleus* of the thalamus [5]. In this way, the crossing fibers of the trigeminal lemniscus decussate in the medulla and join the STT to be integrated in thalamic relays to convey pain and temperature sensation from the contralateral face.

Central Mechanisms: Thalamocortical – Ascending Nociceptive Pathways, Higher Cortical Processing, and Descending Modulation

The primary relay which transmits nociceptive cutaneous and temperature input from the periphery to the CNS is the *spinothalamic tract (STT)*. Discriminative cutaneous and temperature nociception project from Rexed laminae I, II, and V and decussate ventral to the central canal via the *anterior white commissure*. These axons then form the contralateral white matter of the lateral and anterior STTs and rise to synapse in the VPL nucleus of the thalamus [5]. The VPL nucleus of the thalamus serves as the main cortical relay center for somatosensory input related to pain, temperature, and itch from the contralateral side of the body. The anterior and lateral STTs, along with ascending fibers which terminate in the reticular formation (spinoreticular fibers), *periaqueductal grey (PAG)* (spino-periaqueductal fibers), and hypothalamus (spinohypothalamic fibers), are together considered the *anterolateral system (ALS)* [18]. The ALS stands in contrast to the medial pain pathway that is primarily responsible for transmitting nociceptive information to limbic structures, such as the prefrontal and insular cortices, and the anterior cingulate cortex. The limbic system is what generates many autonomic and affective responses to pain by integrating input from a wide array of collateral systems, including the spinoamygdalar, spinoreticular, and spinohypothalamic tracts [5].

The postsynaptic dorsal column pathway (PSDC) is primarily responsible for relaying visceral nociceptive input [5]. The dorsal column tract is classically considered the main thoroughfare for primary afferent neurons carrying touch, pressure, proprioception, and vibratory sensation; however, animal and human studies support the presence of a visceral nociceptive tract in the dorsal columns in which second-order neurons ascend ipsilaterally to synapse at the gracile and cuneate nuclei [19]. After synapsing in the gracile and cuneate nuclei, relay fibers of the PSDC decussate in the medulla oblongata via the medial lemniscus and ascend to synapse in the thalamus where the signals are then integrated with other forebrain and cortical structures. The functional importance of the PSDC pathway is evidenced by the ability to relieve visceral cancer pain in humans by performing a limited, midline myelotomy of the dorsal columns [20].

Although the PSDC pathway and the STT terminate in thalamic relay centers, they both provide abundant supply to important parallel medullary, pontine, and midbrain integration sites (see Fig. 1.6). Such integrating sites include the rostral ventral medulla (RVM), the PAG, amygdala, and limbic systems [5]. The spinohypothalamic and spinoamygdalar pathways receive innervation from ascending fibers which originate primarily in Rexed laminae I and X [21]. These pathways contribute to the emotional and motivational responses to pain through the generation of anxiety, arousal, and attention. Autonomic alterations also result from these midbrain pathways via changes in sympathetic outflow, heart rate, and blood pressure. The PAG and the nucleus raphe magnus (NRM) are primary sites influencing the descending inhibition of pain transmission [22]. The PAG and the NRM are part of the larger reticular system which balances excitatory and inhibitory nociceptive processing [23]. The spinoreticular pathway is in part made up of neurons which project from the spinal cord to the RVM, NRM, and the A7 catecholaminergic center of the pons. The spinoreticular tracts contribute to descending modulation of pain, cortical and limbic projection, stress responses, and other "anti-nociceptive" reflexes such as the escape response [5]. The complex interactions of these brainstem centers with higher-order cortical areas are illustrated by Fig. 1.6, along with contributions from the STT and PSDC pathway.

The RVM is one important area of the brainstem which receives nociceptive input and exerts both descending inhibitory and excitatory influence on pain transmission. The RVM is composed of the midline raphe system which contains the serotonergic neurons of the NRM, as well as non-serotonergic neurons. The NRM has primarily been implicated in the inhibition of nociceptive transmission via projections down the dorsolateral funiculus to the spinal cord level [24]. Enkephalinergic connections between the NRM and the dorsolateral pons help to potentiate descending control of pain transmission. The noradrenergic neurons of the dorsolateral

Fig. 1.6 The relationship of ascending nociceptive tracts in the brainstem. The primary ascending nociceptive tracts include the spinothalamic tract and the postsynaptic dorsal column pathway. Both tracts supply innervation to brainstem integration sites which contribute to autonomic, affective, neurohormonal, and modulatory responses to pain. The VPL thalamic nucleus is the main cortical relay center for the localization of pain, whereas the medial thalamus projects to the anterior cingulate cortex which produces affective and motivational responses to pain [5]

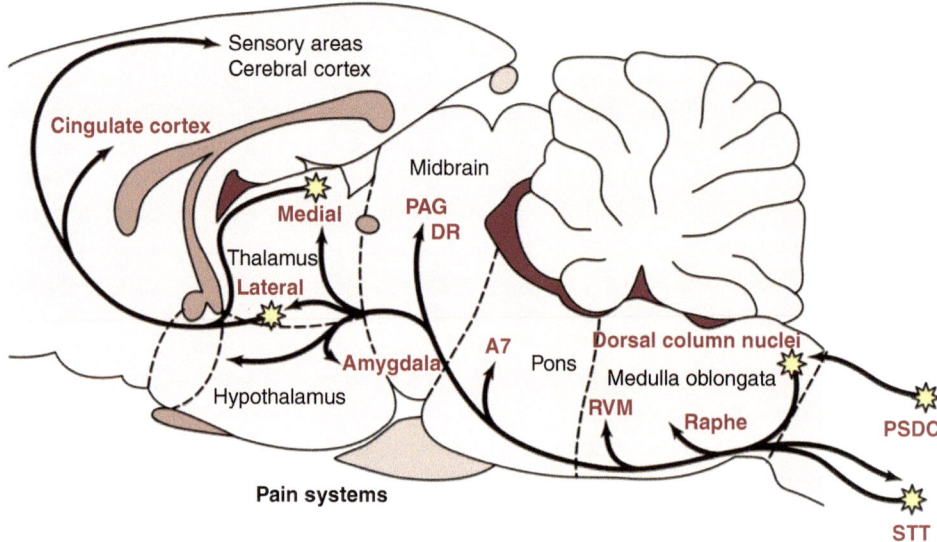

pons receive input from the PAG and the RVM, all of which act to further inhibit the transmission of ascending nociception [25]. Cholinergic transmission in the PAG of the midbrain provides descending connections to both the RVM and dorsolateral pons. The PAG has been found to potentiate opioid analgesia and decrease nociceptive transmission by the activation of projection neurons which descend to laminae III–V in the spinal cord and promote activity of cholinergic interneurons [26].

Somatic nociception is relayed through the VPL thalamic nucleus to the somatosensory cortex, where higher cortical processing plays a discriminative role in the localization of pain. The discriminatory role of the VPL nucleus contrasts with midline thalamic nuclei, which integrate noxious visceral input, as well as the ventromedial nuclei, which receive noxious input from the face and tooth pulp [27]. Cortical projections from the thalamus to the anterior cingulate cortex play a role in an individual's emotional response to pain, whereas the insular cortex and frontal cortex contribute to the memory and learning response to nociception [28]. Overall, excitatory and inhibitory feedback connections between nociceptive tracts in the thalamus, brainstem, and cortex work together to balance the level of perceived pain intensity.

References

1. Merskey H, Bogduk N. Part III: pain terms, a current list with definitions and notes on usage. In: Classification of chronic pain. 2nd ed. Seattle: IASP Press; 1994. p. 209–14.
2. Woolf C, Qiufu M. Nociceptors – noxious stimulus detectors. Neuron. 2007;55:353–64.
3. Das V. Chapter 1: An introduction to pain pathways and pain "targets". Prog Mol Biol Transl Sci. 2015;131:1–30.
4. Fenton B, Shih E, Zolton J. The neurobiology of pain perception in normal and persistent pain. Pain Manag. 2015;5(4):297–317.
5. Westlund K. Chapter 8: Pain pathways: peripheral, spinal, ascending, and descending pathways. In: Benzon H, Rathmell J, Wu C, Turk D, Argoff C, Hurley R, editors. Practical management of pain. 5th ed. Philadelphia: Mosby; 2013. p. 87–98.
6. Tracey W. Nociception. Curr Biol. 2017;27:129–33.
7. Chung K, Lee W, Carlton S. The effects of dorsal rhizotomy and spinal cord isolation on calcitonin gene-related peptide containing terminals in the rat lumbar dorsal horn. Neurosci Lett. 1988;90:27–32.
8. Dhaka A, Viswanath V, Papapoutian A. Trp ion channels and temperature sensation. Annu Rev Neurosci. 2006;29:135–61.
9. Tao YX, Gu J, Stephens R. Role of spinal cord glutamate transporter during normal sensory transmission and pathological pain states. Mol Pain. 2005;1:30.
10. Ye Z, Wimalawansa S, Westlund K. Receptor for calcitonin gene-related peptide: localization in the dorsal and ventral spinal cord. Neuroscience. 1999;92:1389–97.
11. Dougherty P, Willis W. Enhancement of spinothalamic neuron responses to chemical and mechanical stimuli following combined micro-iontophoretic application of N-methyl-D-aspartic acid and substance P. Pain. 1991;47:85–93.
12. Lidierth M. Long-range projections of A-delta primary afferents in the Lissauer tract of the rat. Neurosci Lett. 2007;425:126–30.
13. Rexed B. The cytoarchitectonic organization of the spinal cord in the cat. J Comp Neurol. 1952;96:415–66.
14. Chernavskii D, Karp V, Rodshtat I. The human autodiagnostic system (Rexed's laminae as diagnostic neuroprocessors). Radiophys Quantum Electron. 1994;37:32–44.
15. Light A, Perl E. Spinal termination of functionally identified primary afferent neurons with slowly conducting myelinated fibers. J Comp Neurol. 1979;186:133–50.
16. Melzack R, Wall P. Pain mechanisms: a new theory. Science. 1965;150:971–9.
17. Magnusson K, Larson A, Madl J. Co-localization of fixative-modified glutamate and glutaminase in neurons of the spinal trigeminal nucleus of the rat: an immunohistochemical and immunoradiochemical analysis. J Comp Neurol. 1986;247:477–90.
18. Haines D. Neuroanatomy: an atlas of structures, sections, and systems. 7th ed. Philadelphia: Lippincott Williams & Wilkins; 2008.
19. Willis W, Al-Chaer E, Quast M, Westlund K. A visceral pain pathway in the dorsal column of the spinal cord. Proc Natl Acad Sci U S A. 1999;96(14):7675–9.

20. Willis W, Westlund K. The role of the dorsal column pathway in visceral nociception. Curr Pain Headache Rep. 2001;5(1):20–6.

21. Cliffer K, Burnstein R, Giesler G. Distributions of spinothalamic, spinohypothalamic, and spinotelencephalic fibers revealed by anterograde transport of PHA-L in rats. J Neurosci. 1991;11:852–68.

22. Basbaum A, Fields H. Endogenous pain control systems: brainstem spinal pathways and endorphin circuitry. Annu Rev Neurosci. 1984;7:309–38.

23. Price D. Central neural mechanisms that interrelate sensory and affective dimensions of pain. Mol Interv. 2002;2:392–403.

24. Holden J, Proudfit H. Enkephalin neurons that project to the A7 catecholamine cell group are located in nuclei that modulate nociception: ventromedial medulla. Neuroscience. 1998;83:929–47.

25. Mayer D, Wolfle T, Akil H. Analgesia from electrical stimulation in the brainstem of the rat. Science. 1971;174:1351–4.

26. Riberio-da-Silva A, Cuello A. Choline acetyltransferase-immunoreactive profiles are presynaptic to primary sensory fibers in the rat superficial dorsal horn. J Comp Neurol. 1990;295:370–84.

27. Rydenhag B, Olausson B, Andersson S. Projection of tooth pulp afferents to the thalamus of the cat. I. Focal potentials and thalamo-cortical connections. Exp Brain Res. 1986;64:37–48.

28. Friedman D, Murray E, O'Neill J. Cortical connections of the somatosensory fields of the lateral sulcus of macaques: evidence for a corticolimbic pathway for touch. J Comp Neurol. 1986;252:323–47.

Pharmacology of Pain Transmission and Modulation

Rishi R. Agarwal, Rishi Gaiha, and David R. Walega

Experimental Models: Limitations

The human experience of pain is a wholly subjective one, depending on the perception of the individual experiencing a noxious stimulus. Unlike other acute and chronic conditions such as myocardial infarction or diabetes for which the degree of severity can be reliably quantified with laboratory values, acute and chronic pain conditions lack similar testing to objectively quantify pain levels. As such, experimental models designed to study pain perception are limited by the inherent lack of consistency between different individuals experiencing the same noxious stimulus. Nevertheless, the evolution of experimental models over the past century has enabled a better understanding of pain transmission and modulation, making possible significant advances in therapies and treatments.

An important and increasingly utilized instrument to characterize mechanisms underlying pathologic pain disorders is quantitative sensory testing (QST), which allows for static and dynamic forms of testing [1, 2]. Examples of static QSTs include: cold and heat pain threshold, pressure pain threshold, and 2-point discrimination. Static QSTs are used for threshold determination and provide insight into the basal state of the nociceptive system. Examples of dynamic QSTs include: mechanical wind-up and conditioned pain modulation. Dynamic QSTs are used to assess the mechanisms of pain processing, such as peripheral and central sensitization.

The development of experimental models of pain and knowledge of safety profiles for various analgesic medications

R. R. Agarwal
Department of Anesthesiology, Northwestern, Chicago, IL, USA

R. Gaiha (✉)
Anesthesiology, Northwestern Hospital, Chicago, IL, USA
e-mail: Rishi.gaiha@northwestern.edu

D. R. Walega
Division of Pain Medicine, Department of Anesthesiology, Northwestern University Feinberg School of Medicine, Chicago, IL, USA

are owed to vivisection. Examples of animal neuropathic pain models include: *progressive tactile hypersensitivity*, which develops months after recovery from sciatic nerve crush in response to repeated intermittent low-threshold mechanical stimulation of the re-innervated sciatic nerve skin territory [3]; *spared nerve injury*, which is characterized by an early and sustained increase in stimulus-evoked pain sensitivity in the intact skin territory of the spared sural nerve after sectioning of the two other terminal branches of the sciatic nerve [3]; and *hot plate testing* that assesses pain behaviors such as paw licking or jumping in response to pain due to heat [4]. An example of an animal visceral pain model is the writhing test, in which noxious substances (e.g., capsaicin, acetic acid, mustard oil) are injected intraperitoneally and visceral pain behaviors such as licking of the abdomen, stretching, and contractions of the abdomen are monitored or measured [5]. A less ideal, and arguably inhumane, animal visceral pain model for irritable bowel syndrome involves the use of an inflated balloon tamp applied inside the rectum of rats [6].

Clearly, findings from animal models of pain and pain behavior do not fully translate into the sensory and emotional experience of pain in humans. As such, pain models that are ethically and morally acceptable to perform on consenting humans were developed based on existing animal models. A simple way to organize both animal and human models of pain is by location of the noxious stimulus applied: skin, muscle, or viscera. Commonly used models of pain applied to skin include calibrated filaments (e.g., von Frey filaments), which quantitatively assess the response to touch by bending when a specific pressure is applied but are not able to specifically evoke pain as they primarily activate *A-beta fibers*, and pressure algometers, which apply standardized pressure and activate *A-delta* and *C-fibers* [7]. A classic model of pain applied to muscle is ischemic stimulation, in which ischemic muscle pain is induced by pneumatic tourniquet inflation [7]. The most ideal model of pain applied to the viscera is chemical stimulation, whereby acidic chemicals are applied to the esophagus, as this model closely resembles clinical inflammation [7].

Y. Khelemsky et al. (eds.), *Academic Pain Medicine*, https://doi.org/10.1007/978-3-030-18005-8_2

Peripheral Mechanisms of Pain Transmission and Modulation

There are three types of primary afferent fibers in the skin that are distinguished by conduction velocity (Table 2.1) [8]. *A-beta fibers* are large and myelinated, have the fastest conduction velocity, and transmit light touch, pressure, and hair movement. *Unmyelinated C fibers* and thinly myelinated *A-delta fibers* transmit nociception.

Table 2.1 Chemicals released during peripheral tissue injury

Substance	Source	Effect
Bradykinin	Macrophages and plasma kininogen	Activates nociceptors
Serotonin	Platelets and mast cells	Activates nociceptors
Histamine	Platelets and mast cells	Produces vasodilation, edema and pruritus Potentiates the response of nociceptors to bradykinin
Prostaglandin	Tissue injury and cyclooxygenase pathway	Sensitize nociceptors
Leukotriene	Tissue injury and lipoxygenase pathway	Sensitize nociceptors
Hydrogen ions	Tissue injury and ischemia	Hyperalgesia
Cytokines (interleukins and tumor necrosis factor α)	Macrophages	Excite and sensitize nociceptors
Adenosine	Tissue injury	Pain and hyperalgesia
Substance P Glutamate	Release by peripheral nerve terminals following injury	Substance P activates macrophages and mast cells Glutamate activates nociceptors
Calcitonin G-related peptide Nerve growth factor	Release by peripheral nerve terminals in dorsal horn Macrophages	Excitatory effect on WDR neurons of the dorsal horn Induces heat hyperalgesia Sensitizes nociceptors

Table 2.2 Primary afferent fibers

Group	Diameter (μm)	Conduction velocity (m/s)	Modalities
A (myelinated)			
A-alpha	15–20	8–120	Large motor, proprioception
A-beta	8–15	30–70	Small motor, touch, pressure
A-gamma	4–8	30–70	Muscle spindle, reflex
A-delta	3–4	10–30	Pain, temperature
B (myelinated)	3–4	10–30	Preganglionic autonomic
C (unmyelinated)	1–2	1–2	Pain, temperature

Unmyelinated C fibers transmit nociception at less than 2 m/s, and are associated with prolonged burning sensations. Thinly myelinated A-delta fibers transmit nociception at 5–20 m/s and are associated with sharp, intense, tingling sensations.

The processes that lead to the perception of pain involve the following steps, in order: transduction, transmission, modulation, and perception. Tissue injury from mechanical, thermal, or chemical stimuli results in the release of numerous chemicals including bradykinin, free hydrogen ions, serotonin, histamine, eicosanoids, nitric oxide, adenosine, and cytokines (Table 2.2) by various cell types such as damaged tissue cells, macrophages, and mast cells in the skin (Fig. 2.1) [9]. These, in turn, either directly activate nociceptors or increase the excitability of (e.g., sensitize) nociceptors. These chemical mediators transduce stimuli at the primary afferent fibers of the peripheral nervous system into action potentials that are then transmitted to the spinal cord via the dorsal root ganglion, which houses the cell bodies of the primary afferent fibers.

Pain modulation in the periphery involves the recruitment of inflammatory cells to the site of damage by pro-inflammatory mediators that not only facilitate the perception of pain, but also act to limit pain transmission. For example, *Substance P* released by primary afferent fiber terminals in response to tissue damage leads to the activation of macrophages and mast cells [10, 11]. Conversely, peripheral opioid receptors on the same primary afferent fibers receiving input from noxious stimuli become upregulated in inflammatory environments, allowing endogenous opioids (e.g., *endorphins*), released by inflammatory cells such as macrophages, monocytes, and lymphocytes, to modulate and dampen the pain response to tissue damage. Release of endogenous endorphins is thought to be the mechanism by which acupuncture works [12]. The mechanisms behind neurotransmitters and neuropeptides involved in pain modulation are discussed below.

Synaptic Transmission of Pain in the Dorsal Horn

The first synapse in somatosensory processing of information from A-delta and C fibers occurs in the spinal dorsal horn if the stimulus originates from the body surface (Fig. 2.2) or the spinal trigeminal nucleus if it originates from the face [13]. These initial synapses in the spinal cord occur on the ipsilateral side as the origin of the stimuli. The second-order neurons with which primary afferent fibers synapse are of two predominant types: wide-dynamic-range (WDR) neurons and nociceptive-specific (NS) neurons. WDR cells receive input from A-beta, A-delta, and C fibers, and are thus activated by both innocuous and nox-

Peripheral sensory nerve ending

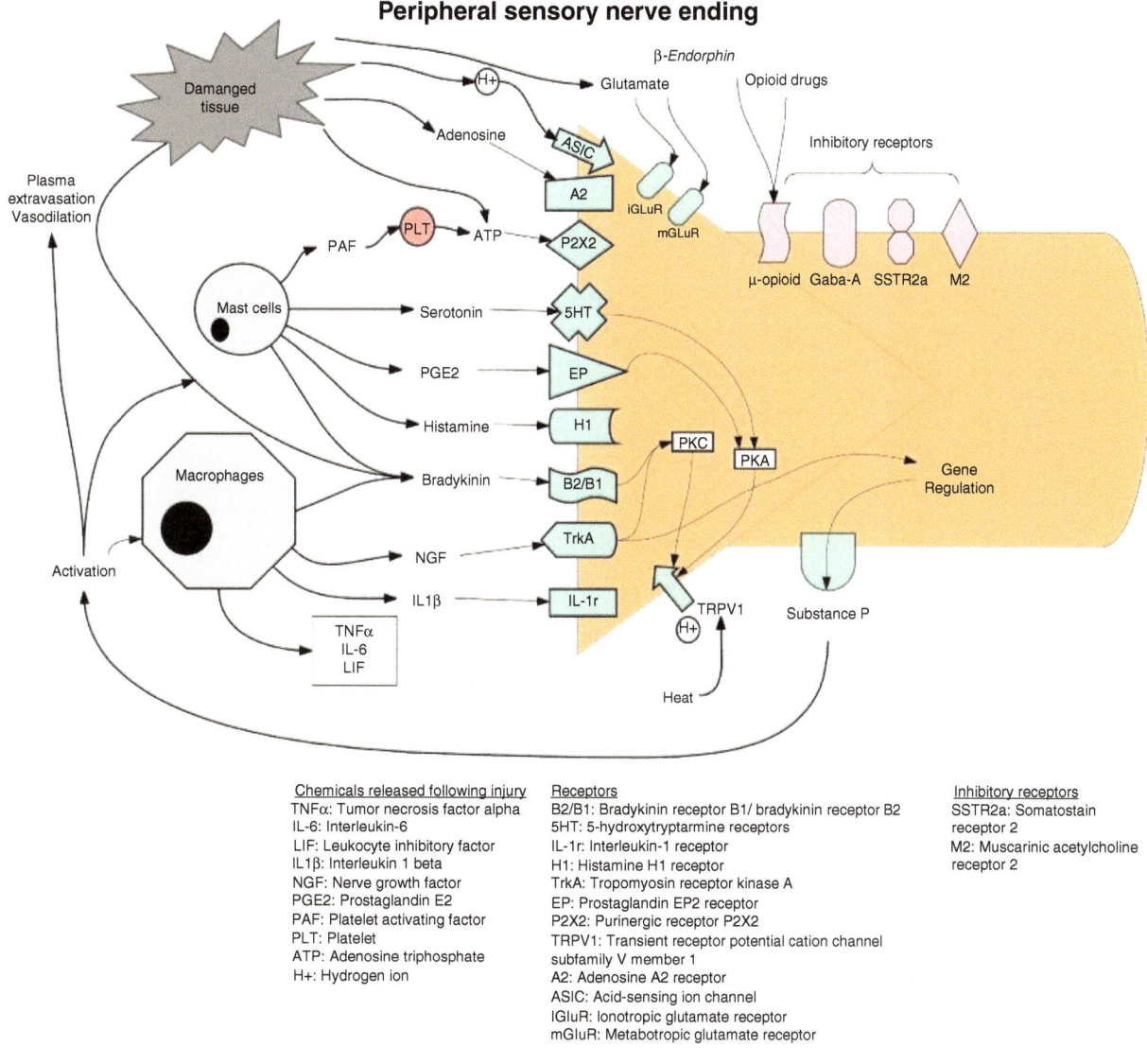

Fig. 2.1 Cell types, neurotransmitters, neuropeptides, and receptors involved in peripheral nociception

ious stimuli. NS neurons receive input solely from A-delta and C fibers.

The ten layers of gray matter of the spinal cord, which includes the ventral, lateral, and dorsal horns, are organized by Rexed's laminae (I–X) [14]. These laminae can help identify where the initial synapses between the primary afferent fibers and second-order neurons occur in the dorsal horn. WDR cells are largely concentrated in laminae III through V, while NS cell bodies are largely concentrated in laminae I and II. The axons of the second-order neurons decussate at 1 or 2 levels above the level of their cell bodies and ascend to the brain via the contralateral anterolateral spinal tracts, where synapses occur with third-order neurons. Third-order neurons are located in the brainstem and diencephalon and transmit nociception to the cerebral cortex.

Central Sensitization: Mechanisms and Implications for Treatment of Pain

The "gate control theory" of neuromodulation was developed by Melzack and Wall in the 1960s as a way to describe the mechanism by which transcutaneous electrical stimulation provides pain relief [15]. The theory suggested that input from low-threshold A-beta primary afferent fibers inhibits the response of WDR cells to nociceptive input from A-delta and primary afferent C fibers. However, present thinking is that the modulation of nociception is likely much more complex than what is explained by the gate control theory and facilitated by numerous neurotransmitters released at the spinal level by intrinsic spinal neurons (e.g., WDR and NS neurons).

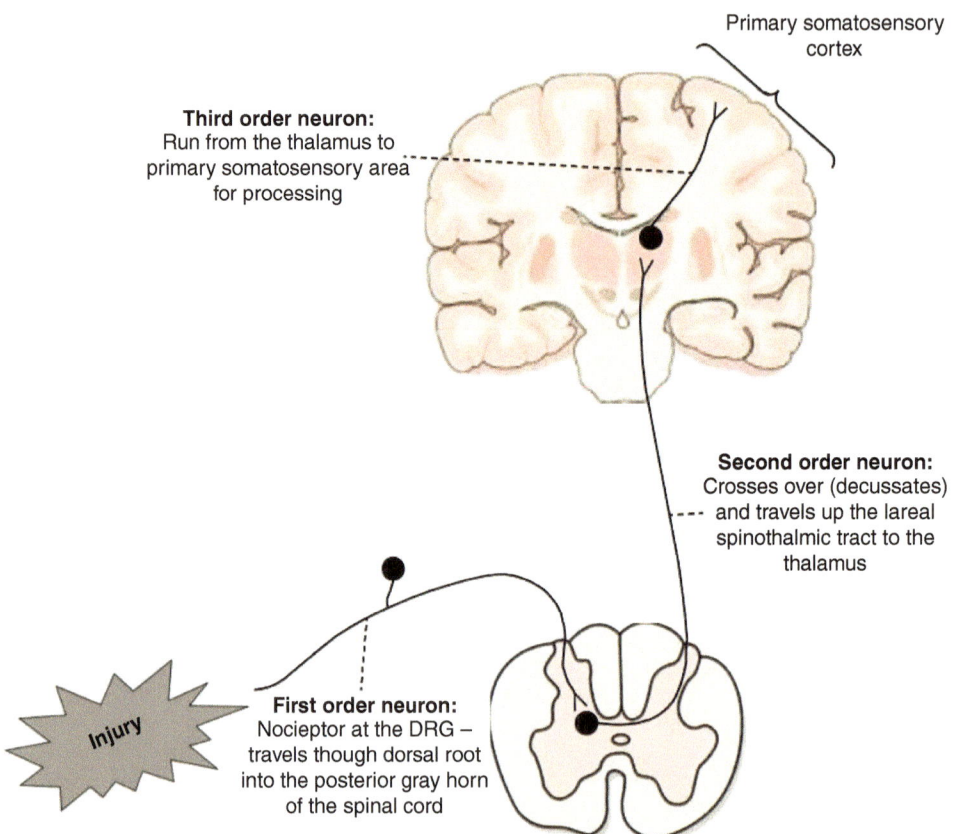

Fig. 2.2 Synapses involved in somatosensory processing

Indeed, high-frequency spinal cord stimulation accomplishes analgesia in patients without causing a paresthesia and thus cannot be explained the gate control theory of neuromodulation [16]. Moreover, descending inputs from the brainstem to the dorsal root ganglion also modulate nociception.

Central sensitization represents a special type of modulation at the spinal level in which the capacity for transmission of nociception is dynamic – exhibiting neuronal plasticity. This plasticity is caused by an alteration in molecular transcriptional activity of second-order neurons following a noxious stimulus of sufficient intensity and duration, like surgical incision, such that the second-order neurons sustain a response to nociceptive stimuli beyond the initiating stimulus [17]. A helpful example which illustrates the concept of central sensitization is the wind-up phenomenon, whereby repeated stimulation of C fibers at frequencies between 0.5 to 1.0 Hz results in a progressive escalation in the number of evoked discharges by primary afferent fibers with a single stimulus. Furthermore, the now sensitized intrinsic spinal neurons display an expanded receptive field size, as well as an increase in the number of spontaneous discharges. Thus, synaptic input from primary afferent fibers that, prior to sensitization, would be subthreshold now generate an augmented action potential output in the newly sensitized second-order neurons.

Specific ligands and receptors are known to be responsible for central sensitization. One well-defined example is the interaction between glutamate and the N-methyl-D-aspartic acid (NMDA) receptor [18]. As detailed earlier, inflammatory cells such as macrophages and mast cells influence the signals transduced by primary afferent fibers in the periphery by the release of various chemicals (Table 2.2). These signals alter the gene transcription patterns in second-order neurons in the dorsal horn, leading to phosphorylation of the NMDA receptor on the synaptic membranes with an increased neuronal responsiveness to the excitatory neurotransmitter glutamate. This increased responsiveness allows the voltage-dependent ion channels to remain open longer due to removal of a magnesium ion from the ion channel when the NMDA receptor is phosphorylated. As a result, second-order neurons in the dorsal horn are activated by subthreshold inputs, and exhibit an increased response to supra-threshold inputs.

Neurotransmitters Involved in Pain Modulation

The neurochemistry of the somatosensory processing system involves three classes of transmitter compounds: excitatory neurotransmitters, inhibitory neurotransmitters, and neuropeptides. These compounds are found in terminals of primary afferent fibers, local circuit neurons, and descending modulatory neurons, and all work to modulate signal transmission of the second-order neurons in the dorsal horn.

The amino acids *glutamate* and *aspartate* are the most ubiquitous excitatory neurotransmitters in the nervous system [19]. Four receptor types for glutamate and aspartate are primarily responsible for excitatory pain modulation: NMDA, kainate, α-amino-3-hydroxy-5-methyl-4-isoxazolepropionic acid (AMPA), and metabotropic receptors. The kainate, AMPA, and metabotropic receptors are collectively referred to as non-NMDA receptors. As detailed earlier, persistent activation of NMDA receptors by glutamate leads to an increase of receptive field size, decreased activation threshold, and prolonged depolarization which in turn causes sensitization of dorsal horn neurons.

The amino acids *glycine* and *gamma-amino-butyric acid (GABA)* are the most ubiquitous inhibitory neurotransmitters in the nervous system [20]. There are two receptor sites for glycine at the spinal level, one of which is on the NMDA receptor. GABA is found in local circuit neurons located in Rexed's laminae I, II, and III. There are three types of GABA receptors: GABAa, which is linked to a chloride channel and is modulated by drugs such as barbiturates, benzodiazepines, propofol, and alcohol; GABAb, which is G-protein-linked complex and is the site of action of the GABAb agonist baclofen; and GABAc, which has no known role in somatosensory modulation. *Norepinephrine* and *serotonin* are other common inhibitory neurotransmitters found in descending pathways, which partially explains the role of serotonin-norepinephrine reuptake inhibitor medications such as duloxetine and venlafaxine, and tricyclic antidepressants such as amitriptyline and in the management of chronic pain [21].

Unlike neurotransmitters, which have rapid onset and termination, neuropeptides have slower onset and longer duration of action. They can, however, similarly be divided into excitatory and inhibitory neuropeptides. *Substance P* is an excitatory neuropeptide found in high concentration in small, unmyelinated afferent C-fiber terminals in the periphery (i.e., skin, muscle, joints), with increased levels leading to vasodilation, inflammation, and pain in response to tissue damage as this neuropeptide activates macrophages and mast cells by elevating intracellular calcium levels [11]. *Calcitonin G-related peptide* (CGRP) is an excitatory neuropeptide that, similarly to *substance P*, is found in high concentration in small, unmyelinated afferent C-fiber terminals at the spinal level, with its release leading to an excitatory effect on WDR neurons [22]. Inhibitory neuropeptides such as *somatostatin* and *endorphins* are found in second-order neurons of the dorsal horn, as well as terminal fibers of descending inputs from different brainstem nuclei. The *endocannabinoids* 2-arachidonoylglycerol (2-AG) and anandamide may also play a role in pain modulation. While patients and clinicians often anecdotally espouse the benefits of *cannabinoids* in treating chronic pain, more research is needed into their potential therapeutic benefits.

References

1. Mackey IG, Dixon EA, Johnson K, Kong JT. Dynamic quantitative sensory testing to characterize central pain processing. J Vis Exp. 2017;120.
2. Hansson P, Backonja M, Bouhassira D. Usefulness and limitations of quantitative sensory testing: clinical and research application in neuropathic pain states. Pain. 2007;129(3):256–9.
3. Decosterd I, Allchorne A, Woolf CJ. Differential analgesic sensitivity of two distinct neuropathic pain models. Anesth Analg. 2004;99(2):457–63.
4. Malmberg AB, Yaksh TL. Effect of continuous intrathecal infusion of omega-conopeptides, N-type calcium-channel blockers, on behavior and antinociception in the formalin and hot-plate tests in rats. Pain. 1995;60(1):83–90.
5. Laird JM, Martinez-Caro L, Garcia-Nicas E, Cervero F. A new model of visceral pain and referred hyperalgesia in the mouse. Pain. 2001;92(3):335–42.
6. Gibney SM, Gosselin RD, Dinan TG, Cryan JF. Colorectal distension-induced prefrontal cortex activation in the Wistar-Kyoto rat: implications for irritable bowel syndrome. Neuroscience. 2010;165(3):675–83.
7. Staahl C, Drewes AM. Experimental human pain models: a review of standardized methods for preclinical testing of analgesics. Basic Clin Pharmacol Toxicol. 2004;95(3):97–111.
8. Meyer RA, Campbell JN. Myelinated nociceptive afferents account for the hyperalgesia that follows a burn to the hand. Sciene. 1981;213(4515):1527–9.
9. Steen KH, Steen AE, Kreysel HW, Reeh PW. Inflammatory mediators potentiate pain induced by experimental tissue acidosis. Pain. 1996;66(2–3):163–70.
10. Carter MS, Krause JE. Structure, expression, and some regulatory mechanisms of the rat preprotachykinin gene encoding substance p, neurokinin a, neuropeptide k, and neuropeptide y. J Neurosci. 1990;10(7):2203–14.
11. Nakanishi S. Substance P precursor and kininogen: their structures, gene organizations, and regulation. Physiol Rev. 1987;67(4):1117–42.
12. Han JS. Acupuncture analgesia. Pain. 1985;21(3):307–10.
13. Cohen SP, Mao J. Neuropathic pain: mechanisms and their clinical implications. BMJ. 2014;348:f7656.
14. Rexed B. The cytoarchitectonic organization of the spinal cord in the cat. J Comp Neurol. 1952;96(3):414–95.
15. Melzack R, Wall PD. Pain mechanisms: a new theory. Science. 1965;150(3699):971–9.
16. Kapural L, Yu C, Doust MW, Gliner BE, Vallejo R, Sitzman BT, Amirdelfan K, Morgan DM, Brown LL, Yearwood TL, Bundschu R, Burton AW, Yang T, Benyamin R, Burgher AH. Novel 10-kHz high-frequency therapy (HF10 therapy) is superior to traditional low-frequency spinal cord stimulation for the treatment of chronic low back and leg pain: the SENZA-RCT randomized controlled trial. Anesthesiology. 2015;123(4):851–60.
17. Woolf CJ. Evidence for a central component of post-injury pain hypersensitivity. Nature. 1983;306(5944):686–8.
18. Cotman CW, Iversen LL. Excitatory amino acids in the brain – focus on NMDA receptors. Trends Neurosci. 1987;10:263–302.

19. Dougherty PM, Li YJ, Lenz FA, Rowland L, Mittman S. Evidence that excitatory amino acids mediate afferent input to the primate somatosensory thalamus. Brain Res. 1996;728(2):267–73.

20. Sivilotti L, Woolf CJ. The contribution of GABAa and glycine receptors to central sensitization: disinhibition and touch-evoked allodynia in the spinal cord. J Neurophysiol. 1994;72(1):169–79.

21. Gassner M, Ruscheweyh R, Sandkuhler J. Direct excitation of spinal GABAergic interneurons by noradrenaline. Pain. 2009;145(1–2):204–10.

22. Ashina H, Newman L, Ashina S. Calcitonin G-related peptide antagonism and cluster headache: an emerging new treatment. Neurol Sci. 2017;38:2089–93.

Development of Pain Systems

3

Michael Miller, Rahul Sarna, and Awss Zidan

Development of Pain Behavior in the Fetus and Newborn

Introduction

Despite a developing, immature nervous system, the human neonate feels pain. In the past, the predominant theory was that infants were not capable of experiencing "true" pain, as the response to a noxious stimulus was believed to be mediated by nociception rather than higher cortical pain processing [1]. Indeed, the inability to communicate, paucity of memory formation, and underdeveloped cerebral processing of the fetus and newborn do suggest that only decorticate pain processing is well-established in early life. However, research has shown that the fetus and neonate possess the spinal and supraspinal neural connectivity required for advanced pain processing; however, the structure and function of this processing differ from the adult nervous system. Additionally, some of these developmental structures and mechanisms of pain processing in the fetus and neonate are not maintained into later stages of pain transmission and perception. Of note, many of the conclusions that are made about human neurodevelopment have been achieved through studies on rats and other mammals.

Defining a Pain Experience

The distinction between pain and nociception should be considered in exploring the nuances of the primitive pain processing system. Pain is defined by the International Association for the Study of Pain as "an unpleasant sensory and emotional experience associated with actual or potential tissue damage, or described in terms of such damage." Nociception is the activation of sensory transduction in nerves by thermal, mechanical, or chemical energy impinging on specialized nerve endings. The nerves involved convey information about tissue damage to the central nervous system [2]. Basic nociception seems more elementary, requiring a noxious peripheral stimulus to create a signal that is propagated along a nerve to ultimately synapse in the central nervous system. The perception of pain is more involved, requiring multiple advanced cortical structures to localize the inciting stimulus, recognize it as painful, and respond accordingly. There is a complex interplay of higher processing centers of the cerebral cortex involving localization of pain, emotional response, memory, and learning, as well as modulation of pain by descending facilitation and inhibition. While these higher centers are not fully developed in the fetal/neonatal period, connections to these maturing areas do exist. The somatosensory cortical response to painful and tactile stimuli has been exhibited in preterm neonates using near-infrared spectroscopy (NIRS). Noxious stimuli have been shown to transmit to the preterm infant cortex from 25 weeks [3]. Bilateral somatosensory cortical activation was seen from unilateral painful stimulation, indicating some degree of cortical pain processing ability in human neonates [4].

Maturation of Pain Behavior

There is ongoing evolution of the fetal and neonatal pain behaviors as the sensory connections are established and refined. This process can be observed clinically by examining the maturation of cutaneous skin reflexes in humans and other mammals. Reflex responses to noxious stimuli require establishment of connections between peripheral receptors, sensory afferents, dorsal horn neurons, and motor neurons. Spinal reflex responses to tactile and noxious skin stimulation are exaggerated in infants compared to the adult. They also exhibit lower thresholds for activation, wider cutaneous

M. Miller (✉) · A. Zidan
Department of Neurology, SUNY Upstate Medical University, Syracuse, NY, USA
e-mail: MillMich@upstate.edu

R. Sarna
Pain Specialists of Austin, Austin, TX, USA

© Springer Nature Switzerland AG 2019
Y. Khelemsky et al. (eds.), *Academic Pain Medicine*, https://doi.org/10.1007/978-3-030-18005-8_3

receptive fields, and less-localized motor responses. Additionally, repeated stimulation results in sensitization of the reflex response. As the infant's pain processing system matures, the threshold for withdrawal increases and the duration of the response decreases [5]. It has been shown in developing rats exposed to intra-plantar injections of formalin that sensitivity was tenfold higher in neonates compared with weanlings [6]. There is also a localization of the reflex response from diffuse, whole body, or limb movements to more focal muscle flexor responses. This reflects "fine-tuning" of neurons and their synaptic connections and a maturation of descending inhibition [7].

Embryology of the Sensory Nervous System

An embryologic nervous system develops in utero from the neural plate. The neural tube gives rise to the brain and spinal cord. The neural crest gives rise to cells that form the primitive dorsal root ganglia, the axons of which will radiate centrally to reach the spinal cord and peripherally to form the beginnings of peripheral nociceptors [8]. Perioral nociceptors first appear at the seventh gestational week. They are present diffusely across the body by 20 weeks [9]. The development of A-fibers first, followed later by polymodal C-fibers, depends on the expression of different classes of *trk* neurotrophin receptors. Nociceptor growth, maturation, and survival are largely dependent upon neurotrophins such as nerve growth factor (NGF), brain-derived neurotrophic factor (BDNF), and glial cell line-derived growth factor (GDNF) [10]. Peripherally, nociceptors mature at different rates; C-fiber nociceptors (which respond in polymodal fashion to chemical, thermal, and mechanical noxious stimuli) are fully mature at birth, while A-δ fiber high-threshold mechanoreceptor activity evolves to the level of adult function over the postnatal period (despite A-δ fiber formation preceding C-fiber formation in utero) [11].

The dorsal horn of the spinal cord also undergoes marked reorganization and growth postnatally, specifically with the localization of A-δ fibers to specific laminae. C-fibers extend their axons to form synapses directly onto laminae I and II; however, the A-δ fibers grow superficially into laminae I and II as well as deeper laminae [12]. They will then regress in the first three postnatal weeks, in an NMDA-dependent process, to their final adult synapses at deeper Rexed laminae, thus removing the competition for synapses at these levels. This NMDA activity-dependent synapse reorganization has been demonstrated in neonatal rats whose lumbar spinal cord dorsal horn was exposed to an NMDA antagonist, which resulted in abnormal laminar synapse formation [13]. The exaggerated reflex response with lower thresholds and wider cutaneous receptive fields may be secondary to primitive A-β-myelinated fibers overlapping in the superficial laminae

before regression to their adult organization in laminae III–V. The predominance of A-β neuronal inputs into the substantia gelatinosa has been demonstrated in immature rats, possibly as a mechanism to maintain neuronal function in lamina II, in which C-fibers are late to develop their synaptic connections [14].

In the adult, pain processing at the spinal cord involves a balance of nociceptive input with descending modulation. In the developing human, due to prolonged maturation of inhibitory pathways, there is a predominance of excitatory stimulation [10]. This contributes to the exaggerated cutaneous reflexes with lower thresholds and longer durations seen in the immature nervous system. It has been shown that though interneurons and neurons that project to higher processing areas do develop at the same time, the upper projection neurons develop ahead of regulatory interneurons [15].

Substance P has been identified in the dorsal root as early as 8 weeks of embryonic age, and enkephalin along with serotonin is present at 12 weeks [16]. NMDA and AMPA glutaminergic receptors are over-expressed in the embryonic dorsal horn and then downregulated to adult levels as development progresses [17]. In the developing central nervous system, GABA, which is an inhibitory neurotransmitter in the adult, carries out an excitatory function. This is an example of the difference in neurologic function between infants and adults. It also highlights the idea that neurologic growth and maturation of synapses is an activity-dependent process that relies on excitatory stimulation [18]. The descending modulatory pathways from the brainstem to the dorsal horn are also in a state of evolution during development. Axons grow from the brainstem to the dorsal horn via the dorsolateral funiculus tract during fetal development, but they do not form synapses on the dorsal horn until later. This represents an underdeveloped system of endogenous pain regulation, suggesting that nociceptive input may result in an exaggerated response [19].

While reflex responses can be studied with relative ease, assessment of behaviors heralding the development of higher pain processing centers is more difficult. The degree to which a fetus or neonate can perceive pain cannot be truly elucidated; however, there is evidence that the synaptic connections are present and functioning. Thalamocortical projections start to form between 23 and 30 weeks of gestational age [20]. Somatosensory-evoked potentials, suggesting the capacity for cortical perception of pain, can be observed by 29 weeks [21]. Cortical synapses develop rapidly in the second postnatal week, and their growth is heavily influenced by sensory experiences, as naturally occurring neural activity influences the development and organization of the primary somatosensory cortex [22, 23]. Further elements of pain perception are quite difficult to follow, and little is known regarding the development of attention, memory formation, and emotional aspects of the pain experience [24].

Physiologic and Behavior Pain Assessment Measures in Infants: Use and Limitations

Introduction

In order for one to treat pain both safely and effectively, one must start with a reliable and thorough pain assessment [25]. The assessment of pain in newborns and infants is often a difficult task for clinicians and caregivers. Due to the inability to verbally report in these patients, clinicians are left to interpret a wide variety of physiological and biobehavioral parameters as surrogates for an infant's pain. Additional barriers, including individual attitudes/beliefs, the myth that neonates/infants do not feel pain, inability to objectify a subjective experience, and concern that treatment of pain will lead to side effects from analgesic medications, make it difficult to assess and treat pain in this vulnerable population [25, 26]. Physiologic and behavioral pain indicators alone are not sufficient to truly understand and assess pain in these patients [25].

Nonetheless, almost 30 different unidimensional, multidimensional, and composite tools exist for the assessment of pain in neonates and infants. The proliferation of such tools has made it easier for clinicians and caregivers to assess the pain; however, these instruments must be carefully employed, as each comes with inherent limitations.

Conceptual and Situational Implications of Pain

Pain has a nociceptive component, but there is also an emotional and cognitive aspect which ultimately means that pain is a subjective experience that can never completely be understood by another [25, 26]. Furthermore, the assessment of pain is further complicated in nonverbal patients, since we still hold verbal report as one of the gold standards of pain assessment [1]. The IASP has released an addendum in 2003, concluding that "the inability to communicate verbally in no way negates the possibility that an individual is experiencing pain and is in need of appropriate pain relieving treatment." While it is clear that an infant can react to a painful stimulus, we do not have a good understanding of whether or not the infant is able to apply coping strategies. It is likely that the infant relies heavily on the caregiver to contextualize the pain experience [25].

By understanding the context in which an infant experiences pain may allow a clinician or caregiver to better evaluate and treat her pain. Three distinct pain scenarios have been described in the literature.

Acute Procedural Precipitated by a specific nociceptive event and is typically self-limited. Usually evidenced by behavioral or physiologic indicators (i.e., facial expression, increased heart rate, etc.). Clinician/caregiver should do their best to predict and prevent acute procedural pain by anticipation of such situations.

Acute Prolonged Less understood and more difficult to treat. Typically has a clearly defined cause (i.e., surgery, burn, etc.), but without a definitive end point. The extended time that the infant experiences pain can result in greater suffering, irritability, and lower future threshold for pain [25]. Prolonged pain may be more difficult to assess as physiologic and behavioral patterns seen in acute procedural pain may be less reliable or absent. Assessment should occur over an extended period of time to better understand resulting behavioral activity and functional impairment [25].

Chronic Pain Pathological pain state without apparent biological value that has persisted beyond the normal tissue healing time [16]. We have little research, tools, and overall understanding in addressing or treating chronic pain states in neonates and infants [25].

Tools for Pain Assessment in Infants

Although several tools exist today, pain assessment can still prove to be difficult in the neonate and infant population. Caregivers and healthcare professionals should always attempt to anticipate pain-associated procedures or conditions and treat pain accordingly in a dynamic fashion with ongoing reassessment [26]. It is important that one is not only treating pain scores but also monitoring the patient's response to treatment along with clear documentation of side effects and vital signs [26]. Although self-report is considered by some to be the gold standard for pain assessment, we must be ready to ascertain behavioral and physiological indicators and be cognizant of influence of psychological, developmental, and cultural factors [26].

There is no single validated indicator of proper and accurate assessment of infant pain; therefore, we are encouraged to use multiple behavioral, biobehavioral, or physiological in order to complete our assessments.

Behavioral Indicators Behavioral indicators are often used to assess neonatal and infant pain, with facial expression, cry, and motor activity being the most common [25]. In 1987, Grunau and Craig described the Neonatal Facial Action Coding System which accounted for the presence or absence of ten objective facial actions (i.e., bulging brows, eye squeeze, etc.) in order to scale the likeliness and severity of a painful condition [27]. It is important to remember that facial expression can be influenced by severity of illness, comorbidities, low birth weight or prematurity, and neurological/physical impairment and furthermore may play a diminished role in persistent or chronic pain states [25, 29].

Cry is another commonly used behavioral indicator, and besides its simple presence or absence has also been studied in terms of amplitude/pitch, latency to cry, duration of expiratory and inspiratory cry, duration of pause, and regulation/rhythm [25]. Procedure-related cries typically occur immediately following a known stimulus and may be more intense or of higher pitch [25], whereas shorter latency and longer duration have been described in chronic or postoperative pain states [12, 13]. It is important to remember that overall, crying is nonspecific in infant populations and can indicate a variety of needs such as hunger, fatigue, or agitation [25].

Physiological Indicators Common physiological indicators used in neonatal/infant pain assessment include heart rate, blood pressure, respiratory rate, skin color, diaphoresis, and vomiting. They have a limited role when used alone as they indicate other situations such as hunger, agitation, fear, anxiety, or physical stress; they can add value when used within context or in combination with behavioral indicators [25, 30]. It is important to remember that autonomic nervous system is developmentally immature in neonates and further blunted in premature or neurologically impaired patient populations, and therefore, the presence or absence of changes in heart rate or blood pressure may not be a sensitive indicator of pain [25].

Biomarkers Biomarkers are widely used, quantitatively and qualitatively, across all aspects of medicine; they also have a role within assessing neonatal pain. Cortisol B endorphins and growth hormone, among others, have been described in the context of pain [1, 28, 31]. Although biomarkers are not typically used as a direct measure of infant pain, it does have a role in describing an infant's reactivity or response to pain [25]. Biomarkers may play additional roles in conveying CNS integrity and understanding health and development [25].

Limitations in Pain Assessment of Infants

- Time consuming for clinicians or caregivers to score and rescore scales.
- Pre-existing individual, cultural, and socioeconomic bias or misconceptions.
- Difficult to generalize a scale to different age populations.
- Some infants may not respond to tissue-damaging events [28].
- Preterm infant's response may be behaviorally blunted or absent (clinical gate).
- Neurologically impaired or cognitively impaired infants.
- Physiologic and behavioral indicators may be nonspecific (sepsis, hunger, anxiety).

Examples of Pain Assessment Tools

Neonatal Facial Coding Scale (NFCS)

The Neonatal Facial Coding Scale (Fig. 3.1) utilizes facial expressions to monitor and assess pain in neonates. This scale can be used in premature infants as well. The absence (0 points) or presence (1 point) of eight different characteristics is summated where a score of 3 or more is considered to be a manifestation of a painful experience.

Faces, Legs, Activity, Cry, and Consolability Scale (FLACC)

The FLACC scale (Fig. 3.2) has five parameters, of which each is scored as 0, 1, or 2. The score ranges from 0 (no pain) to 10 (maximal pain). It can be used in ages 2 months to 7 years old. It is an especially important tool in patient nonverbal populations.

Fig. 3.1 Neonatal Facial Coding System (NFCS)

Facial actions	0 point	1 point
Brow bulge	Absent	Present
Eye squeeze	Absent	Present
Deepening of the nasolabial furrow	Absent	Present
Open lips	Absent	Present
Mouth stretch (horizontal or vertical)	Absent	Present
Tongue tautening	Absent	Present
Tongue protrusion	Absent	Present
Chin quiver	Absent	Present

Maximal score of 8 points, consodering pain ≥ 3.

Fig. 3.2 Faces, Legs, Activity, Cry, and Consolability Scale (FLACC)

Behavioral observation pain rating scale

Categories	Scoring		
	0	1	3
Face	No particular expression or smile; disinterested	Occasional grimace or frown, withdrawn	Frequent to constant frown, clenched jaw, quivering chin
Legs	No position or relaxed	Uneasy, reatless, tense	Kicking, or legs drawn up
Activity	Lying quietly, normal position, moves easily	Squirming, shifting back and forth, tense	Arched, rigid, or jerking
Cry	No crying (awake or asleep)	Moans or whimpers occasional complaint	Crying steadily, screams or sobs, frequent complaints
Consolability	Content, relaxed	Reassured by occasional touching, hugging, or talking to, Distractable	Difficult to console or comfort

Each of the five categories (F) Face; (L) Legs; (A) Activity: (C) Cry: (C) Consolability is scored from 0 to 2, which results in a total score between 0 and 10.

Fig. 3.3 CRIES score

	Date/Time						
Crying – Characteristic cry of pain is high pitched. 0 – No cry or cry that is not high-pitched 1 – Cry high pitched but baby is wasily consolable 2 – Cry high pitched but baby is inconsolable							
Requires O$_2$ for SaO$_2$ < 95% – Babies experiencing pain manifest decreased oxygenation. Consider other causes of hypoxemia, e.g., oversedation, atelectasis, pneumothorax) 0 – No oxygen required 1 – <30% oxygen required 2 – >30% oxygen required							
Increased vital signs (BP* and HR*) – Take BP last as this may awaken child making other assessments difficult 0 – Both HR and BP unchanged or less than baseline 1 – HR or BP inceased but increase in <20% of baseline 2 – HR or BP is increased >20% over baseline.							
Expression – The facial expression most often associated with pain is a grimace. A griamace may be characterized by brow lowering, eyes squeezed shut, deepening naso-labial furrow, or open lips and mouth. 0 – No grimace present 1 – Grimace alone is present 2 – Grimace and non-cry vocalization grunt is present							
Sleepless – Scored based upon the infant's state during the hour preceding this recorded score. 0 – Child has been continuously asleep 1 – Child has awakened at frequent intervals 2 – Child has been awakeconstantly							
Total score							

CRIES Score

The CRIES score (Fig. 3.3) is obtained by adding together a 0, 1, or 2 score for each of five indicators: crying, oxygen saturation, vital signs, facial expression, and sleeping pattern.

A score of 4 or higher is typically considered an indication for medication. The score should be obtained every hour for at least the first 24 hours postoperatively. It is generally used for infants 6 months and younger.

Long-Term Consequences of Neonatal Pain

Effective management of pain is expected for patients of all ages. However, the field of neonatal pain was not recognized until the 1980s due to the preceding convention that memory formation is not well developed in neonates, and hence no long-term consequences can be expected [32]. A strong turn in understanding neonatal pain occurred after a landmark study in 1987 that showed improved survival and short-term outcomes in neonates who received anesthesia for surgery versus paralytics alone. Studying neonatal pain coincided with the advances in care of preterm neonates in neonatal ICU, where numerous pain-provoking procedures are required on daily basis, such as tracheal suctioning, blood drawing, or lines placements. These procedures served as the most feasible and ethical way of studying human pain response at this early age. However, a large source of confounding existed as a result of this methodology due to difficulties of adjusting for factors that are commonly present in NICU infants such as prematurity, infections, and psychological stress from maternal separation, repetitive handling, and alike. Moreover, our current knowledge of the long-term consequences of neonatal pain largely stems from studies of animal models, which need to be cautiously interpreted with regard to humans.

In the periphery, for example, rat pups that had skin-thickness wounds underwent pronounced hyperinnervation (up to 300%) of the tissue. The hyperinnervation persisted long after the wounds had healed. The hyperinnervation effect is maximal when the wound is inflicted in the immediate postnatal period and becomes minimal and transient if the wounds are inflicted later in age [33]. At the spinal level, rat pups exposed to hind paw inflammation expressed increased density of nociceptive fibers in the corresponding segments of spinal cord, and when reaching adulthood, had lower pain threshold in response to stimuli compared to nonexposed pups [34]. The combination of hyperinnervation and increased density of innervation in the dorsal horn of spinal cord is thought to be responsible for the long-term potentiation of painful stimuli [35]. This potentiation is at least partially related to the delayed maturation of supraspinal inhibitory pathways during neonatal period as well [36].

On the contrary, in another series of studies, mice pups that underwent neonatal laparotomy showed reduced nociceptive sensation in adulthood compared to the control group [37]. Studies in humans showed similar controversies. On the one hand, hyperesthesia was reported in children who had undergone cardiac surgeries early in life (not necessarily in neonatal period) [38], while other researchers reported that infants previously operated upon in the same dermatome needed more intraoperative and postoperative analgesia and had higher pain scores than did infants with no prior surgery [39].

Traumatic experience of childhood can undoubtedly cast a lasting impact on later neurobehavioral development, but whether neonatal pain results in long-term effects is a source of debate. A study of preterm neonates (28-week post-conceptual age (PCA)) who spent 4 weeks in NICU found that they were less responsive to heel lances compared to neonates born at 32 weeks and consequently spent no time in NICU. The dampened behavioral responses correlated with the number of pain-provoking procedures in these 4 weeks [40]. Similarly, 4-month-old and an 8-month-old infant and toddlers who were born prematurely or with low birth weight and had prolonged stay in NICU were less responsive to everyday pain compared to their counterparts [41–44]. Limited research suggested that as these children grew older, they had poor adaptation to pain and an increased prevalence of somatization complains [43]. It is prudent to point that the result of the mentioned studies should be interpreted cautiously, as prematurity, low birth weight, and their complications can be all confounding factors for the studied outcome, which is behavioral development. Significant evidence linking neonatal pain and long-term behavior comes from a widely cited study showing that infants circumcised at birth had stronger pain response to subsequent routine vaccination than uncircumcised infants and that pre-treatment of the circumcision site with topical anesthetics resulted in reduction of this pain sensitivity [45]. The conflicting reports on whether neonatal pain dampens or strengthens the pain response later in life indicate that the effect of pain on the development of the nervous system in neonatal period is more complicated than originally thought and that a specific state of potentiation or dampening of the nociceptive system may ensue based on the timing and the nature of the painful experience. It is postulated that painful experiences in late human gestation seem to enhance, whereas painful experiences in early human gestation seem to dampen the behavioral responses to subsequent pain [35].

Analgesia and Prevention of Long-Term Consequences

The term "allostatic load" was developed by some authors to define the cumulative effect of exposure to repeated stress from any source [46], and since pain is an important source of distress in neonatal period, few trials have assessed the role of relieving this allostatic load in preterm neonates by providing preemptive analgesia. A large randomized controlled trial that compared the continuous infusion of morphine versus placebo in preterm ventilated infants found no difference in neurological outcome between both groups [47]. A similarly designed trial also found no difference in the neuropsychological development later in childhood (age

5–6) [48]. This is not to underestimate the importance of humane and appropriate pain management for young children but rather to urge caution in overstating the downstream effects of pain [46].

In conclusion, important steps have been made in understanding the long-term effect of neonatal pain, but we are still far from a complete understanding of this complex subject. The neonatal nervous system, both peripheral and central, is in a state of constant formation and reorganization, and it is likely that nociceptive input may result in long-term sequela. Thus, a concerted effort should be made to provide safe and effective analgesia in this vulnerable patient population.

References

1. Anand KJS. Pain and its effects in the human neonate and fetus. N Engl J Med. 1987;317:1321–9.
2. Fishman S, Ballantyne J, Rathmell J. Bonica's management of pain. Philadelphia: Lippincott, Williams & Wilkins; 2010.
3. Slater R, Cantarella A, Gallella S, et al. Cortical pain responses in human infants. J Neurosci. 2006;26(14):3662–6.
4. Bartocci M, Bergqvist L, Lagercrantz H. Pain activates cortical areas in the preterm newborn brain. Pain. 2006;122:109–17.
5. Fitzgerald M, Howard RF. The neurobiologic basis of pediatric pain. In: Schechter N, Berde C, Yaster M, editors. Pain in infants, children, and adolescents. Philadelphia: Lippincott, Williams & Wilkins; 2003.
6. Teng C, Abbott V. The formalin test: a dose-response analysis at three developmental stages. Pain. 1998;76:337–47.
7. Beggs S, Fitgerald M. Development of peripheral and spinal nociceptive systems. In: Anand KJS, Stevens BJ, McGrath PJ, editors. Pain in neonates and infants. Edinburgh/New York: Elsevier; 2007.
8. Moore KL, Persaud TVN. The developing human: clinically oriented embryology. Philadelphia: Saunders; 2003.
9. Vanhatalo S, van Nieuwenhuizen O. Fetal pain? Brain Dev. 2000;22:145–50.
10. Fitzgerald M. The development of nociceptive circuits. Nat Rev Neurosci. 2005;6:507–20.
11. Fitzgerald M. Cutaneous primary afferent properties in the hindlimb of the neonatal rat. J Physiol. 1987;383:79–92.
12. Fitzgerald M, Butcher T, Shortland P. Developmental changes in the laminar termination of A-fibre cutaneous sensory afferents in the rat spinal cord dorsal horn. J Comp Neurol. 1994;348:225–33.
13. Beggs S, Torsney C, Drew LJ, Fitzgerald M. The postnatal reorganization of primary afferent input and dorsal horn cell receptive fields in the rat spinal cord is an activity-dependent process. Eur J Neurosci. 2002;16:1249–58.
14. Park JS, Nakatsuka T, Nagata K, Higashi H, Yoshimura M. Reorganization of the primary afferent termination in the rat spinal dorsal horn during post-natal development. Brain Res Dev Brain Res. 1999;113:29–36.
15. Bicknell HRJ, Beal JA. Axonal and dendritic development of substantia gelatinosa neurons in the lumbosacral spinal cord of the rat. J Comp Neurol. 1984;226:508–22.
16. Biljani V, Rizvi TA, Wadhwa S. Development of spinal substrate for nociception in man. NIDA Res Monogr. 1988;87:167–79.
17. Kalb RG, Fox AJ. Synchronized overproduction of AMPA, kainate, and NMDA glutamate receptors during human spinal cord development. J Comp Neurol. 1997;384:200–10.
18. Ben-Ari Y. Excitatory actions of GABA during development: the nature of the nurture. Nat Rev Neurosci. 2002;3:728–39.
19. Van Praag H, Frenk H. The development of stimulation produced analgesia (SPA) in the rat. Dev Brain Res. 1991;64:71–6.
20. Lee SL, Ralston HJP, Drey EA, Partridge JC, Rosen M. Fetal pain: a systematic multidisciplinary review of the evidence. JAMA. 2005;294:947–54.
21. Klimach VJ, Cooke RW. Maturation of the neonatal somatosensory evoked response in preterm infants. Dev Med Child Neurol. 1988;30:208–14.
22. Stern EA, Maravall M, Svoboda K. Rapid development and plasticity of layer 2/3 maps in rat barrel cortex in vivo. Neuron. 2001;31:305–15.
23. O'Leary DD, Ruff NL, Dyck RH. Development, critical period plasticity, and adult reorganizations of mammalian somatosensory systems. Curr Opin Neurobiol. 1994;4:535–44.
24. Anand KJS, Carr DB. The neuroanatomy, neurophysiology, and neurochemistry of pain, stress, and analgesia in newborns and children. Pediatr Clin N Am. 1989;36:795–822.
25. Anand KJS, McGrath PJ, Stevens BJ. Pain in neonates. 1st ed. Amsterdam: Elsevier; 2000. Print.
26. American Academy of Pediatrics. Committee on Psychosocial Aspects of Child and Family Health; Task Force on Pain in Infants, Children, and Adolescents. The assessment and management of acute pain in infants, children, and adolescents. Pediatrics. 2001;108(3):793–7. Web.
27. Silva YP, Gomez RS, Maximo TA, Silva ACS. Pain evaluation in neonatology. Rev Bras Anestesiol. 2007;57(5):565–74.
28. Johnston CC, Sherrard A, Stevens B, et al. Do cry features reflect pain intensity in preterm neonates? A preliminary study. Biol Neonate. 1999;76:120–4.
29. Holsti L, Granau R, Oberlander T, et al. Specific newborn individualized developmental care and assessment program movements are associated with acute pain in preterm infants in the neonatal intensive care unit. Pediatrics. 2004;114:65–72.
30. Assessing pain in the NICU – AboutKidsHealth. Aboutkidshealth. ca. N.p., 2017. Web 15 Dec 2016.
31. Anand KJ, Hickey PR. Halothane-morphine compared with high dose sufentanil for anesthesia and postoperative analgesia in neonatal cardiac surgery. N Engl J Med. 1992;326:1–9.
32. Maroney DI. Recognizing the potential effect of stress and trauma on premature infants in the NICU: how are outcomes affected? J Perinatol. 2003;23(8):679–83.
33. Reynolds ML, Fitzgerald M. Long-term sensory hyperinnervation following neonatal skin wounds. J Comp Neurol. 1995;358(4):487–98.
34. Ruda MA, et al. Altered nociceptive neuronal circuits after neonatal peripheral inflammation. Science. 2000;289(5479):628–30.
35. Anand KJS. Pain, plasticity, and premature birth: a prescription for permanent suffering? Nat Med. 2000;6(9):971–4.
36. Ren K, Blass EM, Dubner R. Suckling and sucrose ingestion suppress persistent hyperalgesia and spinal Fos expression after forepaw inflammation in infant rats. Proc Natl Acad Sci. 1997;94(4):1471–5.
37. Sternberg WF, et al. Long-term effects of neonatal surgery on adulthood pain behavior. Pain. 2005;113(3):347–53.
38. Schmelzle-Lubiecki BM, et al. Long-term consequences of early infant injury and trauma upon somatosensory processing. Eur J Pain. 2007;11(7):799–809.
39. Peters JWB, et al. Does neonatal surgery lead to increased pain sensitivity in later childhood? Pain. 2005;114(3):444–54.
40. Johnston CC, Stevens BJ. Experience in a neonatal intensive care unit affects pain response. Pediatrics. 1996;98(5):925–30.
41. Oberlander TF, et al. Biobehavioral pain responses in former extremely low birth weight infants at four months' corrected age. Pediatrics. 2000;105(1):e6.
42. Grunau RE, et al. Pain reactivity in former extremely low birth weight infants at corrected age 8 months compared with term born controls. Infant Behav Dev. 2001;24(1):41–55.

43. Grunau RVE, Whitfield MF, Petrie JH. Pain sensitivity and temperament in extremely low-birth-weight premature toddlers and preterm and full-term controls. Pain. 1994;58(3):341–6.

44. Grunau RVE, et al. Early pain experience, child and family factors, as precursors of somatization: a prospective study of extremely premature and fullterm children. Pain. 1994;56(3):353–9.

45. Taddio A, et al. Effect of neonatal circumcision on pain response during subsequent routine vaccination. Lancet. 1997;349(9052):599–603.

46. Grunau RE, Holsti L, Peters JWB. Long-term consequences of pain in human neonates. Semin Fetal Neonatal Med. 2006;11(4):268–75. WB Saunders.

47. Anand KJS, et al. Effects of morphine analgesia in ventilated preterm neonates: primary outcomes from the NEOPAIN randomised trial. Lancet. 2004;363(9422):1673–82.

48. MacGregor R, et al. Outcome at 5–6 years of prematurely born children who received morphine as neonates. Arch Dis Child Fetal Neonatal Ed. 1998;79(1):F40–3.

Designing, Reporting, and Interpreting Clinical Research Studies About Treatments for Pain: Evidence-Based Medicine

Nisheeth Pandey, Joseph Park, and Sukdeb Datta

Introduction

A thorough understanding of evidence-based medicine is a requirement for any clinician, especially those in rapidly developing specialties such as pain medicine. This understanding is not only important to guide clinical practice but also to empower active contribution to the body of evidence that is required to justify reimbursements for interventions.

Evidence-based medicine is the conscientious, explicit, and judicious use of the current best evidence in making decisions about the care of an individual patient [1]. Evidence-based medicine's intended purpose is to allow the physician to combine their individual clinical acumen with the best available data from systematic research in order to promote high-quality patient care.

Outcome assessment is the end goal of conducting evidence-based research of different therapeutics. Outcome assessment can be performed for several reasons: to trace the progress of an individual, to study the efficacy of a treatment method, to compare the effectiveness of different treatments, or to evaluate the cost-effectiveness of different treatments. In technical terms, outcome assessment aims at establishing four parameters: efficacy (can it work?), effectiveness (does it work?), efficiency (does it produce value?), and safety (do adverse events exist and are they acceptable?) [2].

Once a defined outcome is selected, the choice of research paradigm can be narrowed to appropriately fit the outcome of interest. Two main study designs exist, observational and interventional. A researcher can either observe events occur among different groups or can introduce an intervention for select groups in order to measure its effectiveness. Research design can be further delineated by a number of parameters including the chronology of outcome occurrence and assessment (prospective versus retrospective), the number of interventions and groups (controlled studies versus longitudinal cohorts versus case series) or patient allocation (simple randomized versus restricted randomized versus nonrandomized). The goal of manipulating these additional parameters is to ultimately tailor a study to best elucidate the primary research question at hand and establish validity of the design. The main hindrance to validity is bias, defined as a "systematic deviation from the truth." The probability of biased results in any given study depends on the rigor of its design, thus creating a hierarchy of "levels of evidence" with Level I studies being regarded as those with the highest degree of evidence and least likely to be affected by bias [2].

The major tools used to safeguard from bias in study design are randomization, blinding, and establishment of a control group. Randomization ensures equitable proportions of a varied population are assigned to the different treatment arms, thereby limiting the impact of patient demographics (i.e., age, etc.) in assessing the outcome of interest. Randomization can be simple or restricted. Simple randomization means that no stratification process was applied to the randomization. In a small sample size, this can lead to dissimilar testing groups. Restricted randomization refers to any process used with random assignment to achieve equality between study groups across baseline characteristics of the study population (e.g., block or stratified randomization).

Blinding conceals experimental group allocation of the participants from the researcher. In a double-blind trial, neither the researcher nor the patient is aware of the assignment of allocation and interventions. Allocation concealment is a technique often used to prevent bias by concealing the allocation sequence from those designating participants to intervention groups until the moment of assignment.

Establishment of a control group, either a placebo or an active therapeutic alternative, allows for an estimation of an intervention's effect size and comparison to other available modalities. In placebo-controlled trials, subjects are assigned

N. Pandey
Pain Management, Fayette County Memorial Hospital, Washington Court House, OH, USA

J. Park
Department of Anesthesiology, Icahn School of Medicine at Mount Sinai, New York, NY, USA

S. Datta (✉)
Department of Anesthesiology, Mount Sinai Medical Center, New York, NY, USA

© Springer Nature Switzerland AG 2019
Y. Khelemsky et al. (eds.), *Academic Pain Medicine*, https://doi.org/10.1007/978-3-030-18005-8_4

to the test treatment or an identical appearing treatment that does not contain the test drug. Trade-offs exist between using a placebo control versus an active control. Placebo-controlled studies allow for assessment of the absolute effect size of a treatment; however these studies can raise ethical concerns, as physicians are not providing a known treatment to patients with disease. In addition, placebo controls can affect patient recruitment if patients believe that they will potentially not be receiving real treatment. Active therapeutic controls do not have the same ethical concerns, however these studies are limited in their ability to show the true effect size of the treatment being studies and also require larger sample sizes to show statistically significant differences between the two treatments.

The WHO International Clinical Trial Registry Platform defines a clinical trial as any research study that prospectively assigns human participants or groups of humans to one or more health-related interventions to evaluate effects on health outcome [3]. As the name indicates, randomized controlled trials (RCTs) are generally designed with the use of randomization, control groups, and blinding to minimize bias. RCTs showing either statistically significant differences or lack thereof with narrow confidence intervals constitute Level I evidence for investigational studies comparing therapeutic outcomes. They are regarded as the gold standard for understanding the safety and efficacy of healthcare interventions. RCTs have a number of strengths and they continue to play an important role in the development, evaluation, and regulatory approval of new treatments and interventions. Compared to other research designs, RCTs establish an internal validity by diligently controlling for potential confounding factors. This allows for their ability to provide specific answers to questions related to the efficacy of new treatments compared with alternatives in addition to establishing proper dosing of the treatment being tested [4].

The field of pain management presents unique challenges to producing reliable RCT-based evidence. While the research design allows for the maintenance of internal validity to determine efficacy, RCTs used for the study of pain management can have limitations in predicting effectiveness (external validity) and determining how a therapy will perform in real-life populations. The difficulties in treating pain have stemmed from the difficulties in the development of clinical research trials that can adequately assess the myriad factors affecting the experience of pain. Every facet of pain-related clinical research, from the study design to patient selection to study duration, has been shown to potentially confound results. Only by understanding and addressing these issues can research studies be designed effectively and ultimately improve the management of pain [4].

Many RCTs of current analgesic medications have failed to show statistically significant pain relief over placebo in conditions where efficacy has been demonstrated [5, 6]. In fact, meta-analyses of approved pain treatments demonstrate a less than 30% improvement in pain intensity when compared with placebo [7]. The reason for the failure of RCTs in analgesic studies is still not clear although a number of theories exist. One proposed explanation for the failure of these RCTs is the inclusion of a placebo group and the overestimation of clinical improvement [8]. A large Cochrane review found that trials assessing pain, unlike almost every other outcome measure, had a potentially strong placebo effect [9]. The implication of this is that the treatment effect may be underestimated relative to the "control," which leads to negative trial results. In addition, the length of a study factors into the results since longer studies have shown a tendency toward greater placebo effect. The combination of this information with regulatory changes mandating longer duration of phase 3 trials may be contributing to a large number of failed trials considering some longer-duration trials have shown efficacy early in the course of treatment but eventually may show decreased separation of drug effect from placebo [10].

Another problem with many RCTs is the exclusion of the elderly and those with a history of psychiatric disorder, the two patient populations where pain is most prevalent. Because many studies require subjects be free of co-existing chronic conditions and to not be on other medications, many older patients (especially those >80 years old) find themselves unable to participate [11]. Patients with psychiatric disorders have also been routinely excluded; one review article found roughly 75% of trials involving lower back pain had psychiatric exclusion criteria [12]. The underrepresentation of these populations reduces generalizability and severely diminishes any assessment of benefit and risk of treatment with regard to these patients. Patient drop-out has also plagued many analgesic trials. As many as 30–60% of patients withdraw and fail to provide primary and secondary outcome data [5, 13]. The approach taken in assessing this missing data can have major consequences on the results of the study. For example, many trials consider early dropout due to toxicity a treatment failure, pooling these results with dropouts due to lack of efficacy [14]. Imputing this missing data has been achieved mainly by using the last observation carried forward or baseline observation carried forward methods. These methods may not be ideal for approaching missing primary data [15, 16]. Lack of complete data and the improper handling of this incomplete data may obscure the true outcomes of many RCTs.

Clinical study sites have also drastically changed in recent decades, moving from academic medical centers to private sites where financial incentives may play a role [17]. Rewards for recruiting patients may affect patient selection and conduct of investigators which in turn could lead to flawed conclusions of the trial. Examples of this have been seen in the antidepressant literature, and it is posited that improper recruitment of patients who were not "severely" depressed may have contributed to the "failed" trial [8, 18].   T h e plethora of negative pain trials has provided the impetus to standardize studies and minimize the issues detailed previously involving methodology and patient selection. An important tool that has helped in this pursuit is the Consolidated Standards of Reports Trials (CONSORT) which set guidelines emphasizing an avoidance of bias and transparent reporting of data [19]. The most recent iteration of CONSORT from 2010 includes a 25-item checklist and a flow diagram for participants which focus on protocol design, analysis, and interpretation. The diagram tracks participant progress through the trial. At its core, CONSORT does not aim to shape the design, conduct, or analysis of the trials – it addressed the need for rigorous standards for accurate reporting of what was done.

Following the model of CONSORT, the Standard Protocol Items: Recommendations for Interventional Trials (SPIRIT) were developed [20]. The authors of SPIRIT recognized that guidelines for protocol content were heterogeneous and very rarely included empirical evidence to support recommendations. These deficiencies had the potential to lead to poor trial conduct, amendments to the protocol, and possible inaccurate publications. Thus, SPIRIT guidelines were developed to improve the content and quality of protocols by ensuring that primarily evidence-based recommendations were included in studies. A checklist of 33 items was created with this goal in mind with sections focusing on administrative information, introduction, methods, ethics, and appendices.

Pain-specific guidelines have also been developed. The Initiative on Methods, Measurement, and Pain Assessment in Clinical Trials (IMMPACT) collaborative group has been instrumental in creating guidelines by which studies can be designed [21]. Special importance is placed on four broad areas including participant selection, trial phases and duration, treatment groups and dosing regimens, and types of trials. Another group called the Analgesic Clinical Trial Translations, Innovations, Opportunities, and Networks (ACTTION) was formed with the goal of standardizing data collection and terminology in the hopes of improving the quality of pain trial data across institutions [22].

The challenges of interpreting data from individual trials are further compounded when examining meta-analyses. The Interventional Pain Management techniques Quality Appraisal of Reliability and Risk of Bias Assessment (IPM-QRB) was developed recently as a means of evaluating trials for inclusion in systematic reviews of interventional pain management techniques, specifically involving spine techniques [23]. The Cochrane Review Group's quality assessment and bias assessment for randomized trials has been the most commonly used method of evaluating studies and meta-analyses. However, no instrument had been developed specifically for interventional techniques, hence the development of IPM-QRB. There are 22 items in this tool used to assess trials, including pain-specific considerations such as imaging used, financial conflicts of interest, and selection with diagnostic blocks. Analysis by this group found improved intraclass correlation coefficient among interventional pain trials (0.833) as compared to the widely accepted standard, the Cochrane review instrument (0.407), signifying a much improved standardized means of evaluating pain studies.

New study designs are needed in order to incorporate the psychological, social, clinical, and demographic characteristics of patients with pain. The collaborative efforts of IMMPACT and ACTTION are signs that there is an increased attention to the methodological aspects of pain trials which are paving the way toward more meaningful evaluations and ultimately more effective treatments for pain.

References

1. Sackett DL, Rosenberg WM, Gray JA, Haynes RB, Richardson WS. Evidence based medicine: what it is and what it isn't. BMJ. 1996;312(7023):71–2.
2. Vavken P, Ganal-Antonio AKB, Shen FH, Chapman JR, Samartzis D. Fundamentals of clinical outcomes assessment for spinal disorders: study designs, methodologies, and analyses. Global Spine J. 2015;5(2):156–64.
3. World Health Organization. n.d. Retrieved January 17, 2017, from http://www.who.int/ictrp/en/.
4. IOM (Institute of Medicine). Relieving pain in America: a blueprint for transforming prevention, care, education, and research. Washington, DC: The National Academies Press; 2011.
5. Katz N. Methodological issues in clinical trials of opioids for chronic pain. Neurology. 2005;65(12 Suppl 4):S32–49.
6. XenoPort, Inc. Phase II results for GSK1838262 (XP13512) reported for neuropathic pain associated with diabetic peripheral neuropathy; 2009.
7. Turk DC. Clinical effectiveness and cost-effectiveness of treatments for patients with chronic pain. Clin J Pain. 2002;18(6):355–65.
8. Dworkin RH, et al. Evidence-based clinical trial design for chronic pain pharmacotherapy: a blueprint for ACTION. Pain. 2011;152(3 Suppl):S107–15.
9. Hrobjartsson A, Gotzsche P. Placebo interventions for all clinical conditions. Cochrane Database Syst Rev. 2010;(1):CD003974.
10. Quessy SN, Rowbotham MC. Placebo response in neuropathic pain trials. Pain. 2008;138:479–83.
11. Schmader KE, et al. Treatment considerations for elderly and frail patients with neuropathic pain. Mayo Clin Proc. 2010;85(3 Suppl):S26–32.
12. Humphreys K, Blodgett JC, Roberts LW. The exclusion of people with psychiatric disorders from medical research. J Psychiatr Res. 2015;70:28 32.
13. Galer BS, Lee D, Ma T, Nagle B, Schlagheck TG. MorphiDex (morphine sulfate/dextromethorphan hydrobromide combination) in the treatment of chronic pain: three multicenter, randomized, double-blind, controlled clinical trials fail to demonstrate enhanced opioid analgesia or reduction in tolerance. Pain. 2005;115:284–95.
14. Kim Y. Missing data handling in chronic pain trials. J Biopharm Stat. 2011;21(2):311–25.
15. Molenberghs G, Kenward MG. Missing data in clinical studies. Chichester, UK: John Wiley & Sons, Ltd; 2007.

16. National Research Council. The prevention and treatment of missing data in clinical trials. Washington, DC: The National Academies Press; 2010.
17. IOM (Institute of Medicine). Transforming clinical research in the United States: challenges and opportunities. Washington, DC: The National Academies Press; 2010.
18. Liu KS, Snavely DB, Ball WA, Lines CR, Reines SA, Potter WZ. Is bigger better for depression trials? J Psychiatr Res. 2008;42:622–30.
19. Turner L, Shamseer L, Altman DG, Weeks L, Peters J, Kober T, Dias S, Schulz KF, Plint AC, Moher D. Consolidated standards of reporting trials (CONSORT) and the completeness of reporting of randomised controlled trials (RCTs) published in medical journals. Cochrane Database Syst Rev. 2012;11:MR000030.
20. Chan AW, Tetzlaff JM, Altman DG, Laupacis A, Gøtzsche PC, Krleža-Jerić K, Hróbjartsson A, Mann H, Dickersin K, Berlin JA, Doré CJ, Parulekar WR, Summerskill WS, Groves T, Schulz KF, Sox HC, Rockhold FW, Rennie D, Moher D. SPIRIT 2013 statement: defining standard protocol items for clinical trials. Ann Intern Med. 2013;158:200–7.
21. Dworkin RH, et al. Research design considerations for confirmatory chronic pain trials: IMMPACT recommendations. Pain. 2010;149(2):177–93.
22. Dworkin RH, et al. A standard database format for clinical trials of pain treatments. Pain. 2013;154(1):11–4.
23. Manchikanti L, Hirsch JA, Cohen SP, Heavner JE, Falco FJ, Diwan S, et al. Assessment of methodologic quality of randomized trials of interventional techniques: development of an interventional pain management specific instrument. Pain Physician. 2014;17:E263–90.

Animal Models of Pain and Ethics of Animal Experimentation

5

Arjun Yerasi and Laxmaiah Manchikanti

Introduction

Pain affects up to 100 million Americans. It remains difficult to treat with basic science findings often having limited clinical translatability. Trends over the last 30 years have shifted toward an in increase in the use of animal studies to characterize pain states [1]. Through these animal models, there have been advancements in understanding the anatomical, biochemical, and physiological mechanisms of pain [2].

Measuring Pain Behavior in Animals

A unique challenge to developing animal pain models is the inability to obtain subjective pain information. Unlike research involving human subjects where patient pain surveys can augment behavioral response data, animal models must rely solely on evaluating objective responses to stimuli [3]. As such, appropriate animal models must utilize specific noxious stimuli and subsequent outcomes that are clinically measurable and consistent with the pain experience of individual disease states [4]. Many behavioral tests measure the latency to withdraw from such stimuli with longer times suggesting higher nociceptive tolerance. These tests utilize various nociceptive stimuli including thermal, mechanical, chemical, and electrical to elicit both reflexive and non-reflexive responses [5].

Thermal Stimuli

One of the first developed methods of thermal testing is the *Tail-Flick Test*, where heat is applied to the tail provoking a rapid withdrawal movement [6]. The reaction time is measured and referred to as the "tail-flick latency." The tail-flick is a spinal reflex whose latency is modified by supraspinal mechanisms. A variation of this test involves directly immersing the tail in hot water.

The *Hot-Plate Test* involves placing a rat or mouse into a cylindrical container with a metal plate underneath heated to a specific temperature [7, 8]. Supraspinally mediated behaviors including a rapid response of paw-licking and a more elaborated response of jumping are observed [9]. A modification of the Tail-Flick Test involves applying heat to the plantar hind paws of the rodent known as the *Paw-Flick Test* or *Hargreaves Test* [10]. This modification allows the opportunity to test an experimental and control paw in the same subject.

Mechanical Stimuli

The application of mechanical nociceptive stimuli dates back to the late nineteenth century with the work of Maximilian von Frey. He used animal hair as aesthesiometer to study cutaneous sensory mechanoreceptors [11]. Subsequent experiments used nylon monofilaments eponymously named *von Frey filaments* to study neuropathy-induced cutaneous allodynia and hyperalgesia. Filaments of various diameters applied to skin produce a range of forces that can be tested with the "up down" method to quantify the pain withdrawal threshold of the subject [12]. Another commonly used approach to assess acute mechanical pain is the *Randall-Selitto Paw Pressure Test*, which utilizes a conical blunt tipped stylus applied at increasing pressures [13]. One can successively observe the reflex withdrawal of the paw, a more complex movement where the animal tries to release the trapped limb, and finally a vocal reaction [14].

A. Yerasi (✉)
Department of Anesthesiology, Perioperative and Pain Medicine, Icahn School of Medicine at Mount Sinai, New York, NY, USA
e-mail: arjun.yerasi@mountsinai.org

L. Manchikanti
Pain Management Center of Paducah, Paducah, KY, USA

University of Louisville, Louisville, KY, USA

© Springer Nature Switzerland AG 2019
Y. Khelemsky et al. (eds.), *Academic Pain Medicine*, https://doi.org/10.1007/978-3-030-18005-8_5

Chemical Stimuli

Multiple tests have been developed that use irritant chemical agents as nociceptive stimuli. They differ from traditional tests that attempt to determine the nociceptive threshold and instead aim to quantitatively measure behavior following a stimulus with a potency that varies over time [5].

The *formalin test* involves injecting dilute solution of formalin into the dorsal paw of an animal and rating behavior with 0 describing an unaffected animal; 1 indicating avoidance of placing weight on the injected paw and limping; 2 indicating an elevated paw; and 3 including licking, biting, or shaking the paw [15]. There appears to be a biphasic behavioral reaction with an early phase of frequent flicking and licking beginning immediately after injection and lasting for 5 minutes, followed by a second phase after 15–30 minutes. The first phase is a direct response to activation of peripheral nociceptors, while the second phase likely involves inflammation with peripheral and central sensitization [14].

The *writhing test* involves intraperitoneal injection of irritants producing behavior characterized by abdominal contractions, trunk twisting and turning, motor incoordination, hind limb extension, and decreased motor activity [16]. The original test used phenylbenzoquinone with subsequent studies using various chemical agents including acetic acid, hydrochloric acid, bradykinin, acetylcholine, adrenaline, adenosine triphosphate, tryptamine, potassium chloride, and oxytocin. The test is thought to mimic the pain of peritonitis through activation of both visceral and somatic nerve fibers [14].

Nociceptive Stimuli and Avoidance Behavior

Numerous experiments have built on the methods developed in these tests to assess cognitive function through the learned behavior of stimulus avoidance. A variation of the hot plate test, known as the *Thermal Escape Test*, uses a two-chamber box where floor temperature can be varied and latency to withdrawal and preference for escaping can be assessed. This design allows for the comparison between latencies for innate behaviors like licking and guarding and learned escape behavior [4]. In the *Conditioned Place Avoidance* model, animals are preconditioned by placement in a box with different chambers with varying stimuli (both noxious and neutral). The following day, their chamber preference is assessed in the absence of stimuli, a model thought to mimic averseness to an unpleasant condition [4]. The *Place Escape Avoidance* model assesses the unpleasantness of a stimulus by measuring deviation from a previously preferred chamber when a new noxious stimulus (i.e., von Frey filament, etc.) is applied to that chamber. Through experiments like these, regions of the brain involved in pain behavioral responses have been discovered. For example, rodents with electrolytic lesions to the anterior cingulate cortex (ACC) did not escape the chamber with the noxious stimulus despite displaying the same paw withdrawal reflex, suggesting that ACC lesions selectively alter the negative affective response without removing the sensory response [17].

Animal Models of Pain

Many animal models of pain have been developed using the methods of measuring pain described in this chapter. These models aim to replicate both the physical, cognitive, and psychosocial dimensions of clinical pain conditions. By understanding the underlying processes that contribute to the overall experience of pain, researchers can begin to evaluate therapeutics and possibly translate findings to the human realm.

Neuropathic Pain Models

Neuropathic pain results from damage to the nervous system. Depending on the location of injury or dysfunction, pain can be classified as central or peripheral; however, often both locations contribute to the development and maintenance of pain.

Pain After Peripheral Nerve Injury

The most common approach to producing peripheral neuropathy in animals is through traumatic nerve injury by transection or compression. The neuroma or axotomy-autotomy model developed by Wall et al. involves complete transection of the sciatic and saphenous nerves of rats to denervate the limb [18]. The resultant autotomy or self-mutilative behavior is thought to either represent the reaction to pain from the neuroma or possibly the animal's attempt to remove what it deems a foreign appendage [19]. The chronic constriction or Bennet-Xie model involves loose ligation of the sciatic nerve with sutures to produce constriction of the nerve without complete transection [20]. This constriction is thought to simulate conditions with nerve entrapment like lumbar disc herniation. The animal experiences mechanical and thermal hyperalgesia and allodynia to cold and tactile stimuli that lasts for months [21]. Similarly, the partial sciatic nerve ligation or Seltzer model involves ligation of one-third to one-half of the sciatic nerve [22]. Some of the observed behaviors include paw licking and guarding with the development of allodynia and hyperalgesia, even on "mirror sites" on the opposite limb [19]. Interestingly, these behaviors are abolished by chemical sympathectomy suggesting that this model can mimic complex regional pain syndrome (CRPS) type II [19, 23]. Other models attempt to isolate certain parts of the sciatic nerve. The spinal nerve ligation model involves ligation of L5 and L6 spinal nerves distal to the dorsal root ganglion, while the spared nerve injury model involves lesions of the terminal branches (tibial and common peroneal nerves) [24, 25]. This allows for the study of more consistent and localized nerve damage.

Pain After Spinal Ganglia and Dorsal Root Injury

Radicular pain has been modeled using injury to the dorsal root ganglion and dorsal nerve roots. The chronic constriction of DRG (CCD) model produces neuropathy after placing rods into the intervertebral foramen at L4 and L5 to result in reversible compression of the DRG [26]. Cutaneous hyperalgesia, guarding, and ataxia in the paw ipsilateral to injury are observed [27]. Experiments using dorsal root transection create similar behavior, but find less excitation of DRG neurons and spontaneous ectopic activity [28]. By injecting an immune activator zymosan near the DRG, the molecular and cellular changes associated with inflammation such as glial activation and an increase in pro-inflammatory cytokine levels can be studied [29].

Central Neuropathic Pain

Central neuropathic pain arises from injury to the spinal cord or brain. Such injury creates changes at the molecular and cellular levels that alter neuronal excitability and modulate the way the CNS processes nociceptive information. Most animal models use direct injury to the spinal cord or injection of toxic material into the brain and spinal cord [30]. The most widely used model to produce central neuropathic pain called the contusion model involves dropping a weight on the surgically exposed spinal cord to produce hind-limb paralysis [31]. Other models of mechanical injury such as spinal cord hemisection, a model of Brown-Sequard syndrome, have also been developed [32]. Chemical injury through injection of excitotoxic substances, like the AMPA–metabotropic receptor agonist quisqualic acid and ischemic spinal vessel injury through exposure of injected erythrosin B dye to an argon laser, produce similar outcomes of mechanical and thermal hypersensitivity and excitatory behavior [33, 34]. Cortical central pain can be induced by injecting picrotoxin into the somatomotor cortex of rodents while thalamic syndrome has been modeled by injecting collagenase into the ventral posterolateral nucleus of the rat thalamus producing a small hemorrhagic stroke [35, 36].

Diabetic Neuropathic Pain

Distal symmetric sensory polyneuropathy is a common finding in patients with diabetes. Experiences of pain can vary from hyperalgesia and allodynia to sensation loss, depending on the time course and severity of disease. Rodent models have been able to mimic certain aspects of diabetic neuropathy, but often cannot replicate the entire progressive disease process. Rodent models include biobreeding of diabetic prone animals (e.g., leptin gene mutations), streptozotocin-induced destruction of insulin-secreting islet of Langerhans pancreatic cells, and high fat/caloric diets as methods to produce type 1 and type 2 diabetes [37]. Evoked pain measures of pressure and thermal hyperalgesia, tactile allodynia, and hypoalgesia with increased disease duration have all been observed in these models. Yet limitations exist, such as the short lifespan and rapid onset of symptoms in rodents, easy reversibility by treatments that do not work for humans, and reliance on evoked rather than spontaneous measures of pain [37].

Inflammatory Pain Models

Inflammation and tissue injury are involved in many pain conditions. Animal models use injections of noxious substances in skin, joints and muscles to simulate both acute and chronic pain processes.

Cutaneous and Subcutaneous Inflammation

Many chemical irritants have been used to study aspects of inflammatory pain. Complete Freund's adjuvant (CFA) produces significant tissue edema with primary and secondary thermal hyperalgesia and mechanical allodynia peaking around 5 hours and lasting for 1–2 weeks [38]. Carrageenan produces similar dose dependent responses, but with a shorter onset and lasting only 1–2 days [38]. Mustard oil, which activates TRPA1, an excitatory ion channel of primary afferent neuroreceptors and formalin both produce nocifensive behavior and are used as short-term acute inflammation models with onset within minutes and duration of only 1 hour [39]. Capsaicin which activates TRPV1, a heat-sensitive cation channel on nociceptor terminals, produces a visual flare reaction whose area is smaller than the area of hyperalgesia to stroking stimulation, which is in turn smaller than that for punctate stimuli [40].

Arthritic Pain

Models of arthritic pain have been developed with techniques that cause joint inflammation and tissue damage. Many of irritants described above can also be injected into joint spaces. CFA injected into the base of a rat's tail induces a rheumatoid-like polyarthritis with systemic findings of skin lesions, bone and cartilage destruction, and lymphadenopathy [41]. Injection of CFA into the knee space produces a chronic inflammation lasting several weeks while injection of kaolin and carrageenan results in an acute reaction lasting one day [42]. Both produce monoarticular joint swelling, lowered limb withdrawal thresholds, decreased weight bearing, thermal hyperalgesia, and mechanical allodynia. Models of surgically-induced arthritis subject animals to anterior cruciate ligament ligation and meniscectomy. Histopathologic findings of subchondral bone sclerosis, osteophyte formation, chondrocyte reduction, and cartilage reduction mimic the pathophysiology observed in humans [43].

Muscle Pain

Muscle pain or deep tissue pain differs from subcutaneous pain in that it tends to be dull, aching, poorly localized, and exhibits referral. Similar to the other inflammatory models described, muscle pain has generally been studied through the injection of chemical irritants. Intramuscular application of carrageenan induces local inflammation with leukocyte accumulation that is designed to mimic myositis and muscle strains in humans. Behavioral findings include decreased limb grip strength, increased mechanical and thermal hyperalgesia, and decreased voluntary activity [39, 44]. Injection of acidic saline into the gastrocnemius produces widespread secondary mechanical hyperalgesia that is not associated with inflammation, modeling the pain of fibromyalgia [45]. Another type of muscle pain, delayed onset muscle soreness, has been studied by inducing eccentric contraction to the extensor digitorum longus of rats and observing mechanical hyperalgesia [46].

Cancer Pain Models

Pain is a very debilitating symptom experienced by many patients with cancer, affecting nearly all those with advanced stage disease. Among the etiologies for this pain are tumor compression of soft tissue, bone, nerves, and vasculature, the release of inflammatory cytokines and chemical mediators, bone metastases leading to destruction and fracture, and side effects of chemotherapy/radiotherapy [47]. The first model used to study cancer pain involved injecting fibrosarcoma cells into the femurs of mice [48]. Using this model for bone cancer pain, researchers studied the histopathology of tumor-mediated bone destruction, neurochemical changes in the spinal cord and tumor environment, the progression of spontaneous and evoked pain behaviors, as well as the role of therapeutics like opioids and COX-2 inhibitors. A model to study cancer invasion of peripheral nerves involved injection of sarcoma cells in close proximity of the sciatic nerve of mice. Findings included a slow progression of neuropathy with spontaneous pain behavior, thermal hyperalgesia, mechanical allodynia, histological damage to myelinated and unmyelinated nerves, and upregulation of various spinal cord neurotransmitters [49].

Many non-bone cancer models have also been developed. One such model initiated pancreatic cancer cell growth in mice and observed visceral pain behavior as well as cellular changes of increases in microvascular density, macrophages that expressed nerve growth factor, and the density of sensory and sympathetic fibers that innervated the pancreas [50]. A model of orofacial pain involving squamous cell carcinoma injection into the gingiva observed maxillary and mandibular nerve hypersensitivity and upregulation of trigeminal ganglia proteins [51]. Treatment-associated pain has been studied by inducing peripheral neuropathy through injection of chemotherapeutic agents like cisplatin, vincristine, and paclitaxel [47].

Postoperative Pain Models

Persistent postoperative pain remains a challenging problem for many patients following surgery and often leads to functional impairment and decreased quality of life. Various incisional animal models have been developed to study this subject. In the plantar incision model, a longitudinal incision is made under anesthesia on the plantar paw of a rat through skin, fascia, and muscle. Observations of decreased withdrawal thresholds to von Frey filaments and paw pressures are noted in the following days with gradual return to baseline [52]. Incisions made on hairy skin and the gastrocnemius produce similar findings, as well as secondary hyperalgesia in areas distant to the incisional site, suggesting that there exists a component of central sensitization with surgical incisions [53, 54]. The long-lasting and severe pain of post-thoracotomy pain syndrome has been reproduced in rats by making pleural incisions with nerve ligation. This produces increased mechanical and cold hypersensitivity, as well as pain response to pinch, lasting for 27 days [55].

Ethics of Animal Experimentation

A chapter on the animal models of pain would not be complete without a discussion of the ethical considerations of animal experimentation. The increasing role of animal studies in biomedical research over the last few decades has generated considerable debate on this topic. Issues regarding the justifiability of using animals for experiments and weighing the costs against the benefits of such use raise questions about complex scientific, philosophical, and moral values. It is generally recognized that the well-being of animals should be taken into account from a moral perspective independent of their usefulness to human beings [56]. As such, the Three R's (Replacement, Reduction, and Refinement) have served as a general framework to guide the ethical use of animals in research [57]. Replacement involves finding methods or comparatively substitutable subjects to avoid animal use. Strategies include experimenting on tissue and cell cultures, developing computer and epidemiologic models, or "relative replacement" with less sentient species. Reduction refers to minimizing the number of animals used per study. This can be achieved through improving experimental techniques,

techniques of analysis of data such as the use of meta-analyses, and encouraging collaboration among researchers. Refinement refers to methods to minimize potential pain or distress. Approaches may include non-invasive techniques, adequate anesthesia and analgesia, and appropriate housing and environments.

However, there are no universal standard policies. Specific compliance requirements often vary by country and organization, with the Animal Welfare Act serving as the primary US regulation. There has been a push in the scientific community to improve the reporting of animal research with the voluntary adoption of the ARRIVE (Animals in Research: Reporting in Vivo Experiments) guidelines by many scientific journals [58]. Through steps such as these, animal investigators can gain an understanding of the ethical consideration involved in their work.

Conclusion

Animal models provide unique challenges and opportunities for understanding the mechanisms and treatment strategies for pain conditions. Through validated measures of evoked and spontaneous behavior, we can begin to understand the multidimensional experience of pain. However, as animal models may not always fully represent human pain conditions, care must be taken when applying experimental conclusions to clinical practice.

References

1. Mogil JS, Simmonds K, Simmonds MJ. Pain research from 1975 to 2007: a categorical and bibliometric meta-trend analysis of every research paper published in the journal – Pain. Pain. 2009;142:48–58.
2. Mogil JS, Davis KD, Derbyshire SW. The necessity of animal models in pain research. Pain. 2010;151:12–7.
3. Burma NE, Leduc-Pessah H, Fan CY, Trang T. Animal models of chronic pain: advances and challenges for clinical translation. J Neurosci Res. 2017;95:1242–56.
4. Gregory N, Harris AL, Robinson CR, Dougherty PM, Fuchs PN, Sluka KA. An overview of animal models of pain: disease models and outcome measures. J Pain. 2013;14:1255–69.
5. Le Bars D, Gozariu M, Cadden SW. Animal models of nociception. Pharmacol Rev. 2001;53:597–652.
6. D'Amour FE, Smith DL. A method for determining loss of pain sensation. J Pharmacol Exp Ther. 1941;172:74–9.
7. Woolfe G, MacDonald AL. The evaluation of the analgesic action of pethidine hydrochloride (Demerol). J Pharmacol Exp Ther. 1944;80:300–7.
8. Eddy NB, Leimbach D. Synthetic analgesics: II. Dithenylbutenyl and dithienyl-butylamines. J Pharmacol Exp Ther. 1953;107:385–93.
9. Espejo EF, Mir D. Structure of the rat's behaviour in the hot plate test. Behav Brain Res. 1993;56:171–6.
10. Hargreaves K, Dubner R, Brown F, Flores C, Joris J. A new and sensitive method for measuring thermal nociception in cutaneous hyperalgesia. Pain. 1988;32:77–88.
11. von Frey M. Untersuchunger über die Sinnesfunctionen der menschlichen Haut. Bandes der Abhandlungen der mathematisch-physischen Classe der Königl. Sächsischen Gesellschaft der Wissenschaften. 1896;23:175–266.
12. Chaplan SR, Bach FW, Pogrel JW, Chung JM, Yaksh TL. Quantitative assessment of tactile allodynia in the rat paw. J Neurosci Methods. 1994;53(1):55–63.
13. Randall LO, Selitto JJ. A method for measurement of analgesic activity on inflamed tissue. Arch. Int. Pharmacodyn. Ther. 1957;111:409–19.
14. Xie W. Assessment of pain in animal. In: Ma Z, Zhang JM, editors. *Animal models of pain*. New York: Humana Press; 2011. p. 1–22.
15. Dubuisson D, Dennis SG. The formalin test: a quantitative study of the analgesic effects of morphine, meperidine and brain stem stimulation in rats and cats. Pain. 1977;4:161–74.
16. Siegmund E, Cadmus R, Lu G. A method for evaluating both non-narcotic and narcotic analgesics. Proc. Soc. Exp. Biol. Med. 1957;95:729–31.
17. Lagraize SC, Labuda CJ, Rutledge MA, Jackson RL, Fuchs PN. Differential effect of anterior cingulate cortex lesion on mechanical hypersensitivity and escape/avoidance behavior in an animal model of neuropathic pain. Exp Neurol. 2004;188: 139–48.
18. Wall PD, Devor M, Inbal R, Scadding JW, Schonfeld D, Seltzer Z, Tomkiewicz MM. Autotomy following peripheral nerve lesions: experimental anesthesia dolorosa. Pain. 1979;7:103–11.
19. Qu L, Ma C. Animal models of pain after peripheral nerve injury. In: Ma Z, Zhang JM, editors. *Animal models of pain*. New York: Humana Press; 2011. p. 69–80.
20. Bennett GJ, Xie YK. A peripheral mononeuropathy in rat that produces disorders of pain sensation like those seen in man. Pain. 1988;3:87–107.
21. Ma C. Animal models of pain. Int Anesthesiol Clin. 2007;45:121–31.
22. Seltzer Z, Dubner R, Shir Y. A novel behavioral model of neuropathic pain disorders produced in rats by partial sciatic nerve injury. Pain. 1990;43:205–18.
23. Shir Y, Seltzer Z. Effects of sympathectomy in a model of causalgiform pain produced by partial sciatic nerve injury in rats. Pain. 1991;45:309–20.
24. Kim SH, Chung JM. An experimental model for peripheral neuropathy produced by segmental spinal nerve ligation in the rat. Pain. 1992;50:355–63.
25. Decosterd I, Woolf CJ. Spared nerve injury: an animal model of persistent peripheral neuropathic pain. Pain. 2000;87:149–58.
26. Hu SJ, Xing JL. An experimental model for chronic compression of dorsal root ganglion produced by intervertebral foramen stenosis in the rat. Pain. 1998;77:15–23.
27. Song XJ, Hu SJ, Greenquist KW, Zhang JM, Lamotte RH. Mechanical and thermal hyperalgesia and ectopic neuronal discharge after chronic compression of dorsal root ganglia. J Neurophysiol. 1999;82:3347–58.
28. Yoon YW, Na HS, Chung JM. Contributions of injured and intact afferents to neuropathic pain in an experimental rat model. Pain. 1996;64:27–36.
29. Xie WR, Deng H, Li H, Bowen TL, Strong JA, Zhang JM. Robust increase of cutaneous sensitivity, cytokine production and sympathetic sprouting in rats with localized inflammatory irritation of the spinal ganglia. Neuroscience. 2006;142:809–22.
30. Colleoni M, Sacerdote P. Murine models of human neuropathic pain. BBA-Mol. Basis Dis. 2010;1802:924–33.
31. Allen AR. Surgery of experimental lesion of spinal cord equivalent to crush injury of fracture dislocation of spinal column. JAMA. 1911;57:878–80.
32. Christensen MD, Everhart AW, Pickelman JT, Hulsebosch CE. Mechanical and thermal allodynia in chronic central pain following spinal cord injury. Pain. 1996;68:97–107.

33. Yezierski RP, Liu S, Ruenes GL, Kajander KJ, Brewer KL. Excitotoxic spinal cord injury: behavioral and morphological characteristics of a central pain model. Pain. 1998;75:141–55.

34. Watson BD, Prado R, Dietrich WD, Ginsberg MD, Green BA. Photochemically induced spinal cord injury in the rat. Brain Res. 1986;367:296–300.

35. Oliveras JL, Montagne-Clavel J. Picrotoxin produces a "central" pain-like syndrome when microinjected into the somato-motor cortex of the rat. Physiol Behav. 1996;60:1425–34.

36. Wasserman JK, Koeberle PD. Development and characterization of a hemorrhagic rat model of central post-stroke pain. Neuroscience. 2009;161:173–83.

37. Dobretsov M, Backonja MM, Romanovsky D, Stimers JR. Animal models of diabetic neuropathic pain. In: Ma Z, Zhang JM, editors. *Animal models of pain*. New York: Humana Press; 2011. p. 147–69.

38. Iadarola MJ, Brady LS, Draisci G, Dubner R. Enhancement of dynorphin gene expression in spinal cord following experimental inflammation: stimulus specificity, behavioral parameters and opioid receptor binding. Pain. 1988;35:313–26.

39. Zhang RX, Ren K. Animal models of inflammatory pain. In: Ma Z, Zhang JM, editors. *Animal models of pain*. New York: Humana Press; 2011. p. 23–40.

40. Sumikura H, Andersen OK, Drewes AM, Arendt-Nielsen L. Spatial and temporal profiles of flare and hyperalgesia after intradermal capsaicin. Pain. 2003;105:285–91.

41. De Castro Costa M, De Sutter P, Gybels J, Van Hees J. Adjuvant-induced arthritis in rats: a possible model of chronic pain. Pain. 1981;10(2):173–85.

42. Sluka KA, Westlund KN. Behavioral and immunohistochemical changes in an experimental arthritis model in rats. Pain. 1993;55:367–77.

43. Hayami T, Pickarski M, Zhuo Y, Wesolowski GA, Rodan GA, Duong LT. Characterization of articular cartilage and subchondral bone changes in the rat anterior cruciate ligament transection and meniscectomized models of osteoarthritis. Bone. 2006;38:234–43.

44. Kehl LJ, Fairbanks CA. Experimental animal models of muscle pain and analgesia. Exerc. Sport Sci. Rev. 2003;31:188–94.

45. Sluka KA, Kalra A, Moore SA. Unilateral intramuscular injections of acidic saline produce a bilateral, long-lasting hyperalgesia. Muscle Nerve. 2001;24:37–46.

46. Taguchi T, Matsuda T, Tamura R, Sato J, Mizumura K. Muscular mechanical hyperalgesia revealed by behavioural pain test and c-Fos expression in the spinal dorsal horn after eccentric contraction in rats. J Physiol. 2005;564:259–68.

47. Pacharinsak C, Beitz A. Animal models of cancer pain. Comp Med. 2008;58:220–33.

48. Schwei MJ, Honore P, Rogers SD, Salak-Johnson JL, Finke MP, Ramnaraine ML, Clohisy DR, Mantyh PW. Neurochemical and cellular reorganization of the spinal cord in a murine model of bone cancer pain. J Neurosci. 1999;19:10886–97.

49. Shimoyama M, Tanaka K, Hasue F, Shimoyama N. A mouse model of neuropathic cancer pain. Pain. 2002;99:167–74.

50. Lindsay TH, Jonas BM, Sevcik MA, Kubota K, Halvorson KG, Ghilardi JR, Kuskowski MA, Stelow EB, Mukherjee P, Gendler SJ, Wong GY, Mantyh PW. Pancreatic cancer pain and its correlation with changes in tumor vasculature, macrophage infiltration, neuronal innervation, body weight, and disease progression. Pain. 2005;119:233–46.

51. Nagamine K, Ozaki N, Shinoda M, Asai H, Nishiguchi H, Mitsudo K, Tohnai I, Ueda M, Sugiura Y. Mechanical allodynia and thermal hyperalgesia induced by experimental squamous cell carcinoma of the lower gingiva in rats. J Pain. 2006;7:659–70.

52. Brennan TJ, Vandermeulen EP, Gebhart GF. Characterization of a rat model of incisional pain. Pain. 1996;64:493–501.

53. Duarte AM, Pospisilova E, Reilly E, Hamaya Y, Mujenda F, Strichartz GR. Reduction of post-incisional allodynia by subcutaneous bupivacaine: findings with a new model in the hairy skin of the rat. Anesthesiology. 2005;103:113–25.

54. Pogatzki EM, Niemeier JS, Brennan TJ. Persistent secondary hyperalgesia after gastrocnemius incision in the rat. Eur J Pain. 2002;6:295–305.

55. Nara T, Saito S, Obata H, Goto F. A rat model of postthoracotomy pain: behavioural and spinal cord NK-1 receptor assessment. Can J Anaesth. 2001;48:665–76.

56. Ohl F, Meijboom F. Ethical issues associated with the use of animal experimentation in behavioral neuroscience research. Curr Top Behav Neurosci. 2015;19:3–15.

57. Russell WMS, Burch RL. The principles of humane experimental technique. London: Methuen; 1959.

58. Kilkenny C, Browne WJ, Cuthill IC, Emerson M, Altman DG. Improving bioscience research reporting: the ARRIVE guidelines for reporting animal research. PLoS Biol. 2010;8:e1000412.

Taxonomy of Pain Systems

Anuj Malhotra

International Association for the Study of Pain (IASP) Classification of Chronic Pain Syndromes: Basis and Application

The need for taxonomy for chronic pain was expressed in 1979 by Bonica, who observed: "The development and widespread adoption of universally accepted definitions of terms and a classification of pain syndromes are among the most important objectives and responsibilities of the IASP." A list of pain terms was first published in 1979 in *Pain* [1] based on terms already established in the literature. The original list was adopted by the first Subcommittee on Taxonomy of IASP and published in 1986 with subsequent revisions in 1994 and 2011 [2].

Initial efforts focused on definitions for common pain states to allow specialists from different disciplines to better define the conditions being treated. This is a distinction of the IASP's guiding principle in standardizing definitions: The terms have been developed for use in clinical practice rather than for experimental work. As such, they can be of use for studies of epidemiology, etiology, prognosis, and treatment but may be of less use for basic science research.

In addition to singular term definitions, the IASP introduced a multidimensional Scheme for Coding Chronic Pain. The system is the result of consensus expert opinion and computational cross-checking to ensure no overlap between diagnoses. In an attempt to create distinct classifications, some commonly used terms were not included, such as atypical facial pain and chronic pain syndrome. These omissions have been the source of some controversy, particularly given the difficulty reconciling coding inconsistencies with the International Classification of Diseases (ICD-10). The resulting IASP system relies on five axes to determine a five-digit descriptor to provide a common reference point for pain syndromes.

Application and Definition of Pain Terms

Below is a list of pain terminology defined by the IASP, reflecting the most recent revisions by the 2011 IASP Taxonomy Working Group [2]. In addition, definitions for additional common pain syndromes and terms not addressed have been included and marked with "*" to reflect that these are not IASP-defined terms.

- Pain: An unpleasant sensory and emotional experience associated with actual or potential tissue damage:
    - *Acute pain: Pain due to local tissue damage, may be nociceptive or neuropathic, generally self-limited, and resolves with tissue healing
    - *Chronic pain: Pain beyond the expected duration of tissue healing, most commonly defined as persisting 3 or 6 months beyond the inciting event
    - *Persistent postsurgical pain: Pain beyond the expected duration of tissue healing, clinically defined as persisting 2 months after surgery [3]
- *Addiction: Compulsive behavior, commonly substance abuse, despite evidence of physical or psychological harm to the user
- Allodynia: Pain due to a non-painful stimulus
- Analgesia: Absence of pain in response to painful stimulation
- Anesthesia dolorosa: Pain in an area which is anesthetized/without sensation
- *Cancer pain: Pain associated with malignancy or treatments for malignancy
- *Catastrophizing: A negative cognitive-affective response to anticipated or actual events, commonly pain, resulting in feelings of helpless and distortion of threat, associated with poor pain-related outcomes
- Causalgia (complex regional pain syndrome, Type II): A syndrome of sustained neuropathic pain, allodynia, and hyperpathia *after nerve injury*, not confined to the nerve distribution, often combined with vasomotor and sudomotor dysfunction and trophic changes

A. Malhotra (✉)
Department of Anesthesiology Perioperative and Pain Medicine, Icahn School of Medicine at Mount Sinai, New York, NY, USA

© Springer Nature Switzerland AG 2019
Y. Khelemsky et al. (eds.), *Academic Pain Medicine*, https://doi.org/10.1007/978-3-030-18005-8_6

- *Deafferentation pain: Pain due to loss of sensory input to the central nervous system
- *Dependence: Physical requirement to maintain homeostasis, manifested by withdrawal if the required substance is withheld
- Diffuse noxious inhibitory control: Mechanism by which dorsal horn-wide dynamic range neurons responsive to stimulation from one location of the body may be inhibited by noxious stimuli applied to another location in the body
- Dysesthesia: An unpleasant abnormal sensation
- Hyperalgesia: Increased pain from a painful stimulus
- Hyperesthesia: Increased sensitivity to normal stimulation
- Hyperpathia: An abnormally painful reaction to a repetitive stimulus, related to temporal summation
- Hypoalgesia: Diminished pain in response to a painful stimulus
- Hypoesthesia: Decreased sensitivity to stimulation
- Neuralgia: Pain in the distribution of a nerve or nerves
- Neuritis: Inflammation of a nerve or nerves
- Neuropathic pain: Pain caused by a lesion or disease of the somatosensory nervous system:
  - Central neuropathic pain: Pain caused by a lesion or disease of the central somatosensory nervous system
  - Peripheral neuropathic pain: Pain caused by a lesion or disease of the peripheral somatosensory nervous system
- Neuropathy: A disturbance of function in a nerve:
  - Mononeuropathy: Dysfunction in one nerve
  - Mononeuropathy multiplex: Dysfunction in multiple nerves
  - Polyneuropathy: Diffuse involvement, often bilateral
- Nociception: The processing of noxious stimuli
- Nociceptive pain: Pain that arises from actual or threatened damage and is due to the activation of nociceptors
- Noxious stimulus: A stimulus that is damaging or threatens damage
- Pain threshold: The minimum intensity of a stimulus that is perceived as painful
- Pain tolerance level: The maximum intensity of a pain-producing stimulus that a subject is willing to accept
- Paresthesia: An abnormal sensation
- *Phantom pain: Pain referred to an amputated limb
- *Reflex sympathetic dystrophy (complex regional pain syndrome, type I): A syndrome of neuropathic pain, allodynia, and hyperpathia after a noxious event *without defined nerve injury*, not limited to a single nerve distribution, with a distal predominance, and often combined with vasomotor and sudomotor dysfunction and trophic changes
- *Residual limb pain (stump pain): Pain at the site of amputation

- Sensitization: Increased responsiveness of nociceptive neurons to their normal input and lowered response threshold
- Central sensitization: Increased responsiveness of nociceptive neurons in the central nervous system to normal or subthreshold stimuli
- Peripheral sensitization: Increased responsiveness and reduced threshold of nociceptive neurons in the periphery to stimulation
- *Somatic pain: Pain carried along sensory fibers, usually discrete
- *Tachyphylaxis: Rapid decrease in response to repeated doses of a medication
- *Tolerance: Requirement for higher doses of a substance to achieve the same response
- *Withdrawal: Symptoms related to cessation of a substance, often manifested as the opposite effects of the substance being withheld

IASP Scheme for Coding Chronic Pain Diagnoses

The IASP multiaxial coding schema for chronic pain is comprehensive and well-researched; however despite best attempts, inter-observer variability has been noted in validation studies [4]. The axes are arranged as follows, with each assigned a digit in the final code:

1. Region affected – if more than one region is affected, then these can be coded separately.
   (a) Head, face, and mouth 000
   (b) Cervical region 100
   (c) Upper shoulder and upper limbs 200
   (d) Thoracic region 300
   (e) Abdominal region 400
   (f) Lower back, lumbar spine, sacrum, and coccyx 500
   (g) Lower limbs 600
   (h) Pelvic region 700
   (i) Anal, perineal, and genital region 800
   (j) More than three major sites 900
2. System – identify the body system most likely to be responsible for the pain.
   (a) Nervous system (anatomic) 00
   (b) Nervous system (psychological and social) 10
   (c) Respiratory and cardiovascular systems 20
   (d) Musculoskeletal system and connective tissue 30
   (e) Cutaneous and subcutaneous and associated glands (including the breast) 40
   (f) Gastrointestinal system 50
   (g) Genitourinary system 60
   (h) Other organs or viscera (including lymphatic, hemopoietic) 70

(i) More than one system 80

(j) Unknown 90

3. Temporal characteristics of pain – pattern of occurrence.

   (a) Not recorded, not applicable, or not known 0

   (b) Single episode, limited duration 1

   (c) Continuous or nearly continuous, non-fluctuating 2

   (d) Continuous or nearly continuous, fluctuating severity 3

   (e) Recurring irregularly 4

   (f) Recurring regularly 5

   (g) Paroxysmal 6

   (h) Sustained with superimposed paroxysms 7

   (i) Other combinations 8

   (j) None of the above 9

4. Patient's statement of pain intensity and time since onset of pain – combination measure of intensity and duration of pain.

   (a) Not recorded, not applicable, or not known 0.0

   (b) Mild

      (i) <1 month 0.1

      (ii) 1–6 months 0.2

      (iii) >6 months 0.3

   (c) Medium

      (i) <1 month 0.4

      (ii) 1–6 months 0.5

      (iii) >6 months 0.6

   (d) Severe

      (i) <1 month 0.7

      (ii) 1–6 months 0.8

      (iii) >6 months 0.9

5. Etiology – inciting event.

   (a) Genetic or congenital disorders 0.01

   (b) Trauma, operation, burns 0.01

   (c) Infective, parasitic 0.02

   (d) Inflammatory, immune reactions 0.03

(e) Neoplasm 0.04

(f) Toxic, metabolic, radiation 0.05

(g) Degenerative, mechanical 0.06

(h) Dysfunctional (including psychophysiological) 0.07

(i) Unknown or other 0.08

(j) Psychological origin 0.09

As some syndromes yield the same five-digit code, there is sometimes the need for addition of a lower-case letter in the sixth place (a, b, c). If the code is for spinal (S), radicular (R), or combined (C) pain, then one of these uppercase letters may appear. Codes can be referenced in the IASP Classification of Chronic Pain, Second Edition, Revised [2].

Codes for well-defined syndromes are codified with appropriate modifiers to be adjusted per the clinician, for example, phantom limb pain of the leg will be listed as 603. X7a with the X to be replaced based on axis IV, intensity, and duration. Examples of coding for other common diagnoses include chronic, severe, and cervical spondylosis, 133.96cS; subacute, mild, and hip osteoarthritis, 638.26b; and chronic and moderate fibromyalgia, 933.68a.

References

1. Pain terms: a list with definitions and notes on usage. Recommended by the IASP Subcommittee on Taxonomy. Pain. 1979;6(3):249.
2. IASP. Classification of chronic pain. 2nd ed. Revised. E-book. http://www.iasp-pain.org/PublicationsNews/Content.aspx?ItemNumber=1673&navItemNumber=677.
3. Werner MU, Kongsgaard UE. Defining persistent post-surgical pain: is an update required? Br J Anaesth. 2014;113(1):1–4.
4. Fishman S, Ballantyne J, Rathmell J, editors. Bonica's management of pain. 4th ed. Filadelfia: Wolters Kluwer; 2009.

Assessment and Psychology of Pain

Will Tyson and Anuj Malhotra

Pain as a Subjective, Multidimensional Experience

Common Definition of Pain

The International Association for the Study of Pain defines pain as "an unpleasant sensory or emotional experience associated with actual or potential tissue damage, or described in terms of such damage" [1]. Unlike other chronic diseases, such as hypertension, hyperlipidemia, or diabetes mellitus, there is no single objective measurement to best characterize the extent of the problem or to evaluate treatment outcomes. Measuring a patient's pain must correlate objective data with the patient's subjective reporting to provide a comprehensive outcome which represents the pain state.

Pain Versus Nociception

Measurement of pain is complicated by the fact that nociception is often confused with the subjective experience of pain. Nociception involves peripheral nerve signals generated by specialized receptors (nociceptors) in response to noxious stimuli. Pain requires a functioning central nervous system to interpret these signals and produce a subjective experience. There is often a wide variability in how much subjective pain a given stimulus or injury will cause. This variability is influenced by genetics, mood, beliefs, early life experiences with pain, sex, ethnicity, and many other factors [2].

Chronic pain can be associated with a global reduction in a patient's quality of life, encompassing domains such as sleep disturbance, impaired social and physical function, depression, and anxiety. Moreover, there appears to be rela-

tive independence between pain and these coexisting stressors. Therefore, to capture the pain experience, it is necessary to also define and characterize these related domains.

Introspection and Measures of Subjective Experience: Basic Concepts and Self-Report

For an individual to adequately report their current level of pain, he or she must first be able to internally evaluate it and express it. Self-reported expression of pain is one of the best means to directly evaluate a patient's current pain state for both research and clinical purposes. This expression can be in the form of a simplified unidimensional scale, a comprehensive multidimensional rating scale, or via surrogate measures.

Unidimensional Rating Scales

Unidimensional rating scales measure pain as a single quality varying only in intensity and report a single outcome score. These methods are most effectively used in clinics and acute settings to provide information about current pain and need for rescue analgesics, such as postoperatively [3].

Verbal Rating Scale

The Verbal Rating Scale (VRS) utilizes a series of categorical descriptors ordered in increasing intensity (i.e., none, mild, moderate, and severe). The advantages of the VRS are that it is easy to administer and report, particularly for elderly patients [4]. The major disadvantages are that it has fewer response choices (shortened scale) and the categorical options limit statistical analysis. It has demonstrated ability to distinguish treatment effect, test–retest reliability, and convergent validity in cancer pain, analgesic trials, and evoked pain studies [4, 5].

W. Tyson
Icahn School of Medicine at Mount Sinai, New York, NY, USA

A. Malhotra (✉)
Department of Anesthesiology Perioperative and Pain Medicine, Icahn School of Medicine at Mount Sinai, New York, NY, USA

© Springer Nature Switzerland AG 2019
Y. Khelemsky et al. (eds.), *Academic Pain Medicine*, https://doi.org/10.1007/978-3-030-18005-8_7

Visual Analog Scale

The Visual Analog Scale (VAS) is typically a 10-cm line anchored at one end by a label stating "no pain" and at the other end by a label stating "worst pain." The patient chooses a point on the line to indicate their level of pain and the interpreting clinician measures the length of the line on a 101-point scale [6]. The advantages of VAS are that there is good evidence for responsiveness, validity, test–retest reliability, and the scores can be treated as ratio data [7]. Limitations relate to its time consuming process and elderly patients may have difficulty with it [8].

Numerical Rating Scale

The Numerical Rating Scale (NRS) is the most used univariable instrument for measuring pain. It consists of a rating scale from 0 to 10, with 0 signifying "no pain" and 10 signifying "worst pain." Patients may respond orally or by circling the appropriate number. A similar scale with 0 to 100 is also used. The NRS minimizes patient and provider burden during data collection and demonstrates excellent compliance. In contrast to VAS, it can be administered via a phone interview; however, scores cannot be treated as ratio data. It demonstrates sensitivity to change, test–retest reliability, and correlates well with other measures of pain intensity [5].

Patient Global Impression of Change (PGIC)

The Patient Global Impression of Change (PGIC) represents an attempt to capture pain improvement more broadly using a single item measure. The patient is asked to rate their current status compared to a previous time point from best to worst (i.e., very much improved, much improved, minimally improved, same, minimally worse, much worse, or very much worse). This scale lacks sensitivity but is applicable to many conditions and treatments [9].

Rescue Medication Use

Need for rescue analgesic medications can be used as a surrogate for pain, even though it is not a true pain outcome scale. It is particularly useful when medication use is triggered by meeting or exceeding a set pain score (i.e., medication Z to be administered for NRS >5) [3].

Multidimensional Measures

Chronic pain reporting requires a more comprehensive global assessment than univariable measures can provide.

This assessment should evaluate several aspects of pain (quality, intensity, location), disability, emotional affect, and effect on quality of life. This complex approach to the pain experience is much more likely to reflect the impact of pain.

Brief Pain Inventory

The Brief Pain Inventory (BPI) was developed by the Pain Research Group of the World Health Organization (WHO) Collaborating Centre for Symptom Evaluation in Cancer Care to measure both the sensory dimension of pain (intensity) and the reactive dimension (interference in patient's life) [10]. The BPI has been used mostly for cancer pain and consists of a 17-item scale that traditionally takes less than 15 minutes to complete. It has been validated in multiple languages and demonstrates good sensitivity to pharmacologic treatment effects. The BPI interference scale, in particular, has been validated as a measure of physical functioning in multiple domains.

McGill Pain Questionnaire

The McGill Pain Questionnaire (MPQ) was developed to specify the qualities of pain. Pain is scaled in three dimensions (sensory, affective, and evaluative) and the questionnaire consists of 20 sets of words for each dimension with each having from two to six descriptors that vary in intensity. Multiple studies have supported the reliability and validity of the MPQ for specific pain syndromes [11] and it is available in multiple languages. It takes approximately 15 minutes to complete. The Short-Form McGill Pain Questionnaire (SF-MPQ) was developed for research purposes and consists of 15 words from the sensory and affective categories from the standard long form with a four-point rating scale for each, a pain intensity VAS score, and overall assessment of pain VRS score [12].

West Haven–Yale Multidimensional Pain Inventory

The West Haven–Yale Multidimensional Pain Inventory (WHYMPI) best assesses adaptation to chronic pain [13]. It can yield clinically useful information regarding pain-coping styles, such as adaptive copers, interpersonally depressed, or dysfunctional copers. It is composed of 52 items with 12 subscales, including perceived interference of pain, response from significant others, pain intensity, emotional affect, perceived control, and participation in social or work activities. Patients respond to the questions on a seven-point scale. The WHYMPI has been validated for diverse pain syndromes and is sensitive to treatment effects. The WHYMPI interference scale correlates with physical functioning and is an alternative to the BPI [14].

Medical Outcome Study 36-Item Short-Form Health Survey

The 36-Item Short-Form Health Survey (SF-36) is a frequently used measure of function and quality of life in a variety of patient populations [15]. It consists of eight subscales including physical function, limitations due to physical problems, social function, pain, limitations due to emotional problems, general mental health, vitality, and general health perceptions. It takes approximately 10 minutes to complete, and scores can be compared across multiple populations. While widely used, it features only two questions related to pain and there are concerns about insensitivity to change when measuring an individual patient.

The Treatment Outcomes of Pain Survey (TOPS)

The Treatment Outcomes of Pain Survey (TOPS) is an extension of the SF-36 specifically designed for patients with chronic pain [16]. TOPS derived many of its questions from other previously discussed measures, including the SF-36, WHYMPI, and BPI. It consists of 120 items with a 61-item follow-up and addresses pain symptoms, function, perceived disability, objective disability, satisfaction with treatment, fear avoidance, coping, life control, limitations, demographics, and substance abuse history. The scale scores are quite comprehensive and have been found sensitive to change with good validity; however, adherence is limited by increased questionnaire length.

Oswestry Disability Index

The Oswestry Disability Index (also known as the Oswestry Low Back Pain Disability Questionnaire, ODI) is an extremely important tool that researchers and disability evaluators use to measure a patient's permanent functional disability. The test is considered the 'gold standard' of low back functional outcome tools. The ODI shows moderate correlation with pain measures such as a VAS ($n = 94$, $r = 0.62$) and the MPQ. The ODI has been used to validate the Pain Disability Index, the Low Back Outcome Score, Manniche, the Aberdeen score, a new German language scale, the Curtin Scale, and a functional capacity evaluation [17].

Emotional Measures

A relationship between pain and emotional distress exists and there is evidence of relative independence [18, 19]. Emotional assessment instruments, either as part of a broader multidimensional pain measure or as a specialized emotion scale, can elucidate the interplay of emotion and pain and help guide therapy.

Commonly, anxiety, depression, and fear are found to coexist and can significantly affect pain and treatment outcomes. Measurements of depression include: the Beck Depression Inventory (BDI) [20], Zung Self-Rating Depression Scale [21], and Hamilton Rating Scale for Depression [22]. Anxiety and fear measures include the Pain Anxiety Symptoms Scale [23], State-Trait Anxiety Inventory [24], and Fear-Avoidance Beliefs Questionnaire (FABQ) [25]. Of these, the BDI has been most extensively studied, demonstrating internal consistency (Cronbach alpha 0.73–0.95), test–retest reliability (Pearson's r 0.80–0.90), and convergent validity (Pearson r mean = 0.60).

Measurement of Pain in Special Populations: Challenges and Limitations

Measurement of Pain in Children or Patients with Significant Impairment

Measurement of pain in children or patients with significant impairment can be significantly more difficult than measuring pain in adults with normal functional ability. Children and patients with significant impairment often are not capable of understanding common pain rating measures. Therefore some simplified options based on traditional pain rating scales have been developed [3]. The Colored Analog Scale (CAS) replaces a VAS with gradually increasing red coloring to indicate increasing intensity of pain. The Wong-Baker FACES Pain Rating Scale replaces a VAS with varying facial expressions from crying to smiling. A major disadvantage of these scales, however, is difficulty separating pain from other sources of sadness, anxiety, or anger.

For nonverbal adults or infants in whom self-report is not possible, facial action, body movement, tone, cry, state/sleep, and consolability often serve as proxies for pain [26]. These measures may be clinically beneficial, but they are unlikely to meet the scientific standard for reporting [26, 27].

Indirect Pain Measurement: Observations

Certain physiologic variables have been suggested as surrogates for pain, including autonomic activity such as skin conductance [28] and heart rate [29], or biomarkers of pain intensity [30]. Caution should be used when interpreting these peripheral measures as they can be influenced by forms of arousal other than pain and can be modulated by non-analgesic medications. Physical function tests, such as range of motion and strength, have been used as proxies for pain, including the timed "Up and Go" test for osteoarthritis [31], loaded forward-reach test for low back pain [32], and grip strength for rheumatoid arthritis [33]. Physical function tests have been shown to only modestly predict self-reported pain scores, which suggests that other factors may heavily influence the subjective experience of pain.

Recent attempts to objectively measure pain have focused on the central nervous system using neuroimaging. Studies suggest that brain imaging may be used to objectively distinguish the presence of evoked painful stimuli [34] as well as the presence of chronic low back pain [34, 35]. Despite these promising reports, there is significant additional research that needs to be done in order to validate the use of neuroimaging more widely. The monetary and time cost associated with neuroimaging dictate that it will primarily be used to help guide further research and understanding of brain mechanisms involved in pain as opposed to daily clinical practice.

Outcome Measures in Clinical Studies of Pain: Basic Issues and Requirements

In addition to the clinical need to provide and document appropriate care for pain, there is clearly an impetus to provide the evidence necessary to guide and justify appropriate treatments. The National Institutes of Health funded the Patient-Reported Outcomes Measurement Information System (PROMIS) with the goal of developing valid, reliable, and standardized questionnaires to measure patient-reported outcomes. These assessment instruments were developed to yield calibrated item banks measuring domains such as pain, fatigue, physical function, depression, anxiety, and social function. These banks can be used to produce short forms or computerized adaptive tests for researcher and clinician use [36].

Further efforts have involved academia, pharmaceutical companies, and government agencies to define and standardize outcome measures. The Initiative on Methods, Measurement, and Pain Assessment in Clinical Trials (IMMPACT) consortium, comprised of members from these diverse backgrounds, granted most weight to the following criteria and core domains [37].

IMMPACT Criteria

Reliability

The instrument must demonstrate test–retest reliability when a patient's status does not change over time. It should have inter-rater reliability, i.e., clinicians observing the same patient should provide similar scores. There should be internal reliability if the scale contains multiple items measuring the same domain, meaning the scores should correlate.

Validity

The scale must measure what it is intended to measure. The scale should display convergent validity in that it must agree with other similar indicators and discriminate validity in that it must be distinguishable from related conditions.

Appropriateness

The scale's content must be in keeping with the measured outcome and relevant to the patient population being studied. The outcome measure must be scaled to the target patient population so that scores do not aggregate in a restricted area of the scale and should be at intervals to allow statistical flexibility.

Responsiveness

The scale must display the ability to detect changes over time and to distinguish between treatments. This requisite is of particular interest for clinical trials, wherein a treatment effect is investigated.

Burden

The scale must be easy to administer, complete, and score. Desire for additional data must be balanced with time constraints and patient adherence.

IMMPACT Core Domains

IMMPACT has defined six core outcome domains that should be considered when designing clinical trials: pain, physical functioning, emotional functioning, participant ratings of improvement, symptoms and adverse events, and participant disposition [38]. IMMPACT has defined specific validated measures for each of the core outcome domains in the follow-up IMMPACT-II including NRS, use of rescue analgesics, WHYMPI interference scale, BPI interference items, BDI, Profile of Mood States, PGIC, passive capture of adverse events, participant disposition, and tailored measures specific to the study population [37].

Clinical vs Statistical Significance

Outcome measures for pain provide a metric by which treatments and progression can be compared. Ideally, an intervention should produce both a clinically and statistically significant difference versus alternative treatment or placebo;

however, as sample size increases, statistical significance increases regardless of clinical effect. In order to interpret the results of a clinical trial, the clinically relevant effect size must first be determined. Studies suggest that for pain, a 30% reduction, corresponding with a PGIC of "much improved" or "very much improved," two-point reduction on NRS [39, 40], or 35-mm reduction on VAS represents a satisfactory result for the patient [41].

References

1. Merskey H. Psychological approaches to the treatment of chronic pain. Postgrad Med J. 1984;60(710):886–92.
2. Kim H, Neubert JK, San Miguel A, Xu K, Krishnaraju RK, Iadarola MJ, et al. Genetic influence on variability in human acute experimental pain sensitivity associated with gender, ethnicity and psychological temperament. Pain. 2004;109(3):488–96.
3. Malhotra A, Mackey S. Outcomes in pain medicine: a brief review. Pain Ther. 2012;1(1):5. https://doi.org/10.1007/s40122-012-0005-4.
4. Gagliese L, Melzack R. Chronic pain in elderly people. Pain. 1997;70(1):3–14.
5. Gilron I, Jensen MP. Clinical trial methodology of pain treatment studies: selection and measurement of self-report primary outcomes for efficacy. Reg Anesth Pain Med. 2011;36(4):374–81.
6. Miller MD, Ferris DG. Measurement of subjective phenomena in primary care research: the visual analogue scale. Fam Pract Res J. 1993;13(1):15–24.
7. Price DD, McGrath PA, Rafii A, Buckingham B. The validation of visual analogue scales as ratio scale measures for chronic and experimental pain. Pain. 1983;17(1):45–56.
8. Revill SI, Robinson JO, Rosen M, Hogg MI. The reliability of a linear analogue for evaluating pain. Anaesthesia. 1976;31(9):1191–8.
9. Younger J, McCue R, Mackey S. Pain outcomes: a brief review of instruments and techniques. Curr Pain Headache Rep. 2009;13(1):39–43.
10. Cleeland CS, Ryan KM. Pain assessment: global use of the brief pain inventory. Ann Acad Med Singap. 1994;23(2):129–38.
11. Melzack R, Torgerson WS. On the language of pain. Anesthesiology. 1971;34(1):50–9.
12. Melzack R. The short-form McGill pain questionnaire. Pain. 1987;30(2):191–7.
13. Kerns RD, Turk DC, Rudy TE. The West Haven-Yale Multidimensional Pain Inventory (WHYMPI). Pain. 1985;23(4):345–56.
14. Dworkin RH, Turk DC, Wyrwich KW, Beaton D, Cleeland CS, Farrar JT, et al. Interpreting the clinical importance of treatment outcomes in chronic pain clinical trials: IMMPACT recommendations. J Pain. 2008;9(2):105–21.
15. Mchorney CA, Johne W, Anastasiae R. The MOS 36-item short-form health survey (SF-36). Med Care. 1993;31(3):247–63.
16. Rogers WH, Wittink H, Wagner A, Cynn D, Carr DB. Assessing individual outcomes during outpatient multidisciplinary chronic pain treatment by means of an augmented SF-36. Pain Med. 2000;1(1):44–54.
17. Fairbank JCT, Pynsent PB. The Oswestry disability index. Spine. 2000;25(22):2940–53.
18. Rogers WH, Wittink HM, Ashburn MA, Cynn D, Carr DB. Using the "TOPS," an outcomes instrument for multidisciplinary outpatient pain treatment. Pain Med. 2000;1(1):55–67.
19. De Gagné TA, Mikail SF, D'Eon JL. Confirmatory factor analysis of a 4-factor model of chronic pain evaluation. Pain. 1995;60(2):195–202.
20. Beck AT. An inventory for measuring depression. Arch Gen Psychiatry. 1961;4(6):561.
21. Zung WW. A self-rating depression scale [Internet]. PsycTESTS Dataset. 1965; https://doi.org/10.1037/t04095-000.
22. Hamilton M. Hamilton rating scale for depression [Internet]. PsycTESTS Dataset. 1960; https://doi.org/10.1037/t04100-000.
23. McCracken LM, Zayfert C, Gross RT. The pain anxiety symptoms scale: development and validation of a scale to measure fear of pain. Pain. 1992;50(1):67–73.
24. Spielberger CD. State-trait anxiety inventory. In: The Corsini encyclopedia of psychology. Hoboken: Wiley; 2010.
25. Waddell G, Newton M, Henderson I, Somerville D, Main CJ. A Fear-Avoidance Beliefs Questionnaire (FABQ) and the role of fear-avoidance beliefs in chronic low back pain and disability. Pain. 1993;52(2):157–68.
26. Hummel P, van Dijk M. Pain assessment: current status and challenges. Semin Fetal Neonatal Med. 2006;11(4):237–45.
27. Li D, Puntillo K, Miaskowski C. A review of objective pain measures for use with critical care adult patients unable to self-report. J Pain. 2008;9(1):2–10.
28. Storm H. Skin conductance and the stress response from heel stick in preterm infants. Arch Dis Child Fetal Neonatal Ed. 2000;83(2):F143–7.
29. Tousignant-Laflamme Y, Marchand S. Autonomic reactivity to pain throughout the menstrual cycle in healthy women. Clin Auton Res. 2009;19(3):167–73.
30. Okuse K. Pain signalling pathways: from cytokines to ion channels. Int J Biochem Cell Biol. 2007;39(3):490–6.
31. Stratford PW, Kennedy DM, Woodhouse LJ. Performance measures provide assessments of pain and function in people with advanced osteoarthritis of the hip or knee. Phys Ther. 2006;86(11):1489–96.
32. Smeets RJ, Hijdra HJM, Kester ADM, Hitters MW, André Knottnerus J. The usability of six physical performance tasks in a rehabilitation population with chronic low back pain. Clin Rehabil. 2006;20(11):989–97.
33. Goodson A, McGregor AH, Douglas J, Taylor P. Direct, quantitative clinical assessment of hand function: usefulness and reproducibility. Man Ther. 2007;12(2):144–52.
34. Brown JE, Chatterjee N, Younger J, Mackey S. Towards a physiology-based measure of pain: patterns of human brain activity distinguish painful from non-painful thermal stimulation. PLoS One. 2011;6(9):e24124.
35. Ung H, Brown JE, Johnson KA, Younger J, Hush J, Mackey S. Multivariate classification of structural MRI data detects chronic low back pain. Cereb Cortex. 2014;24(4):1037–44.
36. Gershon RC, Rothrock N, Hanrahan R, Bass M, Cella D. The use of PROMIS and assessment center to deliver patient-reported outcome measures in clinical research. J Appl Meas. 2010;11(3):304–14.
37. Dworkin RH, Turk DC, Farrar JT, Haythornthwaite JA, Jensen MP, Katz NP, et al. Core outcome measures for chronic pain clinical trials: IMMPACT recommendations. Pain. 2005;113(1–2):9–19.
38. Turk DC, Dworkin RH, Allen RR, Bellamy N, Brandenburg N, Carr DB, et al. Core outcome domains for chronic pain clinical trials: IMMPACT recommendations. Pain. 2003;106(3):337–45.
39. Farrar JT, Berlin JA, Strom BL. Clinically important changes in acute pain outcome measures: a validation study. J Pain Symptom Manage. 2003;25(5):406–11.
40. Farrar JT, Young JP Jr, LaMoreaux L, Werth JL, Poole RM. Clinical importance of changes in chronic pain intensity measured on an 11-point numerical pain rating scale. Pain. 2001;94(2):149–58.
41. Kvien TK, Heiberg T, Hagen KB. Minimal clinically important improvement/difference (MCII/MCID) and patient acceptable symptom state (PASS): what do these concepts mean? Ann Rheum Dis. 2007;66(Suppl 3):iii40–1.

Placebo and Pain

Thomas Palaia, Christopher Curatolo, and Stelian Serban

Definition and Incidence

In Latin, placebo translates to "I shall please" and was used in the eighth century as part of a psalm sung at funerals. The term was initially used in medicine in the late eighteenth century to indicate a commonplace method or medicine. By the early nineteenth century, it was used to refer to any medicine adapted more to please than to benefit the patient. Modern usage typically refers to a drug or therapy that simulates medical treatment, but has no specific action on the condition being treated [1]. It is important to note, however, that placebo can also refer to the response experienced by the patient and not only the word for a seemingly inert stimulus.

Beecher, in his landmark 1955 JAMA study entitled "The powerful placebo," quantified the placebo effect at 35% based on 15 uncontrolled observational studies [2]. While later studies have estimated this number as both higher and lower, the Beecher placebo effect size is the most commonly cited number.

Historic Aspects of Placebo

In 1782, a French scientific commission is credited as the first to use placebos in a scientific study. The commission, whose participants included Benjamin Franklin, was charged with investigating the validity of animal magnetism. During their study, the potential power of a placebo response was noted when a woman fainted after she drank water that she thought was magnetized [3].

Also frequently cited are trials by John Haygarth in 1799 and 1801, when implanted metal rods (known as Perkins tractors), thought to alleviate symptoms of several diseases secondary to electromagnetic properties of the metal, were compared to implanted wood rods. Four of five patients treated noted relief. When the procedure was repeated with Perkins tractors, the same four of five patients found relief [4]. This foreshadowed the concept that certain patients may be "placebo responders," while others are not.

Placebo Response: Mechanisms and Interpretation

How can a seemingly "inert" substance or intervention exert a biological action? Several theories exist about why placebo effects occur and they are summarized in Table 8.1.

A patient's expectations of a given treatment play an integral role in the response to placebo. These expectations are typically based on automatic emotional and physiological responses to a particular stimulus. An example is a patient who is keenly aware that a fellow is performing a supervised interventional procedure with the attending. The patient may have a decreased response to this treatment because she perceives the fellow as less skilled than the attending. Simply, low expectation on the part of the patient may lead to a lower placebo response. Conversely, high expectations may lead to a high placebo response, which may be additive to non-placebo treatments. When it comes to clinical trials, it has been shown that patients who believe they are in the treatment arm

T. Palaia
Department of Anesthesiology, Mount Sinai Medical Center, New York, NY, USA

C. Curatolo · S. Serban (✉)
Department of Anesthesiology, Perioperative and Pain Medicine, Icahn School of Medicine at Mount Sinai, New York, NY, USA
e-mail: stelian.serban@mountsinai.org

Table 8.1 Psychotherapeutic theories for the placebo effect

Expectation[a]
Conditioning[a]
Learning
Alteration in the emotional state of the individual/therapist/patient interaction

[a]Likely most important in placebo analgesics

© Springer Nature Switzerland AG 2019
Y. Khelemsky et al. (eds.), *Academic Pain Medicine*, https://doi.org/10.1007/978-3-030-18005-8_8

of a study (regardless of whether they are) experience a larger clinical effect than the actual treatment alone [5].

Conditioning also likely contributes significantly to the placebo response. An example is a patient who receives an opioid analgesic and time after time receives pain relief. If that patient's opioid is subsequently replaced with a placebo, they may continue to experience pain relief [6]. There is likely much overlap between expectation and conditioning, with the most profound placebo responses occurring when both conditioning and expectancy are involved.

While direct experience is a potent method of creating a placebo trigger, social observations and/or learning can also be a potent source of placebo. If someone learns of and believes an analgesic treatment is beneficial, they are more likely to experience analgesia following that treatment, even if it is a placebo.

Provider-patient interactions resulting in an alteration in the emotional state of the patient have also been implicated as a theory to explain the placebo response. While anxiety, histrionism, dependence, and other features have been suggested historically, they have not borne out in further studies. Placebo responders, however, seem to respond as a result of altering their emotional state in response to a provider. For example, a provider whom the patient views to be as competent, confident, and prestigious may elicit a stronger placebo response. This helps to explain why some studies performed by prestigious and expert practitioners with positive results fail to be reproduced at other centers.

There is likely a highly complex neuro-psycho-physiologic interaction responsible for the placebo effect. Patients who expect and have experienced certain physiological responses to medications and procedures are more likely to experience them with a placebo. Laska et al. noted the critical role that anticipation plays in the placebo response [7]. In one study, patients who received postoperative opioids for 2 days and were given placebo on their third postoperative day experienced similar reductions in their respiratory rate [8]. Subjects who habitually drink coffee and experience an increase in heart rate following consumption may have an increase in their heart rate following decaffeinated coffee if they think they're having regular, caffeinated coffee.

Naloxone, an endogenous opioid antagonist, was able to reverse the analgesic properties of placebo [9]. Other studies found no reversal of placebo analgesia with naloxone, which has led to the hypothesis that placebo analgesia can be mediated by both endogenous opioid and non-opioid mechanisms [10, 11]. Additional mechanisms of the placebo effect include the release of other endogenous neurotransmitters. For example, placebo administration in Parkinson's disease patients led to increases in dopamine in the ventral and dorsal striatum with objective improvements in motor function [12, 13].

Studies using PET scan found activation of similar neural pathways when patients were subjected to placebo injection versus remifentanil when patients were conditioned with simple verbal cues [14]. Furthermore, decreased activation was shown on fMRI in the dorsolateral prefrontal cortex, orbitofrontal cortex, prefrontal cortex, superior parietal cortex, and periaqueductal gray following both opioid and placebo administration. These are opioid receptor-rich areas of the brain and support the hypothesis that the placebo response may involve descending inhibitory pathways activated by opioids [15]. PET imaging utilizing a μ-opioid receptor-selective radiotracer depicted that placebo can induce activation of the μ-receptor in the dorsolateral prefrontal cortex, pregenual rostral anterior cingulate cortex, anterior insular cortex, and nucleus accumbens. This suggests that cognitive factors, such as expectation of pain relief, are capable of modulating physical states through activation of μ-receptors [16].

Quite thought provoking is the potential presence of a somatotopic placebo response to topical therapies whose effect is blocked in the presence of naloxone. This was illustrated in a study in which topical capsaicin cream was applied to three out of four remote body parts and a placebo cream was applied on the remaining site. Patients were told the cream was a "powerful local anesthetic," and this resulted in pain relief in only the area of application in the majority of patients. This effect, which was blocked if patients were pretreated with naloxone, indicates that placebo-activated endogenous pathways may not act on the entire body, but only on the part where expectancy is directed [17].

Role of Placebo in Clinical Trials

After World War II, a great debate began about the use of placebo for clinical trials. At the suggestion of Henry Beecher in his 1955 study, the possible effect of placebo was too large to be ignored in clinical trials. Placebo groups were quickly included in the current gold standard – double blinded, randomized placebo controlled studies in order to determine whether a plausible placebo component of experimental treatments could account for a significant difference in treatment modalities. The inclusion of placebo treatment in the contemporary research paradigm has not only increased the sensitivity in demonstrating a significant clinical difference between two treatments but also has elucidated the importance of the patient-clinician interaction, patient expectations, and the context of treatment.

As Polston aptly notes, however, "a major problem with the use of placebos is that negative study results can occur not because of lack of efficacy in the studied intervention, but because of a large placebo response" [3]. This is more likely to occur with studies using subjective measures. It is possible that eliminating placebo responders from clinical trials may improve the accuracy and validity of trials. While many methods of identifying placebo responders have been suggested, it has been noted that a prior placebo responder has the same probability of placebo response in future placebo challenges. Attempts to minimize this by using enrichment trials or multi-dosing strategies have been ineffective or have increased the placebo response since the perception of more treatment results in an augmented placebo response.

Role of Placebo in Clinical Trials: Response Bias

Response bias, in the context of clinical trials that use placebo, refers to patient responses that aim to be socially acceptable or please study clinicians. It includes a wide range of cognitive biases that influence the responses of participants away from an accurate or truthful response. These biases are most prevalent in the types of studies and research that involves self-reporting (e.g., surveys).

Ethics of Placebo in Clinical Trials and Clinical Practice

The introduction of placebo into controlled studies after World War II included calls to protect placebo recipients from harm. Some have called for elimination of placebos from clinical research, arguing that comparisons should involve not placebo but the accepted standard of care. Additionally, it has been asserted that the deception involved in placebo violates patient autonomy and individual rights and could jeopardize the patient-clinician relationship. Ultimately, it should be ensured that placebo is not known to be inferior to the proposed comparison modality. It is essential that patients express complete understanding upon entering a clinical trial that they may receive placebo in lieu of the modality being studied.

Open-Hidden Paradigm

The open-hidden paradigm describes two methods of drug delivery in a trial. In open administration, the patient is aware they are receiving a drug. This allows the patient to employ expectation and context. Hidden administration, however, involves an unaware patient receiving a drug, blinding them to expectation. This separates the physiological response from the psychological response. Several studies have examined this and compared covert (or hidden) administration of a treatment to open treatment [18, 19]. The main finding is that the treatment is less effective when the treatment is given covertly, despite no placebo being employed. Some think of this difference in effect as the placebo response, again reinforcing the idea that placebo is a response and not limited to simply a specific definition of an inert treatment. The increased effectiveness of open treatments suggests the importance of several notions, which include patients understanding the treatments they are being given as well as the potential impact of the patient-provider relationship.

Placebo as Treatment Modality

Placebo treatments are effective in a significant proportion of patients. Certain patients respond at much higher rates than others. While certain traits and characteristics were thought to predict "placebo responders," this has shown harder to elucidate in clinical studies. There are likely many psychological, cultural, and social factors that influence the context and response to treatment.

Nocebo Effect

Nocebo refers to negative side effects expected only for patients in the active treatment arm yet experienced by patients receiving placebo treatments. When surreptitious administration of decaffeinated coffee to a habitual coffee drinker still results in tachycardia, a nocebo effect has occurred. The same is true for patients with back pain whose pain increases when a test they feel they need (e.g., imaging) does not occur. This effect is thought to be the result of similar cognitive and conditioning mechanisms as the positive effects seen with placebo treatments. Similar to the placebo response, it is likely not the result of gender, race, education, or social factors.

Conclusion

In summary, placebo refers to both a seemingly inert substance used in clinical trials and a highly individual and complex neuro-psycho-physiologic response experienced by patients. It is most likely the result of expectancy and conditioning on the part of the patient, but also may involve a social learning component, as well as a positive emotional interaction between the provider and patient. Placebo treatments are effective in a significant percentage of patients. The mechanism may be mediated via endogenous opioid pathways, as well as opioid-independent pathways. Finally, nocebo refers to negative side effects expected only for patients in the active treatment arm yet experienced by patients receiving placebo treatments.

References

1. The powerful placebo: from ancient priest to modern physician. BMJ. 1998;316(7141):1396B.
2. Beecher HK. The powerful placebo. J Am Med Assoc. 1955;159(17):1602–6.
3. Polston GR. Pain medicine & management: just the facts. 2nd ed. New York: McGraw-Hill Education; 2015.
4. de Craen AJ, Kaptchuk TJ, Tijssen JG, Kleijnen J. Placebos and placebo effects in medicine: historical overview. J R Soc Med. 1999;92(10):511–5.
5. McRae C, Cherin E, Yamazaki TG, Diem G, Vo AH, Russell D, et al. Effects of perceived treatment on quality of life and medical outcomes in a double-blind placebo surgery trial. Arch Gen Psychiatry. 2004;61(4):412–20.
6. Amanzio M, Benedetti F. Neuropharmacological dissection of placebo analgesia: expectation-activated opioid systems versus conditioning-activated specific subsystems. J Neurosci. 1999;19(1):484–94.
7. Laska E, Sunshine A. Anticipation of analgesia. A placebo effect. Headache. 1973;13(1):1–11.
8. Benedetti F, Amanzio M, Baldi S, Casadio C, Maggi G. Inducing placebo respiratory depressant responses in humans via opioid receptors. Eur J Neurosci. 1999;11(2):625–31.
9. Levine JD, Gordon NC, Fields HL. The mechanism of placebo analgesia. Lancet. 1978;2(8091):654–7.
10. Gracely RH, Dubner R, Wolskee PJ, Deeter WR. Placebo and naloxone can alter post-surgical pain by separate mechanisms. Nature. 1983;306(5940):264–5.
11. Vase L, Robinson ME, Verne GN, Price DD. Increased placebo analgesia over time in irritable bowel syndrome (IBS) patients is associated with desire and expectation but not endogenous opioid mechanisms. Pain. 2005;115(3):338–47.
12. de la Fuente-Fernandez R, Phillips AG, Zamburlini M, Sossi V, Calne DB, Ruth TJ, et al. Dopamine release in human ventral striatum and expectation of reward. Behav Brain Res. 2002;136(2):359–63.
13. de la Fuente-Fernandez R, Ruth TJ, Sossi V, Schulzer M, Calne DB, Stoessl AJ. Expectation and dopamine release: mechanism of the placebo effect in Parkinson's disease. Science. 2001;293(5532):1164–6.
14. Petrovic P, Kalso E, Petersson KM, Ingvar M. Placebo and opioid analgesia-- imaging a shared neuronal network. Science. 2002;295(5560):1737–40.
15. Wager TD, Rilling JK, Smith EE, Sokolik A, Casey KL, Davidson RJ, et al. Placebo-induced changes in FMRI in the anticipation and experience of pain. Science. 2004;303(5661):1162–7.
16. Zubieta JK, Bueller JA, Jackson LR, Scott DJ, Xu Y, Koeppe RA, et al. Placebo effects mediated by endogenous opioid activity on mu-opioid receptors. J Neurosci. 2005;25(34):7754–62.
17. Benedetti F, Arduino C, Amanzio M. Somatotopic activation of opioid systems by target-directed expectations of analgesia. J Neurosci. 1999;19(9):3639–48.
18. Benedetti F, Amanzio M, Maggi G. Potentiation of placebo analgesia by proglumide. Lancet. 1995;346(8984):1231.
19. Colloca L, Lopiano L, Lanotte M, Benedetti F. Overt versus covert treatment for pain, anxiety, and Parkinson's disease. Lancet Neurol. 2004;3(11):679–84.

Epidemiology

Michael Andreae

Use of Data from Epidemiological Studies of Pain

Epidemiology is concerned with patterns, causes, and effects of health and disease in large populations with a goal of disease surveillance and public health interventions as opposed to individual treatment decision, as may be seen in Table 9.1 by the outcome measures of interest [1].

Often we have to accept simplified measures focusing on the presence and absence of disease, as opposed to continuous more sophisticated constructs, for example, limiting ourselves to investigating the presence or absence of chronic pain after surgery [2] as opposed to employing multidimensional scales like the Brief Pain Inventory [3]. The latter, while more meaningful, are also more resource intensive.

The goal of epidemiology in pain medicine is to identify risk factors in order to attenuate them and/or to gauge the burden of disease in order to inform public resource allocation. Figure 9.1 [4] illustrates how risk factors for chronic pain formation can be related to the individual (e.g., genetic predisposition to developing persistent pain after surgery) pain therapies received [2] and the environment (surgical insult, stressful family situation, or spousal depression) [5].

The sources of data in epidemiology are often questionnaires, surveys, and surveillance efforts that can compromise data integrity due to low response rates, loss to follow-up, and questionnaire fatigue. These are often resistant to methods designed to improve response rates, like incentives and personalized reminders, especially when physicians are surveyed [6]. Another source of data increasingly used in epidemiology are electronic medical records and registries, but data in both are often incomplete. As data is not missing at random (because tests are done preferentially when indicated), significant bias may be present [7].

M. Andreae (✉)
Department of Anesthesiology, Penn State Milton S. Hershey Medical Center, Hershey, PA, USA
e-mail: mandreae@pennstatehealth.psu.edu

Measurement of Disease Burden in a Population

When we compare burden of disease across populations, it is critical to distinguish prevalence from incidence. Prevalence renders a snapshot picture in a defined population at a given moment in time. It is the *proportion* of individuals who have the disease at a particular time point, that is, how widespread it is. In contrast, incidence counts the number of new cases within a specified period; hence, incidence is a *rate over time*, indicating the risk of contracting the disease; in other words, incidence measures how contagious a condition is. For example, the annual attack rate (incidence) in an influenza epidemic is estimated at 10% per annum in adults, but at no point in time will 10% of the population have influenza (prevalence), because influenza lasts only a few days and one patient recovers before the next patient is affected.

Observational Studies: Uses and Limitations

In an attempt to prove causality by demonstrating a statistical association between a predictor (e.g., independent variable) and an outcome (e.g., dependent variable), three study designs are employed in epidemiological pain research: cohort, case-control, and cross-sectional. Their temporal directionality [8] is illustrated in Fig. 9.2 [9]. Figure 9.3 displays an algorithm useful in identifying clinical study designs. In the cohort design, one starts from the exposure and moves forward in time to the disease. The opposite is true for case-control studies, where one starts with the disease (the case), finds a control, and then goes backward in time to define the exposure. In cross-sectional studies, predictor variables and outcome measures are obtained in the same moment. Association observed in cross-sectional studies is insufficient proof for causality. Cohort and case-control studies, by demonstrating temporality, strengthen the inferences according to the Bradford Hill criteria [10], but

Table 9.1 Overview of outcome measure, with corresponding statistical models and representation

Outcome data type	Effect estimate	Example	Statistical model	Tabular/graphical representation
Dichotomous	Relative risk	Persistent postoperative pain (yes/no)	Chi-square	Point estimate with confidence intervals
Dichotomous	Odds ratio	Persistent postoperative pain (yes/no)	Logistic regression	Table of regression coefficients
Time to event	Hazard ratio	Time to cancer recurrence (days)	Cox regression	Kaplan-Meier curves or Cox hazard ratios
Rare events	Relative risk	Number of infections after spinal (n)	Poisson regression	Table of regression coefficients

In this overview of epidemiological measures, we tabulate frequently used outcomes with the corresponding effect estimates, the statistical test, and the typical tabular or graphical representation [1]. The choice of statistical modeling will be contingent on the data type of interest, e.g., a Cox model for time to event data

Fig. 9.1 The hardwired genetic makeup of an individual interacts with the environment, for example, in the development of persistent pain after surgery [5]. (Adapted from Denk et al. [4])

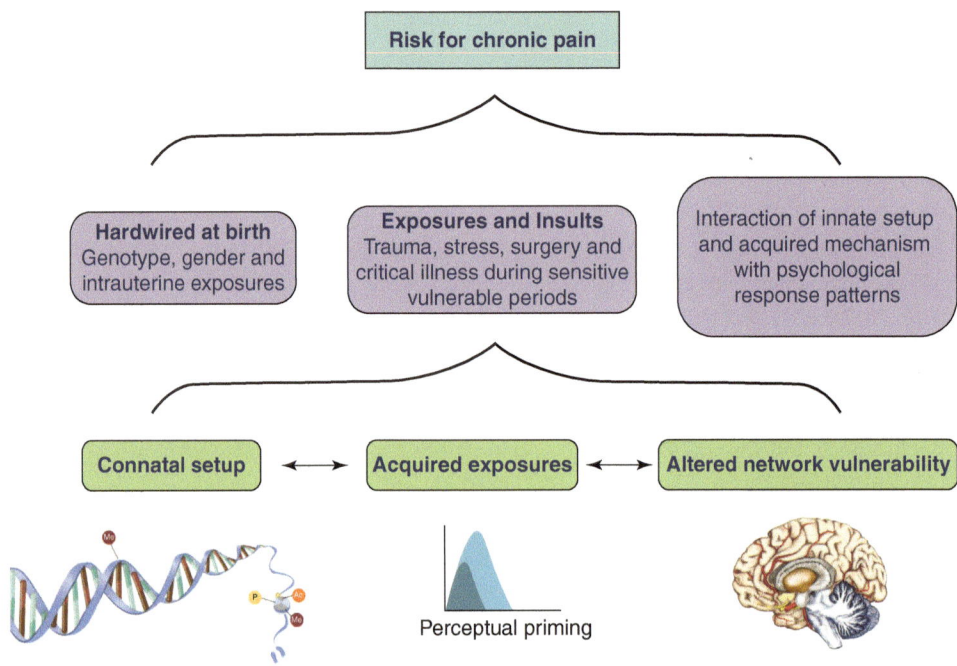

Fig. 9.2 Cohort studies move forward in time ascertaining outcomes as they occur. This is in contrast with case-control studies which go back in time to obtain the predicting risk factor in the past in the cases and the controls. Cross-sectional studies are a snapshot capturing risk exposure and outcome simultaneously but without establishing temporality. (Adapted from Grimes and Schulz [9])

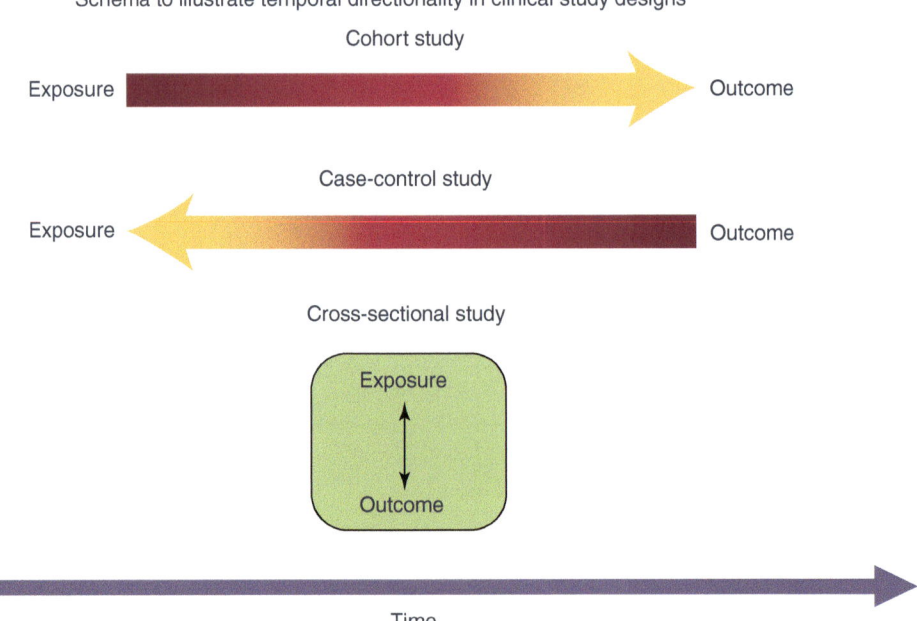

Fig. 9.3 Assigning the exposure to the factor of interest can control for *unknown* confounders, especially if group allocation is randomized, while cross-sectional, case-control, and cohort studies can only attempt to control for confounders *known* to the investigator and measured precisely. (Adapted from Grimes and Schulz [9])

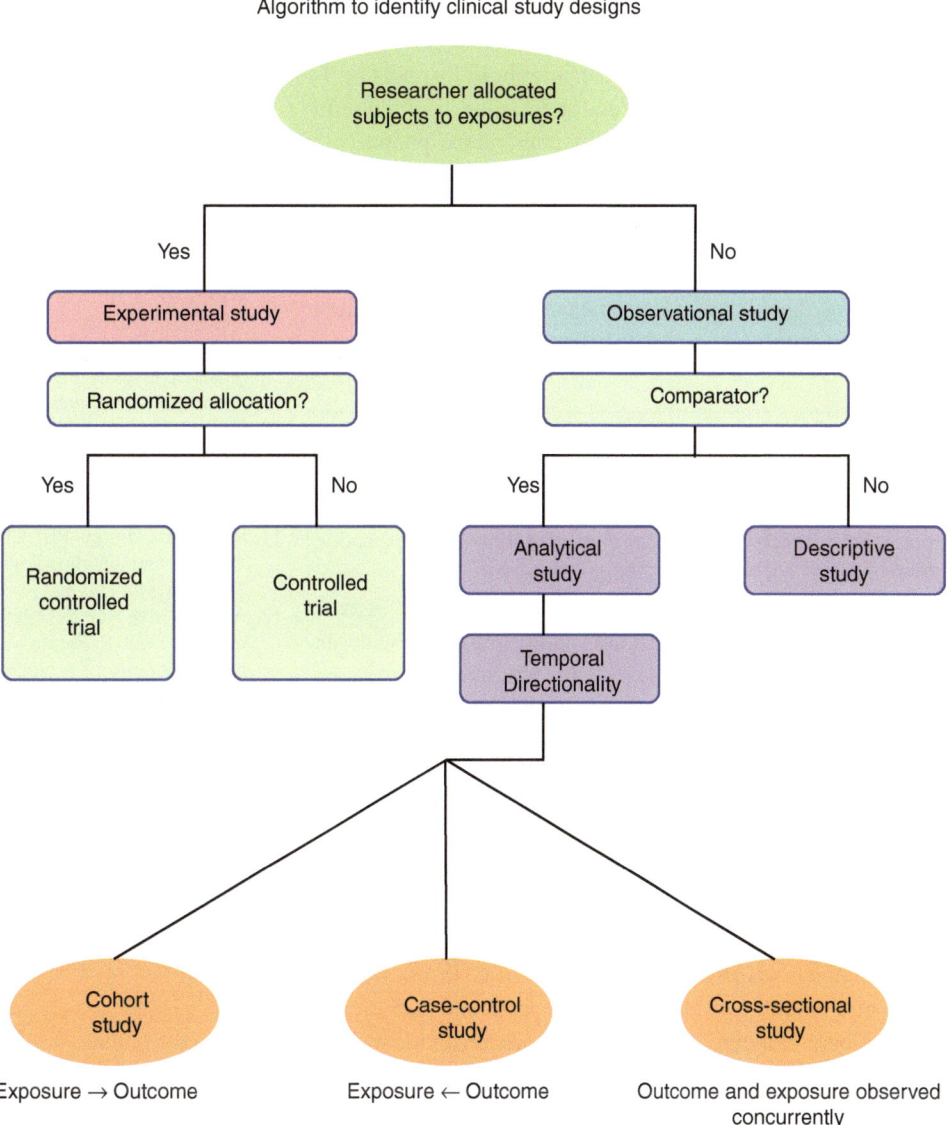

consistency, coherence with animal experiments, dose dependency, and findings in quasi-experimental designs are also sought.

Case-control studies start with patients who have the disease and try to find suitable control cases. Case-control studies seek to ascertain the predictor (e.g., the risk factors investigated) in the past, which can be fraught with recall bias. For example, female physicians asked about prenatal radiation exposure after the birth of a child with birth defects are more likely to recall exposure during training. Matching cases with controls is rarely perfect, giving rise to a plethora of biases, such as sampling and selection bias [11].

Controlling for bias is challenging, in particular, when we attempt to study healthcare disparities, which is still rampant in pain and perioperative medicine in the USA [12, 13]. Statistical inference in observational studies is based on the fictitious counterfactual theory of causation, consid-

ering what the outcome would have been, had the subject not been assigned the exposure [14]. This counterfactual approach is compelling in randomized studies where the assignment to the treatment or exposure is not associated with any potential confounders, but proves to be less useful in health disparity research [15]. We can make inferences about bias, by observing that psychiatric case descriptions randomly assigned a black phenotype are more often adjudicated by psychiatrists as paranoid schizophrenia than identical cases randomly assigned a white phenotype [16]. In contrast, observational studies of discrimination are less compelling. Todd showed that after controlling for known confounders like gender or pain, black patients received less analgesia administered in the emergency room than their white counterparts did [17]. However, patient characteristics known to the treating emergency room physician, but unknown to the analyst, may have acted as a confounder and create a spurious association between race and outcome [18]. Indeed, Kaufman argued that the counterfactual approach to statistical inference cannot hold for innate differences [19], because we cannot imagine of randomly assigning race, arguably a socially constructed phenotypic categorization devoid of scientific support [20]. Kaufman showed how inappropriate use of logistic regression can reinforce racial discrimination by reinforcing stereotypical assumptions. This, in essence, may lead to erroneously attributing healthcare disparities to individual patient choices or immutable genetic differences [18].

Cohort Studies

Different from case-control studies, cohort studies follow patients forward in time and register outcomes as they occur. For example, an investigator may observe the occurrence of drug addiction over a year in a cohort of sickle cell disease patients treated in the pain clinic with opioids or without. The investigator does not allocate the treatment or exposure of interest randomly (the major shortcoming of observational studies), in contrast to randomized designs as illustrated in Fig. 9.3.

Allocating treatment randomly can reduce the risk of bias by eliminating confounding by those factors not considered or unknown to the investigator [11]. Otherwise, these unmeasured and/or unknown variables (i.e., ethnicity, insurance status, provider treating the individual, etc.) may confound the association between the risk factor (in our example opioid treatment) and the outcome occurrence (addiction), inducing a spurious association that may not reflect causality [8].

It is imperative to critically appraise the legitimacy of evidence purporting causality prior to incorporating it into our clinical decision-making [21–23].

References

1. Ressing M, Blettner M, Klug SJ. Data analysis of epidemiological studies: part 11 of a series on evaluation of scientific publications. Dtsch Arztebl Int. 2010;107(11):187–92.
2. Andreae MH, Andreae DA. Regional anaesthesia to prevent chronic pain after surgery: a Cochrane systematic review and meta-analysis. Br J Anaesth. 2013;111(5):711–20.
3. Younger J, McCue R, Mackey S. Pain outcomes: a brief review of instruments and techniques. Curr Pain Headache Rep. 2009;13(1):39–43.
4. Denk F, McMahon SB, Tracey I. Pain vulnerability: a neurobiological perspective. Nat Neurosci. 2014;17(2):192–200.
5. Schreiber KL, Martel MO, Shnol H, Shaffer JR, Greco C, Viray N, Taylor LN, McLaughlin M, Brufsky A, Ahrendt G, Bovbjerg D, Edwards RR, Belfer I. Persistent pain in postmastectomy patients: comparison of psychophysical, medical, surgical, and psychosocial characteristics between patients with and without pain. Pain. 2013;154:660.
6. Cunningham CT, Quan H, Hemmelgarn B, Noseworthy T, Beck CA, Dixon E, Samuel S, Ghali WA, Sykes LL, Jetté N. Exploring physician specialist response rates to web-based surveys. BMC Med Res Methodol. 2015;15:32.
7. Sterne JA, White IR, Carlin JB, Spratt M, Royston P, Kenward MG, Wood AM, Carpenter JR. Multiple imputation for missing data in epidemiological and clinical research: potential and pitfalls. BMJ. 2009;338:b2393.
8. Sessler DI, Imrey PB. Clinical research methodology 2: observational clinical research. Anesth Analg. 2015;121(4):1043–51.
9. Grimes DA, Schulz KF. An overview of clinical research: the lay of the land. Lancet. 2002;359(9300):57–61.
10. Hill AB. The environment and disease: association or causation? Proc R Soc Med. 1965;58:295–300.
11. Sessler DI, Imrey PB. Clinical research methodology 1: study designs and methodologic sources of error. Anesth Analg. 2015;121(4):1034–42.
12. Andreae MH, Nair S, Gabry JS, Goodrich B, Hall C, Shaparin N. A pragmatic trial to improve adherence with scheduled appointments in an inner-city pain clinic by human phone calls in the patient's preferred language. J Clin Anesth. 2017;42:77–83.
13. Andreae MH, Gabry JS, Goodrich B, White RS, Hall C. Antiemetic prophylaxis as a marker of health care disparities in the National Anesthesia Clinical Outcomes Registry. Anesth Analg. 2018;126(2):588–99.
14. Rubin DB. Causal inference using potential outcomes: design, modeling, decisions. J Am Stat Assoc. 2005;100(469):322–31.
15. Benn EK, Goldfeld KS. Translating context to causality in cardiovascular disparities research. Health Psychol. 2016;35(4):403.
16. Loring M, Powell B. Gender, race, and DSM-III: a study of the objectivity of psychiatric diagnostic behavior. J Health Soc Behav. 1988;29(1):1–22.
17. Todd KH, Deaton C, D'Adamo AP, Goe L. Ethnicity and analgesic practice. Ann Emerg Med. 2000;35(1):11–6; May;154(5):660–8.
18. Robinson WR, Gordon-Larsen P, Kaufman JS, Suchindran CM, Stevens J. The female-male disparity in obesity prevalence among black American young adults: contributions of sociodemographic characteristics of the childhood family. The American journal of clinical nutrition. 2009;89(4):1204–12.
19. Kaufman JS, Long AE, Liao Y, Cooper RS, McGee DL. The relation between income and mortality in U.S. blacks and whites. Epidemiology. 1998;9(2):147–55.
20. Witzig R. The medicalization of race: scientific legitimization of a flawed social construct. Ann Intern Med. 1996;125(8):675–9.
21. Edlund MJ, Steffick D, Hudson T, Harris KM, Sullivan M. Risk factors for clinically recognized opioid abuse and dependence among veterans using opioids for chronic non-cancer pain. Pain. 2007;129(3):355–62.
22. Sackett DL, Rosenberg WM, Gray JA, Haynes RB, Richardson WS. Evidence based medicine: what it is and what it isn't. BMJ. 1996;312(7023):71–2.
23. Cohen-Cole E, Fletcher JM. Is obesity contagious? Social networks vs. environmental factors in the obesity epidemic. J Health Econ. 2008;27(5):1382–7.

Psychosocial and Cultural Aspects of Pain

10

Ravi Prasad and Laura Wandner

Pain as a Biopsychological Experience

Definition

Biomedical characterizations of pain posit that the existence and severity of pain can be attributed to a specific organic pathology: identifying and correcting the latter should result in eradication of the pain symptoms [1]. While the simplicity of such cause-and-effect models can be attractive, they fail to take into consideration the role of psychological factors in the onset, maintenance, and exacerbation of pain [2] and may thus limit a patient's response to treatment [3]. The International Association for the Study of Pain (IASP) defines pain as "an unpleasant sensory and emotional experience associated with actual or potential tissue damage, or described in terms of such damage" [4]. Biopsychological characterizations such as this expand on biomedical models by recognizing that the experience of pain possesses both physiologic and psychological underpinnings. Concurrently addressing the physical, behavioral, and psychological components of pain has been shown to improve functioning and decrease pain-related distress and could potentially reduce the financial burden associated with pain treatment [3].

Measurement

As pain has both biologic and psychological dimensions, it is important to ensure that the contributions of each are measured as a part of the clinical evaluation. A multidisciplinary evaluation process is one in which clinicians from different specialty areas (i.e., pain physician, psychologist, etc.) assess a patient from the perspective of their specific discipline. The impressions and recommendations of each evaluator are then incoprporated into a comprehensive treatment plan that addresses the direct, indirect, and interactive impact of the assessed variables.

A pain physician evaluates all biologic aspects of a patient's predicament to determine the role(s) that injection therapies, surgery, implantable devices, and/or pharmacologic treatment may play in the treatment plan. Data gathered from physical exam findings, imaging studies, lab results, and patient self-report inform this medical decision making process.

A pain psychologist assimilates data from self-report assessment devices and a comprehensive clinical interview to identify the nature and extent to which psychological and behavioral factors may be influencing a pain condition. Information about pain perception, substance use/abuse, early life experiences, academic and vocational histories, current physical functioning, past and present psychiatric distress, situational stressors, and coping strategies is used to facilitate development of a treatment plan.

Limiting the evaluation to the medical evaluation alone is consistent with a purely biomedical pathway. A biopsychological approach integrates the findings of both the physician and the psychologist when conceptualizing the etiology and treatment of pain conditions. As there are individual differences in the affective, cognitive, behavioral, and physiologic responses to pain, treatment plans should be specifically tailored to each patient and his/her environment. Once a treatment pathway has been established, it is important to continue to measure specific areas of functioning (i.e., emotional distress, pain perception, functional activity, etc.) to assess the efficacy of treatment. The treatment plan should be modified as needed to maximize outcomes.

Coping Styles

Definition

Coping is broadly defined as the use of behavioral and cognitive techniques to manage physical and emotional stress

R. Prasad (✉)
Division of Pain Medicine, Stanford University, Redwood City, CA, USA
e-mail: rprasad@stanford.edu

L. Wandner
Walter Reed National Military Medical Center, Bethesda, MD, USA

© Springer Nature Switzerland AG 2019
Y. Khelemsky et al. (eds.), *Academic Pain Medicine*, https://doi.org/10.1007/978-3-030-18005-8_10

[5]. Individuals experiencing pain often use a combination of coping strategies. Pain coping strategies can be conceptualized into three main groups: (1) cognitive vs. behavioral strategies; (2) active vs. passive coping strategies; and (3) problem-focused vs. emotion-focused strategies [5].

One conceptualization of pain coping differentiates cognitive from behavioral strategies. Various types of cognitive strategies can be adopted by patients to manage pain (e.g., diverting attention, focusing on or reinterpreting pain sensations, coping self-statements, suppression of pain-related thoughts, and praying/hoping). There also are a number of behavioral strategies to manage pain (e.g., behavioral activation, time-based pacing, relaxation exercises, use of pain behaviors) [5].

Another conceptualization of coping differentiates active from passive pain coping strategies. Active coping refers to strategies that patients use to control pain or to function despite pain by using their own resources. Passive coping involves patients relinquishing control of pain to others. Studies have linked active coping strategies to positive effects, better psychological adjustment, and decreased depression, while passive strategies generally are linked to poor outcomes such as increased pain and depression [5].

Coping also can be classified into problem-focused versus emotion-focused strategies. Problem-focused approaches involve patients' direct attempts to deal with pain, whereas emotion-focused approaches involve patients managing their emotional reactions to pain. There is some evidence that suggests that emotion-focused coping is associated with higher pain intensity ratings and worse functioning in individuals with chronic pain [5].

Patients typically use different coping strategies when they experience differences in pain intensity, when they adjust from acute to chronic pain, when they experience changes in psychological well-being, and with changes in physical functioning. For example, multiple studies have found that ignoring strategies are associated with less pain, whereas praying, hoping, and catastrophizing (magnification and rumination of pain-related information) are associated with higher pain levels [5].

Expectations, Coping, Cultural, and Environmental Factors

Sex/Gender

Epidemiological researchers have found that pain is more commonly reported by women than men and that the prevalence of some chronic pain conditions is more common in women than in men [6, 7]. One study found that for ten different anatomical regions, a greater percentage of women than men reported pain in the past week and women also were more likely to report chronic widespread pain than men [8].

It appears that coping style contributes to sex differences in experimental as well as clinical settings. Men have been found to more frequently use behavioral distraction and problem-focused strategies to manage pain, whereas women have a tendency to use a range of coping techniques (e.g., social support, positive self-statements, emotion-focused techniques, cognitive reinterpretation, and attentional focus) [6]. Research has found that women, more so than men, use catastrophizing as a strategy to manage pain, which is associated with higher pain intensity and pain-related disability [6, 7]. With regard to coping styles, catastrophizing has been found to partially mediate sex differences in pain sensitivity, but variables such as masculinity-femininity personality traits likely contribute to this finding. Women also have been found to use more adaptive coping strategies, especially when coping with laboratory pain, such as using attentional focus or reinterpreting pain sensation strategies, while some research suggests that men find distraction more efficient [9].

Race

A large body of research suggests that Blacks report higher levels of clinical pain across a range of painful conditions than Hispanics or Whites [5, 10]. Such differences have implications that could explain racial/ethnic differences in treatment response. For example, patients presenting with higher pain intensity levels/disability also are more likely to exit treatment with higher pain intensity levels/disability. Patients who have perceived that their pain has been discounted in previous appointments may augment symptom reports in order to reduce the likelihood of being discounted again. This makes it difficult to interpret the association between race/ethnicity and self-reported pain and/or disability in a clinical sample [11]. Evidence suggests that many Blacks and Hispanics and other minorities lack trust in the medical system. Relative to non-Hispanic Whites, Blacks are almost three times and Hispanics over two times more likely to believe racism is a significant healthcare problem [11]. Given these high levels of distrust, it is not surprising that Blacks and Hispanics feel high levels of stereotype threat in medical encounters and do not expect significant benefit from treatment. These expectations may contribute to the persistently low rates of surgery for knee and joint replacement among minorities [11].

Blacks and Hispanics appear to demonstrate higher levels of post-treatment disability than non-Hispanic Whites for conditions that include chronic low back pain and other chronic pain conditions. In addition to increased disability, Blacks and Hispanics demonstrate more affective distress in response to chronic pain as well as greater levels of pain-related disability [10, 11]. Other psychological factors also might impact pain-related disability. For example, Blacks and

Hispanics are more likely than Whites to use passive coping strategies such as prayer, while Whites are more likely to use active coping-self statement and perceive themselves as having greater pain control [5, 10]. Evidence also suggests that Black and Hispanic individuals have a more external locus of control orientation, have a lower overall sense of self-efficacy, and report greater feelings of helplessness. Because passive strategies are minimally effective for pain management, individuals who frequently use them might conclude that they have little control over their pain. This could possibly lead to and/or reinforce the belief of helplessness toward pain [5]. Similarly, research has suggested that Blacks are more likely to catastrophize than other ethnic groups, and pain catastrophizing contributes to poorer pain adjustment and a sense of learned helplessness [5, 11, 12]. Catastrophizing may also function to solicit assistance or empathetic responses from others, including family members, friends, and medical providers. This understanding of the communal model of coping posits that catastrophizing strategies are used to secure social or interpersonal resources, as well as to induce others to alter their expectations, reduce performance demands, or manage interpersonal conflict. The communal model of coping is consistent with the collectivistic orientation that is characteristic of many Black cultures [5].

Some may think that having more tools in one's coping toolbox is preferable to having fewer; however, the results from a meta-analysis suggest that use of maladaptive coping was a more important indicator of pain adjustment than was adaptive coping. Since Blacks use pain-coping strategies more frequently overall, they also are more likely to engage in maladaptive strategies more frequently, which may offset any gains from adaptive coping and account for their increased pain and impairment compared to Whites [5].

Age

The literature suggests that individuals interpret their health-related symptoms within the context of their life stage and overall physical health. Older adults may have a number of attitudes about health and disability that are relevant to their perception of pain. It is important to be mindful of some of these beliefs because some beliefs might be helpful while others might be barriers to effective pain management [13]. Some research has suggested that older adults compare their experiences to those of their peers, particularly those who are more ill peers, and may conclude that they are better off than others they know. Findings have also suggested that many older adults perceive pain and disability as "normal" or "expected" in aging; however, pain severe enough to impact function is not a normal part of aging, and this is a social expectation vs. a medical reality. This belief is highlighted in one study where 40% of adults in the sample reported it

was "definitely true" that one is expected to have more aches and pains with aging, but 94% of participants also stated that it was "very" or "somewhat" important that someone with aches and pains should talk to a doctor about treatment [14].

Generally, research has suggested an increase in the use of "adaptive" coping strategies across domains in later life [13]. Studies have shown that older adults often may have fewer coping strategies, but they use them as effectively, or more effectively, than younger adults. Older adults also have a tendency to use the same strategies for managing stressors across various life domains, that is, older adults find strategies that work and use them in multiple settings [13]. Several pain studies have suggested that adults use different coping strategies across the life span. For example, older adults with persistent pain are more likely to use emotion-focused coping strategies. One study found that younger people used twice as many "cognitive" strategies (e.g., imagery) for managing pain as did older adults. But findings are equivocal in one community sample of 280 patients with persistent pain; age was negatively correlated with a variety of emotion- and problem-focused strategies [15], suggesting less frequent use of coping strategies across the board in older adults. There also is some preliminary evidence that older adults use certain pain coping strategies (e.g., resting and pacing themselves) consistently on a daily basis, regardless of temporary flare-ups in pain, whereas younger adults may be more likely to use their coping strategies when their pain worsens [16].

Some barriers that can impact treating pain in older adults are cognition, hearing, and communication impairment. The literature suggests that older adults are more likely than younger adults to underreport or minimize pain, particularly if they perceive that the pain symptoms are manageable. Older adults are also more likely to try and adapt by limiting their physical and social activities instead of seeking treatment. Older adults with stoic attitudes present with lower levels of affective distress relative to their pain levels. However, stoicism also may limit reporting of important symptoms to family and healthcare providers, which can delay the diagnosis or treatment of a chronic illness. Research also suggests that some older adults are reluctant to discuss their pain due to fear of a diagnosis that is progressive and/or fear of losing their independence. There also could be a fear of being labeled "a hypochondriac" and wanting to be considered a "good patient" [13].

There is recent research suggesting that children have different coping styles. Studies have found that youths with pain have been found to be higher catastrophizers than adolescents. Adaptive responses to stress and pain have been reported to increase as children age. It has been hypothesized that as more opportunities to apply coping strategies arise, a greater number of coping responses are learned [17]. It also is possible that pain catastrophizing may not be due to maladaptive cognitive coping strategies, which has been speculated in adults, but rather, a developmentally normal process related to limited coping resources. Thus, as children mature into adolescents and early adults, a wider array of cognitively complex resources may help minimize the effect of pain catastrophizing on children's functional outcomes and disability. The research suggests that adolescents may use more active and accommodative coping methods compared to children, which may be due to the development of cognitive resources and executive functions needed to enact these strategies [17].

Education

Higher levels of education appear to protect against pain-related disability. One possible reason for this is that the association between higher levels of education and higher levels of health literacy. For example, health literacy is associated with higher levels of function in patients with rheumatologic diagnoses. Similarly, low back pain patients with higher levels of education demonstrate lower levels of fear-avoidance beliefs and pain-related disability than do patients with lower levels of education [11].

Cultural, Environmental, and Racial Variations in the Experience and Expression of Pain

Stereotypes

Stereotyping is an intuitive process, of which people often are unaware, which can bias judgments. Stereotypes represent a shorthand way to characterize a group of people that share a given attribute, such as race or ethnicity. Such biases are difficult to study: explicit biases are commonly disavowed, even as implicit biases continue to operate – generally reflecting culturally derived associations that are less amenable to conscious control [11].

Judgments about pain are influenced by features of the patient, the situation, and the provider. This may be a function of uncertainty inherent in pain assessment which introduces considerable ambiguity into provider judgments of pain and treatment decisions. Like a projective test, providers can project onto patients their attitudes, beliefs, and opinions, making clinical judgments vulnerable to the influence of stereotyping [11]. Pain studies researching stereotypes are important because pain is subjective, treatment guidelines are not always well defined, and there is not always a "correct" way to treat a patient. In a few studies, subjects viewed a series of pained facial expressions, estimated the level of pain that patients experienced and then rated whether demographic characteristics influenced their judgments. While

respondents denied any influence of demographic characteristics, analyses showed that demographic characteristics did influence judgments (pain ratings and recommendations for pain management) [18–21].

Race

There has been longstanding interest in the racial/ethnic differences in pain sensitivity. Much of the research reveals that Blacks and Hispanics demonstrate lower pain thresholds and tolerance than Whites. Recent experimental research has attempted to understand this finding. For example, there is evidence that differences in pain perception may be mediated by higher levels of negative affect among Blacks relative to Whites. Alternatively, Blacks may approach pain inductions with a higher level of vigilance, and vigilance may mediate perceptions of pain severity, threshold, or tolerance [11, 22, 23]. Studies examining Hispanics' pain experience have found that they report fewer pain conditions but report higher pain sensitivity and severity, but are more likely to work in jobs that predispose them to pain [10]. However, only limited pain research has been conducted on Hispanics and would benefit from future studies examining individual (i.e., age, work satisfaction, personal acculturation, etc.) and sociocultural reasons (i.e., social support, collectivistic culture, familial pain models, etc.) for these seemingly contradictory findings. Results from a race expectation of pain questionnaire found that a sample of participants believed that the typical White person is more sensitive to pain and more willing to report pain than other minority groups which may help explain some of the variability in assessment and treatment practices of patients [24].

Sex/Gender

Gender-specific beliefs and expectations about pain, which are partly acquired by social learning, have been proposed as potential factors contributing to differences in pain perception in women and men. "Gender role" broadly refers to a socially accepted set of characteristics ascribed to each sex. With regard to pain, the feminine role is stereotypically associated with greater willingness to report pain, whereas the expected masculine role is more related to stoicism [9]. Studies have found that gender role expectations probably play a significant role, explaining some of the differences in experimental pain perception in female and male participants.

The masculinity-femininity trait (emotional vulnerability) and perceived identification according to typical male/female stereotypes (willingness to report pain) seems to alter pain tolerance, pain intensity, and pain unpleasantness [9]. In a study, both men and women believed that men are less willing to report pain, have a higher pain endurance and lower pain sensitivity than the typical woman and such gender role expectations may contribute to sex differences in experimental pain [25]. Pain studies have found that sex differences in pain sensitivity may be influenced by sex-related expectations regarding performance on the pain task, suggesting that gender-related motivation may influence pain expression [6]. Another [26] study examined self-reported pain intensity ratings. Subjects were either told that (1) a typical male or female could tolerate pain for 30 s, or (2) a typical male or female could tolerate pain for 90 s, or (3) they received no information about performance. The study found that when given no information, male subjects reported having higher pain tolerance and lower pain intensity than females. However, this difference in pain perception disappeared when they received information about expected performance (30 or 90 s).

Age

Social context is important among older adults, especially those who live with pain and disability. Changes in social support network size and organization are among the best documented effects in the literature, with good evidence that older adults report fewer friends and social support than do younger people. Older adults' well-being is more tied to having a few close friends or family members than to having a broad network of support. The smaller social support networks seen in older people may be the result of intentionally "downsizing" on their part in which they reduce the energy spent on maintaining contact with peripheral social partners. This process of "downsizing" is more pronounced from early to middle adulthood and may be especially true of older adults with decreasing physical capacities, since they may lack the energy and resources to maintain a large group of friends. It is important to note that the perspective that older adults intentionally reduce their networks, rather than have them reduced by external factors, is not without controversy [13].

Results from an age expectation of pain questionnaire showed that a sample of participants believed that the typical older adult is more sensitive to pain and more willing to report pain than other minority groups which, similar to race, may help explain some of the variability in assessment and treatment practices of patients [24].

Limited English Proficiency/Communication with Providers

High levels of patient-provider communication have been found to increase patient engagement in self-management and increase feedback to providers regarding treatment effectiveness [27]. However, one factor that can negatively impact communication involves language skills, especially limited English proficiency (LEP). While only limited research has examined LEP and pain care, there is abundant evidence that LEP is in general a barrier to adequate healthcare, and is assumed to also impact adequate pain management [11]. While language proficiency is an obvious factor that can adversely affect communication, nonspecific factors associated with race/ethnicity also are important. For example, minority patients have been found to be less active in their communications when the encounter is race-discordant, more active with race-concordant providers, and more likely to report more distressing pain to a race-concordant observer [11]. Several studies of primary care physicians examined clinically implicit race bias and its associations with provider communication and patient satisfaction. Among other results, the data showed that high racial bias was associated with less patient-centered dialogue toward Blacks and with Black patient perceptions of providers as less respectful [11].

Income

Higher levels of education are associated with higher levels of income. Income has been found to be linked with the likelihood of experiencing a recent pain episode. People with incomes at 400% of the poverty level are 1.76 times more likely to report low back pain and 1.59 times more likely to report neck pain than people with incomes below the poverty level [11]. There also is data suggesting that the effects of race and socioeconomic status (SES) on pain adjustment may differ over time. Workers' compensation claimants with low back pain exhibit patterns of adjustment that reflects differing relative contributions of race and SES over time. Data collected 2 years post-settlement showed that Blacks received lower levels of care and demonstrated poorer outcomes than non-Hispanic Whites. The contribution of race to those differences was significantly greater than that of SES. At 6 years post-settlement, however, the opposite result was obtained: SES accounted for substantially greater variance in clinical adjustment than did race. The pattern reflects a greater contribution of race during the time frame of most active treatment studies, and greater contribution of SES thereafter, likely reflecting differential access to resources.

Role of Family in Promoting Illness and Well Behavior

Individuals living with pain do not exist in a vacuum; their pain affects their life but their life can also affect their pain. This bidirectional relationship emphasizes the need for addressing the role of the social system in the experience of pain and pain-related behaviors.

Solicitous Responses

Although often well-intentioned, family members who react to patients' verbal and nonverbal expressions of pain with overly protective responses may unwittingly be contributing to the pain problem itself. Solicitous responses from spouses/significant others of individuals living with pain may include offering physical assistance, providing medication, completing tasks for the partner, or encouraging rest.

They have been associated higher levels of reported pain, disability, and pain behaviors [28, 29] and are negatively associated with pain acceptance, the latter a finding that remained significant after adjusting for patient age, education, pain level, and significant other support [30]. Furthermore, solicitous responses have also been linked with medication dosing. More specifically, researchers have found that the higher levels of solicitous behaviors are associated with increased dosing of opioids [31]. These findings persisted even after controlling for age, gender, ethnicity, education level, employment status, pain duration, pain severity, and depression.

Punitive Responses

Punitive responses to pain, characterized by verbal and/or nonverbal expressions of negative emotion in response to patients' pain behaviors, are similarly associated with poorer outcomes. This category of social reaction is related to lower physical health-related quality of life, work-related fear-avoidance, pain interference, and affective distress [32]. As with solicitous responses, they are also linked with higher levels of pain-related disability [33] and negatively associated with pain acceptance [30].

Positive Reinforcement and Confidence

Facilitative reponses to well behavior is associated with lower levels of pain behavior [34]. Such reactions include encouragement and reinforcement of activity and healthy actions. Spousal confidence in a patients' ability to manage health issues has also been associated with a number of positive health outcomes, including functional improvements in stroke survivors and increased compliance with dietary and exercise regimens among diabetics [35, 36]. In the realm of pain, spousal confidence was predictive of improvements in depression, perceived health, and lower extremity function, and illness severity among a group of arthritis patients [37].

Common Emotional Problems and Psychiatric Disorders Associated with Pain

Fear Avoidance

Patients living with pain may avoid engaging in activity secondary to fear that it might worsen their condition. Pain-related fear often leads to somatic hypervigilance and hypersensitivity to painful stimuli, which further reinforces the avoidant behaviors [38]. Activity avoidance can ultimately lead to impairment in physical functioning due to guarded movement and/or deconditioning. This self-perpetuating process is known as the fear-avoidance cycle, and it is strongly associated with self-reported disability [39].

Catastrophization

Catastrophization is an exaggerated perception that a situation is significantly worse than it actually is. It can manifest through magnification of the predicament (e.g., "This pain is so bad it will kill me!"), perseveration on the situation, and/or a sense of helplessness regarding the ability to influence one's outcome. The pervasive expectation of inescapable pain can lead to adoption of an avoidant coping strategy, which can place a patient in a fear-avoidance cycle. Pain catastrophizing is associated with increased pain intensity and interference and poorer psychological functioning [40].

Perceived Injustice

Most commonly seen in patients with pain conditions secondary to an industrial injury, perceived injustice refers to a cognitive appraisal of an injury in terms of the severity and irreparability of the loss, a sense of blame, and unfairness regarding the situation. It is predictive of depression and disability, and contributes to both catastrophization and pain behavior [41, 42].

Anxiety

Anxiety is characterized by pervasive worry and difficulty shifting attention away from such stressful thoughts. Beyond these cognitive processes, it may also have somatic manifestations such as dizziness, shortness of breath, increased heart rate, and/or shakiness.

Anxiety can trigger activation of the sympathetic nervous system, and aspects of the subsequent physiologic arousal can subsequently exacerbate pain, leading to a vicious cycle in which anxiety and pain are influencing each other. Fear avoidance and catastrophization are both strongly associated with anxiety.

Depression

While dysphoria may accompany pain conditions, major depressive episodes are marked by a constellation of symptoms that may include pervasive feelings of sadness; anhedonia; impairment in attention, concentration, and/or memory; loss of energy or motivation; appetite changes; weight gain/loss; sleep disturbance; and possible suicidality. The presence of a pain condition can lead to the development of depression [43] but some studies have found that the presence of depression may increase the likelihood of developing chronic pain [44, 45]. Like anxiety, the presence of untreated or undertreated depression can result in a worsening of physical pain.

References

1. Fishman S, Ballantyne J, Rathmell JP, Bonica JJ. Bonica's management of pain. 4th ed. Baltimore: Lippincott, Williams & Wilkins; 2010. xxxiii, 1661 p.
2. Gatchel RJ, Okifuji A. Evidence-based scientific data documenting the treatment and cost-effectiveness of comprehensive pain programs for chronic nonmalignant pain. J Pain. 2006;7:779–93.
3. Malladi N. Interdisciplinary rehabilitation. Phys Med Rehabil Clin N Am. 2015 May;26(2):349–58.
4. Bonica JJ. The need of a taxonomy. Pain. 1979;6(3):247–8.
5. Meints SM, Miller MM, Hirsh AT. Differences in pain coping between black and white americans: a meta-analysis. J Pain. 2016;17(6):642–53.
6. Bartley EJ, Fillingim RB. Sex differences in pain: a brief review of clinical and experimental findings. Br J Anaesth. 2013;111(1):52–8.
7. Fillingim RB, King CD, Ribeiro-Dasilva MC, Rahim-Williams B, Riley JL III. Sex, gender, and pain: a review of recent clinical and experimental findings. J Pain. 2009;10(5):447–85.
8. Gerdle B, Bjork J, Coster L, Henriksson K, Henriksson C, Bengtsson A. Prevalnce of widespread pain and associations with work status: a population study. BMC Musculoskelet Disord. 2008;9:102.
9. Racine M, Tousignant-Laflamme Y, Kloda LA, Dion D, Dupuis G, Choiniere M. A systematic literature review of 10 years of research on sex/gender and pain perception – part 2: do biopsychosocial factors alter pain sensitivity differently in women and men? Pain. 2012;153:619–35.
10. Hollingshead NA, Ashburn-Nardo L, Stewart JC, Hirsh AT. The pain experience of Hispanic Americans: a critical literature review and conceptual model. J Pain. 2016;17(5):513–28.
11. Tait RC, Chibnall JT. Racial/ethnic disparities in the assessment and treatment of pain. Am Psychol. 2014;69(2):131–41.
12. Sullivan MJ, Rodgers WM, Kirsch I. Catastrophizing, depression and expectancies for pain and emotional distress. Pain. 2001;91(1–2):147–54.
13. Molton IR, Terrill AL. Overview of persistent pain in older adults. Am Psychol. 2014;69(2):197–207.
14. Sarkisian CA, Hays RD, Mangione CM. Do older adults expect to age successfully? The association between expectations regarding gaining and beliefs regarding healthcare seeking among older adults. J Am Geriatr Soc. 2002;50(11):1837–43.
15. Lachapelle DL, Hadjistavropoulos T. Age-related differences among adults coping with pain: evaluation of a developmental life-context model. Can J Behav Sci. 2005;37:123–37.
16. Molton IR, Jensen MP, Ehde DM, Carter GT, Kraft G, Cardenas DD. Coping with persistent pain among younger, middle-aged, and older adjults living with neurological injury and disease. J Aging Hum Dev. 2008;62:39–59.
17. Feinstein AB, Sturgeon JA, Barnall BD, Dunn AL, Rico T, Kao MC, Bhandari RP. The effect of catastrophizing on outcomes: a developmental perspective across children, adolescents, and young adults with chronic pain. J Pain. 2017;18(2):144–54.
18. Hirsh AT, George SZ, Robinson ME. Pain assessment and treatment disparities: a virtual human technology investigation. Pain. 2009;143:106–13.
19. Hirsh AT, Alquadah AF, Stutts L, Robinson ME. Virtual human technology: capturing sex, race, and age influences individual pain decision policies. Pain. 2009;140:231–8.
20. Stutts LA, Hirsh AT, George SZ, Robinson ME. Investigating patient characteristics on pain assessment using virtual human technology. Eur J Pain. 2010;14:1040–5.
21. Wandner LD, Stutts LA, Alquadah AF, Jason JG, Scipio CD, Hirsh AT, Robinson ME. Virtual human technology: patient demographics and healthcare training factors in pain observation and treatment recommendations. J Pain Res. 2010;3:241–7.
22. Campbell CM, Edwards RR, Fillingim RB. Ethnic differences in responses to multiple experimental pain stimuli. Pain. 2005;113:20–6.
23. Campbell CM, France CR, Robinson ME, Logan HL, Geffken GR, Fillingim RB. Ethnic differences in the nociceptive flexion reflex (NFR). Pain. 2008;134:91–6.
24. Wandner LD, Scipio CD, Hirsh AT, Torres CA, Robinson ME. The perception of pain in others: how gender, race, and age influence pain expectations. J Pain. 2012;13(3):220–7.
25. Robinson ME, Riley JL III, Myers CD, Papas RK, Wise EA, Waxenberg LB, Fillingim RB. Gender role expectations of pain: relationship to sex differences in pain. J Pain. 2001;2:251–7.
26. Robinson ME, Gagnon CM, Riley JL III, Price DD. Altering gender role expectations: effects on pain tolerance, pain threshold, and pain ratings. J Pain. 2003;4:284–8.
27. Dorflinger L, Kerns RD, Auerback SM. Providers' roles in enhancing patients' adherence to pain self management. Transl Behav Med. 2013;3:39–46.
28. Turk DC, Kerns RD, Rosenberg R. Effects of marital interaction on chronic pain and disability: examining the down side of social support. Rehabil Psychol. 1992;37:259–74.
29. Romano JM, Turner JA, Jensen MP, Friedman LS, Bulcroft RA, Hops H, Wright SF. Chronic pain patient-spouse behavioral interactions predict patient disability. Pain. 1995;63(3):353–60.
30. McCracken LM. Social context and acceptance of chronic pain: the role of solicitous and punishing responses. Pain. 2005;113(1–2):155–9.
31. Cunningham JL, Hayes SE, Townsend CO, Laures H, Hooten WM. Associations between spousal or significant other solicitous responses and opioid dose in patient with chronic pain. Pain Med. 2012;13(8):1034–9.
32. McGeary CA, Blount TH, Peterson AL, Gatchel RJ, Hale WJ, McGeary DD. Interpersonal responses and pain management within the US Military. J Occup Rehabil. 2016;26(2):216–28.
33. Alschuler KN, Otis JD. Significant others' responses to pain in veterans with chronic pain and clinical levels of post-traumatic stress disorder symptomatology. Eur J Pain. 2013;17(2):245–54.

34. Raichle KA, Romano JM, Jensen MP. Partner responses to patient pain and well behaviors and their relationship to patient pain behavior, functioning, and depression. Pain. 2011;152(1):82–8.

35. Molloy GJ, Johnston M, Johnston DW, Pollard B, Morrison V, Bonetti D, Joice S, MacWalter R. Spousal caregiver confidence and recovery from ambulatory activity limitations in stroke survivors. Health Psychol. 2008;27:286–90.

36. Johnson MD, Anderson JR, Walker A, Wilcox A, Lewis VL, Robbins DC. Common dyadic coping is indirectly related to dietary and exercise adherence via patient and partner diabetes efficacy. J Fam Psychol. 2013;27:722–30.

37. Gere J, Martire LM, Keefe FJ, Stephens MAP, Schulz R. Spouse confidence in self-efficacy for arthritis management predicts improved patient health. Ann Behav Med. 2014;48:337–46.

38. Gatchel RJ, Nesblett R, Kishino N, Ray CT. Fear-avoidance beliefs and chronic pain. J Orthop Sports Phys Ther. 2016;46(2):38–43.

39. Crombez G, Vlaeyen JWS, Heuts PHTG, Lysens R. Pain-related fear is more disabling than pain itself: evidence on the role of pain-related fear in chronic back pain disability. Pain. 1999;80:329–39.

40. Hirsh AT, Bockow TB, Jensen MP. Catastrophizing, pain, and pain interference in individuals with disabilities. Am J Phys Med Rehabil. 2011;90:713–22.

41. Sullivan MJL, Adams H, Martel MO, Scott W, Wideman T. Catastrophizing and perceived injustice. Spine. 2011;36(25S):S244–9.

42. Scott W, Trost Z, Milioto M, Sullivan MJL. Barriers to change in depressive symptoms following multidisciplinary rehabilitation for whiplash: the role of perceived injustice. Clin J Pain. 2015;31(2):145–51.

43. Greist JH, Greden JF, Jefferson JW, Trivedi MH. Depression and pain. J Clin Psychiatry. 2008;69(12):1970–8.

44. Currie S, Wang J. More data on major depression as an antecedent risk factor for first onset of chronic back pain. Psychol Med. 2005;35(9):1275–82.

45. Larson S, Clark M, Eaton W. Depressive disorder as a long-term antecedent risk factor for incident back pain: a 13-year follow-up study from the Baltimore Epidemiological Catchment Area sample. Psychol Med. 2004;34(2):211–9.

Sex and Gender Issues in Pain

Priya Pinto

Definition of Sex and Gender

Distinguishing between sex and gender involves a complex understanding of the terms, and acceptance that there is fluidity to these definitions. This distinction is not universal, and often, these terms are used interchangeably. "Sex" is defined as a sum of the structural and functional differences, by which male and female are distinguished, or the phenomena or behavior dependent on these differences. In brief, it is the anatomy of an individual's reproductive system and secondary sexual characteristics. "Gender," in contrast, is an individual's identity of themselves, as differentiated by social and cultural roles and behavior. It may be masculine, feminine, or a category outside this binary classification and is based on personal awareness or identity. In some circumstances, an individual's assigned sex and gender may not align. They might identify as transgender, non-binary, or gender-nonconforming [1]. There remains major gaps in the literature looking at pain in these populations.

Epidemiology of Pain in Relation to Age and Reproductive History

Chronic Nonmalignant Pain

Females exhibit a higher prevalence of pain among all body sites [2–5] as well as for all individual musculoskeletal sites [2]. The sex difference is consistent across all age categories with the biggest difference between 45 and 54 years and the 55–64 age ranges [6]. Other epidemiological studies support the fact that close to 50% of chronic pain issues are more prevalent in women than men [7, 8]. In addition to a higher prevalence, women also seem to experience stronger and longer lasting pain than men [4, 9]. In terms of musculoskel-

etal pain, women tend to have more widespread pain [10]. Among patients with fibromyalgia, women have significantly more "tender points" and more symptoms of fatigue [11]. A recent study suggests that in women, reproductive changes over time can affect pain sensitivity. Decreased estrogen has been known to lead to decreased headaches but has also been found to increase the intensity of other painful conditions such as osteoporosis and osteoarthritis [12]. On the other side, increased estrogen levels, including in postmenopausal females on estrogen, has been shown to increase both the incidence, as well as the severity of pain related to fibromyalgia and temporomandibular joint disease [13, 14]. Pain prevalence in females appears to increase with age. A handful of studies show either increased or no difference in pain prevalence with increasing age in men [15].

In pediatrics, chronic pain seems to be experienced more often by girls than boys and with greater intensity [16]. Studies also suggest that some syndromes such as migraines with or without aura develop at a younger age in boys, but girls are more likely to report the symptoms [17]. In many studies, girls are more likely to report symptoms of pain such as headaches [18], upper limb pain [19] and abdominal pain [18].

Cancer Pain

In cancer, studies have not shown any differences between the sexes in terms of intensity or prevalence [20, 21]. However, females were more likely to have additional symptoms of depression and fatigue along with pain. Female patients admitted to a cancer hospital are also more likely to have cancer-related than non-cancer-related pain and the pain is more likely to be severe [20].

Post-procedural Pain

Women appear to experience more severe post-procedural pain [22, 23]. Women report more pain than men in the

P. Pinto (✉)
Division of Palliative Medicine and Bioethics, NYU Winthrop Hospital, Mineola, NY, USA

© Springer Nature Switzerland AG 2019
Y. Khelemsky et al. (eds.), *Academic Pain Medicine*, https://doi.org/10.1007/978-3-030-18005-8_11

postoperative period following oral surgery [24, 25] and orthopedic surgery [26, 27]. Women also display greater post-colonoscopy discomfort than men [28].

Nociceptive Responses and Pain Perception

Pain perception and responses to pain have been measured in animal and human models using a variety of stimuli (e.g., chemical, mechanical, thermal). These studies have looked at the time and intensity of pain sensation, tolerance, and other measures. Females and males have comparable thresholds for cold and ischemic pain, while pressure pain thresholds are lower in females than in males. In animal and human models alike, females have been noted to experience pain with a greater intensity and response [8, 29] and have a lower threshold for pain as compared to males [30]. Many studies have looked at the issues of anatomical as well as hormonal differences as a reason of these findings [31]. Interestingly, pain responses may vary based on type of pain stimulus [32, 33].

Pressure Pain

When stimulated with pressure (e.g., algometers or von Frey filaments), females exhibit a lower threshold, as well as lower tolerance for pain [33]. Similarly, when exposed to suprathreshold mechanical stimulation, females report greater pain sensitivity compared to men (e.g., hyperalgesia) and an associated greater autonomic response [34]. There appear to be differences in the pertinent neuroanatomic pathways. For example, during a painful rectal stimulus with pressure, males displayed activation of the left thalamus/ventral striatum, while women females were observed to experience deactivation of the midcingulate cortex [35].

Electrical Pain

Some studies employing fMRI have demonstrated a greater activation of the primary sensory and prefrontal cortices in females than in males with electrical stimulation [36, 37], while others failed to show any differences in pain response [38].

Ischemic Pain

While there are differences in areas of the brain stimulated by ischemic pain, there are no noted differences in pain thresholds or pain tolerance between sexes in response to ischemic pain [33, 39, 40]. Several studies do support the differences in patterns of response. Where men show activation of the parietal cortices, the contralateral secondary somatosensory cortex, the prefrontal cortex and the insula, women show activation in the ipsilateral perigenual and ventral cingulate cortex [39].

Heat/Cold Pain

Females appear to have lower thresholds than males, as well as lower pain tolerance when exposed to cold or hot stimuli [31, 33].

Analgesic Response

The analgesic response (response to pain therapy) appears to be different between the sexes. Females are prescribed more opioids and adjuvants than males. However, it is unclear if this is related to prescribing behaviors, noted differences in pain tolerance or differences in how females respond to treatment [41, 42]. There is some evidence that females utilize less opioids in the postoperative period despite having similar pain scores [43]. This may be partially explained by the fact that females exhibit a greater analgesic response to administration of morphine [44]. Multiple mechanisms may explain sex differences in opioid analgesia, including hormonal effects, pharmacokinetics and pharmacodynamics, genetic influences, balance of analgesic/antianalgesic processes, and psychological factors.

Multi-modal and interdisciplinary pain programs have been found to be successful in reducing pain in both males and females. However, while females tend to report significantly more pain and intensity after 3 months of the treatment program [45], they also have more pronounced improvements in pain-related disability as compared with males [46].

Biologic Contributions to Pain Response

Females have a higher average nerve fiber density in their skin as compared to males [47]. Increased innervation could result in nociceptive hypersensitivity as seen in some animal models [48].

The influence of sex hormones represents a significant source of pain-related variability that likely impacts men and women differently. This is not surprising given the distribution of sex hormones and their receptors in areas of the peripheral and central nervous systems associated with pain. As noted earlier, estrogen plasma levels can impact the incidence of recurrent pain in women. In addition, pain levels can vary significantly during different phases of the menstrual cycle, indicating that rapid estrogen changes, as well as high estrogen and progesterone levels, can worsen the experience of pain [49, 50]. Clinically, this is evident because intensity of pain varies with each stage of the menstrual cycle especially in conditions such as irritable bowel syndrome, temporomandibular joint (TMJ) pain, primary headache, and fibromyalgia [29]. In addition, during pregnancy, migraine frequency declines and TMJ pain is reduced [50].

Psychosocial Contribution to Pain

Pain is a multidimensional sensation, with cognitive, emotional and psychosocial components. Studies support that men and women use different strategies to cope with pain [29]. Women seek out social support and use more emotion focused techniques to assist in self managing their pain, while men tend to use behavioral modification and distraction [51, 52]. Women also tend to have more anxiety in association with pain [53]. Catastrophizing is the tendency to exaggerate the magnitude of pain, and alters the feeling of a painful stimulus, possibly increasing its reported intensity. Women seem more likely to engage in this behavior when in pain [54–56]. Empathy is also an important phenomenon in pain perception and women are known to be more empathetic than men [57]. Society and its expected gender roles also seem to impact the experience of pain. Society expects that men and boys should minimize their response to pain [58]. Family relations will also play a role, as it appears that girls are more likely to respond to maternal influences [59].

Role in Treatment Seeking, Delivery, and Effectiveness of Treatment

Women are more likely than men to seek medical care and report pain [31]. Because of these differences, there have been many studies assessing factors that might affect this gender-specific characteristic. While there are clearly differences in the way pain is treated in men vs women, it is unclear which gender derives an advantage from this disparity [60]. Providers are more likely to provide pain management to a patient of the same gender, and females are more likely to be recommended opioids [61–63].

References

1. American Psychological Association. APA dictionary of psychology. 2nd ed. Washington, DC: Author; 2015.
2. Picavet HS, Schouten JS. Musculoskeletal pain in the Netherlands: prevalences, consequences and risk groups, the DMC3-study. Pain. 2003;102(1–2):167–78.
3. Wijnhoven HA, De Vet HC, Picavet HS. Prevalence of musculoskeletal disorders is systematically higher in women than in men. Clin J Pain. 2006;22(8):717–24.
4. Wijnhoven HA, de Vet HC, Picavet HS. Sex differences in consequences of musculoskeletal pain. Spine. 2007;32(12):1360–7.
5. Chopra A, Saluja M, Patil J, Tandale HS. Pain and disability, perceptions and beliefs of a rural Indian population: a WHO-ILAR COPCORD study. WHO-International League of Associations for Rheumatology. Community Oriented Program for Control of Rheumatic Diseases. J Rheumatol. 2002;29(3):614–21.
6. Guo HR, Chang YC, Yeh WY, Chen CW, Guo YL. Prevalence of musculoskeletal disorder among workers in Taiwan: a nationwide study. J Occup Health. 2004;46(1):26–36.
7. Berkley KJ. Sex differences in pain. Behav Brain Sci. 1997;20(3):371–80.
8. Mogil JS. Sex differences in pain and pain inhibition: multiple explanations of a controversial phenomenon. Nat Rev Neurosci. 2012;13(12):859.
9. Heitkemper MM, Cain KC, Jarrett ME, Burr RL, Hertig V, Bond EF. Symptoms across the menstrual cycle in women with irritable bowel syndrome. Am J Gastroenterol. 2003;98(2):420–30.
10. Leveille SG, Zhang Y, McMullen W, Kelly-Hayes M, Felson DT. Sex differences in musculoskeletal pain in older adults. Pain. 2005;116(3):332–8.
11. Wolfe F, Ross K, Anderson J, Russell IJ, Hebert L. The prevalence and characteristics of fibromyalgia in the general population. Arthritis Rheum. 1995;38(1):19–28.
12. Meriggiola MC, Nanni M, Bachiocco V, Vodo S, Aloisi AM. Menopause affects pain depending on pain type and characteristics. Menopause. 2012;19(5):517–23.
13. Marcus DA. Interrelationships of neurochemicals, estrogen, and recurring headache. Pain. 1995;62(2):129–39.
14. Dao TT, LeResche L. Gender differences in pain. J Orofac Pain. 2000;14(3):169.
15. Abdulla A, Adams N, Bone M, Elliott AM, Gaffin J, Jones D, Knaggs R, Martin D, Sampson L, Schofield P. Guidance on the management of pain in older people. Age Ageing. 2013;42:i1–57.
16. Perquin CW, Hazebroek-Kampschreur AA, Hunfeld JA, Bohnen AM, van Suijlekom-Smit LW, Passchier J, van der Wouden JC. Pain in children and adolescents: a common experience. Pain. 2000;87(1):51–8.
17. Stewart WF, Linet MS, Celentano DD, Natta MV, Ziegler D. Age- and sex-specific incidence rates of migraine with and without visual aura. Am J Epidemiol. 1991;134(10):1111–20.
18. Sundblad GM, Saartok T, Engström LM. Prevalence and co-occurrence of self-rated pain and perceived health in school-children: age and gender differences. Eur J Pain. 2007;11(2):171–80.
19. Zapata AL, Moraes AJ, Leone C, Doria-Filho U, Silva CA. Pain and musculoskeletal pain syndromes in adolescents. J Adolesc Health. 2006;38(6):769–71.
20. Reyes-Gibby CC, Aday LA, Anderson KO, Mendoza TR, Cleeland CS. Pain, depression, and fatigue in community-dwelling adults with and without a history of cancer. J Pain Symptom Manag. 2006;32(2):118–28.
21. Bartley EJ, Fillingim RB. Sex differences in pain: a brief review of clinical and experimental findings. Br J Anaesth. 2013;111(1):52–8.
22. Fillingim RB, Maixner W. Gender differences in the responses to noxious stimuli. Pain Forum. 1995;4(4):209–21. Elsevier.
23. Robinson ME, Wise EA, Riley JL III, Atchison JW. Sex differences in clinical pain: a multisample study. J Clin Psychol Med Settings. 1998;5(4):413–24.
24. Averbuch M, Katzper M. Baseline pain and response to analgesic medications in the postsurgery dental pain model. J Clin Pharmacol. 2000;40(2):133–7.

25. Coulthard P, Haywood D, Tai MA, Jackson-Leech D, Pleuvry BJ, Macfarlane TV. Treatment of postoperative pain in oral and maxillofacial surgery. Br J Oral Maxillofac Surg. 2000;38(6):588–92.

26. Taenzer AH, Clark C, Curry CS. Gender affects report of pain and function after arthroscopic anterior cruciate ligament reconstruction. Anesthesiology. 2000;93(3):670–5.

27. Thomas T, Robinson C, Champion D, McKell M, Pell M. Prediction and assessment of the severity of post-operative pain and of satisfaction with management. Pain. 1998;75(2–3):177–85.

28. Froehlich F, Thorens J, Schwizer W, Preisig M, Köhler M, Hays RD, Fried M, Gonvers JJ. Sedation and analgesia for colonoscopy: patient tolerance, pain, and cardiorespiratory parameters. Gastrointest Endosc. 1997;45(1):1–9.

29. Fillingim RB, King CD, Ribeiro-Dasilva MC, Rahim-Williams B, Riley JL. Sex, gender, and pain: a review of recent clinical and experimental findings. J Pain. 2009;10(5):447–85.

30. Craft RM, Mogil JS, Aloisi AM. Sex differences in pain and analgesia: the role of gonadal hormones. Eur J Pain. 2004;8(5):397–411.

31. Melchior M, Poisbeau P, Gaumond I, Marchand S. Insights into the mechanisms and the emergence of sex-differences in pain. Neuroscience. 2016;338:63–80.

32. Riley JL III, Robinson ME, Wise EA, Myers CD, Fillingim RB. Sex differences in the perception of noxious experimental stimuli: a meta-analysis. Pain. 1998;74(2–3):181–7.

33. Racine M, Tousignant-Laflamme Y, Kloda LA, Dion D, Dupuis G, Choinière M. A systematic literature review of 10 years of research on sex/gender and experimental pain perception–part 1: are there really differences between women and men? Pain. 2012;153(3):602–18.

34. Ellermeier W, Westphal W. Gender differences in pain ratings and pupil reactions to painful pressure stimuli. Pain. 1995;61(3):435–9.

35. Berman SM, Naliboff BD, Suyenobu B, Labus JS, Stains J, Bueller JA, Ruby K, Mayer EA. Sex differences in regional brain response to aversive pelvic visceral stimuli. Am J Phys Regul Integr Comp Phys. 2006;291(2):R268–76.

36. Moulton EA, Keaser ML, Gullapalli RP, Maitra R, Greenspan JD. Sex differences in the cerebral BOLD signal response to painful heat stimuli. Am J Phys Regul Integr Comp Phys. 2006;291(2):R257–67.

37. Straube T, Schmidt S, Weiss T, Mentzel HJ, Miltner WH. Sex differences in brain activation to anticipated and experienced pain in the medial prefrontal cortex. Hum Brain Mapp. 2009;30(2):689–98.

38. Hobson AR, Furlong PL, Sarkar S, Matthews PJ, Willert RP, Worthen SF, Unsworth BJ, Aziz Q. Neurophysiologic assessment of esophageal sensory processing in noncardiac chest pain. Gastroenterology. 2006;130(1):80–8.

39. Derbyshire SW, Jones AK, Creed F, Starz T, Meltzer CC, Townsend DW, Peterson AM, Firestone L. Cerebral responses to noxious thermal stimulation in chronic low back pain patients and normal controls. NeuroImage. 2002;16(1):158–68.

40. Bragdon EE, Light KC, Costello NL, Sigurdsson A, Bunting S, Bhalang K, Maixner W. Group differences in pain modulation: pain-free women compared to pain-free men and to women with TMD. Pain. 2002;96(3):227–37.

41. Holdcroft A, Berkley KJ. Sex and gender differences in pain and its relief. In: McMahon SB, Wall KM, editors. Melzack's textbook of pain. 2006;1181–97.

42. Miaskowski C, Gear RW, Levine JD. Sex-related differences in analgesic responses. In: Fillingim RB, editor. Sex, gender, and pain. Seattle: IASP Press; 2000;209–30.

43. Miaskowski C, Levine JD. Does opioid analgesia show a gender preference for females? Pain Forum. 1999;8(1):34–44. Churchill Livingstone.

44. Niesters M, Dahan A, Kest B, Zacny J, Stijnen T, Aarts L, Sarton E. Do sex differences exist in opioid analgesia? A systematic review and meta-analysis of human experimental and clinical studies. Pain. 2010;151(1):61–8.

45. Keogh E, McCracken LM, Eccleston C. Do men and women differ in their response to interdisciplinary chronic pain management? Pain. 2005;114(1–2):37–46.

46. Pieh C, Altmeppen J, Neumeier S, Loew T, Angerer M, Lahmann C. Gender differences in outcomes of a multimodal pain management program. Pain. 2012;153(1):197–202.

47. Mowlavi A, Cooney D, Febus L, Khosraviani A, Wilhelmi BJ, Akers G. Increased cutaneous nerve fibers in female specimens. Plast Reconstr Surg. 2005;116(5):1407–10.

48. Chakrabarty A, McCarson KE, Smith PG. Hypersensitivity and hyperinnervation of the rat hind paw following carrageenan-induced inflammation. Neurosci Lett. 2011;495(1):67–71.

49. Korszun AN, Young EA, Engleberg NC, Masterson LO, Dawson EC, Spindler KA, McCLURE LA, Brown MB, Crofford LJ. Follicular phase hypothalamic-pituitary-gonadal axis function in women with fibromyalgia and chronic fatigue syndrome. J Rheumatol. 2000;27(6):1526–30.

50. Hellström B, Anderberg UM. Pain perception across the menstrual cycle phases in women with chronic pain. Percept Mot Skills. 2003;96(1):201–11.

51. Unruh AM, Ritchie J, Merskey H. Does gender affect appraisal of pain and pain coping strategies? Clin J Pain. 1999;15(1):31–40.

52. Thompson T, Keogh E, French CC, Davis R. Anxiety sensitivity and pain: generalisability across noxious stimuli. Pain. 2008;134(1–2):187–96.

53. Ramírez-Maestre C, Esteve R. The role of sex/gender in the experience of pain: resilience, fear, and acceptance as central variables in the adjustment of men and women with chronic pain. J Pain. 2014;15(6):608–18.

54. Jensen MP, Turner JA, Romano JM, Lawler BK. Relationship of pain-specific beliefs to chronic pain adjustment. Pain. 1994;57(3):301–9.

55. Keefe FJ, Lefebvre JC, Egert JR, Affleck G, Sullivan MJ, Caldwell DS. The relationship of gender to pain, pain behavior, and disability in osteoarthritis patients: the role of catastrophizing. Pain. 2000;87(3):325–34.

56. Edwards RR, Haythornthwaite JA, Sullivan MJ, Fillingim RB. Catastrophizing as a mediator of sex differences in pain: differential effects for daily pain versus laboratory-induced pain. Pain. 2004;111(3):335–41.

57. Eisenberg N, Shea CL, Carlo G, Knight GP. Empathy-related responding and cognition: a "chicken and the egg" dilemma. In: Handbook of moral behavior and development, vol. 2; 2014. p. 63–88.

58. Robinson ME, Riley JL, Myers CD, Papas RK, Wise EA, Waxenberg LB, Fillingim RB. Gender role expectations of pain: relationship to sex differences in pain. J Pain. 2001;2(5):251–7.

59. Chambers CT, Craig KD, Bennett SM. The impact of maternal behavior on children's pain experiences: an experimental analysis. J Pediatr Psychol. 2002;27(3):293–301.

60. LeResche L. Defining gender disparities in pain management. Clin Orthop Relat Res. 2011;469(7):1871–7.

61. Alqudah AF, Hirsh AT, Stutts LA, Scipio CD, Robinson ME. Sex and race differences in rating others' pain, pain-related negative mood, pain coping, and recommending medical help. J Cyber Ther Rehabil. 2010;3(1):63.

62. Wandner LD, Stutts LA, Alqudah AF, Craggs JG, Scipio CD, Hirsh AT, Robinson ME. Virtual human technology: patient demographics and healthcare training factors in pain observation and treatment recommendations. J Pain Res. 2010;3:241.

63. Hirsh AT, George SZ, Robinson ME. Pain assessment and treatment disparities: a virtual human technology investigation. Pain. 2009;143(1–2):106–13.

Opioids

Kristoffer Padjen, Scott Maddalo, Patrick Milord,
Chaim Goldfeiz, Robert Otterbeck,
and Christopher Gharibo

Introduction

Opioids have long been a mainstay of therapy for pain. This is particularly true for acute, often postsurgical pain, as well as cancer pain and other palliative indications. In recent years, the use of opioids has increased dramatically with prescription rates approaching one opioid prescription per US resident [1]. Despite being one of the oldest and most frequently utilized pharmaceutical classes, opioid use continues to be wrought with controversy. From 1999 to 2014, drug overdose deaths in the United States have increased dramatically. In 2014 alone, approximately 61% of the 47,055 drug overdose deaths involved an opioid [1, 2]. This has brought into question the role of opioid medications in pain management, particularly in the context of chronic nonmalignant pain states. In 2016, the Centers for Disease Control published a set of guidelines to assist physicians in prescribing opioids for patients with chronic pain (Table 12.1).

Nociceptive Signaling

Molecular characterization has revealed that opioid receptors are functionally G-protein-coupled receptors. These receptors, which are located both pre- and postsynaptically, may be activated by either endogenous ligands (e.g., endorphins, enkephalins, and dynorphins) or opioids [4–9]. Activation of presynaptic receptors leads to inhibition of voltage-gated *calcium* channels, resulting in a decrease in neurotransmitter release [10, 11]. Postsynaptic activation increases *potassium* conductance and leads to hyperpolarization of the membrane [12, 13]. The major subtypes of opioid receptors (e.g., mu (μ), kappa (κ), and delta (δ)) are found in the brain (i.e., rostral

ventromedial medulla, periaqueductal gray, mesencephalic reticular formation, amygdala, etc.) spinal cord (dorsal horn (substantia gelatinosa/Rexed lamina II), dorsal root ganglia (DRG), as well as peripheral tissues [14–16]. Listed in Table 12.2 are the major subtypes of opioid receptors.

Adverse Effects

Multiple adverse effects are associated with opioid use. These include but are not limited to constipation, respiratory depression, nausea, vomiting, pruritus, and urinary retention. Constipation and respiratory depression are both common and of significant concern and are expanded upon below. It should be noted that tolerance, as manifested by physical dependence and withdrawal, may develop quickly. Rather than being seen as a side effect, tolerance occurs with such frequency that it should be regarded as an expected result of any extended opioid therapy. Tolerance is defined as an increasing dose of a medication or substance that is required to achieve an effect (whether desired or not). Physical dependence is a state in which an individual requires continued use of a medication/substance in order to avoid withdrawal. Withdrawal is a syndrome of unpleasant signs and symptoms precipitated by the acute discontinuation of a substance. Opioid withdrawal tends to be associated with dysphoria, diarrhea, nausea, and diaphoresis. Physical dependence should be differentiated from addiction which is both a physical and psychological pathology. Addiction is characterized by the continued and compulsive use of a substance *despite harm*.

Patients receiving opioids very frequently complain of constipation. Opioid-induced constipation varies from patient to patient but is dose-dependent and significant problems with this side effect may limit opioid use, even in the acute setting. Unlike other opioid adverse effects where tolerance will develop with prolonged exposure, opioid-induced constipation frequently does not improve with time [17]. Constipation results from the binding of

K. Padjen (✉) · S. Maddalo · P. Milord · C. Goldfeiz
R. Otterbeck · C. Gharibo
Department of Anesthesiology, NYU Langone Medical Center,
New York, NY, USA
e-mail: Kristoffer.Padjen@nyumc.org

© Springer Nature Switzerland AG 2019
Y. Khelemsky et al. (eds.), *Academic Pain Medicine*, https://doi.org/10.1007/978-3-030-18005-8_12

Table 12.1 Centers for Disease Control Guideline for Prescribing Opioids for Chronic Pain [3]

Nonpharmacologic therapy and nonopioid pharmacologic therapy are preferred for chronic pain. Clinicians should consider opioid therapy only if expected benefits for both pain and function are expected to outweigh risks to the patient. If opioids are used, they should be combined with nonpharmacologic therapy and nonopioid pharmacologic therapy, as appropriate.

Before starting opioid therapy for chronic pain, clinicians should establish treatment goals with all patients, including realistic goals for pain and function and should consider how opioid therapy will be discontinued if benefits do not outweigh risks. Clinicians should continue opioid therapy only if there is clinically meaningful improvement in pain and function that outweighs risks to patient safety

Before starting and periodically during opioid therapy, clinicians should discuss with patients known risks and realistic benefits of opioid therapy and patient and clinician responsibility for managing therapy

When starting opioid therapy for chronic pain, clinicians should prescribe immediate-release opioids instead of extended-release/long-acting opioids

When opioids are started, clinicians should prescribe the lowest effective dosage. Clinicians should use caution when prescribing opioids at any dosage, should carefully reassess evidence of individual benefits and risks when considering increasing dosage to ≥50 morphine milligram equivalents (MME) per day, and should avoid increasing dosage to ≥90 MME/day or carefully justify a decision to titrate dosage to ≥90 MME/day

Long-term opioid use often begins with the treatment of acute pain. When opioids are used for acute pain, clinicians should prescribe the lowest effective dose of immediate-release opioids and should prescribe no greater quantity than needed for the expected duration of pain severe enough to require opioids. Three days or less often will be sufficient; more than 7 days will rarely be needed

Clinicians should evaluate benefits and harms with patients within 1–4 weeks of starting opioid therapy for chronic pain or of dose escalation. Clinicians should evaluate benefits and harms of continued therapy with patients every 3 months or more frequently. If benefits do not outweigh harms of continued opioid therapy, clinicians should optimize other therapies and work with patients to taper opioids to lower dosages or to taper and discontinue opioids

Before starting and periodically during continuation of opioid therapy, clinicians should evaluate risk factors for opioid-related harms. Clinicians should incorporate into the management plan strategies to mitigate risk, including considering offering naloxone when factors that increase risk for opioid overdose, such as history of overdose, history of substance use disorder, higher opioid dosages (≥50 MME/day), or concurrent benzodiazepine use, are present

Clinicians should review the patient's history of controlled substance prescriptions using state prescription drug monitoring program (PDMP) data to determine whether the patient is receiving opioid dosages or dangerous combinations that put him or her at high risk for overdose. Clinicians should review PDMP data when starting opioid therapy for chronic pain and periodically during opioid therapy for chronic pain, ranging from every prescription to every 3 months

When prescribing opioids for chronic pain, clinicians should use urine drug testing before starting opioid therapy and consider urine drug testing at least annually to assess for prescribed medications as well as other controlled prescription drugs and illicit drugs

Clinicians should avoid prescribing opioids pain medication and benzodiazepines concurrently whenever possible

Clinicians should offer or arrange evidence-based treatment for patients with opioid use disorder

Table 12.2 Major opioid receptor subtypes

Receptor subtype	Location	Action
μ₁	Brain, spinal cord	Analgesia
μ₂	Brain, spinal cord	Analgesia, GI transit, respiratory depression, itching
Δ	Brain	Analgesia, cardioprotection, thermoregulation
K	Brain, spinal cord	Analgesia, feeding, diuresis, neuroendocrine
NOP	Brain, spinal cord	Anxiety, depression, appetite, development of tolerance

the opioid molecule to gastrointestinal mu opioid receptors [18]. Opioids induce or exacerbate delayed gastric emptying and decrease gastrointestinal motility regardless of the route of administration [19, 20]. Prophylactic treatment and management of opioid-induced constipation routinely include laxatives, gastrointestinal motility stimulants, and stool bulking agents. Methylnaltrexone, a naloxone derivative, has been shown to effectively reverse opioid-induced constipation without compromising the analgesic effect of opioid pain medications [21].

Perhaps, the most important and most feared adverse effect of opioids is fatal respiratory depression. Opioids decrease the drive to breath partially by decreasing the brain's responsiveness to carbon dioxide. This can be particularly dangerous in patients in which respiration may already be compromised such as those with sleep apnea or those with severe asthma [22]. Additional caution is required when treating patients at the extremes of age and patients with pre-existing dementia or delirium. Combination of opioids and other sedating drugs, such as benzodiazepines or alcohol has the potential to cause severe respiratory depression [23].

Table 12.3 Common opioids

Name	Brand name(s)	Route(s)	Onset	Peak	Metabolism	Metabolites
Morphine	MSIR, Roxanol, MS-Contin, Oramorph-SR, Kadian, Embeda, Duramorph	IV, IM, PO, epidural, intrathecal, Per Rectum	PO 15–30 min; IV < 5 min	PO < 60 min, IV 20 min	2D6,3A4	Morphine-3-glucuronide, Morphine-6-glucuronide (active metabolite: caution accumulation in renal failure)
Codeine	Tylenol #3 Tylenol #4	PO	30–60 min	1 hr	2D6	Morphine
Oxycodone	Percocet, Roxicodone, OxyIR, Endocet, Roxicet, Percodan, Endodan	PO	10–15 min (IR)	1.5–2 hr (IR), 4–5 hr (CR)	2D6,3A4	Oxymorphone, noroxycodone
Meperidine	Demerol	IV, IM, PO	Rapid	30–60 min	2B6, 3A4, 2C19	Normeperidine (caution with MAOI inhibitors and accumulation)
Oxymorphone	Nurmorphan, Opana IR and ER	IV, PO	5–10 min	30 min	3A4	Oxymorphone-3-glucorinide, 6-OH-oxymorphone
Hydromorphone	Dilaudid Exalgo (ER)	IV, PO, epidural, intrathecal	15–30 min PO, 5 min IV	30–60 min PO, 15–30 min IV	2D6	Hydromorphone-3-glucoronide
Methadone	Dolophine	IV, PO	30–60 min PO, 10–20 min IV	1–7.5 hr	2D6, 3A4, 2B6	Methadol, EDDP, EMDP
Fentanyl	Sublimaze, Duragesic	IV, IM, PO, Transdermal, Transmucosal, Intranasal	Rapid	30–60 min IV	3A4	Norfentanyl
Hydrocodone	Norco, Hycet, Vicoprofen	PO	10–20 min	1 hr	2D6,3A4	Hydromorphone, norhydrocodone
Tramadol	Ultram	IV, IM, PO, rectal	1 hr	1.5 hr	2D6,3A4	O-desmethyltramadol
Tapentadol	Nucynta	PO	30 min	4–6 hr	2D6, 2C9, 2C19	N-desmethyltapentadol and hydroxyl-tapentadol
Buprenorphine	Suboxone (combined with naloxone)	IV, sublingual, buccal, transdermal	40 min	4–6 hr	3A4	Norbuprenorphine

Metabolism

The analgesic properties and many of the side effects from opioids are the result of their metabolites. Most opioids are metabolized by glucuronidation or by the P450 (CYP) system. Urine drug testing allows monitoring of patients about to begin or continuing on opioid therapy. Table 12.3 lists common metabolites of major opioids which may be used in the analysis of urine drug screening. CDC guidelines advise physicians to perform urine drug screening at the initiation of opioid therapy and at least annually while taking opioids (see Table 12.1).

Specific Opioids

Opioids are classified as either naturally occurring, semi-synthetic, or fully synthetic. Morphine and codeine are naturally occurring opioids (previously known as opiates), with all other opioids routinely utilized being either semi-synthetic or fully synthetic (see Table 12.4). Morphine is considered the prototypical μ-opioid receptor agonist against which all other opioids are compared. To allow easier comparison of opioids, the term morphine equivalent dosing (MED) was created. Table 12.5 displays equianalgesic doses of opioids commonly used in medical practice. Safely converting dosages between opioids is important since patients can develop tolerance or suffer intolerable side effects. When transitioning between opioids, the initial equianalgesic dose of the new opioid should be 25–50% less than of the original opioid due to *incomplete cross-tolerance* to the respiratory depressive effects of these medications. Table 12.3 lists the properties of commonly prescribed opioids [24–37].

Table 12.4 Common naturally occurring, semisynthetic, and synthetic opioids

Naturally occurring	Semisynthetic	Synthetic
Morphine	Diamorphine (Heroin)	Meperidine
Codeine	Hydromorphone	Fentanyl
Thebaine	Hydrocodone	Methadone
	Oxycodone	Tramadol
	Oxymorphone	Tapentadol
	Buprenorphine	Levorphanol
		Butorphanol
		Pentazocine

Table 12.5 Opioid conversions

Drug	Parenteral (mg)	Oral (mg)
Morphine	10	30
Hydromorphone	1.5	7.5
Oxycodone	10	20
Hydrocodone	–	30–45
Oxymorphone	1	10
Meperidine	75	300
Codeine	100	200
Tramadol	100	120
Fentanyl	0.1	–
Methadone	10	20
Buprenorphine	0.3	0.4 (sublingual)

References

1. Rudd RA, Aleshire N, Zibbell JE, Gladden RM. Increases in drug and opioid overdose deaths—United States, 2000–2014. MMWR Morb Mortal Wkly Rep. 2016;64:1378–82.
2. Rudd RA, Seth P, David F, Scholl L. Increases in drug and opioid-involved overdose deaths — United States, 2010–2015. MMWR Morb Mortal Wkly Rep. ePub: 16 December 2016. https://doi.org/10.15585/mmwr.mm655051e1.
3. Dowell D, Haegerich TM, Chou R. CDC guideline for prescribing opioids for chronic pain – United States, 2016. JAMA. 2016;315(15):1624–45.
4. Messlinger K. Functional morphology of nociceptive and other fine sensory endings (free nerve endings) in different tissues. In: Kumazawa T, Kruger L, Mizumura K, editors. The polymodal receptor—a gateway to pathological pain. Progress in brain research, vol. 113. Amsterdam: Elsevier; 1996. p. 273–98.
5. Cervero F. Sensory innervation of the viscera: peripheral basis of visceral pain. Physiol Rev. 1994;74:95–138.
6. Ness TJ, Gebhart GF. Visceral pain: a review of experimental studies. Pain. 1990;41:167–234.
7. Mense S. Nociception from skeletal muscle in relation to clinical muscle pain. Pain. 1993;54:241–89.
8. Schaible HG, Grubb BD. Afferent and spinal mechanisms of joint pain. Pain. 1993;55:5–54.
9. Heppelmann B, Messlinger K, Neiss WF, et al. Ultrastructural three-dimensional reconstruction of group III and group IV sensory nerve endings ("free nerve endings") in the knee joint capsule of the cat: evidence for multiple receptive sites. J Comp Neurol. 1990;292:103–16.
10. Carlton SM, Zhou S, Coggeshall RE. Localization and activation of substance P receptors in unmyelinated axons of rat glabrous skin. Brain Res. 1996;734:103–8.
11. Coggeshall RE, Zhou S, Carlton SM. Opioid receptors on peripheral sensory axons. Brain Res. 1997;764:126–32.
12. Barash PG, Cullen BF, Stoelting RK. Handbook of clinical anesthesia. 6th ed. Philadelphia: Lippincott Williams & Wilkins; 2009. Chapter 19
13. Keiffer BL. Opioids: first lessons from knockout mice. Trends Pharmacol Sci. 1999;20:19–26.
14. Hassan AHS, Ableitner A, Stein C, et al. Inflammation of the rat paw enhances axonal transport of opioid receptors in the sciatic nerve and increases their density in the inflamed tissue. Neuroscience. 1993;55:185–95.
15. Stein C, Pfluger M, Yassouridis A, et al. No tolerance to peripheral morphine analgesia in presence of opioid expression in inflamed synovia. J Clin Invest. 1996;98:793–9.
16. Besse D, Lombard MC, Zajac JM, et al. Pre- and post-synaptic distribution of mu, delta and kappa opioid receptors in the superficial layers of the cervical dorsal horn of the rat spinal cord. Brain Res. 1990;521:15–22.
17. Wirz S, Wittmann M. Gastrointestinal symptoms under opioid therapy: a prospective comparison of oral sustained-release hydromorphone, transdermal fentanyl, and transdermal buprenorphine. Eur J Pain. 2009;13(7):737–43.
18. Thomas J, Karver S, Cooney GA, et al. Methylnaltrexone for opioid-induced constipation in advanced illness. N Engl J Med. 2008;358:2332–43.
19. Thorn SE, Wickbom G, Philipson L, et al. Myoelectricactivity in the stomach and duodenum after epidural administration of morphine or bupivacaine. Acta Anaesthesiol Scand. 1996;40:773–8.
20. Mahajan G, Wilsey B, Fishman SM. Opioid therapy: adverse effects including addiction. In: Benzon HT, Raja SN, Molloy RE, et al., editors. Essentials of pain and regional anesthesia. Philadelphia: Elsevier Churchill Livingstone; 2005. p. 94–105.
21. Candy B, Jones L, Goodman ML, Drake R, Tookman A. Laxatives or methylnaltrexone for the management of constipation in palliative care patients. Cochrane Database Syst Rev. 2011;1:CD003448.
22. Golembiewski J. Morphine and hydromorphone for postoperative analgesia: focus on safety. J Perianesth Nurs. 2003;18(2):120–2.
23. Centers for Disease Control and Prevention. J Pain Palliat Care Pharmacother. 2016;14(2):138–40.
24. Inturrisi CE. Clinical pharmacology of opioids for pain. Clin J Pain. 2002;18(4 Suppl):S3–13.
25. Christrup LL. Morphine metabolites. Acta Anaesthesiol Scand. 1997;41:116–22.
26. Tiseo PJ, Thaler HT, Lapin J, et al. Morphine-6-glucuronide concentrations and opioid-related side effects: a survey in cancer patients. Pain. 1995;61:47–54.
27. Lurcott G. The effects of the genetic absence and inhibition of CYP2DA on the metabolism of codeine and its derivatives, hydrocodone and oxycodone. Anesth Prog. 1998;45(4):154–6.
28. Ercoli N, Lewis MN. The Time-Action curves of morphine, codeine, dilaudid, and Demerol by various methods of administration. J Pharmacol Exp Ther. 1945;84(4):301–17.
29. Kirchheiner J. Pharmacokinetics of codeine and its metabolite morphine in ultra-rapid metabolizers due to CYP2D6 duplication. Pharmacogenomics J. 2007;4(7):257–75.
30. Pasternak G. Pharmacological mechanisms of Opioid Analgesics. Clin Neuropharmacol. 1993;16(1):1–18.
31. Angst MS, Drover DR. Pharmacodynamics of orally administered sustained- release hydromorphone in humans. Anesthesiology. 2001;94(1):63–7.
32. Kaplan HL, Busto UE. Inhibition of cytochrome P450 2D6 metabolism of hydrocodone to hydromorphone does not importantly affect abuse liability. J Pharmacol Exp Ther. 1997;281(1):103–8.
33. Kullgren J, Le V. Incidence of hydromorphone-induced neuroexcitation in hospice patients. J Palliat Med. 2013;12(10):1205–9.

34. American Pain Society. Principles of analgesic use in the treatment of acute pain and cancer pain. 4th ed. Glenview: American Pain Society; 1999.
35. Mahajan G, Fishman SM. Major opioids in pain management. In: Benzon HT, Raja SN, Molloy RE, et al., editors. Essentials of pain and regional anesthesia. Philadelphia: Elsevier Churchill Livingstone; 2005. p. 94–105.
36. Fukada K. Chapter 27. Opioids. In: Miller RD, Eriksson I, Fleisher L, et al., editors. Miller's anesthesia. 7th ed. Philadelphia: Churchill-Livingstone; 2009.
37. Benzon HT, Raja SN, Liu SS, et al. Essentials of pain medicine. 4th ed. Philadelphia: Elsevier; 2018. Chapter 42.

Nonsteroidal Anti-inflammatory Drugs (NSAIDs)

13

Ricardo Maturana, Andrew So, and Karina Gritsenko

Introduction

Nonsteroidal anti-inflammatory drugs (NSAIDs) are broadly used for their analgesic, antipyretic, and anti-inflammatory properties. Inflammation is an attempt by the body to recruit cells of the immune system in order to overcome pathologic processes, remove harmful factors, and restore normal structure to damaged tissues [1]. NSAIDs work by inhibiting the function of prostaglandin endoperoxide synthases. Prostaglandin endoperoxide H synthases (PGHS), also known as cyclooxygenases, play a crucial role in the inflammatory pathway leading to the production of prostaglandins [2]. It is by preventing the formation of these pro-inflammatory mediators that NSAIDs impart their medical benefits, as well as adverse effects.

Cyclooxygenase Enzymes and Prostaglandins

Prostaglandins and thromboxane (TXA2) are eicosanoids produced from phospholipase-released arachidonic acid, a 20-carbon polyunsaturated fatty acid, by the cyclooxygenases (COX) [1]. COX-1 and COX-2 are enzymes that contain both cyclooxygenase and peroxidase activity with distinct functions and locations in the body [3]. The difference in function, expression and production of these enzymes determine the effect of their inhibition by nonsteroidal anti-inflammatory medications. COX-1, is constitutively expressed throughout the body and is involved in essential homeostatic and physiologic functions including thromboxane synthesis for platelet aggregation, vasodilation during contractile conditions, renal

vasodilation in response to low blood flow in the kidneys, and cytoprotection in the gastric mucosa [4, 5]. COX-2, is induced by pathological processes, traumatic stimuli, hormones, and growth factors playing a significant role in inflammation, pain, immune response, and some neoplasias [4]. COX-1 and COX-2 are involved in the production of multiple prostanoids (prostaglandins, thromboxanes, and prostacyclins) including prostaglandin E2, prostacyclin (PGI2), prostaglandin D2, and prostaglandin F2alpha (Fig. 13.1). Prostaglandin E2 (PGE2), is one of the most abundant prostaglandins involved in increased circulation and tissue permeability, as well as pain perception in the spinal cord and brain [6]. Prostacyclin (PGI2) is involved in cardiovascular homeostasis, vasodilation, inhibition of platelet aggregation, leukocyte adhesion, vascular smooth muscle cells proliferation, and mediation of nociceptive pain during active inflammation [1]. Prostaglandin D2 is found in mast cells and plays a role in type I allergic reactions and atopic conditions. PGF2 alpha is involved in multiple physiologic roles including ovulation, initiation of parturition, renal function, brain injury response, myocardial dysfunction, pain, and chronic inflammation [1]. One of the major thromboxanes, TxA2, is another arachidonic acid metabolite mainly derived from platelet COX-1 and is involved in platelet adhesion and aggregation, smooth muscle contraction, allergies, and neovascularization [7].

Chemical Properties of NSAIDs and COX Selectivity

NSAIDs possess high lipophilic and weak acid qualities mimicking the properties of arachidonic acid [8]. Structurally, some NSAIDs lack functional acidic groups and some present with polar lipophilic tails, both needing to be metabolized in order to become effective COX inhibitors [8].

Aspirin, acetylsalicylic acid (ASA), is a salicylate that irreversibly inhibits COX-1 and COX-2 enzymes in a time-dependent fashion through acetylation with more potent modification of the COX-1 enzyme compared to COX-2 [9]. Aspirin causes more analgesia at lower doses while requiring

The original version of this chapter was revised. The correction to this chapter can be found at https://doi.org/10.1007/978-3-030-18005-8_49

R. Maturana · A. So
Albert Einstein College of Medicine, Montefiore Medical Center, Bronx, NY, USA

K. Gritsenko (✉)
Department of Anesthesiology, Montefiore Medical Center and Albert Einstein College of Medicine, Bronx, NY, USA
e-mail: KGRITSEN@montefiore.org

Fig. 13.1 Biosynthetic pathway of prostanoids. (Arterioscler Thromb Vasc Biol. Author manuscript; available in PMC 2012 May 1. Published in final edited form as: Ricciotti and FitzGerald [1])

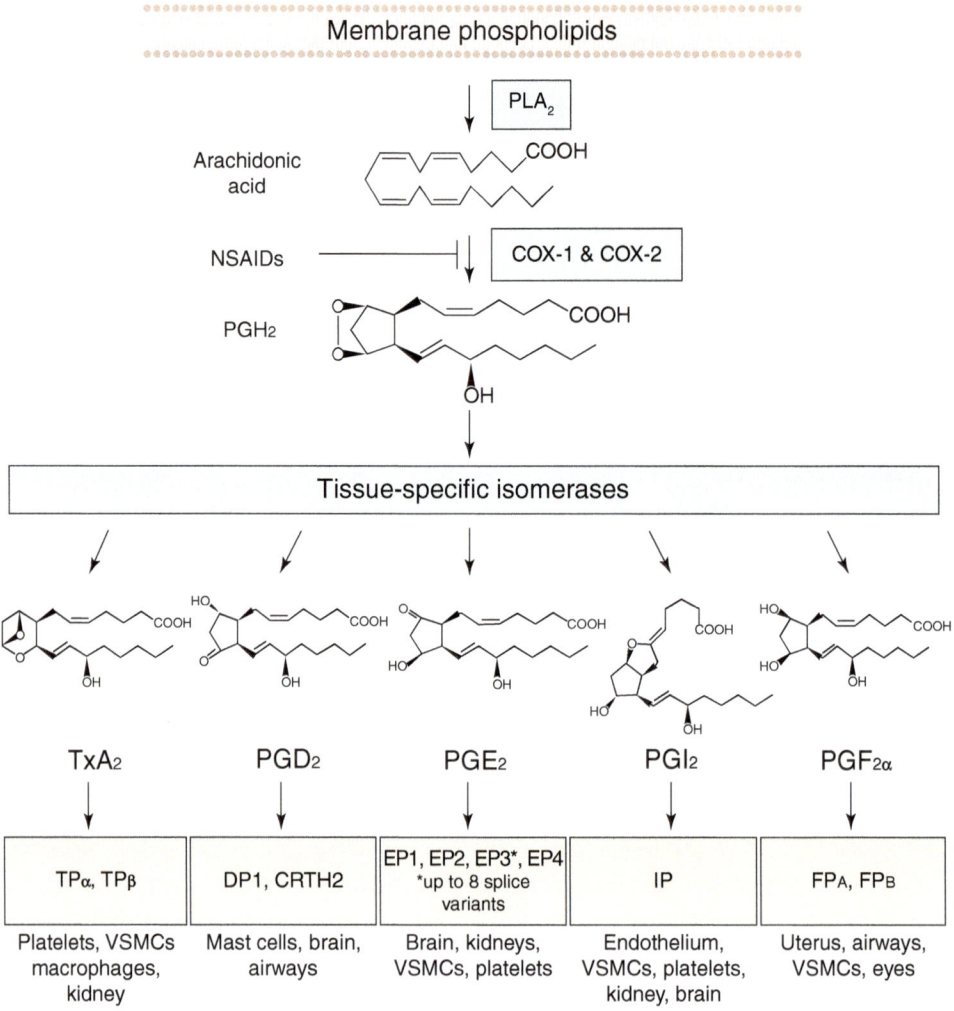

higher doses to see anti-inflammatory effects secondary to its poor lipophilic yet high acidic function [8]. Irreversible inactivation of COX-1 in platelets by aspirin leads to lowered thromboxane production for the entire life span of these cells [10]. Elimination of salicylates is first order at low doses and zero order at higher doses with renal excretion, increased by alkalization of urine [11].

Other NSAID categories include acetic acid, fenamic acid, enolic acid, and propionic acid derivatives as well as the selective COX-2 inhibitors, also known as coxibs (Table 13.1). Propionic acid derivatives include ibuprofen, naproxen, and fenoprofen. Ibuprofen is the most commonly used NSAID in the United States with a half-life similar to fenoprofen of approximately 2 hours where naproxen has a longer half-life between 12 and 15 hours [12]. The more commonly known acetic acid derivatives include indomethacin, diclofenac, sulindac, and ketorolac. Indomethacin, indole-acetic acid, is comparable with aspirin in analgesic properties, popularly known for its use in the treatment of patent ductus arteriosus, but with a more toxic profile than aspirin [13]. Diclofenac has a short half-life of 1–2 hours with

high first-pass metabolism, more selectivity for COX-2 than COX-1, and can be applied topically [12]. Sulindac is a prodrug related to indomethacin [14]. Ketorolac is a commonly used for post-operative pain, as it may be administered via the IV and IM routes.

Enolic acid derivatives include lornixacam, meloxicam, piroxicam, and tenoxicam. They possess long half-lives and almost a tenfold selectivity for the COX-2 enzyme [12]. Cyclooxygenase-2 selective inhibitors have reduced gastrointestinal adverse effects while still maintaining similar renal risks as nonselective COX inhibitors [11]. Figure 13.2 outlines the cyclooxygenase selectivity of commonly prescribed NSAIDs. The only selective COX-2 inhibitor used in the United States is celecoxib. Celecoxib was among the first COX-2 inhibitor used to treat inflammatory pathology in humans. Its anti-inflammatory and analgesic effects are similar to naproxen. The sulfone group in celecoxib is responsible for selective binding to COX-2 [15]. Recent research has also proposed the benefits of celecoxib as means of decreasing the development of colorectal cancer and breast cancer prevention [16, 17] (Table 13.2).

Table 13.1 Classes of NSAIDs

Salicylates	Acetic acid derivatives	Fenamic acid derivatives	Enolic acid derivatives	Propionic acid derivatives	Selective COX-2 inhibitors
Aspirin (acetylsalicylic acid) *Diflunisal* (Dolobid) *Salsalate* (Mono-Gesic, Salflex, Disalcid, Salsitab)	*Diclofenac* (Voltaren, Cataflam, Voltaren-XR) Etodolac (Lodine, Lodine XL) *Indomethacin* (Indocin, Indocin SR, Indocin IV) *Ketorolac* (Toradol, Sprix) *Sulindac* (Clinoril)	*Meclofenamic acid* (Meclomen) *Mefenamic acid* (Ponstel) *Tolfenamic acid* (Clotam Rapid, Tufnil)	*Lornoxicam* (Xefo) *Meloxicam* (Mobic) *Piroxicam* (Feldene) *Tenoxicam* (Mobiflex)	*Dexketoprofen* (Keral) *Fenoprofen* (Nalfon) *Ibuprofen* (Advil, Brufen, Motrin, Nurofen, Medipren, Nuprin) *Ketoprofen* (Actron, Orudis, Oruvail, Ketoflam) *Naproxen* (Aleve, Anaprox, Midol Extended Relief, Naprosyn, Naprelan) Duraprox)	*Celecoxib* (Celebrex)

Fig. 13.2 Selectivity of NSAIDs for COX-1 and COX-2 enzymes. CXO cyclooxygenase, CV cardiovascular, GI gastrointestinal, NSAID Nonsteroidal anti-inflammatory drugs. (Perry [39])

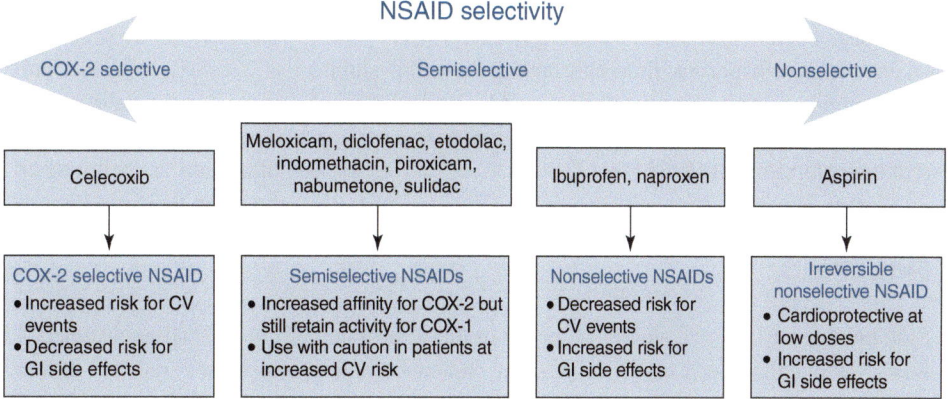

Table 13.2 Dosing of common NSAIDs

Drug	Dose (mg)	Frequency (hours)	Max daily dose (mg)
Ibuprofen	200–400	4–6	2400
Naproxen	250–500	6–8	1500
Ketorolac	30–60 IM, 30 IV followed by 15–30	6	150 first day, 120 after
Aspirin	500–1000	4–6	4000
Sulindac	150	12	400
Celecoxib	200–400	12–24	400
Diclofenac	50–75	8	150
Meloxicam	7.5–15	12–24	15
Nabumetone	500–750	12–24	2000

Distribution, Metabolism, and Excretion of NSAIDs

Oral absorption of NSAIDs is generally rapid. High binding to albumin may explain potential interactions between NSAIDs and other drugs [8]. The liver plays the major role in the metabolism of NSAIDs through various pathways including oxidation and conjugation to inactive metabolites. The liver is another source of drug interaction where NSAIDS can cause induction or inhibition of hepatic drug metabolism. They are mainly excreted as phase-II glucuronides and as sulfate conjugates by the kidneys, with urine pH alkalization increasing the rate of excretion [8].

Contraindications and Interactions

NSAIDs, like many other drugs, can induce hypersensitivity reactions. It is important to remain vigilant of these reactions as they can become life threatening [18, 19].

Exposure to NSAIDs late in pregnancy is associated with the closure of fetal ductus arteriosus, while the risks of exposure in early pregnancy are unclear [20]. The American Congress of Obstetricians and Gynecologist (ACOG) recommend the consideration of low-dose aspirin in women at risk of preeclampsia a with thorough patient-to-patient medical analysis prior to use [21]. The association between Reye's syndrome, a rapidly progressive encephalopathy and liver failure, and aspirin has been long-standing. Consequently, it is recommended that individuals younger than 19 should not receive aspirin during fever-causing or viral illnesses [22]. The use of aspirin in children younger than 3 years old is also contraindicated.

NSAIDs may play a significant role in the incidence of myocardial infarction and other serious vascular events. Different drugs in this class appear to have distinct risk profiles [23]. Caution should be used when prescribing NSAIDs to patients with liver disease. They should also be avoided in patients with pre-existing renal disease and congestive heart failure [24].

Significant adverse effects including GI bleeds have been reported with concomitant use of NSAIDs and warfarin [25]. Administration of NSAIDS with other anti-coagulants and anti-platelet medications is also not recommended. NSAIDs have also been implicated in causing kidney injury when taken with cyclosporine, thus care and monitoring should be taken when combining these drugs [26]. Serum levels of lithium and methotrexate may be are elevated during concurrent consumption with NSAIDs [27].

Side Effects

Side effects are most frequently observed in the gastrointestinal system and include gastritis, bleeding, and exacerbation of inflammatory bowel diseases. Endoscopic studies have shown that gastric duodenal ulcers due to NSAIDs use have a prevalence rate among users of 14–25% [28, 29]. COX-1 enzymes are present in the gastric mucosal lining and serve to produce prostaglandins, which play a role in maintaining an effective mucus barrier [28]. To mitigate these effects, proton pump inhibitors or histamine channel blockers (H2) are often co-prescribed. COX-2 inhibitors may also be considered, as their selectivity appears to result in a lower probability of GI injury [30].

NSAIDs are also known to produce adverse side effects to the renal system. Unlike frequently observed GI side effects, renal side effects tend to be more rare and transient in nature [31]. Most notably, NSAIDs have shown to cause renal impairment and acute renal injury that results from inhibition of vasodilatory renal prostaglandins, which leads to a decrease in renal blood flow. Renal injury is normally associated with patients with renal insufficiency and diabetes mellitus, as well as with individuals who suffer from intravascular volume depletion of any etiology, as these patients depend on renal blood flow controlled by vasodilator prostaglandins. It should also be noted that the elderly population are at higher risk of renal impairment given the prolonged half-lives of the drug in these patients [32]. Additionally, via inhibition of prostaglandin synthesis, NSAIDS may cause increased sodium and potassium retention, resulting in the elevation of blood pressure, which may also contribute to

the cardiovascular risk profile. NSAIDs should be avoided or used cautiously for patients taking diuretics, as this combination may potentiate renal injury [33].

NSAIDS have also been observed to cause liver injury. The severity of NSAIDS on the hepatic system can range from asymptomatic transient transaminasemia to as severe as fulminant hepatic failure. Studies have shown that approximately 10% of total drug-induced hepatotoxicity is due to NSAID ingestion [34]. Hepatic injury is most common among patients with previous hepatic injury and known dysfunction. Patients who are also taking known hepatic toxic agents are among the highest-risk individuals for NSAID-induced liver injury [35]. While the exact mechanism behind hepatic injury is not completely understood, some studies suggest the involvement of oxidative stress from accumulated metabolites.

NSAIDs play a significant effect on the cardiovascular system and they must be considered carefully when administering to patients with cardiovascular risk factors. COX-2 inhibition is believed to shift the prothrombotic balance favoring the formation of clots increasing the risks of acute myocardial infarcts [36]. Some COX-2 selective inhibitors were withdrawn from the market after studies revealed an increased incidence of acute myocardial infarction. Large cohort studies revealed that all NSAIDs are associated with increased risks of infarcts and ischemia particularly with higher doses [37]. The FDA has intensified warnings against liberal use of NSAIDs in all patient populations as they increase the changes of heart attack or stroke. These risks are seen in patients without cardiovascular risks, but more so in patients with known history of cardiovascular disease [38].

Conclusion

NSAIDs remain a mainstay of analgesic therapy for a variety of indications. As their use can produce a variety of deleterious effects on multiple organ systems, careful patient selection and a thorough discussion of the risks and benefits is essential when utilizing this class of medications.

References

1. Ricciotti E, FitzGerald GA. Prostaglandins and inflammation. Arterioscler Thromb Vasc Biol. 2011;31(5):986–1000. https://doi.org/10.1161/ATVBAHA.110.207449.
2. Smyth EM, Grosser T, Wang M, Yu Y, FitzGerald GA. Prostanoids in health and disease. J Lipid Res. 2009;50:S423–8.
3. Smith WL, DeWitt DL, Garavito RM. Cyclooxygenases: structural, cellular, and molecular biology. Annu Rev Biochem. 2000;69:145–82.
4. Dubois RN, Abramson SB, Crofford L, Gupta RA, Simon LS, Van De Putte LB, Lipsky PE. Cyclooxygenase in biology and disease. FASEB J. 1998;12:1063–73.

5. Rouzer CA, Marnett LJ. Cyclooxygenases: structural and functional insights. J Lipid Res. 2009;50(Suppl):S29–34. https://doi.org/10.1194/jlr.R800042-JLR200.
6. Funk CD. Prostaglandins and leukotrienes: advances in eicosanoid biology. Science. 2001;294:1871–5.
7. The thromboxane/endoperoxide receptor (TP): the common villain, Nakahata N. Thromboxane A2: physiology/pathophysiology, cellular signal transduction and pharmacology. Pharmacol Ther. 2008;118:18–35.
8. Mehanna AS. NSAIDs: chemistry and pharmacological actions. Am J Pharm Educ. 2003;67(2):Article 63. https://doi.org/10.5688/aj670263.
9. Meade EA, Smith WL, DeWitt DL. Differential inhibition of prostaglandin endoperoxide synthase (cyclooxygenase) isozymes by aspirin and other non-steroidal anti-inflammatory drugs. J Biol Chem. 1993;268:6610–4.
10. Blobaum AL, Lawrence J, Marnett J. Structural and functional basis of cyclooxygenase inhibition. Med Chem. 2007;50(7):1425–41. https://doi.org/10.1021/jm0613166. Publication Date. March 7, 2007. Copyright 2007 American Chemical Society.
11. Katzung & Trevor's pharmacology: examination & board review 11e. Chapter 36: NSAIDs, Acetaminophen, & Drugs Used in Rheumatoid Arthritis & Gout. Copyright © 2015, 2013, 2010, 2008, 2005, 2002 by McGraw-Hill Education. All rights reserved. Printed in the United States of America.
12. Nonsteroidal anti-inflammatory drugs and cyclooxygenase-2 inhibitors. Steven D. Waldman. Pain Management, Second Edition. Chapter 121, 884–889. Copyright 2011, 2007 by Saunders, an imprint of Elsevier Inc. All rights reserved.
13. Mehta SK, Younoszai A, Pietz J, Achanti BP. Pharmacological closure of the patent ductus arteriosus. Images Paediatr Cardiol. 2003;5(1):1–15.
14. Yin T, Wang G, Ye T, Wangb Y. Sulindac, a non-steroidal anti-inflammatory drug, mediates breast cancer inhibition as an immune modulator. Sci Rep. 2016;6:19534. Published online 2016 Jan 18. https://doi.org/10.1038/srep19534.
15. Davies NM, McLachlan AJ, Day RO, Williams KM. Clinical pharmacokinetics and pharmacodynamics of Celecoxib. A selective Cyclo-Oxygenase-2 inhibitor. Clin Pharmacokinet. 2000;38(3):225–42.
16. Koki AT, Leahy KM, Masferrer JL. Potential utility of COX-2 inhibitors in chemoprevention and chemotherapy. Expert Opin Investig Drugs. 1999;8:1623–38.
17. Davies G, Martin LA, Sacks N, Dowsett M. Cyclooxygenase-2 (COX-2), aromatase and breast cancer: a possible role for COX-2 inhibitors in breast cancer chemoprevention. Ann Oncol. 2002;13:669–78.
18. Doña I, Blanca-López N, Cornejo-García JA, Torres MJ, Laguna JJ, Fernández J, et al. Characteristics of subjects experiencing hypersensitivity to non-steroidal anti-inflammatory drugs: patterns of response. Clin Exp Allergy. 2011;41:86–95.
19. Kowalski ML, Makowska JS. Seven steps to the diagnosis of NSAIDs hypersensitivity: how to apply a new classification in real practice? Allergy Asthma Immunol Res. 2015 Jul;7(4):312–20. Published online 2015 Apr 21. https://doi.org/10.4168/aair.2015.7.4.312.
20. Antonucci R, Zaffanello M, Puxeddu E, Porcella A, Cuzzolin L, Pilloni MD, Fanos V. Use of non-steroidal anti-inflammatory drugs in pregnancy: impact on the fetus and newborn. Curr Drug Metab. 2012;13(4):474–90.
21. Practice advisory on low-dose aspirin and prevention of preeclampsia: updated recommendations. This practice advisory was developed by the American College of Obstetricians and Gynecologists in collaboration with Christopher M. Zahn, MD; Joseph R. Wax, MD; and T. Flint Porter, MD. July 11, 2016.
22. National Reye's Syndrome Foundation. Reye's syndrome bulletin, 2005. Accessed 20 Aug 2009.
23. Trelle S, Reichenbach S, Wandel S, Hildebrand P, Tschannen B, Villiger PM, Egger M, Jüni P. Cardiovascular safety of non-steroidal anti-inflammatory drugs: network meta-analysis. BMJ. 2011;342:c7086. Epub 2011 Jan 11.
24. Patino FG, Olivieri J, Allison JJ, et al. Nonsteroidal antiinflammatory drug toxicity monitoring and safety practices. J Rheumatol. 2003;30(12):2680–8.
25. Battistella M, Mamdami MM, Juurlink DN. Risk of upper gastrointestinal Hemorrhage in Warfarin users treated with nonselective NSAIDs or COX-2 inhibitors. Arch Intern Med. 2005;165(2):189–92. https://doi.org/10.1001/archinte.165.2.189.
26. Altman RD, Perez GO, Sfakianakis GN. Interaction of cyclosporine A and nonsteroidal anti-inflammatory drugs on renal function in patients with rheumatoid arthritis. Am J Med. 1992;93(4):396–402.
27. Becker DE. Adverse drug interactions. Anesth Prog. 2011;58(1):31–41. https://doi.org/10.2344/0003-3006-58.1.31.
28. Russell RI. Non-steroidal anti-inflammatory drugs and gastrointestinal damage---problems and solutions. Postgrad Med J. 2001;77(904):82–8.
29. Buttgereit F, Burmester GR, Simon LS. Gastrointestinal toxic side effects of nonsteroidal anti-inflammatory drugs and cyclooxygenase-2–specific inhibitors. Am J Med. 2001;110(3):13–9.
30. Sostres C, Gargallo CJ, Lanas A. Nonsteroidal anti-inflammatory drugs and upper and lower gastrointestinal mucosal damage. Arthritis Res Ther. 2013;15(Suppl 3):S3.
31. Harirforoosh S, Jamali F. Renal adverse effects of nonsteroidal anti-inflammatory drugs. Expert Opin Drug Saf. 2009;8(6):669–81.
32. Schlondorff D. Renal complications of nonsteroidal anti-inflammatory drugs. Kidney Int. 1993;44(3):643–53.
33. Weir MR. Renal effects of nonselective NSAIDs and coxibs. Cleve Clin J Med. 2002;69(Suppl 1):SI53–8.
34. Bessone F. Non-steroidal anti-inflammatory drugs: what is the actual risk of liver damage? World J Gastroenterol. 2010;16(45):5651.
35. García Rodríguez LA, Pérez Gutthann S, Walker AM, Lueck L. The role of non-steroidal anti-inflammatory drugs in acute liver injury. BMJ. 1992;305(6858):865–8.
36. Balancing Risks and Benefits: cardiovascular Safety of NSAIDs. Jul 22, 2016. Prashant Vaishnava, MD. American College of Cardiology.
37. Bally M. Risk of acute myocardial infarction with NSAIDs in real world use: Bayesian meta-analysis of individual patient data. BMJ. 2017;357:j1909. https://doi.org/10.1136/bmj.j1909.
38. FDA strengthens warning For NSAIDs. Jul 10, 2015 ACC News Story. American College of Cardiology.
39. Perry LA. Cardiovascular risk associated with NSAIDs and COX-2 inhibitors. US Pharm. 2014;39(3):35–8.

Antidepressants and Anticonvulsants

14

Chukwuemeka Okafor and Melinda Aquino

Antidepressants

Tricyclic Antidepressants (TCA)

TCA: Introduction

Tricyclic antidepressants (TCAs), named for their chemical structure, have been used for the treatment of depression since the early 1950s. Discovery of their effectiveness as analgesics dates back to the late 1980s. These drugs are subdivided into several groups based on the number of substitutions of the side chain amine. The major groups are the tertiary (e.g., amitriptyline, imipramine, trimipramine, doxepin, and clomipramine) and secondary amines (desipramine, protriptyline, nortriptyline) [1]. Chemical structures of TCAs are depicted in Fig. 14.1.

TCA: Pharmacodynamics

All tricyclics work at nerve synapses to block the reuptake of norepinephrine, serotonin, or both. How TCAs affect pain isn't entirely clear, but the consensus thought is that their role in pain modulation results from augmentation of descending serotonergic and noradrenergic inhibitory pathways in the dorsal horn of the spinal cord. It appears that analgesic effects may be independent of their antidepressant benefits. As such, their role may be in the restoration of normal nerve transmission pathways and less so in the frank inhibition of pain [2].

In addition to affecting noradrenergic (NE) and serotonergic (5HT-3) receptors, TCAs exhibit activity at other receptor types, such as N-methyl-D-aspartate (NMDA), opioid,

adenosine, calcium, sodium, muscarinic, cholinergic, histaminergic, and nicotinic (Fig. 14.2). This receptor cross-reactivity is more pronounced with tertiary than with secondary amines, making tertiary TCAs more effective analgesics; however, undesirable side effects, such as sedation, orthostatic hypotension, and urinary retention, among others, are also more frequent and severe with the use of this class of medications.

TCA: Pharmacokinetics

Most TCAs are absorbed well orally and have long half-lives. They are typically administered at night in order to avoid daytime sedation, as well as to capitalize on their soporific effects (usually greater with tertiary amines), which are beneficial for patients with nighttime pain and resulting insomnia. TCAs undergo hepatic metabolism by the CYP2D6 system, so care must be taken when co-administering with inducers and inhibitors of this system. Patient variables such as ethnicity and genetic polymorphisms also affect TCA metabolism. It is important to note that renal clearance of active TCA metabolites (more of an issue with tertiary amines) is decreased with aging, which results in a high risk of side effects in the elderly.

TCA: Indications

There are a variety of pain syndromes for which TCAs have found to be beneficial, including headache, radicular pain, neuropathic pain, fibromyalgia, and phantom limb pain. Their most widespread and accepted use has been for neuropathic pain syndromes (i.e., postherpetic neuralgia, diabetic neuropathy, etc.). It is important to note that as with many medications, most of the analgesic indications for TCAs are considered off-label.

TCA: Adverse Effects

Common side effects include sedation, fatigue, orthostatic hypotension, and anticholinergic effects (i.e., dry mouth, constipation, etc.). Sympathomimetic effects including agitation, tachycardia, sweating can also be seen with their

The original version of this chapter was revised. The correction to this chapter can be found at https://doi.org/10.1007/978-3-030-18005-8_49

C. Okafor
Forbes Hospital, Pittsburgh, Pennsylvania, USA

M. Aquino (✉)
Montefiore Medical Center, Albert Einstein College of Medicine, Bronx, NY, USA
e-mail: maquino@montefiore.org

Fig. 14.1 Chemical structures of tricyclic antidepressants

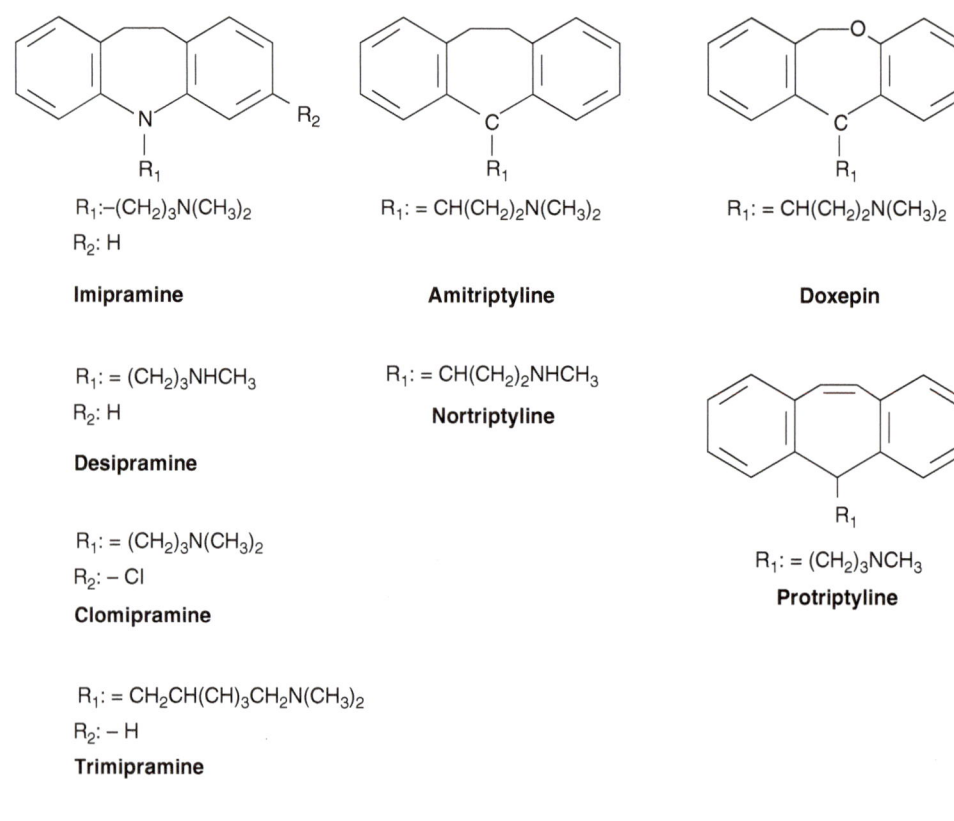

$R_1: -(CH_2)_3N(CH_3)_2$
R_2: H

Imipramine

$R_1: = CH(CH_2)_2N(CH_3)_2$

Amitriptyline

$R_1: = CH(CH_2)_2N(CH_3)_2$

Doxepin

$R_1: = (CH_2)_3NHCH_3$
R_2: H

Desipramine

$R_1: = CH(CH_2)_2NHCH_3$

Nortriptyline

$R_1: = (CH_2)_3NCH_3$

Protriptyline

$R_1: = (CH_2)_3N(CH_3)_2$
$R_2: - Cl$

Clomipramine

$R_1: = CH_2CH(CH)_3CH_2N(CH_3)_2$
$R_2: - H$

Trimipramine

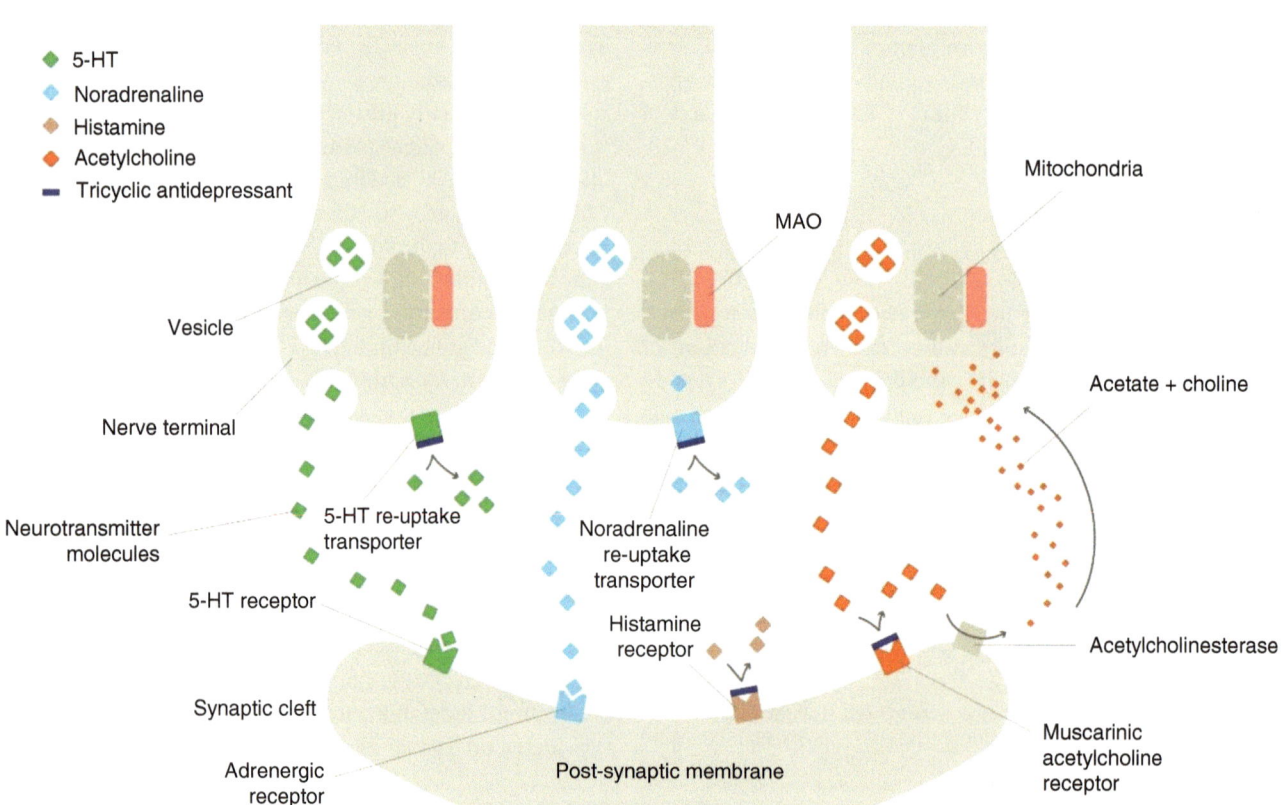

- ◆ 5-HT
- ◆ Noradrenaline
- ◆ Histamine
- ◆ Acetylcholine
- ▬ Tricyclic antidepressant

Mitochondria

MAO

Acetate + choline

Vesicle

Nerve terminal

Neurotransmitter molecules

5-HT re-uptake transporter

Noradrenaline re-uptake transporter

Acetylcholinesterase

5-HT receptor

Histamine receptor

Muscarinic acetylcholine receptor

Synaptic cleft

Adrenergic receptor

Post-synaptic membrane

Fig. 14.2 Select receptor types affected by TCAs

Table 14.1 Pharmacologic properties of SNRIs

Properties of SNRis	Venlafaxine	Desvenlafaxine	Duloxetine	Milnacipran	Mirtazapine
Therapeutic dose range	75–375 md/day	50 mg/day	60–120 mg/day	25–200 mg/ day	15–45 mg/ day
Biotransformation	CYP2D6	CYP3A4	CYP2D6, CYP1A2	CYP2D6, CYP2C9	CYP2D6,CYP3A4, CYP1A2
Half-life	4 h	9–10 h	12.5 h	12 h	20–40 h
Elimination route	Renal	Renal	Renal, urine (72%), feces (19%)	Renal	Renal, urine (75%), feces (15%)
NE/5HT affinity ratio	15:7	13:8	9:3	2:1	–
5HT/NE selectivity	30	3 × higher (NE binding)	10	1	300
Efficacy	SKRI action	Better efficacy at low doses	May require higher than approved doses	Better efficacy at higher doses	Dose-dependent
Hepatic side effects	Elevated liver enzymes	–	Complicated by alcohol consumption	Elevated liver enzymes	Hepatic insufficiency
Cardiac side effects	+	QTc interval prolongation	–	–	–
Sexual dysfunction	Loss of libido, anorgasmia	Delayed ejaculation	Loss of libido, anorgasmia	Decrease in sexual desire and ability	Not cause significant sexual dysfunction

Shelton [4]

NE norepineprine, *5HT* serotonin

administration. Tertiary amines are more likely to produce these side effects mainly because of their antagonism at histaminergic, cholinergic, and muscarinic receptors. Nortriptyline, a second-generation TCA, has been found to be as efficacious as tertiary TCAs, but better tolerated in the elderly population with fewer adverse effects. Initiation of therapy and dose titration must be monitored and handled with extreme care in patients with a history of cardiovascular disease. An array of cardiac conduction abnormalities have been known to accompany TCA therapy. Before starting a TCA, a baseline ECG should be considered to screen for any underlying cardiac conduction abnormalities.

TCA: Medication Interactions

TCAs may interact with other medications that cause an increase in serotonin, which may result in serotonin syndrome. Typically, serotonin syndrome presents as a triad of altered mental status, autonomic dysfunction, and neuromuscular excitation. Common medications responsible for this interaction with TCAs include selective serotonin reuptake inhibitors (SSRIs), serotonin and norepinephrine reuptake inhibitors (SNRI), tramadol, and other medications which alter the metabolism of TCAs.

Serotonin and Norepinephrine Reuptake Inhibitors (SNRIs)

SNRI: Introduction

Although a number of neurotransmitters likely modulate the ascending and descending pain pathways, serotonin (5-HT) and norepinephrine (NE) are likely the major mediators in descending inhibitory pathways. Inhibition of serotonin and norepinephrine reuptake in descending inhibitory pathways potentiates their activity and results in attenuation of ascending nociceptive input. The drugs in this class most commonly used to treat pain include duloxetine, venlafaxine, milnacipran, and desvenlafaxine.

SNRI: Pharmacodynamics

The various SNRIs are differentiated based on their relative abilities to inhibit the reuptake of serotonin and norepinephrine. Pharmacologic properties of SNRIs are listed in Table 14.1. The onset of clinically significant reuptake inhibition in serotonin before that of norepinephrine may play a role in the delayed onset of pain suppression seen with this class of medications. Interestingly, milnacipran lacks the sequential order of inhibition that is seen in the older generation of SNRI's [3].

SNRI: Pharmacokinetics

SNRIs have relatively short half-lives compared to most antidepressants. They are metabolized in the liver although their metabolism is not specific to one particular enzyme (Table 14.1) [4]. The only SNRI with an active metabolite is venlafaxine, with its metabolite being desvenlafaxine.

SNRI: Indications

SNRIs have been found to be efficacious in the treatment of fibromyalgia, diabetic neuropathy, as well as pain related to osteoarthritis. Duloxetine is currently the only antidepressant FDA approved for musculoskeletal pain. In addition, it is approved for the management of diabetic peripheral neuropathic pain and fibromyalgia. Venlafaxine has been shown to be better for chronic postsurgical pain in mastectomy than gabapentinoids [5]. Milnacipran is FDA approved for the treatment of fibromyalgia [6].

Adverse Effects

In general, SNRIs appear to be better tolerated than TCAs. Despite this, nausea, somnolence, and dizziness were repeatedly reported in patients taking duloxetine. Like most drugs

Table 14.2 Common side effects of SNRIs

Venlafaxine	Duloxetine	Milnacipran	Desvenlafaxine
Nausea	Nausea	Anxiety	Nausea
Sweating	Increased sweating	Excessive sweating	Hyperhidrosis
Somnolence	Somnolence	Vertigo	Somnolence
Anorexia	Decreased appetite	Hot flush	Decreased appetite
Tremor	Constipation	Dysuria	Constipation
Nervousness	Fatigue		Anxiety
Dry mouth	Dry mouth		Insomnia
Dizziness			Dizziness
Abnormal dreams			Specific male sexual function disorders
Abnormal Ejaculation			

Shelton [4]

Adverse reactions as defined as occurring in ≥5% of SNRI-treated patients and at least twice the rate for placebo for venlafxine, duloxetine, and desvenlafaxine; as defined by the European Medicines Agency for milnacipran

SNRI serotonin-norepinephrine reuptake inhibitor

that inhibit 5-HT reuptake, SNRIs can produce sexual dysfunction ranging from difficulty becoming aroused, disinterest in sex, genital anesthesia, and anorgasmia [7]. The cardiovascular adverse effects are less common with SNRIs compared to TCAs although venlafaxine has been shown to increase blood pressure and heart rate with higher doses. Interestingly, a case of Takotsubo cardiomyopathy as a result of duloxetine administration has been reported in the literature [8]. Table 14.2 summarizes common side effects of SNRIs.

Anticonvulsants

Introduction

Anticonvulsants, also referred to as antiepileptic drugs (AEDs), have been in use for almost a century. This nomenclature is nonspecific as there is no uniform structure or mechanism of action within this group. The drugs that are used to cease or prevent seizures have a wide array of structures, mechanisms, and sites of action. Accepted use of AEDs in the realm of pain management goes back the 1960s, but reports of these medications used in trigeminal neuralgia date back to the 1940s. Their efficacy has mostly been seen in chronic neuropathic pain states in which pain is described as burning, lancinating, and electric shock-like in quality [9]. The primary means by which this class is thought to relieve pain is by decreasing aberrant neuronal signals [10]. AEDs impart their effects in the peripheral nervous system (PNS), as is the case with carbamazepine, central nervous system (CNS) (i.e., clonazepam, valproic acid, etc.), or dual action on both CNS and PNS as seen with gabapentinoids.

Pharmacokinetics

In general, AED absorption through the gastrointestinal system is rapid with peak plasma concentrations being seen after 1–4 hours. Oxcarbazepine must be converted to an active metabolite, 10-OH-carbamazepine. AEDs are mostly considered to have a low volume of distribution, with few drugs being heavily protein bound throughout the body. Gabapentin is considered to have close to no protein binding. It is important to note that, the CNS concentration does not necessarily correlate with the concentration of the unbound drug in the plasma [11].

Pharmacodynamics

As mentioned earlier, AEDs encompass a broad range of medications. When considering the structures of these drugs and how/where they act, the group may be subdivided even further.

Gabapentin and pregabalin are both GABA analogs with similarities in structure and mechanism of action. It is important to note that these medications do not act on the GABA receptor. Instead, gabapentinoids block the alpha-2 subunit of voltage-dependent calcium channels on the neuronal cells of the spinal cord [12]. The main difference between the two is that pregabalin has a higher affinity for the binding site and better systemic absorption.

Older AEDs such as phenytoin and carbamazepine exert a blockade on sodium channels to reduce the neuronal excitability and discharge that has been proposed to cause neuropathic pain. Lamotrigine is another drug that has its effect at sodium channels and also suppresses the neuronal release of glutamate, an excitatory neurotransmitter (NT). Valproic acid works to elevate the level of GABA (an inhibitory neurotrasmitter) in the CNS and therefore treats pain that related to the pathological overexcitation of the nervous system [13].

Indications

Although some drugs in this class are FDA approved for the treatment of neuropathic pain syndromes, many are used off-label. Carbamazepine, gabapentin, and pregabalin are currently the only three AEDs approved by the FDA and European Medicines Agency for the treatment of neuropathic pain. Some of the pain syndromes treated with AEDs include painful diabetic neuropathy, postherpetic neuralgia, and HIV-related neuropathic pain. Carbamazepine is well established as first-line treatment for trigeminal neuralgia, with treatment response rates as high as 70% [13].

Adverse Effects

Side effects such as sedation, ataxia, vertigo and even diplopia have been associated with the use of carbamazepine, phenytoin, and gabapentin. Phenytoin's other unique side effects are gingival hyperplasia, as well as peripheral neuropathy both seen in the setting of long-term use [14]. Although uncommon, carbamazepine has been found to cause chronic diarrhea as well as syndrome of inappropriate antidiuretic hormone secretion (SIADH). Serious skin reactions, including Stevens Johnson syndrome are possible with carbamazepine and oxcarbazepine, especially in Asian populations. Other rare reactions to these medications include aplastic anemia and agranulocytosis; therefore, monitoring of blood counts is recommended. Valproic acid carries the risk of nausea, vomiting, and tremor [14]. Gabapentin and pregabalin can cause peripheral edema. Many anticonvulsants have a warning of possible psychological effects including changes in mood and suicidal ideation [15].

Drug Interactions

Drug interactions are very common as many of these medications inhibit or induce liver enzymes involved in the metabolism of many other medications. Carbamazepine is considered one of the most active AEDs in regards to drug interactions. One of its most significant interactions is its ability to cause a significant reduction in the anticoagulant effect of warfarin. Oxcarbazepine, a structural derivative of carbamazepine, is a reasonable substitute in a poly AED user. In one study, after patients were switched from carbamazepine to oxcarbazepine, the mean increase in serum concentration of associated drugs was 25% for phenytoin and 20–30% for valproic acid [11].

Gabapentin neither induces nor inhibits microsomal liver enzymes. Contributing to its favorable profile is the fact most drugs play no role in its pharmacokinetics or pharmacodynamics. One exception is its moderate decrease in absorption when co-administered with antacids [11].

Summary

Antidepressants and anticonvulsants are useful as both primary and adjuvant analgesics. It is critical to review the specific side effect profiles of these medications, carefully select appropriate patients, and closely monitor for adverse reactions – especially for the medications known to (rarely) produce life-threatening complications.

References

1. DeBattista C. Antidepressant agents. In: Katzung BG, Trevor AJ, editors. Basic & clinical pharmacology. 13th ed. New York: McGraw-Hill; 2015.
2. Verdu B. Antidepressants for the treatment of chronic pain. Drugs. 2008;68(18):2611–32.
3. Kasper S, Pail G. Milnacipran: a unique antidepressant? Neuropsychiatr Dis Treat. 2010;6(Suppl I):23–31. https://doi.org/10.2147/NDT.S11777.
4. Shelton R. Serotonin norepinephrine reuptake inhibitors: similarities and differences. Prim Psychiatry. 2009;15:5(Suppl 4):25–35.
5. Roe M, et al. Pharmacology in the management of chronic pain. Anaesth Intensive Care Med. 2016;17(11):548–51.
6. Derry S, Gill D, Phillips T, Moore RA. Milnacipran for neuropathic pain and fibromyalgia in adults. Cochrane Database Syst Rev. 2012;(3):Art. No.: CD008244. https://doi.org/10.1002/14651858.CD008244.pub2.
7. Celikyurt IK, Mutlu O, Ulak G. Serotonin Noradrenaline Reuptake Inhibitors (SNRIs), Effects of antidepressants, Dr. Ru-Band Lu (Ed.), InTech, 2012. https://doi.org/10.5772/37999.
8. Selke KJ, Dhar G, Cohn JM. Takotsubo cardiomyopathy associated with titration of duloxetine. Tex Heart Inst J. 2011;38(5):573–6.
9. Park HJ, Moon DE. Pharmacologic management of chronic pain. Korean J Pain. 2010;23(2):99–108. https://doi.org/10.3344/kjp.2010.23.2.99.
10. Aronoff GM, Gallagher RM, Patel JG. Pharmacological management of chronic pain: a review. In: Tollison CD, et al., editors. Practical pain management. 3rd ed. Philadelphia: Lippincott Williams and Wilkins; 2002.
11. Perruca E. The clinical pharmacokinetics of the new antiepileptic drugs. Epilepsia. 1999;40(Suppl):S7–S13.
12. Sidhu HS, Sadhotra A. Current status of the new antiepileptic drugs in chronic pain. Front Pharmacol. 2016;7:276. https://doi.org/10.3389/fphar.2016.00276.
13. Ryder S-A, Stannard CF. Treatment of chronic pain: antidepressant, antiepileptic and antiarrhythmic drugs. Contin Educ Anaesth Crit Care Pain. 2005;5(1):18–21.
14. Rose MA, Kam PCA. Gabapentin: pharmacology and its use in pain management. Anaesthesia. 2002;57:451–62.
15. Dinakar P. Principles in pain management. In: Daroff RB, Jankovic J, et al., editors. Bradley's neurology in clinical practice. 7th ed. Philadelphia: Elsevier Health Sciences; 2015.

Miscellaneous Analgesic Agents

15

Shawn Amin, Christy Anthony, Vincent Reformato,
and Andrew G. Kaufman

Introduction

Classic adjuvant pain medications such as tricyclic antidepressants (TCA), Serotonin Norepinephrine Reuptake Inhibitors (SNRI), and Antiepileptic Drugs (AED) are discussed in a separate chapter. This chapter will focus on additional agents that may be used in analgesic regimens.

Although most of these medications are not FDA approved for the treatment of specific pain disorders, off-label use is commonly accepted [1]. Table 15.1 lists medications covered in this chapter. Their frequency of use in clinical practice varies dramatically. For example, muscle relaxants, steroids, local anesthetics, and NMDA antagonists enjoy widespread use, while neuroleptics, analeptics, and monoamine oxidase inhibitors (MAOIs) are seldomly employed in contemporary practice.

Neuroleptic Agents

Typical

- Chlorpromazine (Thorazine), Chlorprothixene (Taractan), Levomepromazine (Nozinan), and Thioridazine (Mellaril)
- *Mechanism of Action* – Dopamine D_2 receptor antagonist, central H_1 receptor antagonism, M_1 antagonism, and α_1 adrenergic antagonism.
- *Indications* – Psychotic disorders, anxiety disorders, Tourette's disease, Huntington disease, and autism.

S. Amin
Anesthesiology – Department of Pain Medicine, Rutgers
University – New Jersey Medical School, Newark, NJ, USA

C. Anthony
Department of Anesthesiology and Pain Management, University
Hospital, Rutgers – NJMS, Newark, NJ, USA

V. Reformato · A. G. Kaufman (✉)
Department of Anesthesiology, Rutgers, New Jersey Medical
School, Newark, NJ, USA
e-mail: kaufmaga@njms.rutgers.edu

Table 15.1 Miscellaneous analgesic medications

Class of drug	Subclasses	Examples of Agents
Neuroleptic agents	Typical	Chlorpromazine, thioridazine
	Atypical	olanzapine, risperidone, quetiapine
Antihistamines	First-generation H_1 antagonists	Diphenhydramine, carbinoxamine
	Second-generation H_1 antagonists	Cetirizine, loratadine
	H_2 receptor antagonists	Ranitidine, famotidine
Analeptic drugs		doxapram, prethcamide, pentylenetetrazole, nikethamide
Corticosteroids		Prednisone, betamethasone, hydrocortisone
Muscle relaxants/ antispasticity		Baclofen, cyclobenzaprine, methocarbamol, carisoprodol, tizanidine, chlorzoxazone
NMDA antagonists		Ketamine, methadone, memantine, dextromethorphan
Local anesthetics	Amides	Bupivacaine, lidocaine, mepivacaine
	Esters	Procaine, benzocaine, chloroprocaine
Sympatholytic drugs		Clonidine, alpha-methyldopa
Monoamine oxidase inhibitors	Nonselective	Isocarboxazid
	Selective MAO-A	Moclobemide
	Selective MAO-B	Selegiline
Others		Orphenadrine

- *Metabolism – Pharmacokinetics* – Variable T1/2 depending on the route of administration and form of drug; highly lipophilic drugs remain in the system for long after dosing is discontinued. Phase I and II liver metabolism and renal and bile excretion
- *Adverse Effects*– Weight gain, orthostatic hypotension, neuroleptic malignant syndrome (NMS), extrapyramidal

side effects (Parkinson's-like symptoms), akathisia, tardive dyskinesia, hyperprolactinemia, and QTc prolongation leading to ventricular arrhythmias/sudden cardiac death.
- *Drug Interactions* – Avoid with other D_2 receptor antagonists.

Atypical

- Olanzapine (Zyprexa), Clozapine (Clozaril), Risperidone (Risperdal), Quetiapine (Seroquel), and Aripiprazole (Abilify)
- *Mechanism of Action:* Potent $5HT_2$ antagonism and weaker D_2 antagonism (less EPS)
- *Indications*: Bipolar disorder, schizophrenia, and major depressive disorder
- *Metabolism:* Excreted in the urine
- *Adverse Effects:* Weight gain, extrapyramidal symptoms (EPS), and NMS

Antihistamines

First-Generation H₁ Receptor Antagonists

- Diphenhydramine (Benadryl), Carbinoxamine (Palgic), and Clemastine (Tavist)
- *Mechanism of Action* – competitive inhibition of histamine receptor, inhibition of muscarinic anticholinergic receptors
- *Indication* – allergic reaction, motion sickness, vertigo, and sedation
- *Metabolism – Pharmacokinetics* – T1/2 ~ 4–8 hrs, liver metabolism, renal excretion
- *Adverse Effects* – sedation, impaired motor skills, dizziness, tinnitus, blurred vision, diplopia, loss of appetite, nausea, vomiting, epigastric distress, constipation, or diarrhea
- *Drug Interactions* – any CYP450 induction or inhibition

Second-Generation H₁ Receptor Antagonists

- Cetirizine (Zyrtec), Loratadine (Claritin), Terfenadine (Seldane), and Quifenadine (Phencarol)
- *Mechanism of Action* – reversible inhibition of H_1 receptors, decreased CNS penetration
- *Indication* – allergic reaction, motion sickness, vertigo, sedation
- *Metabolism – Pharmacokinetics* – T1/2 ~ 4–8 hrs, liver metabolism, renal excretion

- *Adverse Effects* – decreased sedation and CNS effects (less pronounced CNS effects, such as sedation
- *Drug Interactions* – any CYP450 induction or inhibition

H₂ Receptor Antagonists

- Ranitidine (Zantac) and Famotidine (Pepcid)
- *Mechanism of Action* – reversible inhibition of H_2 receptors on the basolateral membrane of parietal cells in the stomach.
- *Indication* – GERD, PUD.
- *Metabolism* – thirty percent excreted unchanged, caution in patients with renal failure.
- *Adverse Effects* – diarrhea, headache, drowsiness, fatigue, muscular pain, constipation, confusion, delirium, and slurred speech.
- *Drug Interactions* – absorption may be enhanced by food or decreased by antacids.

Analeptic Drugs [2]

Doxapram (Dopram), Prethcamide (Micoren), Pentylenetetrazole (Cardiazol), and Nikethamide (Coramine)

Doxapram

- *Mechanism of Action* – K^+ channel inhibitor of carotid chemoreceptors →respiratory stimulation
- *Indication* – opioid-induced respiratory depression and COPD
- *Metabolism – Pharmacokinetics* – onset of action 20–30 seconds, peak effect 1–2 minutes, and duration 5–12 min. Rapidly metabolized to ketodoxapram (active metabolite)
- *Adverse Effects* – anxiety, panic attacks, sympatho-excitation, sweating, and convulsions. Not to be used in neonates (preparation with benzyl alcohol)
- *Drug Interactions* – MAOIs, sympathomimetics, and theophylline (increased sympathomimesis)

Prethcamide [3]

- *Mechanism of Action* – Central and peripheral respiratory stimulant that acts on central receptors in the brainstem and peripheral chemoreceptors; it is a mixture of equal parts of crotethamide and cropropamide. It may also increase catecholamine release.

- *Indication* – Respiratory depression.
- *Metabolism* – Hepatic metabolism (N-demethylation) with urinary excretion.
- *Adverse Effects* – Dyspnea in severe asthmatics, muscular, GI, CNS (should be avoided in patients with epilepsy or other convulsive disorders, recent strokes, and increased ICP), and CV (patients with uncontrolled HTN, ischemic heart disease, pheochromocytoma).
- *Drug Interactions* – Can cause cardiac arrhythmias when used with anesthetics, synergistic pressor effects when used with sympathomimetics or MAOIs, and may mask residual effects of NMBDs.

Corticosteroids

Glucocorticoids: Prednisone (Deltasone), Betamethasone (Celestone), Hydrocortisone (Solu-Cortef), Methylprednisolone (Solu-Medrol, Depomedrol), and Dexamethasone (Decadron, Dexasone)

Mechanism of Action
- Anti-inflammatory, mediated cellularly via alteration of gene expression and enzymatic inhibition
- Phospholipase inhibition – prevents the formation of arachidonic acid →inflammatory mediators LTB-4, LTC-4, LTD-4, and LTE-4
- Diminished function and availability of lymphocytes (altered chemotactic/chemoattractant mechanism)
- Inhibition of IL-1 and TNF
- Stabilizes membrane permeability → decreases fluid movement
- Prevents lysosomal enzyme release

- *Indication* – injected locally (i.e., epidural, intra-articular, etc.), systemic (IV or PO)
- *Metabolism* – liver, metabolized by conjugation with a sulfate or glucuronic acid, and are secreted in the urine
- *Adverse Effects*
  - Local reactions: tendon rupture, cartilage damage, crystal-induced arthritis, and pericapsular calcification
  - Systemic reactions: fluid and electrolyte imbalances (edema/congestive heart failure), bone demineralization (osteoporosis/fractures), gastrointestinal (GI) disease (nausea/vomiting/diarrhea/peptic ulcer disease), impaired glucose metabolism, mood swings, nervousness, appetite stimulation, psychosis, and adrenal-cortical insufficiency (chronic use)
- *Drug Interactions* – recommend that the practitioner look up each individual medication to research drug/drug interaction

Muscle Relaxants/Antispasticity Drugs

- Baclofen (Kemstro, Gablofen, Lioresal) [4]
  - *Mechanism of action:* In the CNS (along the spinal cord) by activating GABA$_B$ receptors [5].
  - *Indications*: Muscle spasm, amyotrophic lateral sclerosis (ALS), cerebral palsy, multiple sclerosis, and trigeminal neuralgia [6].
  - *Metabolism:* Oral half-life is 2–4 hours. Minimal biotransformation and so baclofen is predominantly excreted renal unchanged.
  - *Adverse Effects*: Sedation, urinary retention, hypotension, constipation [5], and withdrawal symptoms similar to benzodiazepine withdrawal [7].
  - *Drug Interactions*: Baclofen has an additive effect with imipramine and may cause short-term memory loss with antidepressants.
- Cyclobenzaprine (Amrix, Fexmid, Flexeril)
  - *Mechanism of Action*: Structurally related to TCAs and acts centrally to reduce tonic somatic motor activity.
  - *Indications*: Acute pain from muscle spasm, TMJ, and fibromyalgia (off-label) [5]
  - *Metabolism*: Hepatically metabolized to inactive metabolites, which are excreted renally. Also the drug undergoes enterohepatic recycling and excreted in feces via bile.
  - *Adverse Effects*: Drowsiness, dry mouth, dizziness, urinary retention, constipation, and withdrawal with chronic use [5].
  - *Drug Interactions:* May cause seizure when co-administered with tramadol and serotonin syndrome when given with MAOI, SSRI, tramadol, and other serotonergic agents.
- Tizanidine (Zanaflex) [8]
  - *Mechanism of Action*: Spinal and supraspinal alpha-2-agonist, which causes inhibition to excitatory spinal interneuron that regulates motor neurons.
  - *Indications:* Muscle spasticity, MS, and spinal cord injury.
  - *Metabolism*: Approximately 95% of an administered dose is metabolized. The primary cytochrome P450 isoenzyme involved in tizanidine metabolism is CYP1A2. Tizanidine metabolites are not known to be active; their half-lives range from 20 to 40 hours.
  - *Adverse Effects*: Sedation, drowsiness, hypotension, dry mouth, and transaminitis.
  - *Drug Interactions*: Increased effect with oral contraceptives. CYP1A2 inhibitors lead to increased levels of tizanidine.

- Methocarbamol (Robaxin)
  - *Mechanism of Action:* unknown, depresses CNS activity (central muscle relaxant), onset is 30 minutes with PO administration.
  - *Indications:* muscle spasms.
  - *Metabolism:* phase I and phase II hepatic metabolism, urine excretion, half-life 1–2 hours.
  - *Adverse Effects*: sedation, ataxia, nausea/vomiting, flushing, blurred vision, tachycardia, bradycardia, mood changes, fever, and hypersensitivity.
  - *Drug Interactions*: decreases seizure threshold.
- Chlorzoxazone (Lorzone, Parafon) [9]
  - *Mechanism of Action*: exact mechanism unknown, inhibits polysynaptic spinal reflexes→ increased muscle mobility and reduces spasticity. Take up to 1 hour for effects to manifest and usually last for up to 6 hours
  - *Indications:* muscle spasm
  - *Metabolism*: hepatic metabolism via glucuronidation, with renal excretion; half-life 1 hour
  - *Adverse Effects:* sedation, malaise, dyspepsia, anaphylaxis, hepatotoxicity, and GI bleeding
  - *Drug Interactions*: weak CYP3A4 inhibitor, but acts as a substrate for CYP2E1
- Carisoprodol (Soma) [13, 14]
  - *Mechanism of Action*: exact mechanism unknown, central muscle relaxant that is believed to interrupt neuronal communication, resulting in the alteration of pain perception. It should only be used for short periods (<1 month), as there is no evidence of effectiveness with prolonged use.
  - *Indications*: muscle spasm.
  - *Metabolism:* hepatic, via CYP2C19 into active metabolite: meprobamate. Half-life of meprobamate is 10 hours. Rapid onset, with a 4–6 hour duration. Urinary excretion of active metabolite.
  - *Adverse Effects*: sedation, headache, anaphylaxis, angioedema, orthostatic hypotension, seizures, erythema multiforme, and *abuse/addiction*.
  - *Drug Interactions:* acts as a substrate for CYP2C19.
- Metaxalone (Skelaxin)
  - *Mechanism of Action*: exact mechanism unknown, depresses CNS activity
  - *Indications*: muscle spasm
  - *Metabolism:* CYP450 hepatic metabolism, and urine excretion
  - *Adverse Effects:* sedation, malaise, nausea/vomiting, jaundice, anxiety, anaphylaxis, hemolytic anemia, and leukopenia
  - *Drug Interactions:* acts a substrate for the following enzymes: CYP1A2, CYP2C19, CYP2C8, CYP2C9, CYP2D6, CYP2E1, and CYP3A4

NMDA Antagonists

- Ketamine (Ketalar)
  - *Mechanism of Action:* NMDA antagonist, mu and kappa agonist, norepinephrine-serotonin-dopamine, and alpha-2-agonist. Provides dissociative anesthesia by acting on the limbic system and cortex.
  - *Indications*: Chronic opioid use, high tolerance/addiction, and anesthesia.
  - *Metabolism*: Hepatic, norketamine is an active metabolite.
  - *Adverse Effects*: Salivation, respiratory depression(at high doses), dysphoria, hallucinations, and sympathetic activation.
  - *Drug Interactions*: Ketamine is a CYP3A enzyme substrate. Mixing with diazepam or barbiturates may cause precipitation of drug.
- Methadone (Dolophine, Methadose) [15, 16]
  - *Mechanism of Action:* Levomethadone (R enantiomer) mu-opioid-receptor agonist, *dextromethadone (S enantiomer) NMDA receptor antagonist.*
  - *Indications:* Chronic opioid use – maintenance therapy, opioid detoxification in high tolerance/addiction.
  - *Metabolism:* Hepatic CYP3A4 and CYP2D6.
  - *Adverse Effects:* Sedation, dizziness, diarrhea or constipation, flushing, perspiration, dry mouth, hypotension, hallucinations, urinary retention, seizures, and QT prolongation potentially leading to Torsades de pointes.
  - *Drug Interactions:* Ketamine is a CYP3A enzyme substrate. Mixing with diazepam or barbiturates may cause precipitation of drug.

Local Anesthetics and Membrane-Stabilizing Drugs

- Amides: Bupivacaine (Marcaine), lidocaine (Xylocaine), mepivacaine (Carbocaine), prilocaine (Citanest), and ropivacaine (Naropin)
- Esters: Procaine (Novocaine), benzocaine (Topex, Orajel, Cepacol), and chloroprocaine (Nesacaine)
- *Mechanism of Action*: Block intracellular voltage-gated sodium channels decreasing nerve conduction
- *Indications*: Peripheral nerve block, sympathetic block, neuraxial, topical application, and IV infusion
- *Metabolism*: Amides – hepatic metabolism. Esters – plasma cholinesterase
- *Adverse Effects*: Seizures, tinnitus, cardiovascular collapse, apnea, and methemoglobinemia
- *Drug Interactions*: (Dapsone, quinine) may cause methemoglobinemia for benzocaine, prilocaine, and lidocaine in susceptible patients

Sympatholytic Drugs

- Clonidine (Catapres) and Alpha-Methyldopa (Dopamet, Aldomet)
  - *Mechanism of Action*: Alpha-2-agonist.
  - *Indications:* Alcohol and opiate withdrawal, ADHD, and hypertension.
  - *Metabolism:*. Metabolized hepatically and excreted in the urine and feces. Clonidine onset is 2–4 hours and lasts 6–10 hours.
  - *Adverse Effects:* Drowsiness, orthostatic hypotension, dry mouth, and rebound hypertension upon abrupt discontinuation.
  - *Drug Interactions:* May increase serum concentrations of cyclosporine, TCAs antagonize the cardiovascular effects of clonidine. Clonidine can prolong the blockade of local anesthetics.

Monoamine Oxidase Inhibitors

- Nonselective: Isocarboxazid (Marplan)
- Selective MAO-A inhibitors: Moclobemide (Aurorix)
- Selective MAO-B inhibitors: Selegiline (Zelapar, Deprenyl)

- *Mechanism of Action* – Inhibit catabolism of serotonin and norepinephrine and irreversibly bind both MAO-A and MAO-B (some selective and reversible agents exist, though not FDA approved).
- *Indication* – Major depression, Parkinson's disease (MAO-B selective selegiline).
- *Metabolism – Pharmacokinetics* – Metabolized by acetylation, some slow acetylators show increased plasma concentrations. Takes up to 2 weeks for MAO activity to recover due to irreversible binding; thus new MAO must be synthesized.
- *Adverse Effects* – Hypertensive crisis with overabundance of tyramine leading to adrenergic tone in the periphery.
- *Drug Interactions* – As above; serotonin syndrome with SSRIs, SNRIs, TCAs, bupropion, opioid agonists, alcohol, and anesthetic agents.

Other

- Orphenadrine (Norflex) [17]
- *Mechanism of Action* – considered and anticholinergic central muscle relaxant (nonselective mACHR antagonist), also inhibits histamine H_1 and NMDA receptors.
- *Indication* – muscle spasms/myalgias, and Parkinson's disease.

- *Metabolism* – orphenadrine is a derivative of diphenhydramine, available in various formulations mixed with aspirin, ibuprofen, acetaminophen, or codeine. It undergoes hepatic metabolism, primarily urine excretion, and some fecal excretion. Half-life 14 hours.
- *Adverse Effects* – palpitations, urinary hesitancy/retention, nausea/vomiting, constipation, sedation, and hallucinations.
- *Drug Interactions* – anticholinergic effects and CNS depression.

References

1. Gilman A, Gilman A, Goodman L. Goodman and Gilman's The pharmacological basis of therapeutics. New York: Pergamon; 1992.
2. Bleul U, Bylang T. Effects of doxapram, prethcamide and lobeline on spirometric, blood gas and acid–base variables in healthy newborn calves. Vet J. 2012;194(2):240–6.
3. tid. O, Epilepsy or other convulsive disorders p, Dyspnoea C, blockers. C, Stimulants R. prethcamide: indication, dosage, side effect, precaution I CIMS India [Internet]. Mims.com. 2018 [cited 5 March 2018]. Available from: http://www.mims.com/india/drug/info/prethcamide/prethcamide?type=full&mtype=generic.
4. Leo R, Baer D. Delirium associated with baclofen withdrawal: a review of common presentations and management strategies. Psychosomatics. 2005;46(6):503–7.
5. Berry H, Hutchinson D. A multicentre placebo-controlled study in general practice to evaluate the efficacy and safety of Tizanidine in acute low-back pain. J Int Med Res. 1988;16(2):75–82.
6. Delgado M, Hirtz D, Aisen M, Ashwal S, Fehlings D, McLaughlin J, et al. Practice parameter: pharmacologic treatment of spasticity in children and adolescents with cerebral palsy (an evidence-based review): report of the Quality Standards Subcommittee of the American Academy of Neurology and the Practice Committee of the Child Neurology Society. Neurology. 2010;74(4):336–43.
7. Malanga G, Reiter R, Garay E. Update on tizanidine for muscle spasticity and emerging indications. Expert Opin Pharmacother. 2008;9(12):2209–15.
8. Saper J, Lake A, Cantrell D, Winner P, White J. Chronic daily headache prophylaxis with Tizanidine: a double-blind, placebo-controlled, multicenter outcome study. Headache. 2002;42(6):470–82.
9. Desiraju R, Renzi N, Nayak R, Ng K. Pharmacokinetics of Chlorzoxazone in Humans. J Pharm Sci. 1983;72(9):991–4.
10. Backer R, Zumwalt R, McFeeley P, Veasey S, Wohlenberg N. Carisoprodol concentrations from different anatomical sites: three overdose cases. J Anal Toxicol. 1990;14(5):332–4.
11. D G. Carisoprodol toxicity. - PubMed - NCBI [Internet]. Ncbi.nlm.nih.gov. 2018 [cited 5 March 2018]. Available from: https://www.ncbi.nlm.nih.gov/pubmed/?term=Goldberg+Carisoprodol+Toxicity.
12. Olsen H, Koppang E, Alvan G, Morland J. Carisoprodol elimination in humans. Ther Drug Monit. 1994;16(4):337–40.
13. TOTH P, URTIS J. Commonly used muscle relaxant therapies for acute low back pain: a review of carisoprodol, cyclobenzaprine hydrochloride, and metaxalone. Clin Ther. 2004;26(9):1355–67.
14. Skelaxin (by Cardinal Health) [Internet]. Drugs-Library.com. 2018 [cited 5 March 2018]. Available from: http://www.bing.com/cr?IG=DC13866D43374747B69AF890EABE3953&CID=0701C67FEFB56B6228A8CDD6EE1A6A99&rd=1&h=Nw

qa4BJ-YOh4yjhBaR27wdfAnjopgu5vxz4mF-ELP7U&v=1&r=
http%3a%2f%2fwww.drugs-library.com%2fdrugs%2fskelaxin.
html&p=DevEx,5327.1.

15. Trafton J, Ramani A. Methadone: a new old drug with promises and pitfalls. Curr Pain Headache Rep. 2009;13(1):24–30.

16. Layson-Wolf C, Goode J, Small R. Clinical use of methadone. J Pain Palliat Care Pharmacother. 2002;16(1):29–59.

17. Clarke B. Acute poisoning with orphenadrine. Lancet. 1985;325(8442):1386.

Psychological Treatments

Isaac Cohen

Cognitive and Behavioral Strategies: Application to Specific Pain Syndromes

The International Association for the Study of Pain (IASP) defines pain as "An unpleasant sensory and emotional experience associated with actual or potential damage, or described in terms of such damage" [1]. This definition of pain acknowledges that pain is a multidimensional sensory-perceptual phenomenon. The traditional Western biomedical model posits that pain is due to clearly identifiable tissue injury and presents a dichotomy of pain being either physical or psychological. In practice, this dichotomy is rarely absolute. The biopsychosocial model of illness is more consistent with the IASP definition, incorporating psychological and social elements to understand pain from a broader perspective. The implication is that optimal patient care will be delivered by physicians aware of and skilled in the assessment and management of psychosocial components of illness.

The rationale for psychological treatment is to address cognitive, emotional, and social elements to mitigate suffering and improve function. The main objectives for psychological treatment are to diminish stress, reduce medication intake, decrease healthcare utilization, and increase physical activity and resumption of life responsibilities such as functioning at home and return to work.

Reactions to pain are mediated by cognitive processes that enable people to perceive and interpret reality. Thoughts can influence and elicit mood and behavioral responses. Errors in cognition or unhelpful cognitions produce negative interpretations of the pain experience that persist even in spite of evidence to the contrary. A large body of literature demonstrates associations between pain beliefs and adherence to treatment, function and treatment outcomes [2–7]. Several studies have demonstrated that disability is more strongly associated with psychosocial variables than biomedical factors [8]. Studies show that those with high fear-avoidance beliefs may have higher levels of distress, greater utilization of healthcare resources, functional impairment, and increased opioid usage [9, 10]. Collectively, these studies underscore the importance of cognitions and emotions in the pain experience. During history taking, the clinician should look for pain fears and beliefs in the patient's narrative, such as pain indicates physical harm or that one is disabled because of the pain. The Fear-Avoidance Beliefs Questionnaire (FABQ) [11] and Tampa Scale of Kinesiophobia (TSK) [12] are examples of standardized assessment tools used in practice and research to quantify pain-related fears and beliefs. Cognitive therapy (e.g., cognitive restructuring) teaches patients to identify their thoughts and beliefs about pain and evaluate whether these cognitions are accurate or helpful and how to challenge and replace inaccurate or unhelpful beliefs with ones that are more accurate and balanced.

For example, "I cannot function when I am in pain" can be changed to "I am going to continue to live my life in spite of my pain." There is variability in the nature, mode, and context of cognitive interventions, and debate exists as to the efficacy of different approaches.

The goal of behavioral therapy is to restore functioning by modifying overt pain behaviors that can interfere with recovery. Behavioral therapy is most appropriate when pain behaviors are judged to be in excess of what would be expected by findings on physical examination and imaging. Pain behaviors are the outward expressions of pain and suffering, reflecting attitudes and beliefs of an individual toward nociceptive input. Pain behaviors are influenced by anxiety, family, cultural, and environmental elements. Simple pain behaviors may include verbal expressions or non-verbal expressions such as grimacing, posturing, and limping. More complex behaviors include functional limitations, changes in social interaction, or seeking health care. The perpetuation of pain behaviors contributes to suffering and disability by limiting one's activity and functioning. According to the operant

I. Cohen (✉)
Frank H. Netter School of Medicine, Quinnipiac University, Hamden, CT, USA

© Springer Nature Switzerland AG 2019
Y. Khelemsky et al. (eds.), *Academic Pain Medicine*, https://doi.org/10.1007/978-3-030-18005-8_16

Table 16.1 Behavioral coping strategies

Technique	Description
Relaxation	Deep breathing, positive self-statements, guided imagery
Guided imagery	Using imagination to create pleasant experiences and promote sense of well-being
Meditation	Focusing on one thing at a time, mindfulness of thoughts
Self-help organizations	Providing sense of not being alone, decreasing social isolation

conditioning model, these behaviors might initially be responses to nociceptive biological stimuli, but subsequently may come under the control of environmental consequences (contingencies). Behaviors that are positively reinforced tend to increase in frequency and be maintained over time, whereas behaviors that are not reinforced or punished (negative reinforcement) are likely to decrease in frequency or be extinguished.

The basic assumption of the operant model is that change in pain behaviors can occur via manipulation of contingencies. The patient should be questioned about the impact of pain on activities and how significant others respond to these pain behaviors. Positive reinforcement for pain behaviors is often provided by family, friends, co-workers, and healthcare providers. Positive reinforcement may include responses such as a spouse expressing concern, injured worker receiving financial benefits, or physician prescribing desired pain medication. Healthcare providers and family members should ignore pain behaviors to decrease their frequency and provide positive reinforcement for engaging in well behaviors. In addition to extinction of pain behaviors, patients can be provided with helpful behavioral coping strategies (Table 16.1).

Specific Conditions

Low Back Pain/Neck Pain

Individuals with chronic low back and neck pain often harbor strong pain beliefs, fear of activities and believe that exercise may increase pain or cause further injury. Many healthcare providers may have similar concerns: they do not perceive persons with spinal pain as having the potential to perform normal or strenuous activities, and are cautious about recommending exercises that may be stressful or elicit pain [13]. For successful rehabilitation of the chronic neck or back pain, patient must focus on lessening pain behaviors and encouraging self-management and a wellness lifestyle. The cognitive-behavioral approach requires that the treatment team have firm beliefs that the potential for normal function exists in spite of pain and consistently express this to patients. Team members must understand pain-related ill-

ness behaviors and the impact of psychosocial factors on reported pain and disability. All members of the healthcare team need to present a united front in the belief that functioning is not necessarily dictated by pain levels and that patients can function in the presence of pain. Patients are reassured that pain intensity does not indicate disease severity and that it is "safe" for individuals with neck and low back pain to exercise. Pain behaviors are ignored to decrease their frequency, and wellness behaviors (i.e., increasing activities in spite of pain, completion of exercises, etc.) are positively reinforced with praise and encouragement.

Goals for physical therapy should be stated at the outset as concrete, objective, measurable, and functional. Aggressive, quota-based, non-pain contingent physical therapy addresses impairments in strength, flexibility, and endurance while enabling a graded exposure to fearful activities. Improving exercise performance is fed back to the patient to improve self-efficacy and reinforce that wellness can be acquired despite ongoing symptoms. Studies support that significant reductions of pain and improved function are possible with the above approach [14–16].

Fibromyalgia

Fibromyalgia (FM) is a relatively common syndrome of chronic idiopathic widespread pain, accompanied by other clinical manifestations such as sleep disturbance, fatigue, irritable bowel syndrome, headaches, cognitive dysfunction, and mood disorders [17]. Currently, there are no curative treatments for patients with fibromyalgia. The multifaceted nature of this condition suggests that a multimodal treatment program may be necessary to achieve optimal outcomes. It has been shown that the inclusion of cognitive-behavioral therapy as part of the treatment regimen for patients with FM improves physical functioning [18]. Stress management, pacing oneself with activities, and coping strategies are strategies that are commonly employed. A systematic review and meta-analysis of randomized controlled trials of cognitive-behavioral therapy for fibromyalgia concluded that cognitive-behavioral therapy improves coping with pain and reduces depressed mood and health-seeking behavior [19]. Furthermore, a Cochrane review of CBT therapy in FM showed a small incremental benefit over control interventions in reducing pain, negative mood, and disability at the end of treatment and 6-month follow-up [20].

Postoperative Pain

An integral component of clinical pathways for various surgeries, preoperative patient education provides patients with appropriate information to assist in postoperative recovery. The patient gains a better understanding of their physical condition and self-care using the experience and guidance of the multidisciplinary team. Preoperative patient education typically consists of group classes covering a host of topics encompassing the surgical procedure and its benefits, symptom management, operative risks, and discharge planning. There are potential benefits in terms of shortened length of stays and less patient dissatisfaction from unmet expectations [21]. Although numerous studies have suggested the preoperative patient education as being effective in reducing length of stay of orthopedic patients [22], the literature remains divided on the effect of preoperative education on pain level and functional ability. One review found that knowledge, anxiety, pain, length of stay, performance of exercise and mobilization, self-efficacy, patient compliance, adherence, and empowerment were all improved as a result of patient education. In contrast, a more recent review was unable to determine if pre-op education offers benefits over usual care in terms of anxiety, pain, function, and adverse events, but acknowledged that education can a useful adjunct with low risk of adverse effects, particularly in those with depression, anxiety, or unrealistic expectations [23].

Burn Pain

Non-pharmacologic treatments have been reported to be effective in reducing burn pain in both children and adults and may serve as useful adjuncts to pharmacologic analgesia. Research suggests that attention to pain plays a role in pain perception. Cognitive techniques for diverting attention away from pain include hypnotherapy and distraction [24–27]. Examples of distraction techniques include deep breathing, videos, listening to music, or playing video games. The success of these treatments has led to the innovative use of virtual reality (VR) as a distraction technique. VR diverts attention away from pain by immersing patients in pleasant, rich and engaging computer generated environments. In recent studies, the use of VR has been found to be effective in reducing pain and distress in burn patients undergoing joint range of motion exercises in physical/occupational therapy or burn care [25–31].

Temporomandibular Joint Pain (TMJ)

TMJ is characterized by pain in the face, jaw, head, or ear that originates from the temporomandibular joint. In many cases, the anatomic etiology of pain cannot be identified, and pain is thought to be caused by stress or habits that result in increased muscle tension and jaw clenching. Patients should be counseled on behavior modification techniques such as stress reduction, sleep hygiene, elimination of habits (i.e., teeth clenching, pencil chewing, etc.), and avoidance of extreme mandibular movement (i.e., excessive jaw opening during yawning, brushing teeth or flossing, etc.). Increased levels of Electromyography (EMG) activity over muscles have been decreased using biofeedback in patients who are jaw clenchers or exhibit bruxism (teeth grinding). A Cochrane review supports the use of cognitive-behavior therapy and biofeedback in both short-term and long-term pain management in patients with symptomatic TMJ when compared to usual management [32].

Integration of Approaches

Cognitive-Behavioral Treatments

Cognitive-behavioral therapy (CBT) acknowledges the importance of both cognitions and behaviors in the acquisition and maintenance of pain behaviors. Cognitive-behavioral treatment focuses on cognitions, affective factors, and coping mechanisms. There is increasing literature correlating changes in patients' pain beliefs with changes in functioning [4, 33]. These studies provide empirical support for the hypothesis that cognitions play a key role in adjustment to chronic pain, and that behaviors can impact cognition. CBT employs a wide range of cognitive and behaviorally focused interventions addressing beliefs about pain that interfere with functioning and provides effective strategies for managing stress and pain. CBT techniques are most often employed in conjunction with other treatment modalities in an interdisciplinary approach to pain management. Patients with minimal pain beliefs may respond well to focused CBT provided by the clinician in the office, whereas patients strongly entrenched in their beliefs may benefit from a more structured cognitive-behavioral treatment program or working with other healthcare providers such as physical therapists or psychologists familiar in employing this approach.

Combined Behavioral and Drug Treatments

Combined behavioral and drug treatments should be considered in the setting of comorbid psychiatric disorders. Chronic pain and psychiatric disorders frequently coexist, and individuals with chronic pain are more likely to have depression or anxiety than the general population [34]. The association between depression and chronic pain has received much research attention. Relative to depression, anxiety disorders have received less attention in the chronic pain literature, likely reflecting the greater prevalence of depression than anxiety in this population. The prevalence of depression in chronic pain patients ranges from 12% to 72% of patients in specialist pain settings, depending on case definitions and populations studied [35–38]. The prevalence of anxiety in pain disorders ranges from 16.5% to 35%, with estimates again varying with case definitions and populations studied [38–40]. Patients with chronic pain may have a preexisting psychiatric disorder or report the onset of depression or anxiety after experiencing pain [41–43]. The coexistence of depression has been shown to incur additive adverse effects on patient outcomes, including poor functioning and reduced response to treatment [44–48]. The presence of anxiety has been shown to lead to more frequent reports of pain [49]. If depression and anxiety modify the relationship between chronic pain and outcomes, this suggests that improved detection and treatment of these underlying conditions may reduce the burden of chronic pain on both the individual and society. Psychiatric disorders should thus be sought after and addressed to maximize health and functioning of patients. Selective integration of anxiolytic or antidepressant medications may potentially augment CBT. Oftentimes, medications can serve dual purposes by treating the underlying psychiatric disorder and pain condition. For example, antidepressants may address both depression and neuropathic pain [50].

Economic Benefits of Integrating Treatment

There is great interest in determining the cost-effectiveness of CBT given its clinical effectiveness. The cumulative evidence to date suggests, but not definitive for, the cost-effectiveness of CBT for various pain conditions across different settings. For low back pain, numerous European studies from the employer, societal, and national healthcare perspectives have found cost-effectiveness in various circumstances [51–54]. In fibromyalgia patients, a 6-month multicenter Spanish RCT revealed significantly lower costs per patient in the CBT group than those receiving drug therapy or treatment as usual [55]. In patients with temporomandibular disorders, an RCT examining the cost-effectiveness of biopsychosocial intervention (cognitive-behavioral skills and biofeedback) in patients at high risk of progressing from acute to chronic TMJ-related pain demonstrated reduced jaw-related healthcare expenditures in the experimental group relative to treatment as usual [56].

Stages of Behavior Changes and Their Effect on Readiness to Adopt Self-Management Strategies for Chronic Pain

Successful cognitive-behavioral treatment for chronic pain requires active participation from the patient and personal motivation to establish and follow through with behavioral changes. The transtheoretical model [57, 58] is an integrative psychosocial model that conceptualizes the process of intentional behavior change into five stages. As opposed to the traditional view of behavior change as a discrete event (i.e., quitting smoking, etc.), the transtheoretical model proposes that people move through a series of stages over time when modifying behavior. The stages are precontemplation, contemplation, preparation, action, and maintenance (Table 16.2). Each stage is accompanied by specific chal-

Table 16.2 Transtheoretical model: stages of behavior change

Stage of behavior change	Description	Clinical approach
Precontemplation	Individual has not yet considered change; often resistant to change when suggested by others	Increase patient awareness of problems/risks with current behaviors
Contemplation	Recognition of a problem or need to change	Elicit from the patient reasons for change and downsides of not changing
Preparation	Commitment to change; initial steps toward behavioral changes	Assist patient in determining most appropriate course of action
Action	Engaging in behaviors directed toward desired change	Assistance by clinician
Maintenance	Continuing with any changes made in action stage	Reviewing progress made; solidifying motivation and commitment as needed

lenges that must be overcome before moving onto the next stage. Although the ultimate responsibility lies with the patient, the clinician can facilitate behavior change by appropriately timing interventions to enhance patient motivation.

Integral to the success of motivational interviewing is assessing the patient's readiness to change the behavior according to the relative progress through the stages.

The interviewer determines the stage that the patient is in, and tailors the approach accordingly. A poorly timed or mismatched intervention would likely be futile or met with resistance. Key principles in motivational interviewing are empathy, pointing out discrepancies between current behaviors and goals, avoiding argumentation, and supporting self-efficacy (the belief in the ability to perform a specific task or behavior). If an individual is not able to sustain these changes over time, they can relapse and re-enter the stages at any point. Relapses are dealt with by addressing obstacles that might have led to the relapse, and minimizing discouragement by reassurance that behavioral change often requires multiple attempts.

Cognitive-Behavioral and Management Interventions: Common Process Factors

The doctor-patient relationship is an important factor in cognitive-behavioral intervention, and communication is paramount to establish rapport. Pain and disability can give rise to numerous and complex emotional reactions, such as anxiety of the unknown, sadness, depression about losses or potential losses, and anger regarding the impact of illness.

The manner in which the physician responds to these emotions will largely determine the overall quality of the doctor-patient relationship. Empathic listening and reassurance are the cornerstones of developing rapport. The need to be validated by the medical community that the pain is real is one of the most important needs. Conveying to the patient "It's all in your head" can be alienating and trigger defensiveness. Refraining from classifying the problem as exclusively either physical or psychological and tactfully explaining that pain is a mind-body problem can be validating constructive and facilitate communication and education. A helpful starting point is explaining how their response to pain plays a role in maintaining their predicament. According to the fear-avoidance model, a vicious cycle can become established when activity is avoided in response to pain, causing deconditioning and fears to set in, leading to further activity avoidance, with the end result being increasing pain and functional decline over time [59, 60]. This paradigm helps explain the downward spiral of how patients become chronic pain patients and presents a scenario that many patients can identify with.

Aligning the patient's expectations with the physician's expectations is important for patient satisfaction with treatment. Often, the source of the patient's pain is not well understood, or cannot be abolished. In those instances, it is helpful to explain that medical science has not been able to find a complete answer to their condition. The expectations for treatment should be prefixed with a discussion of the concepts of "cure" versus "control." Pain often can be controlled to some extent, but not cured, similar to other medical conditions like hypertension or diabetes. Refocusing on symptom management and coping can direct treatment efforts toward more appropriate goals, such as a shift in focus from pain to non-pain aspects of life. A number of studies have shown that greater acceptance of chronic pain is associated with better emotional, physical, and social functioning [61].

Multiple factors can contribute to patients' beliefs about their pain, including past experiences, the Internet, friends and family. Nevertheless, healthcare providers have the strongest influence on patients' beliefs, and studies have shown that people regard their clinicians as the primary source of information and advice, despite the growth of the Internet [62–64]. Ominous terms such as "disc degeneration" can conjure images of progressive pain and dysfunction. Positive expectations can be engendered in patients by reframing anatomic changes in a more positive manner, such as commenting that imaging reveals no evidence of serious or surgical pathology or reveals age-appropriate changes. A healthcare provider's advice to patients concerning appropriate levels of activities may have substantial impact, both positive and negative, on clinical outcomes. For example, advice that is safe to resume normal activities in spite of pain has been demonstrated to decrease disability in randomized controlled trials of acute and subacute low back pain [65, 66]. In subjects with chronic low back pain, effective rehabilitation has been demonstrated using advice that exercise and activity are safe in the presence of chronic back pain [67–69].

References

1. Merskey H, Bogduk N, Part III. Pain terms, a current list with definitions and notes on usage. Classification of chronic pain. 2nd ed. Seattle: IASP task force on taxonomy, IASP press; 1994. p. 209–14.
2. Vlaeyen JW, Kole-Snijders AM, Boeren RG, van Eck H. Fear of movement/(re) injury in chronic low back pain and its relation to behavioral performance. Pain. 1995;62:363–72.
3. Al Obaidi SM, Nelson RM, Al-Awadhi S, Al-Shuwaie N. The role of anticipation and fear of pain in the persistence of avoidance behavior in patients with chronic low back pain. Spine. 2000;25:1126–31.
4. Moseley GL. Evidence for a direct relationship between cognitive and physical change during an education intervention in people with chronic low back pain. Eur J Pain. 2004;8:39–45.
5. Thompson EL, Broadbent J, Bertino MD, Staiger PK. Do pain-related beliefs influence adherence to multidisciplinary rehabilitation? A systematic review. Clin J Pain. 2016;32(2):164–78.
6. Camacho-Soto A, Sowa GA, Perera S, Weiner DK. Fear avoidance beliefs predict disability in older adults with chronic low back pain. PM R. 2012;4:493–7.
7. Alodaibi FA, Minick KI, Fritz JM. Do preoperative fear avoidance model factors predict outcomes after lumbar disc herniation surgery? A systematic review. Chiropr Man Therap. 2013;21:40.
8. Carragee EJ, Alamin TF, Miller JL, Carragee JM. Discographic, MRI and psychosocial determinants of low back pain disability and remission: a prospective study in subjects with benign persistent back pain. Spine J. 2005;5:24–35.
9. Shulman BM. Worklessness and disability: expansion of the biopsychosocial perspective. J Occup Rehabil. 1994;4:113–22.
10. McGrail MP, Calasanz M, Christianson J, et al. The Minnesota health partnership and coordinated health care and disability prevention: the implementation of an integrated benefits and medical care model. J Occup Rehabil. 2002;12:43–54.
11. Waddell G, Newton M, Henderson I, Somerville D, Main CJ. A fear-avoidance beliefs questionnaire (FABQ) and the role of fear-avoidance beliefs in chronic low back pain and disability. Pain. 1993;52:157–68.
12. Kori SH, Miller RP, Todd DD. Kinesiophobia: a new view of chronic pain behavior. Pain Manag. 1990;3:35–43.
13. Rainville J, Carlson N, Polatin P, Gatchel RJ, Indahl A. Exploration of physicians' recommendations for activities in chronic low back pain. Spine. 2000;25:2210–20.
14. Rainville J, Hartigan C, Martinez E, et al. Exercise as a treatment for chronic low back pain. Spine J. 2004;4:106–15.
15. Brox JI, Reikeras O, Nygaard O, et al. Lumbar instrumented fusion compared with cognitive intervention and exercises in patients with chronic low back pain after previous surgery for disc herniation: a prospective randomized controlled study. Pain. 2006;112:145 55.
16. Fairbank J, Frost J, Wilson-MacDonald J, et al. Randomized controlled trial to compare surgical stabilization of the lumbar spine with an intensive rehabilitation program for patients with chronic low back pain: the MRC spine stabilization trial. BMJ. 2005;330:1239–45.
17. Clauw DJ. Fibromyalgia: a clinical review. JAMA. 2014;311(15):1547–55.
18. Williams DA. Psychological and behavioral therapies in FM and related syndromes. Best Pract Res Clin Rheumatol. 2003;17:649–65.

19. Bernardy K, Fuber N, Kollner V, Hauser W. Efficacy of cognitive behavioral therapies in fibromylagia syndrome – a systematic review and metaanalysis of randomized controlled trials. J Rhematol. 2010;37(10):1991–2005.

20. Bernardy K, Klose P, Busch AJ, Choy EH, Hauser W. Cognitive behavioral therapies for fibromyalgia. Cochrane Database Syst Rev. 2013;10(9):CD009796. https://doi.org/10.1002/14651858. CD009796.pub2.

21. Moulton LS, Evans PA, Starks I, Smith T. Pre-operative education prior to elective hip arthroplasty surgery improves postoperative outcome. Int Orthop. 2015;39(8):1483–6.

22. Majid N, Lee S, Plummer V. The effectiveness of orthopedic patient education in improving patient outcomes: a systematic review protocol. JBI Database System Rev Implement Rep. 2015;13(1):122–33.

23. McDonald S, Page MJ, Beringer K, Wasiak J, Sprowson A. Preoperative education for hip or knee replacement. Cochrane Database Syst Rev. 2014;13(5):CD003526. https://doi. org/10.1002/14651858.CD003526.pub3.

24. Patterson DR. Practical applications of psychological techniques in controlling burn pain. J Burn Care Rehabil. 1992;13:13–8.

25. Van der Does AJ, Van Dyck R, Spijker RE. Hypnosis and pain in patients with severe burns: a pilot study. Burns Incl Therm Inj. 1988;14:399–404.

26. Patterson DR, Questad KA, de-Lateur BJ. Hypnotherapy as an adjunct to narcotic analgesia for the treatment of pain for the burn debridement. Am J Clin Hypn. 1989;31:156–63.

27. Everett JJ, Patterson DR, Burns GL, et al. Adjunctive interventions for burn pain control: comparison of hypnosis and ativan: the 1993 Clinical Research Award. J Burn Care Rehabil. 1993;14:676–83.

28. Hoffman HG, Patterson DR, Carrougher GJ. Use of virtual reality for adjunctive treatment of adult burn pain during physical therapy. A controlled study. Clin J Pain. 2000;16(3):244–50.

29. Hoffman HG, Patterson DR, Carrougher GJ, et al. Effectiveness of virtual reality-based pain control with multiple treatments. Clin J Pain. 2001;17(3):229–35.

30. Schmitt YS, Hoffman HG, Blough DK, et al. A randomized, controlled trial of immersive virtual reality analgesia, during physical therapy for pediatric burns. Burns. 2011;37(1):61–8.

31. Carrougher GJ, Hoffman HG, Nakamura DY, et al. The effect of virtual reality on pain and range of motion in adults with burn injuries. J Burn Care Res. 2009;30(5):785–91.

32. Aggarwal VR, Lovell K, Peters S, et al. Psychological interventions for the management of chronic orofacial pain. Cochrane Database Syst Rev. 2011;(11):CD008456.

33. Jensen MP, Romano JM, Turner JA, et al. Patient beliefs predict patient functioning: further support for a cognitive-behavioural model of chronic pain. Pain. 1999;81(1–2):95–104.

34. Mc Williams LA, Cox BJ, Enns M. Mood and anxiety disorders associated with chronic pain: an examination in a nationally representative sample. Pain. 2003;106(1–2):127–33.

35. Ho PT, Li CF, Ng YK, Tsui SL, Ng KF. Prevalence of and factors associated with psychiatric morbidity in chronic pain patients. J Psychosom Res. 2011;70:541–7.

36. Poole H, White S, Blake C, Murphy P, Bramwell R. Depression in chronic pain patients: prevalence and measurement. Pain Pract. 2009;9:173–80.. Proctor SL, Estroff TW, Empting LD, Shearer-Williams S, Hoffmann NG. Prevalence of substance use and psychiatric disorders in a highly select chronic pain population. J Addict Med. 2013;7:17–24.

37. Sagheer MA, Khan MF, Sharif S. Association between chronic low back pain, anxiety and depression in patients at a tertiary care centre. J Pak Med Assoc. 2013;63:688–90.

38. Fishbain DA, Cutler RB, Rosomoff HL, Rosomoff RS. Comorbid psychiatric disorders and chronic pain. Curr Rev Pain. 1998;2:1–10.

39. McWilliams LA, Cox BJ, Enns MW. Mood and anxiety disorders associated with chronic pain: an examination in a nationally representative sample. Pain. 2003;106(1–2):127–33.

40. McWilliams LA, Goodwin RD, Cox BJ. Depression and anxiety associated with three pain conditions: results from a nationally representative sample. Pain. 2004;111(1–2):77–83.

41. Kinney RK, Gatchel RJ, Polatin PB, Fogarty WT, Mayer TG. Prevalence of psychopathology in acute and chronic low back pain patients. J Occup Rehabil. 1993;3(2):95–103.

42. Atkinson JH, Slater MA, Patterson TL, Grant I, Garfin SR. Prevalence, onset, and risk of psychiatric disorders in men with chronic low back pain: a controlled study. Pain. 1991;45(2):111–21.

43. Fishbain D, Cutler R, Rosomoff H, et al. Chronic pain-associated depression: antecedent or consequence of chronic pain? A review. Clin J Pain. 1997;13:116–37.

44. Rayner L, Hotopf M, Petkova H, Matcham F, Simpson A, McCracken LM. Depression in patients with chronic pain attending a specialized pain treatment centre: prevalence and impact on healthcare costs. Pain. 2016;157(7):1472–9.

45. Arnow BA, Hunkeler EM, Blasey CM, Lee J, Constantino MJ, Fireman B, Kraemer HC, Dea R, Robinson R, Hayward C. Comorbid depression, chronic pain, and disability in primary care. Psychosom Med. 2006;68:262–8.

46. Sullivan MJ, Adams H, Tripp D, Stanish WD. Stage of chronicity and treatment response in patients with musculoskeletal injuries and concurrent symptoms of depression. Pain. 2008;135:151–9.

47. Lamb SE, Guralnik JM, Buchner DM, et al. Factors that modify the association between knee pain and mobility limitation in older women: the women's health and aging study. Ann Rheum Dis. 2000;59(5):331–7.

48. Burton AK, Tillotson KM, Main CJ, Hollis S. Psychosocial predictors of outcome in acute and subchronic low back trouble. Spine. 1995;20(6):722–8.

49. Ferguson RJ, Ahles TA. Private body consciousness, anxiety and pain symptom reports of chronic pain patients. Behav Res Ther. 1998;36(5):527–35.

50. Mercier A, Auger-Aubin I, Lebeau JP, Schulers M, Boulet P, Hermil JL, VanRoyen P, Peremans L. Evidence of prescription of antidepressants for non-psychiatric conditions in primary care: an analysis of guidelines and systematic reviews. BMC Fam Pract 2013;May 4;14:55. Doi:10.1186/1471-2296-14-55. Saarto T, Wiffen PJ. Antidepressants for neuropathic pain. Cochrane Database Syst Rev. 2007;(4):CD005454.

51. Lamb SE, Hansen Z, Lall R, et al. Group cognitive behavioural treatment for low-back pain in primary care: a randomized controlled trial and cost-effectiveness analysis. Lancet. 2010;375:916–23.

52. Lambeek LC, Bosmans JE, Van Royen BJ, et al. Effect of integrated care for sick listed patients with chronic low back pain: economic evaluation alongside a randomised controlled trial. BMJ. 2010;340:c1035.

53. Hlobil H, Uegaki K, Staal JB, et al. Substantial sick-leave costs savings due to a graded activity intervention for workers with nonspecific subacute low back pain. Eur Spine J. 2007;16:919–24.

54. Schweikert B, Jacobi E, Seitz R, et al. Effectiveness and cost-effectiveness of adding a cognitive-behavioral treatment to the rehabilitation of chronic low back pain. J Rheumatol. 2006;33:2519–26.

55. Luciano J, D'Amico F, Cerda-Lafont M, Penarrubia-Maria M, Knapp M, Cuesta-Vargas A, Serrano-Blanco A, Garcia-Campayo J. Cost-utility of cognitive-behavioral therapy versus U.S. Food and Drug Administration recommended drugs and usual care in the treatment of patients with fibromyalgia: an economic evaluation alongside a 6-month randomized controlled trial. Arthritis Res Ther. 2014;16:451. http://arthritis-research.com/content/16/5/451.

56. Stowell AW, Gatchel RJ, Wildenstein L. Cost-effectiveness of treatments for temporomandibular disorders: biopsychoso-

cial intervention versus treatment as usual. J Am Dent Assoc. 2007;138(2):202–8.

57. Prochaska JO, DiClemente CC, Norcross JC. In search of how people change: applications to the addictive behaviors. Am Psychol. 1992;47:1102–14.

58. Proschaska JO, Redding CA, Evers K. The transtheoretical model and stages of change. In: Glanz K, Rimer BK, Lewis FM, editors. Health behavior and health education: theory, research and practice. 3rd ed. San Francisco: Jossey-Bass, Inc.

59. Lethem J, Slade PD, Troup JDG, Bentley G. Outline of a fear-avoidance model of exaggerated pain perception. Behav Res Ther. 1983;21:401–8.

60. Vlaeyen JW, Linton SJ. Fear avoidance and its consequences in chronic musculoskeletal pain: a state of the art. Pain. 2000;85:317–32.

61. McCracken LM, Vowles KE, Eccleston C. Acceptance-based treatment for persons with complex, long standing pain: a preliminary analysis of treatment outcome in comparison to a waiting phase. Behav Res Ther. 2005;43(10):1335–46.

62. Briggs AM, Jordan JE, Buchbinder R, et al. Health literacy and beliefs among a community cohort with and without chronic low back pain. Pain. 2010;150(2):275–83.

63. Sillence E, Briggs P, Harris PR, Fishwick L. How do patients evaluate and make use of online health information? Soc Sci Med. 2007;64(9):1853–62.

64. Darlow B, Dowell A, Baxter GD, Mathieson F, Perry M, Dean S. The enduring impact of what clinicians say to people with low back pain. Ann Fam Med. 2013;11(6):527–34.

65. Indahl A, Velund L, Reikeraas O. Good prognosis for low back pain left untampered: a randomized clinical trial. Spine. 1995;20:4730–7.

66. Malmivaara A, Hakkinen U, Aro T, et al. The treatment of acute low back pain: bed rest, exercise, or ordinary activity? N Engl J Med. 1995;332:351–5.

67. Hazard RG, Fenwick JW, Kalisch SW, et al. Functional restoration with behavioral support. A one year prospective study of patients with low back pain. Spine. 1989;14:157–61.

68. Mayer TG, Gatchel RJ, Kishino N, et al. Objective assessment of spine function following industrial injury. A prospective study with comparison group and 1-year follow-up. Spine. 1985;10:482–93.

69. Rainville J, Ahern DK, Phalen I, et al. The association of pain with physical activities. Spine. 1992;17:1060–4.

Psychiatric Treatment

17

Ravi Prasad, Amir Ramezani, Robert McCarron,
and Sylvia Malcore

Psychiatric and Psychologic Morbidities of Chronic Pain

The literature reflects significant overlap between mental health symptoms and patients who have chronic pain. This overlap has been demonstrated across studies in multiple countries, including Hong Kong [1], Singapore [2], Canada [3], New Zealand [4], Finland [5], and the United States [6]. Studies have typically noted associations among depression, anxiety, substance use, and somatoform disorders [1, 2, 5]. Psychiatric conditions may also vary across specific pain conditions: for example, migraines are associated with alcohol use disorders, generalized anxiety disorder, and major depressive disorder (MDD); back pain is associated with MDD; and arthritis is associated with MDD and alcohol use disorder [2].

Depression and anxiety have generally shown the highest rates of comorbidity among individuals with chronic pain, with study results for concurrent rates of MDD and chronic back pain ranging from 19.8% [3] to 66.3% [6] and concurrent rates of anxiety disorders and chronic pain ranging from 18% [1] to 62.5% [7]. Concurrent rates of substance abuse have been reported at 12% [5] to 18% [1], and somatoform disorders have been reported in the 30% range [1, 7]. Personality disorders have also reflected higher rates of comorbidity [7, 8]. In addition, lifetime rates of psychiatric conditions in patients who have chronic pain were found to be higher [5, 9]. There are a number of possible underlying factors for the differing reported rates of psychiatric conditions in individuals who have chronic pain, including the lack of reliable structured criteria in studies [1]. In addition, there are a number of potential methodological differences, such as diagnoses/symptom criteria used and sample differences [7]. Methodological issues have continued to persist in more recent studies and will likely continue considering recent changes to the DSM-5 [10]. The DSM-5 reflects a reconceptualization of the mind-body relationship for somatic symptoms and related disorders, and there are significant changes in symptom criteria between DSM-IV and DSM-5 which impact current estimates of comorbidity. It is relevant to note that not all psychiatric conditions have been found to have consistently higher rates in patients who have chronic pain; for example, bipolar disorder shows little association [1].

The cause and effect relationship between psychiatric conditions and chronic pain is not fully understood. Some evidence suggests that the majority of patients with mood disorders had the onset of the disorder *after* the onset of pain (63%), whereas 77% of patients with an anxiety disorder had the diagnosis *prior* to the onset of pain [5]. This may speak to underlying etiology and risk factors for developing chronic pain, as well as adjustment. It is well established that patients who have chronic pain have higher rates of trauma histories [11] and PTSD has been associated with report of somatic symptoms [12]. Abuse history has been associated with mental health symptoms and reported pain [11, 13]. While the relationship between trauma and pain is not fully understood, a centrally mediated process has been proposed [13]. Data from twin studies has also demonstrated that functional somatic syndromes share underlying etiology with anxiety and depression [14].

Psychiatric and Psychological Factors that Impact Treatment Adherence

Psychiatric factors are relevant when considering the management of patients who have chronic pain. Individuals

R. Prasad (✉)
Division of Pain Medicine, Stanford University,
Redwood City, CA, USA
e-mail: rprasad@stanford.edu

A. Ramezani
Physical Medicine & Rehabilitation, University of California,
Davis, Sacramento, CA, USA

R. McCarron
Department of Psychiatry and Human Behavior, University of
California, Irvine School of Medicine, Orange, CA, USA

S. Malcore
Department of Psychiatry and Behavorial Medicine, Spectrum
Health, Grand Rapids, MI, USA

© Springer Nature Switzerland AG 2019
Y. Khelemsky et al. (eds.), *Academic Pain Medicine*, https://doi.org/10.1007/978-3-030-18005-8_17

with chronic pain have been shown to be higher utilizers of healthcare [15], and this has also been shown in patients with psychiatric factors such as depression [16]. The potential underlying factors associated with increased healthcare utilizers may be useful to understand when working with patients who have chronic pain and psychiatric conditions.

There appears to be a relationship between catastrophizing and multiple factors associated with pain, including reported pain levels, illness behaviors, and disability [17]. Psychiatric factors also demonstrate impact on individuals' coping and functioning with chronic pain. There is an association with decreased functioning, decreased quality of life, and increased pain levels in individuals who have comorbid chronic pain with anxiety and depression [18]. Concurrent depression is also related to number of pain complaints and pain severity [6]. Improvements in pain, as well as depression and functional status, have been associated with adherence to self-management methods for chronic pain [19].

Furthermore, while medication is a commonly used method for pain management, this needs to be balanced with potential risks [20]. The risk of opioid misuse has been associated with psychiatric factors in multiple studies [21]. There is a clear need for high-quality research with the goal of better balancing risk versus benefit of prescription medications by having reliable definitions of abuse, misuse, and addiction [22].

Pharmacotherapy for Treatment of Comorbid Conditions

Psychopharmacological treatments are highly effective in treating comorbid psychiatric conditions that commonly present in individuals suffering from chronic pain. Broadly, psychopharmacological treatments include antidepressants, mood stabilizers, anxiolytics, and antipsychotic medications. Antidepressant agents mainly aim to increase effects of serotonin, norepinephrine, and dopamine [23]. Selective serotonin reuptake inhibitors (SSRI) and selective norepinephrine reuptake inhibitors (SNRI) have been shown to decrease the severity and duration of depression, anxiety, and, in some cases, physical pain [24]. Tricyclic antidepressants mainly block the reuptake of serotonin and norepinephrine [23]. Antidepressant medications indirectly modulate opioid systems through serotonin and noradrenergic systems [24], therefore providing analgesia. Table 17.1 provides a list of selected antidepressant medications.

Bipolar disorder often presents with discrete depressive episodes as well, but also includes hypomanic or manic symptoms. Manic or hypomanic episodes also modulate pain sensitivity [25]; therefore, treatment of bipolar disorders can greatly stabilize the treatment of chronic pain. Once a patient has a hypomanic or manic episode, all future mood dysregula-

Table 17.1 Selected Antidepressant Medications

SSRI	Tricyclics	SNRI
Celexa (citalopram)	Anafranil (clomipramine)	Effexor (venlafaxine)
Luvox (fluvoxamine)	Elavil (amitriptyline)	Pristiq (desvenlafaxine)
Paxil (paroxetine)	Norpramin (desipramine)	Cymbalta (duloxetine)
Prozac (fluoxetine)	Pamelor (nortriptyline)	Savella (milnacipran)
Zoloft (sertraline)	Aventyl Sinequan (doxepin)	
	Surmontil (trimipramine)	
	Tofranil (imipramine)	

Table 17.2 Commonly Used Mood Stabilizers and Atypical Antipsychotics

Mood stabilizers (for acute manic symptoms)	Atypical antipsychotics (selected medications for primary psychotic disorders)
Carbamazepine (Tegretol, Carbatrol, Epitol)	Olanzapine (Zyprexa)
Valproic acid (Depakote)	Risperidone (Risperdal)
Lithium	Quetiapine (Seroquel)
	Aripiprazole (Abilify)
	Lurasidone (Latuda)
	Ziprasidone (Geodon)

tion may be treated with a mood stabilizer and/or an atypical antipsychotic medication, either with or without an antidepressant medication (see Table 17.2). Generally, patients who have an established bipolar spectrum disorder should not be treated solely with antidepressant medications. This practice may lack treatment efficacy and possible increase irritability and depression or lead to a mixed manic and depressive episode. One should use caution when prescribing atypical antipsychotic or mood stabilizer medications, as many can quickly result in metabolic derangements, including diabetes, insulin resistance, weight gain, or dyslipidemia. Tardive dyskinesia is a common side effect of some antipsychotic medications. Commonly used mood stabilizers and atypical antipsychotic medications are listed in Table 17.2.

If a patient exhibits psychotic symptoms such as hallucinations or delusions, a referral should be placed to psychiatrist for assessment and possible psychopharmacological intervention. The clinician should be mindful of secondary, general medical causes and nonpsychotic conditions that present with psychotic symptoms (see Table 17.3). Pain medicine providers may consider deferring treatment of psychotic disorders to psychiatrists. Note that the effectiveness of psychopharmacological treatments of pain, depression, mania, and psychotic disorders is optimized when they are combined with psychotherapy interventions [23].

Table 17.3 Common causes of psychotic symptoms

Schizophrenia

Schizoaffective disorder

Bipolar disorder

Severe and untreated depression

Intoxication with an illicit substance

Increase in dose of high potency opioid medications

Delirium (secondary to infection, toxic metabolic dysregulation, etc.)

Major cognitive disorders (e.g., dementia due to Lewy body or late-stage Alzheimer's disease)

Psychotherapy for Depressive Disorders

Psychotherapy interventions have also been shown to improve depression in patients who are experiencing chronic pain. These include cognitive and behavioral therapy (CBT), group therapy, family therapy, and couples therapy. CBT is an evidence-based psychotherapy system that has been empirically shown to improve the symptoms of clinical depression [26, 27] and chronic pain [28]. CBT is widely applied to manage psychiatric symptoms in individuals who are living with chronic conditions. There are a variety of CBT interventions. The following are a few examples of how therapists use CBT interventions when working with individuals who live with chronic pain and clinical depression: identify the effects of unhelpful thinking (e.g., identify catastrophic or all-or-none thinking) on depression and pain sensation; transition unhelpful thinking to goal-oriented thinking (e.g., patient may be invited to complete a thought experiment to see how he or she would feel physically and emotionally if he or she had goal-oriented thinking); help patient fill out dysfunctional thought records and increase functional daily activities via behavioral activation strategies; modify pain behaviors and patient's sick role that reinforce depression, inactivity, and disability; and increase medication management and medication adherence training.

Given that depression and pain can be an isolating experience, group therapies have also been shown to enhance the management of depression and pain [29]. Mindfulness-based group therapies, similar to group CBT, also have efficacious result when managing depression and chronic pain. Mindfulness is defined as the act of bringing awareness to "moment-to-moment" experience in a nonjudgmental and accepting manner [30]. Mindfulness practices are often conducted in a group format. Mindfulness practices that integrate acceptance-based psychotherapy (e.g., acceptance and commitment therapy) and cognitive therapy (e.g., mindfulness-based cognitive therapy) are evidence-based treatments that have been shown to reduce depression, prevent depression relapse, reduce disability/increase function, and reduce pain intensity [31–34].

Patients' functional deficits from depression and chronic pain have devastating effect on their family and partner. Adopting a systems approach to care can greatly enhance the patient's quality of life [35]. The research literature on family therapy has shown positive effects on depression and pain management outcomes. For example, a randomized controlled trial of 68 individuals living with rheumatoid arthritis completed internal family systems therapy. When compared to a control group, individuals who received internal family systems therapy had less pain intensity, better physical functioning, increased compassion for self and others, and less depression [36]. Expanding the system of care to include the partner also improves the patient's quality of life. Regarding couples, review papers and meta-analytic data of couples-oriented interventions with individuals living with chronic conditions showed that couples therapy can help improve soliciting pain roles, enhance health behaviors, reduce high illness-related conflict between partners, increase partner support, and improve marital quality [37]. The same study also showed that couples therapy improved depression and functional abilities as compared to individualized treatments and the treatment as usual groups [37].

Differential Diagnosis of Anxiety Disorders

Patients with chronic pain commonly present with comorbid anxiety disorders [38]. Identification and treatment of anxiety is a critical piece of pain management care, as untreated or undertreated psychiatric distress can exacerbate the underlying pain condition. One of the most tangible mechanisms for this link involves the stress response within the body; as the brain detects the presence of anxiety, it causes activation of the sympathetic nervous system. Aspects of this sympathetic arousal (e.g., increased muscle tension, constriction of blood vessels, changes in respiration, increased heart rate, etc.) concurrently fuel both anxiety and pain.

While attending to anxiety issues is an essential part of pain management treatment, it is also necessary to ensure that a different condition is not erroneously being labeled as anxiety. The diagnostic criteria for anxiety disorders specifically address the importance of ruling out alternative explanations that can account for a patient's clinical presentation [10]. Differential diagnoses should identify if the manifested symptoms can better be attributed to the effects of a substance, a general medical condition, or a concurrent psychiatric disorder.

Effects of a Substance

When assessing whether symptoms are due to the effects of a substance, it is important to appreciate that such an evaluation should encompass all substances that can impact physiologic functioning, not just drugs of abuse. A thorough history should be obtained from the patient regarding use of illicit drugs, prescribed and over-the-counter medications, and other substances (e.g., caffeine, nicotine, alcohol, etc.). This information should be corroborated with data from objective assessments (e.g., blood work, urine drug screen, etc.) and/or feedback from the patient's social support network to facilitate identifying whether the presenting symptoms are signs of substance withdrawal or intoxication. Once such a determination is made, the relationship between the substance and symptoms should be established. The latter includes ascertaining whether the substance is the primary cause of the symptoms, if the substance use is secondary to a primary psychiatric condition, or if the effects of a substance and a psychiatric disorder are concurrently present but independent from one another [39].

Effects of a General Medical Condition

Information from an exhaustive review of medical records, diagnostic testing results (e.g., imaging studies, blood work, etc.), physical exam findings, and clinical interview data from patients and their social support networks should all be synthesized to formulate a patient's medical diagnosis. As there can be significant overlap in the clinical presentations for medical and psychiatric conditions (e.g., asthma and panic, endocrine dysfunction, depression, etc.), the thoroughness of the medical work-up is a critical factor in determining diagnostic accuracy. If the findings from such an evaluation identify the presence of both a medical and psychiatric condition, the relationship between the two conditions should be established. The latter includes identifying whether the medical condition and/or its treatment causes the psychiatric symptoms, the psychiatric condition moderates or mediates the effects of the medical condition, or the two conditions are independent of one another [39].

Effects of a Concurrent Psychiatric Disorder

Symptoms of anxiety may also mirror other psychiatric conditions. For example, the rumination that is commonly seen in depression may mistakenly be attributed to the perseveration associated with anxiety. It is important to maintain some familiarity with other psychiatric conditions that may have presentations similar to anxiety (e.g., depression, mania, delirium, neurocognitive disorders, etc.) and understand the differences among them. Integrating this baseline knowledge with information from a detailed history of symptoms and the context in which they occur can help minimize the likelihood of misdiagnosing psychiatric condition(s).

A factitious disorder is a psychiatric disorder characterized by intentionally feigning or exaggerating symptoms in the absence of clear external reinforcement. It has some similarities to, but is distinctly different from, malingering, where a person intentionally exhibits symptoms for the purpose of secondary gain. In both situations, an individual may present with symptoms of anxiety that are consistent with the associated diagnostic criteria. Examination of contextual factors through the clinical interview can help elucidate the factors that are motivating behavior and can subsequently aid diagnosis.

The DSM-5 identifies nine psychiatric disorders that are characterized by fear and worry and exhibit behavioral or physical manifestations: separation anxiety disorder, selective mutism, specific phobia, social anxiety disorder, panic disorder, agoraphobia, generalized anxiety disorder, substance/medication-induced anxiety disorder, and anxiety disorder due to another medical condition [10]. When diagnosing anxiety, a clinician should be aware of the discrete diagnoses that are encompassed in this larger category and identify which of these best accounts for the symptoms with which the patient presents.

Anger in Chronic Pain Patients and Relation to Perceived Pain

Researchers have extensively examined the role of anger and pain, which helps to shed light on the contributing factors of chronic pain as well as helps to highlight the role of psychological treatment in managing chronic pain. Studies indicate that high anger levels or perceived injustice are associated with higher pain, depression, and disability levels [40–42]. Higher levels of anger also impact spousal relationships [43]. It is worth noting that anger independently contributes to pain sensitivity and intensity above and beyond the contribution of anxiety and depression [41, 42].

Additional researchers have zeroed in on what is specifically helpful for individuals who are experiencing anger and chronic pain. Although initial models of pain and anger would suggest that increased anger expression would contribute to less pain or, vice versa, that anger inhibition would lead to greater pain intensity, at this time the current literature is not conclusive. Furthermore, there is mixed evidence for the notion that chronic pain patients inhibit their anger more than non-chronic pain patients [44]. Some evidence suggests that the lack of appropriate expression of state-related anger may be a key component in the development of chronic pain [44]. Therefore, pain interventions that focus on the practice of healthy and socially appropriate expressions of anger during periods of being provoked in real time could directly improve anger in chronic pain patients.

Opioids in Chronic Non-cancer Pain

Careful consideration needs to be undertaken when using opioid therapy. The clinician may wish to consider the risks and benefits of starting chronic opioid therapy while at the same time consider the lack of evidence for its long-term use for chronic pain and consider the option of starting non-opioid medications in combination with nonpharmacological modalities (spinal cord stimulation, injections, pain psychology treatments options such as biofeedback, CBT, mindfulness-based psychotherapy, etc.). Appropriate documentation and utilization of best practices, and assessment of psychiatric and substance use disorders is essential [45–47]. Table 17.4 lists many of the opioid medications commonly used to treat chronic pain.

Identifying substance use disorder will also assist in making a decision about starting opioid use. In pseudoaddiction, the individual appears as if he or she is overusing or seeking opioids, yet this is driven by an undertreatment of his or her pain condition. Care must be taken in assuming this diagnosis, and consideration must be given to a more likely opioid use disorder, wherein opioids are overused or taken for longer periods of time than the patient or provider intended despite efforts to cut down. This often will follow with a great deal of time spent gaining or recovering from opioids. Cravings, urges to use, and physical tolerance/withdrawal are also present [10].

Reviewing the five "A's" will also help to assess inappropriate opioid use: (1) Analgesia: Is the patient receiving adequate pain relief; (2) Activity: Is there a change in the patient's activities of daily living and psychosocial functioning (e.g., increase in walking); (3) Adverse effects: Does the patient tolerate the side effects that are related to opioid medications such as constipation, cognitive blunting, sedation, nausea, etc.; (4) Aberrant behaviors: Does the patient increase dosage without notification or consultation with the prescribing provider; does the patient use opioid medications for reasons other than pain relief and functional benefits (e.g., use for anxiety and depression management); does the patient divert or sell medications; (5) Affect: does the opioid medication improve the way the patient emotionally feels in life overall [48, 49].

Table 17.4 Opioid medications

Oxycodone (OxyContin, Oxecta, Roxicodone)
Oxycodone/acetaminophen (Percocet, Endocet, Roxicet)
Oxycodone and naloxone (Targiniq ER)
Meperidine (Demerol)
Methadone (Methadose, Dolophine)
Hydrocodone (Hysingla ER, Zohydro ER)
Hydrocodone/acetaminophen (Norco, Vicodin, Lorcet, Lortab)
Hydromorphone (Dilaudid, Exalgo)
Fentanyl (Duragesic, Fentora, Actiq)
Codeine

Somatic Complaints in Chronic Pain

Individuals experiencing chronic pain may experience an overlap of somatic symptom disorders and related conditions (e.g., somatization involving a conversion condition, etc.). Somatization symptoms may mimic medical conditions and, at times, psychological conditions. As a result, clinicians may be in a diagnostic dilemma given the complexity of the symptoms presentation [50–54]. Patients may present with disproportionate functional decline in the absence of biological pathology. For example, a patient with pain in the mid-central tip of her nose remains in bed for weeks as a result of her nose pain. Another example includes a patient who continues to experience ongoing pain-related functional decline even after pain has been treated or managed effectively. For instance, a patient with a successful spinal cord stimulation implant with low-level pain continues to remain at home and not engage in daily activities or return to work. Finally, a patient may present without the emotional distress expected following functional disability. For example, a patient with a recent lower limb amputation as a result of diabetic neuropathy not exhibiting normal levels of sadness and grieving due to the loss of his or her function and body part.

Assessing somatic complaints requires a review of psychiatric systems, evaluation of specific somatic symptom disorders and related conditions, and familiarity with medical conditions that present with psychiatric symptoms. A review of psychiatric symptoms can include assessing for anxiety, OCD, trauma, depression, bipolar disorder, substance use disorders, and psychotic disorders [55]. In assessing somatic symptoms, the first consideration is whether symptoms are intentionally produced for secondary gain (e.g., malingering) or intentionally produced for attention (e.g., factitious). Once these conditions have been ruled out, reviewing somatic symptom and related conditions can further clarify the presence of a somatization process. The following figure helps to review the key symptoms present in somatic symptom disorders (see Fig. 17.1). This figure also helps clinicians to make a decision about which somatic symptom the patient may be experiencing.

Providers may wish to use the CARE MD acronym to assist with treatment [56]. CARE MD stands for the following:

1. Consultation/CBT: brief, time-limited CBT treatment.
2. Assess: start by ruling out potential medical causes and treat psychiatric comorbidity.
3. Regular visits: short and frequent visits that focus on stress and health behaviors with the agreement of the patient to avoid excessive medications or inappropriate use of emergency services.

Fig. 17.1 This figure also helps clinicians to make a decision about which somatic symptom the patient may be experiencing. (Figure adapted from [10, 55])

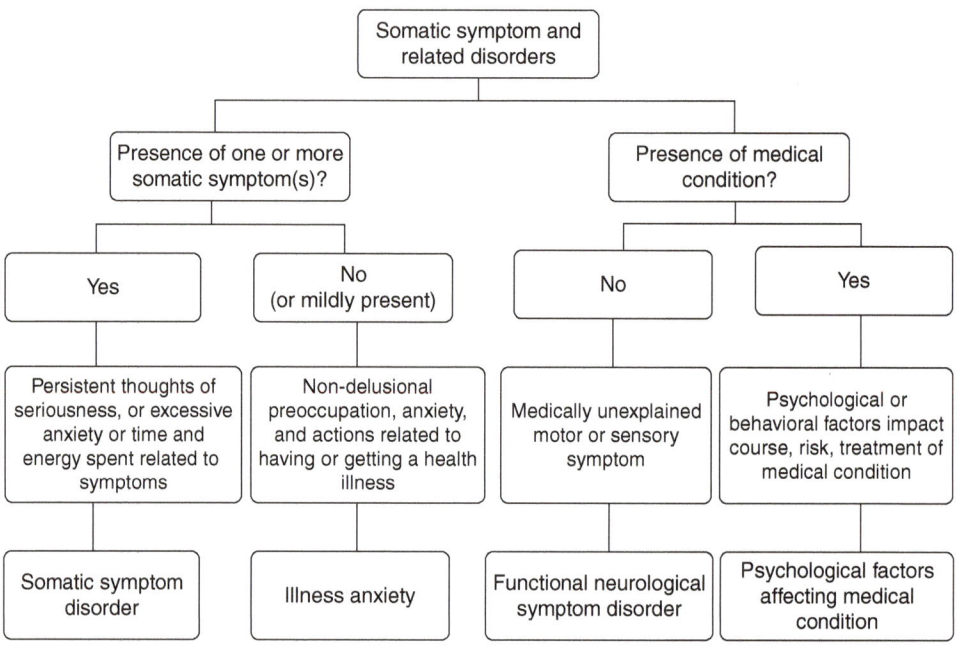

4. Empathy (E): understand the clinical situation and its accompanying emotions from the perspective of the patient.
5. Med-psych (M) interface: help to make mind-body connection.
6. Do no harm (D): Avoid excessive diagnostic medical work-up or interventions.

Note that clarifying diagnostic procedures such as psychological and neuropsychological testing is an exception as these tools can help clarify psychosomatic symptoms and provide objective evidence of current functional, psychological, psychomotor, malingering, or cognitive status. At the same time, clinicians need to exercise their clinical judgment on a case-by-case basis. For example, a patient who has clear somatization with unexplained medical etiology who is requesting another neuropsychological test would likely not benefit from any additional testing.

Role of Family

There is a long history of working with family/partners of patients who have chronic pain [57], highlighting the role of potential reinforcers of pain behavior and working with identified family to address target behaviors and develop alternative behaviors (e.g., not being responsive to pain behavior and reinforcement of adaptive behaviors) [58]. Treatments targeting spouses (e.g., [59]) and parents of individuals with chronic pain (e.g., [60]) have been promising.

Social support has been cited as an important factor in the adjustment of individuals with pain (e.g., [61, 62]). Marital status has been found to be associated with response to spinal cord stimulation [63]. However, it may be that merely being married is not in itself protective, rather being in a nondistressed marriage [64]. Therefore, the status of the marriage and perceived social support factors may be important when assessing a patient who has chronic pain.

Solicitous behaviors by spouses have been associated with pain behaviors of individuals with chronic pain [65]. Furthermore, solicitous reactions by spouses to pain in their partners are associated with increased disability, whereas distraction by spouses leads to decreased disability [66]. The impact of solicitous behaviors may be mediated by other factors, such as spouse's confidence in their partner's management of their condition [67]. Therefore, it may not only be helpful to observe potential interactions between patients and social supports but also obtain information from family members regarding their impressions of the person who has chronic pain.

Pain can have an impact both on patients and their families, such as responsibilities other family members may take on for the patient and the patient not being able to engage in activities with family [68]. However, patients with pain may perceive their pain having a greater impact on family than family members report [69]. Partners of individuals with chronic pain may also have beliefs similar to those with chronic pain, including degree of helpfulness of treatments or need for a cure in order to return to work [70]. Parent(s) of a child being treated for chronic pain often describe knowledge of the child's pain condition as important to them (e.g., treatment options, etiology) [71]. These findings underscore the value of including family members during interventions of patients who have chronic pain [70].

Role of Patient Beliefs and Expectations

Cognitive-behavioral models expand on stimulus-response theories by positing that thought processes mediate the relationship between these two variables. Applied in the realm of pain, cognitive interpretations play a significant role in shaping an individual's emotional, behavioral, and physiologic responses to painful stimuli (see Fig. 17.2).

Consistent with the model described above, evaluating patients' beliefs about their pain can help shape their response to treatment. Patients whose cognitive appraisal of their pain is rooted in fearful thoughts may adopt a coping strategy in which they actively avoid activities and movements that may aggravate their condition [55]. This process can directly influence compliance with treatment recommendations that involve rehabilitation of the part(s) of the body affected by pain. Development of such a fear-avoidance cycle has been associated with somatic hypervigilance, hypersensitivity to painful stimuli, and disability [72, 73].

Treatment expectations can impact clinical outcomes [74] and are also influenced by patients' belief structures. For example, a patient suffering from fibromyalgia who views the condition as an acute process that can be eliminated with pharmacologic therapy may thus perceive any treatment that does not result in complete resolution of pain symptoms as a failure. The patient may subsequently be unreceptive to treatments that focus on interdisciplinary approaches to pain management as this is not in line with his/her expectations. To avoid such circumstances, pain clinicians should take the time to provide education on the nature and course of pain early in the treatment process and continuously revisit the topic as patients progress through their care plans.

Pain acceptance, a process that involves both cognitive and emotional components, refers to learning how to live with a pain condition rather than fighting its presence [75].

Cognitively, it entails recognition of the chronicity of a pain condition and the positive role(s) that self-management strategies can play in improving functioning and quality of life. Low pain acceptance has been associated with higher levels of psychological distress, pain disability, and opioid use [76]. Pain education can help patients formulate more accurate beliefs and expectations regarding their conditions, which in turn can influence the process of achieving pain acceptance.

Sleep Disorders in Chronic Pain

Sleep and chronic pain are intrinsically linked to one another; however, there is not a uniform directionality that has been ascribed to the association. Although there have been some studies that have shown evidence of sleep disturbances increasing the risk of developing a pain disorder, many contemporary perspectives posit a reciprocal relationship between these variables [77]. For this reason, assessment of sleep disturbances should be included in the evaluation of patients presenting with pain and a referral to a sleep specialist should be considered if indicated. The current section will discuss sleep apnea and insomnia, two specific sleep disturbances that are commonly seen in pain populations.

Disruption in respiration while asleep is the defining characteristic of sleep apnea. Obstructive sleep apnea (OSA) is usually the result of an airway blockage, whereas central sleep apnea (CSA) is caused by the brain's failure to regulate the breathing process. Individuals with either type of apnea often feel fatigued during the day secondary to the various forms of sleep interference associated with the altered breathing patterns. Polysomnograms assist with diagnosing sleep apnea, and appropriate treatment may be comprised of surgery, lifestyle changes, use of a dental device, or use of a

Fig. 17.2 The role of cognitions

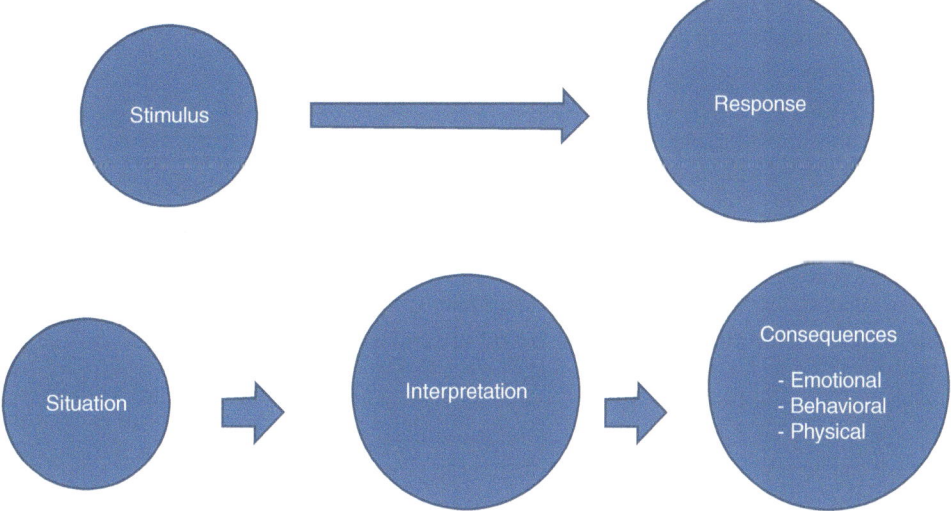

positive airway pressure machine (CPAP or BiPAP). Sleep apnea is particularly important to assess in individuals using opioid medication for pain, as this category of medications by itself is known to cause sleep-disordered breathing and can increase the potential for CSA [78].

Insomnia is characterized by persistent difficulty initiating, maintaining, or returning to sleep [10]. When assessing for this sleep disorder, it is important to identify whether it is a primary disturbance or occurring secondary to another comorbid condition (e.g., depression, etc.) as that will help inform treatment. Insomnia has a bi-directional relationship with pain and has been associated with increased pain sensitivity [79]. This increased sensitivity can contribute to difficulty with sleep onset, thereby triggering the reciprocating relationship. Medications, lifestyle changes, and cognitive behavioral therapy for insomnia (CBTi) are all interventions that can be used to treat insomnia. Participation in CBTi has been shown to result in significant, sustained improvement in sleep maintenance insomnia [80]. Hybrid programs that provide concurrent cognitive behavioral therapy for insomnia and pain have shown improvements in sleep, pain-related disability, mood, and fatigue [81] and may be an efficient approach to addressing these frequently co-occurring disorders.

Work History and Education in Evaluation of Chronic Pain: Frequency of Personality Disorders

Work history and education are major factors that can help identify and assess the patient's premorbid level of functional and the degree to which pain interferes with current functioning [82]. For example, a patient whose work involves repetitive motion, heavy lifting, and rapid posture movements as a result of his/her daily work tasks will have devastating functional decline at work as a result of the onset of hand and back pain. However, the patient whose work does not involve any physical activity and a low cognitive load may have little functional decline at work as a result of pain interference. Assessment of work history and education may include assessing the number of year of formal education; physical activities and emotional factors associated with work tasks; number of sick days taken as a result of chronic pain; presence of sick-role behaviors at work; work-related psychosocial stressors (e.g., negative relationships with supervisor); general like or dislike of work-related tasks, people, and environment; and self-identification of meaningful values and needs fulfilled at work. Evaluation of functional status through the assessment of work history and education is complementary to identification of psychiatric comorbidity, somatic symptom disorders, family dynamics, beliefs/expectations, and sleep-related changes as a result of chronic pain.

Assessment of normal and abnormal personality traits in individuals experiencing chronic pain helps determine appropriate treatment modalities. It has been estimated that 37% of individuals with chronic pain may be experiencing comorbid personality disorders, mainly clusters B (dramatic traits) and C (anxious traits) [83, 84]. Regarding cluster B personality disorders, one study found that borderline traits were associated with increased pain severity, pain-related activity interference, and pain-related affective interference [85]. The emotional dysregulation of personality disorders is thought to impact sensory interpretation and magnification of pain [86]. Certain normal personality traits have also been linked to chronic pain. These include perfectionism and neuroticism [87, 88], particularly in patients experiencing headache disorders. It has been further noted that individuals with such personality traits are more likely to experience pain catastrophizing, fear of movement, and pain-related vigilance [88]. It is worth noting that the personality trait is not necessarily the core issue impacting pain management. It appears that certain personality traits, such as neuroticism, place individuals at risk to cope ineffectively with pain [88]. Therefore, coping skills training can greatly help individual with such personality traits. Also, managing the emotion dysregulation through psychological treatments (e.g., dialectical behavioral therapy) can assist with the management of pain and personality disorder [85].

References

1. Ho PT, Li CF, Ng YN, Tsui SL, Ng NFJ. Prevalence of the factors associated with psychiatric morbidity in chronic pain patients. J Psychosom Res. 2011;70(6):541–7.
2. Subramaniam M, Vaingankar J, Abdin E, Chong SA. Psychiatric morbidity in pain conditions: results from the Singapore mental health study. Pain Res Manag. 2013;18(4):185–90.
3. Currie SR, Wang J. Chronic back pain and major depression in the general Canadian population. Pain. 2004;107(1):54–60.
4. Dominick CH, Blyth FM, Nicholas MK. Unpacking the burden: understanding the relationship between chronic pain and comorbidity in the general population. Pain. 2012;153(2):293–304.
5. Knaster P, Karlsson H, Estlander A, Kalso E. Psychiatric disorders as assessed with SCID in chronic pain patients: the anxiety disorders precede the onset of pain. Gen Hosp Psychiatry. 2012;34:46–52.
6. Ohayon MM, Schatzberg A. Chronic pain and major depressive disorder in the general population. J Psychiatr Res. 2010;44(7):454–61.
7. Fishbain DA, Goldberg M, Meagher BR, Steele R, Rosomoff H. Male and female chronic pain patients categorized by DSM-III psychiatric diagnostic criteria. Pain. 1986;26:181–97.
8. Sansone RA, Sansone LA. Chronic pain syndromes and borderline personality. Innov Clin Neurosci. 2012;9(1):10–4.
9. Radat R, Morgot-Duclot A, Attal N. Psychiatric co-morbidities in patients with chronic peripheral neuropathic pain: a multicenter cohort study. Eur J Pain. 2013;17(10):1547–57.
10. American Psychiatric Association. Diagnostic and statistical manual of mental disorders. 5th ed. Arlington: American Psychiatric Publishing; 2013.
11. Hart-Johnson T, Green CR. The impact of sexual or physical abuse history on pain-related outcomes among blacks and whites with chronic pain: Gender Influence. Pain Med. 2012;13:229–42.

12. Gupta MA. Review of somatic symptoms in post-traumatic stress disorder. Int Rev Psychiatry. 2013;25(1):86–99.

13. Nicol AL, Sieberg CB, Clauw DJ, Hassett AL, Moser SE, Brummett CM. The association between a history of lifetime traumatic events and pain severity, physical function, and affective distress in patients with chronic pain. J Pain. 2016;17(12):1334–48.

14. Kato K, Sullivan PF, Evengård B, Pedersen NL. A population-based twin study of functional somatic syndromes. Psychol Med. 2009;39:497–505.

15. Eriksen J, Sjøgren P, Ekholm O, Rasmussen NK. Health care utilization among individuals reporting long-term pain: an epidemiological study based on Danish national health surveys. Eur J Pain. 2004;8:517–23.

16. Berghöfer A, Roll S, Bauer M, Willich SN, Pfennig A. Screening for depression and high utilization of health care resources among patients in primary care. Community Ment Health. 2014;50:753–8.

17. Sullivan JL, Thorn B, Haythornthwaite JA, Keefe F, Martin M, Bradley LA, Lefebvre JC. Theoretical perspectives on the relation between catastrophizing and pain. Clin J Pain. 2001;17:52–64.

18. Bair MJ, Wu J, Damush TM, Sutherland JM, Kroenke K. Association of depression and anxiety alone and in combination with chronic musculoskeletal pain in primary care patients. Psychosom Med. 2008;70(8):890–7.

19. Nicholas MK, Asghari A, Corbett M, Smeets RJEM, Wood MB, Overton S, Perry C, Tonkin LE, Beeston L. Is adherence to pain self-management strategies associated with improved pain, depression and disability in those with disabling chronic pain? Eur J Pain. 2012;16(1):93–104.

20. Sehgal N, Colson J, Smith HS. Chronic pain treatment with opioid analgesics: benefits versus harms of long-term therapy. Expert Rev Neurother. 2013;13(11):1201–20.

21. Wason AD, Butler SF, Budman SH, Benoit C, Fernandez K, Jamison RN. Psychiatric history and psychologic adjustment as risk factors for aberrant drug-related behavior among patients with chronic pain. Clin J Pain. 2007;23(4):307–15.

22. Cheatle MD. Prescription opioid misuse, abuse, morbidity, and mortality: balancing effective pain management and safety. Pain Med. 2015;16:S3–8.

23. Preston JD, O'neal JH, Talaga MC. Handbook of clinical psychopharmacology for therapists. 8th ed. Oakland: New Harbinger Publications Inc; 2017.

24. Lee YC, Chen PP. A review of SSRIs and SNRIs in neuropathic pain. Expert Opin Pharmacother. 2010;11(17):2813–25.

25. Boggero IA, Cole JD. Mania reduces perceived pain intensity in patients with chronic pain: preliminary evidence from retrospective archival data. J Pain Res. 2016;9:147–52.

26. Beck AT, Rush AJ, Shaw BF, Emery G. Cognitive therapy of depression. New York: Guilford Press; 1979.

27. Kerns RD, Sellinger JJ, Goodin B. Psychological treatment of chronic pain. Annu Rev Clin Psychol. 2011;7:411–34.

28. Jensen MP, Turk DC. Contributions of psychology to the understanding and treatment of people with chronic pain: why it matters to ALL psychologists. Am Psychol. 2014;69(2):105–18.

29. Kanstrup M, Wicksell RK, Kemani M, Wiwe Lipsker C, Lekander M, Holmström L. A clinical pilot study of individual and group treatment for adolescents with chronic pain and their parents: effects of acceptance and commitment therapy on functioning. Walker LS, ed. Children. 2016;3(4):30.

30. Kabat-Zinn J. Full catastrophe living: using the wisdom of your body and mind to face stress, pain and illness. New York: Delacorte; 1990.

31. Cherkin DC, Sherman KJ, Balderson BH, et al. Effect of mindfulness-based stress reduction vs cognitive behavioral therapy or usual care on back pain and functional limitations in adults with chronic low back pain: a randomized clinical trial. JAMA. 2016;315(12):1240–9.

32. McCracken LM, Vowles KE. Acceptance and commitment therapy and mindfulness for chronic pain. Am Psychol. 2014;69(2):178–87.

33. Kuyken W, Hayes R, Barrett B, et al. Effectiveness and cost-effectiveness of mindfulness-based cognitive therapy compared with maintenance antidepressant treatment in the prevention of depressive relapse or recurrence (PREVENT): a randomized controlled trial. Lancet. 2015;386(9988):63–73.

34. Kuyken W, Warren FC, Taylor RS, et al. Efficacy of mindfulness-based cognitive therapy in prevention of depressive relapse: an individual patient data meta-analysis from randomized trials. JAMA Psychiat. 2016;73(6):565–74.

35. Lewandowski W, Morris R, Draucker CB, Risko J. Chronic pain and the family: theory-driven treatment approaches. Issues Ment Health Nurs. 2007;28(9):1019–44.

36. Shadick NA, Sowell NF, Frits ML, et al. A randomized controlled trial of an internal family systems-based psychotherapeutic intervention on outcomes in rheumatoid arthritis: a proof-of-concept study. J Rheumatol. 2013;40(11):1831–41.

37. Martire LM, Schulz R, Helgeson VS, Small BJ, Saghafi EM. Review and meta-analysis of couple-oriented interventions for chronic illness. Ann Behav Med. 2010;40(3):325–42.

38. Bandelow B. Generalized anxiety disorder and pain. Mod Trends Pharmacopsychiatry. 2015;30:153–65.

39. First M. Handbook of differential diagnosis. Arlington: American Psychiatric Publishing; 2014. p. DSM–5.

40. Scott W, McCracken LM, Trost Z. A psychological flexibility conceptualisation of the experience of injustice among individuals with chronic pain. Br J Pain. 2014;8(2):62–71.

41. Berkowitz L. On the formation and regulation of anger and aggression: a cognitive-neoassociationistic analysis. Am Psychol. 1990;45:494–503.

42. Berkowitz L. Pain and aggression: some findings and implications. Motiv Emot. 1993;17:277–93.

43. Schwartz L, Slater MA, Birchler GR, Atkinson JH. Depression in spouses of chronic pain patients: the role of patient pain and anger, and marital satisfaction. Pain. 1991;44(1):61–7.

44. Burns JW, Quartana PJ, Bruehl S. Anger inhibition and pain: conceptualizations, evidence and new directions. J Behav Med. 2008;31(3):259–79.

45. Federation of State Medical Boards. Model policy for the use of opioid analgesics in the treatment of chronic pain. http://www.fsmb.org/Media/Default/PDF/FSMB/Advocacy/pain_policy_july2013.pdf. Published July 2013. Accessed 18 Dec 2015.

46. Chen L, Vo T, Seefeld L, et al. Lack of correlation between opioid dose adjustment and pain score change in a group of chronic pain patients. J Pain. 2013;14(4):384–92.

47. Centers for Disease Control Prevention. CDC grand rounds: prescription drug overdoses-a US epidemic. MMWR Morb Mortal Wkly Rep. 2012;61(1):10.

48. Passik SD, Weinreb HJ. Managing chronic nonmalignant pain: overcoming obstacles to the use of opioids. Adv Ther. 2000;17(2):70–83.

49. Stayner SR, Ramezani A, Prasad R, Mahajan G. Chronic pain management for patients with psychiatric illness. Curr Psychiatr Ther. 2016;15(2):27–33.

50. Engel GL. The need for a new medical model: a challenge for biomedicine. Science. 1977;196(4286):129–36.

51. Engel GL. The clinical application of the biopsychosocial model. Am J Psychiatry. 1980;137(5):535–44.

52. Turk DC, Flor H. Chronic pain: a biobehavioral perspective. In: Gatchel RJ, Turk DC, editors. Psychosocial factors in pain: critical perspectives. New York: Guilford Press; 1999. p. 18–34.

53. Andrasik F, Flor H, Turk DC. An expanded view of psychological aspects in head pain: the biopsychosocial model. Neurol Sci. 2005;26(Suppl 2):s87–91.

54. Ramezani A, McCarron RM, Lashai B, Lenaerts MEP. Head pain and psychiatric illness: applying the biopsychosocial model to care. Curr Psychiatr Ther. 2015;14(9):12–26.

55. Onate J, Xiong G, McCarron R. The primary care psychiatric interview. In: Mc Carron R, Xiong G, Bourgeois J, editors. Lippincott's primary care psychiatry. Lipponcott Philadelphia; 2009. p. 3–4.

56. McCarron RM. Somatization in the primary care setting. Psychiatr Times. 2006;23(6):32–4.

57. Main CJ, Keefe FJ, Jensen MP, Valaeyen JWS, Vowles KE. Fordyce's behavioral methods for chronic pain and illness. Philadelphia: Wolters Kluwer; 2015.

58. Fordyce WE, Fowler RS Jr, Lehmann JF, DeLateur BJ. Some implications of learning in problems of chronic pain. J Chronic Dis. 1968;21:179–90.

59. Abbasi M, Dehghani M, Keefe FJ, Jafari H, Behtash H, Shams J. Spouse-assisted training in pain coping skills and the outcome of multidisciplinary pain management from chronic low back pain treatment: a 1-year randomized controlled trial. Eur J Pain. 2012;16(7):1033–43.

60. Palermo TM, Wilson AC, Peters M, Lewandowski A, Somhegyi H. Randomized controlled trial of an internet-delivered family cognitive-behavioral therapy intervention for children and adolescents with chronic pain. Pain. 2009;146:205–13.

61. Evers AWM, Kraaimaat FW, Geenen R, Jacobs JWG, Bijlsma JWJ. Pain coping and social support as predictors of long-term functional disability and pain in early rheumatoid arthritis. Behav Res Ther. 2003;41(11):1295–310.

62. López-Martínez AE, Esteve-Zarazaga R, Ramírez-Maestre C. Perceived social support and coping responses are independent variables explaining pain adjustment among chronic pain patients. J Pain. 2008;9(4):373–9.

63. Sumner LA, Lofland K. Spinal cord stimulation: subjective pain intensity and presurgical correlates in chronic pain patients. Chronic Illn. 2014;10(2):157–66.

64. Reese JB, Somers TJ, Keefe FJ, Mosley-Williams A, Lumley MA. Pain and functioning of rheumatoid arthritis patients based on marital status: is a distressed marriage preferable to no marriage? J Pain. 2010;11(10):958–64.

65. Romano JM, Jensen MP, Turner JA, Good AB, Hops H. Chronic pain patient-partner interactions: further support for a behavioral model of chronic pain. Behav Ther. 2000;31(3):415–40.

66. Ginting JV, Tripp DA, Nickel JC. Self-reported spousal support modifies the negative impact of pain on disability in men with chronic prostatitis/chronic pelvic pain syndrome. Urology. 2011;78(5):1136–41.

67. Hemphill RC, Marite LH, Stephens MAP, Polenick CA. Spouse confidence and physical function among adults with osteoarthritis: the mediating role of spouse responses to pain. Health Psychol. 2016;35(10):1059–68.

68. Strumin L, Boden LI. Family consequences of chronic back pain. Soc Sci Med. 2004;58(7):1385–93.

69. West C, Usher K, Foster K, Stewart L. Chronic pain and the family: the experience of the partners of people living with chronic pain. J Clin Nurs. 2012;21(23–24):3352–60.

70. McCluskey S, Brooks J, King N, Burton K. The influence of 'significant others' on persistent back pain and work participation: a qualitative exploration of illness perceptions. BMC Musculoskelet Disord. 2011;12:236.

71. Reid K, Lander J, Scott S, Dick B. What do the parents of children who have chronic pain expect from their first visit to a pediatric chronic pain clinic? Pain Res Manag. 2010;15(3):158–62.

72. Gatchel RJ, Nesblett R, Kishino N, Ray CT. Fear-avoidance beliefs and chronic pain. J Orthop Sports Phys Ther. 2016;46(2):38–43.

73. Crombez G, Vlaeyen JWS, Heuts PHTG, Lysens R. Pain-related fear is more disabling than pain itself: evidence on the role of pain-related fear in chronic back pain disability. Pain. 1999;80:329–39.

74. Iversen MD, Daltroy LH, Fossel AH, Katz JN. The prognostic importance of patient pre-operative expectations of surgery for lumbar spinal stenosis. Patient Educ Couns. 1998;34:169–78.

75. LaChapelle DL, Lavoie S, Boudreau A. The meaning and process of pain acceptance. Perceptions of women living with arthritis and fibromyalgia. Pain Res Manag. 2008;13(3):201–10.

76. Martel M, Dionne F, Scott W. The mediating role of pain acceptance in the relation between perceived injustice and pain outcomes in a community sample. Clin J Pain. 2017;33(6):509–16.

77. Finan P, Goodin B, Smith M. The association of sleep and pain: an update and a path forward. J Pain. 2013;14(12):1539–52.

78. Van RE, Antic NA. Opioids and sleep disordered breathing. Chest. 2016;150(4):934–44.

79. Senba E. A key to dissect the triad of insomnia, chronic pain, and depression. Neurosci Lett. 2015;589(4):197–9.

80. Edinger JD, Wohlgemuth WK, Radtke RA, Marsh GR, Quillian RE. Cognitive behavioral therapy for treatment of chronic primary insomnia: a randomized controlled trial. JAMA. 2001;285(14):1856–64.

81. Pigeon W, Moynihan J, Matteson-Rusby S, et al. Comparative effectiveness of CBT interventions for co-morbid chronic pain & insomnia: a pilot study. Behav Res Ther. 2012;50:685–9.

82. Turk DC, Melzak R. Handbook of pain assessment. New York: The Guilford Press; 2013.

83. Reich J, Thompson D. DSM-III personality disorder clusters in three populations. Br J Psychiatry. 1987;150:471–5.

84. Polatin PB, Kinney RK, Gatchel RJ, et al. Psychiatric illness and chronic low-back pain. The mind and the spine—which goes first? Spine. 1993;18:66–71.

85. Reynolds CJ, Carpenter RW, Tragesser SL. Accounting for the association between BPD features and chronic pain complaints in a pain patient sample: the role of emotion dysregulation factors. Personal Disord. 2017, in press (published online).

86. Tragesser SL, Bruns D, Disorbio JM. Borderline personality disorder features and pain: the mediating role of negative affect in a pain patient sample. Clin J Pain. 2010;26(4):348–53.

87. Pompili M, Di Cosimo D, Innamorati M, et al. Psychiatric comorbidity in patients with chronic daily headache and migraine: a selective overview including personality traits and suicide risk. J Headache Pain. 2009;10(4):283–90.

88. Ashina S, Bendtsen L, Buse DC, Lyngberg AC, Lipton RB, Jensen R. Neuroticism, depression and pain perception in migraine and tension-type headache. Acta Neurol Scand. 2017;00:1–7.

Clinical Nerve Function Studies and Imaging

Soo Y. Kim, John S. Georgy, and Yuriy O. Ivanov

Introduction to Electrodiagnosis

Electrodiagnosis (EDX) is a method of evaluating the neuromuscular system by using electrophysiology. Specifically, EDX is used to evaluate the integrity and function of the peripheral nervous system (most cranial nerves, spinal roots, plexi, and nerves), neuromuscular junction, muscles, and the central nervous system (brain and spinal cord) [1]. EDX includes nerve conduction (NCS) and evoked potential (EP) studies, as well as needle electromyography (EMG). NCS and EMG are commonly used to evaluate the peripheral nervous system, whereas EP studies are used for evaluating central nervous system pathology or intraoperative monitoring.

Electromyography

Electromyography (EMG) can be defined as a signal that records the electrical activities generated by depolarization of muscles cells [2]. Needle EMG assesses the size, morphology, and firing characteristics of the electrical signal within the skeletal muscle at rest and during contraction.

While muscle is at rest, the muscle cell membrane is silent except at the neuromuscular junction (NMJ). At the NMJ, acetylcholine vesicles in the nerve ending are released spontaneously and cause endplate potentials. When a needle is inserted into a muscle, mechanical irritation of the muscle membrane causes a brief burst of electrical discharge, which is known as insertional activity. Insertional activity should last only slightly longer than the needle movement. Increased insertional activity may occur in early stages of either neuropathic or myopathic disorders. Decreased insertional activity

is usually seen in chronic end-stage myopathies, when electrically active muscle fibers are replaced by fat or connective tissue [3].

The most common types of abnormal spontaneous activity are fibrillation and positive sharp waves. Abnormal spontaneous activity occurs when the muscle cell membranes become unstable. These small electrical depolarizations which are not enough to create action potentials may be seen in any condition causing denervation, including nerve disease, inflammatory myopathies, and direct muscle trauma [5]. Such findings may be seen after 1 week and may last up to 12 months after an inciting event. Therefore, if the test is done too early, it may be falsely negative and if performed long after the injury, re-innervation may have already occurred.

When a muscle is minimally contracted voluntarily, muscle fiber action potentials (MFAPS) belonging to a single motor unit can be recorded with a needle electrode. As the strength of contraction is slowly increased, motor units are recruited in orderly sequence. Their summated electrical is a motor unit potential (MUP).

The recorded MUP is derived from only muscle fibers that are within the recording radius of the tip of needle electrode (1–3 mm); therefore, it does not reflect the entire muscle and may cause sampling error. Multiple factors influence MUP characteristics, including distance of the recording needle from the fibers, size of the individual muscle fibers, asynchronous firing of fibers within the motor unit, temperature, the degree of effort of muscle contraction, and the type of needle used. The amplitude of the MUP is dependent on the density of the muscle fibers attached to that one motor neuron. Typically, the amplitude is between 200 and 2000 μV for most clinically tested muscles with 1 or 2 upward peaks. As the force of contraction in the muscle increases, an orderly addition of motor units increase which is referred to as recruitment. Recruitment is an important parameter to assess.

In neurogenic disease MUPs have typically high amplitude, long duration, and a greater number of phases-reflecting the remodeling of surviving motor units following loss of a proportion of motor axons [6]. Myopathies are generally

S. Y. Kim (✉) · Y. O. Ivanov
Physical Medicine and Rehabilitation, Montefiore Medical Center, Bronx, NY, USA
e-mail: SOOKIM@montefiore.org

J. S. Georgy
Interventional Pain Medicine, The Spine and Spine and Pain Institute of New York, New York, NY, USA

© Springer Nature Switzerland AG 2019
Y. Khelemsky et al. (eds.), *Academic Pain Medicine*, https://doi.org/10.1007/978-3-030-18005-8_18

characterized by low-amplitude, short-duration motor unit potentials, reflecting muscle fiber splitting and necrosis [6].

Nerve Conduction Study (NCS)

NCS is performed to evaluate the large myelinated nerve fibers, such as sensory and motor nerves. NCS provides data on the speed of conduction and amplitude. Thin myelinated and unmyelinated fibers are not assessed in NCS. This test is performed by giving electrical stimulation proximally and record electrical activities distally. By doing so, it can evaluate any event between the proximal stimulator point and distal recording point. This test is helpful in patients with suspected diseases of the peripheral nervous system and are the mainstay detecting areas of focal nerve damage to myelin sheaths such as entrapment syndromes.

Sensory Conduction Studies

The sensory nerve action potential (SNAP) is obtained by supramaximal electrical stimulation of sensory fibers and recording the nerve action potential certain distance at a point further along the same nerve (Fig. 18.1a). Recording the SNAP orthodromically refers to distal nerve stimulation and recording more proximally (the direction in which physiological sensory conduction occurs). Antidromic testing is the reverse [7]. For each site that is stimulated, the onset latency, peak latency, duration, and amplitude are measured. Sensory nerve conduction velocity (SNCV) can

be calculated with one stimulation alone by taking the measured distance between the stimulator and the active recording electrode and dividing it by the onset latency.

Motor Conduction Studies

Motor conduction studies are performed to assess the functional status in motor fibers of the peripheral nerves by applying the electrical stimulation along the course of a motor nerve while recording the electrical response from its targeted muscle (Fig. 18.1b). The main difference between sensory nerve conduction and motor nerve conduction study is where the recording electrodes are placed. In sensory nerve conduction studies, the recording electrode is placed over the distal nerve itself, whereas the electrode is placed over the innervated muscle in motor nerve conduction studies. The stimulating electrodes are applied over a motor nerve and the recording electrodes over the muscle. Therefore, the motor response is composed of muscle fiber action potentials, and for this reason it is called the compound muscle action potential (CMAP). CMAP represents a summation of motor unit responses beneath the recording electrode and its amplitude proportional to the number of motor axons stimulated. Recording the motor NCV are orthodromically recorded. Measurements taken from the motor responses include the latency, amplitude, duration, and area of the CMAP are measured.

The latency is the time from the stimulus to the initial CMAP deflection from baseline. Latency represents three separate processes: (1) the nerve conduction time from the stimulus site to the neuromuscular junction (NMJ), (2) the time delay across

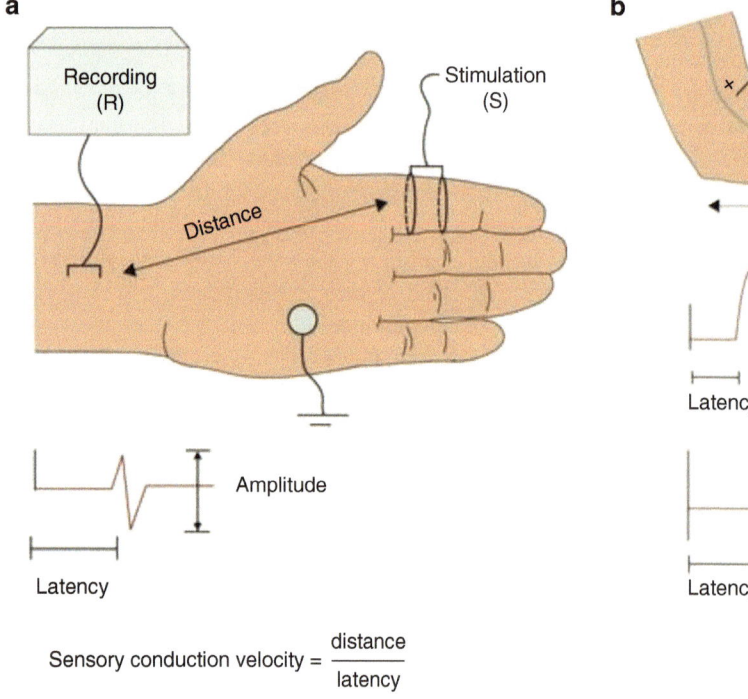

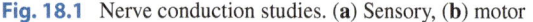

$$\text{Sensory conduction velocity} = \frac{\text{distance}}{\text{latency}}$$

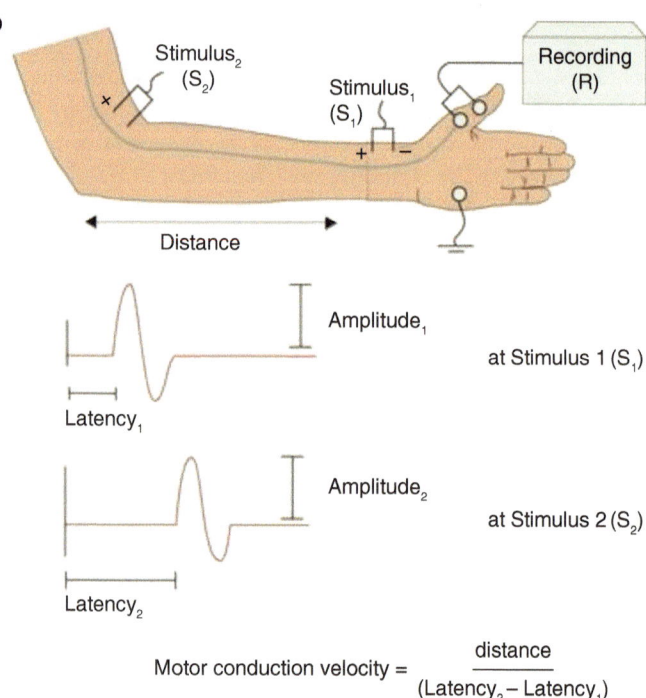

$$\text{Motor conduction velocity} = \frac{\text{distance}}{(\text{Latency}_2 - \text{Latency}_1)}$$

Fig. 18.1 Nerve conduction studies. (**a**) Sensory, (**b**) motor

the NMJ, and (3) the depolarization time across the muscle [7]. There are normal values established for terminal latencies for defined lengths for each of the main motor nerves. Prolonged terminal latencies help detect distal entrapment neuropathies or NMJ disorders. A motor nerve conduction velocity (MNCV) can be calculated by dividing the distance between two sites that have been stimulated (one distal and one proximal) by the difference between terminal latencies.

Understanding Late Potentials

Late potentials are the nerve conduction studies that assess nerve conduction in the more proximal nerve segments such the plexus or the roots. The late responses occur after a CMAP is generated and usually appears more than 10 to 20 milliseconds after stimulation of motor nerves. The two types of late responses are the F-waves and H-reflexes. These two studies provide information when evaluating for cervical or lumbosacral radiculopathies, polyneuropathies, plexopathies, and proximal mononeuropathies.

The H-Reflex

H reflex is a valuable tool is assessing monosynaptic reflex arc activity that directly activates the anterior horn cells in the spinal cord [9]. The H-reflex commonly tested by electrically

stimulating the tibial nerve, recording from the gastrocnemius and soleus muscles. Less frequently, H-reflex of the flexor carpi radialis may be assessed to identify cervical radiculopathies or brachial plexopathies [9]. The response obtained uses the same neural pathway as the ankle-jerk reflex except that it bypasses the muscle spindle. With submaximal stimulation elicited, it measures the latency over the monosynaptic reflex arc through the afferent Ia muscle spindle fibers and efferent α-motor spindle fibers of the S1 root through the dorsal root ganglion and is transmitted across the central synapse to the anterior horn cell which fires it down along the alpha motor axon to the muscle [10]. H-reflex takes relatively a long time in travel designating the term late potential. The clinical significance of this test is that it evaluates the integrity of the reflex arc from the tibial nerve through the spinal cord and back to the gastrocnemius and soleus muscle. Any damage along the tract of the reflex arc including the sciatic nerve or the S1 sensory or motor nerve root can result in loss or slowing of the reflex response. H reflex is delayed or absent in polyneuropathy, tibial neuropathy, sciatic neuropathy, lumbosacral plexopathy, or S1 radiculopathy [11]. (Fig. 18.2)

The F-Response

F-response is the second type of late potential that occurs with impulse first propagating antidromically along the motor nerve axon to the cell body of the anterior horn cells,

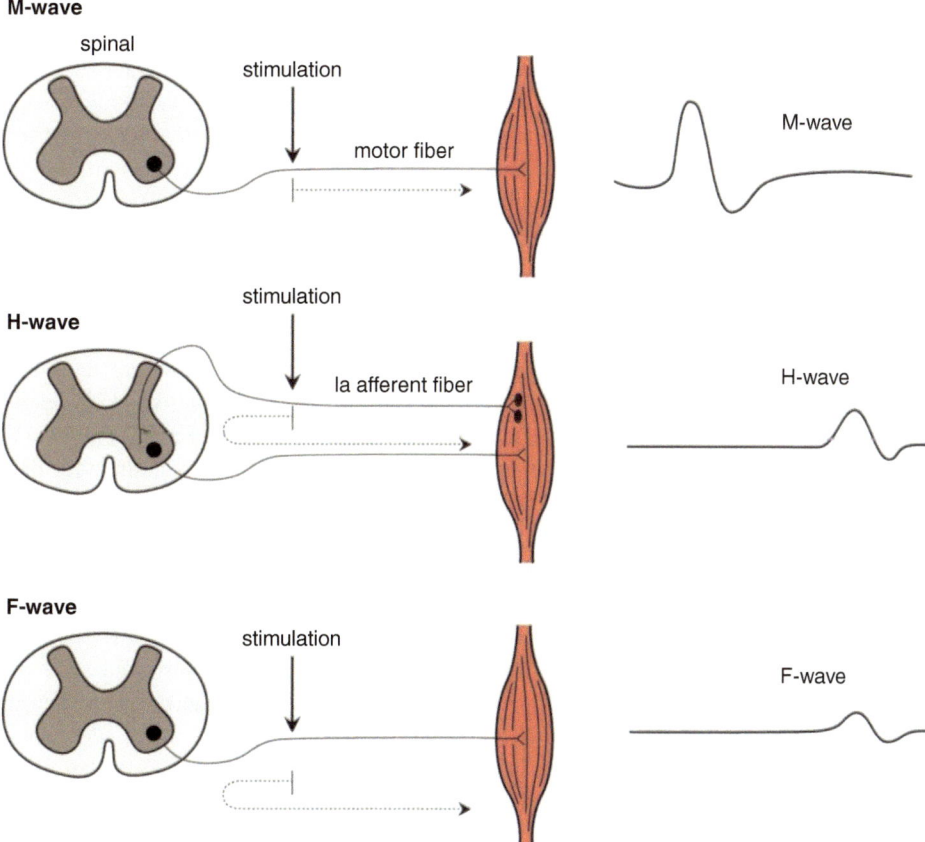

Fig. 18.2 The H-reflex

causing activation of a small variable percentage of anterior horn cells [4]. This results in an orthodromic electrical signal being conducted from the spinal cord to the muscles innervated by the nerve. Several small additional muscle depolarizations occur from motor neurons reactivated known as the F-response. If F-response is prolonged, this indicates some slowing of conduction of the motor axon at the proximal portion of the peripheral nerve, the plexus, or the motor root. Therefore F-response abnormalities can be a sensitive indicator of peripheral nerve pathology such as root pathology seen in plexopathy, radiculopathies, spinal processes, Guillain-Barre syndrome, chronic inflammatory demyelinating polyradiculopathy, and demyelinative peripheral neuropathies [7].

Somatosensory Evoked Potentials

Somatosensory evoked potentials (SEPs) are one type of EP, which is produced by the activation of the large peripheral nerve fibers by mechanical or electrical stimuli. Following either mixed nerve or sensory nerve stimulation, SEPs can be recorded over more proximal portions of the peripheral and central nervous system including peripheral nerves, spinal cord, and/or brain [8]. SEPs are helpful in identifying impaired conduction caused by axonal loss (which may result in a reduced amplitude or absent response) and/or demyelination (which may produce prolonged or absent waveforms) [8]. SSEPs are used predominately in intraoperative monitoring during spinal surgery and instrumentation.

Limitations of Electrodiagnosis

Unfortunately, there are limited electrodiagnostic findings that are distinctly specific for any single diagnosis. For example, fibrillations and PSWs are seen in polyneuropathies, motor neuron disease, inflammatory myopathies, radiculopathies, and entrapment neuropathies [5]. Moreover, negative EMG study does not exclude the pathology of peripheral nervous system. Failing to assess the appropriate nerves and muscles for a given clinical problem may result in a false-negative EMG study. The time course over which a disease process progresses and the time at which electrodiagnostic testing is conducted both play major roles in determining whether the electrodiagnostic testing can provide a reasonably certain diagnosis [5]. Therefore, subsequent examinations are useful if a diagnosis has not been established or to document ongoing recovery.

Final Word on EMG/NCS

Electrodiagnosis is often described as an extension of the clinical history and examination as it can yield physiologic information of nerve dysfunction. It plays a critical role in the assessment of patients with symptoms of and signs of nerve root injury, peripheral nerve disease, and neuropathy. Nerve conduction studies can be exceedingly valuable in localizing lesions and determining the pathological course responsible. It is a valuable tool for confirming diagnosis and helpful in differentiating objective neurological injury from musculoskeletal pain syndromes.

Other Electrodiagnostic Studies

As mentioned before, EDX evaluation is an extension of the physical exam. Whereas nerve conduction studies and electromyography are common diagnostic studies, the next set of tests is used for very specialized assessment of nerve function and pain pathology, and is not commonly done in clinical office settings.

Laser-Evoked Potentials

Laser-evoked potentials (LEPs) are cortical response measurements produced when lasers are used to stimulate thermonociceptors in the skin [12]. Pain pathways are part of the somatosensory system, but the pathways of pain signal processing are via different modalities, at peripheral and central levels [13]. Typically visual and auditory pathways represent one modality only and can thus be easily tested using visual and auditory evoked potentials [14]. Pain pathways, are better studied using LEPs. LEPs currently have two uses, for clinical testing and for research into the pathophysiology of pain pathways. LEP recordings are considered to be the most reliable and widely accepted laboratory tool for assessing nociceptive-pathway function [13].

Specialized infrared lasers are aimed at the patient's skin with the goal of stimulating the heat and pain receptors in order to elicit a cortical response. Two different types are available: CO_2 lasers (wavelength 10.6 μm) and solid-state lasers with shorter wavelengths (1–2 μm). The latter penetrate deeper into the skin, which help reduce superficial burns; however their accuracy is affected by varying skin pigmentations [13]. Patients typically feel pricking (equivalent to getting one hair follicle out) and burning sensations which are a direct result of the laser activation of the Aδ and C fibers respectively. LEP testing is less uncomfortable than NCS and EMG testing and does not require repetitive stimulation with increased signal intensity.

Four electrodes are used to record the cortical potentials with the mean latencies being dependent on the type of laser used. These values are affected by the distance of stimulation from the recording site because there is a higher density of epidermal free nerve endings in proximal vs distal body sites [13]. They are also affected by age (the older the patient, the smaller the LEP amplitude) and patient attention (focusing the patient's attention on a specific task increases the response repetition). LEPs can document lesions of the spinothalamic tract, the lateral aspects of the brainstem, and the thalamocortical projections carrying heat-nociceptive signals. In studying the peripheral nerves, LEPs can distinguish between axonal and demyelinating lesions and large- and small-fiber neuropathies [12]. LEPs are limited in that they can only reliably show decreased transmission of signals and in that they cannot pinpoint the exact location of the lesion.

Quantitative Sensory Testing: Uses and Limitations

Quantitative sensory testing (QST) is a formalized, standardized clinical sensitivity test using calibrated stimuli. The test allows the detection of sensory plus and minus signs such as hypoesthesia or hyperalgesia [15]. The main limitations of traditional physical examination are a result of its qualitative nature and the lack of control and standardization of the stimulus intensity [12]. QST complements the physical exam and decreases its subjective nature to provide reproducible, standardized measurement of the patient's deficits and localize their source.

A historically accepted and standardized method of testing tactile sensation is known as the two-point discrimination test. QST incorporates this and multiple other testing methods. It consists of specially calibrated thermal and mechanical stimuli to test a patient's sensory system, and it is performed in conjunction with a thorough neurological exam. The currently accepted worldwide standard includes a battery of sensory tests that was developed as part of the German Research Network on Neuropathic Pain (DFNS) [15]. The test typically takes 1 hour to complete and subjects patients to hot, cold, vibration, pinprick, and pressure stimuli.

Every patient reacts differently to the same stimuli. Therefore, in order to minimize reporting bias and standardize the results as much as possible, two different algorithms have been used to record and analyze the QST results: method of limits and method of levels. During method of limits testing, the intensity of the stimulus applied to the skin is increased until the subject receives a stimulus or feels it as painful and stops the stimulus by pressing a button. Because it involves reaction time, method of limits is affected by the patient's motor abilities and concentration. In the method of levels, a series of set stimuli are applied to the skin, and the patient has to report (yes or no) whether it is painful or not [12]. This method is not influenced by the patient's reaction time; however it can take a long time.

Although QST is meant to be an objective study, there is still some element of dependence on patient cooperation. QST has great utility for conducting clinical trials but is not very commonly used in the clinical settings. There are, however, conditions when QST is useful, particularly in evaluating neuropathic pain in polyneuropathy and small-fiber neuropathy. In those conditions nerve conduction studies are not suitable as they only test large-fiber function and will be normal, missing the diagnosis [15]. A notable limitation of QST is that it can tell whether or not a lesion exists along the somatosensory pathway, but it cannot localize it [12].

Skin Punch Biopsy: Assessment of Innervation Density

As discussed in previous chapters, small-fiber neuropathy is associated with many specific conditions, and can present as pain or burning in the feet. Traditional sensory nerve conduction studies, which evaluate only the large myelinated fibers, are typically normal in small-fiber neuropathy [12].

Historically, sural nerve biopsy has long been used for the histopathologic diagnosis of most peripheral neuropathies, but it is an invasive procedure performed in the operating room and carries the risks of pain and permanent sensory loss distal to the biopsy site [12]. On top of that, the actual assessment of the nerve fibers is tedious and can only be performed twice, as the entire nerve section has to be obtained for analysis.

Skin biopsy is a safe and inexpensive technique for evaluating small nerve fibers [12]. Decreased nerve-fiber density is typically found in peripheral neuropathies. Innervation density in the biopsy sample can easily be evaluated by measuring the intraepidermal nerve-fiber density under bright-field microscopy. It has been proven as a useful method in quantifying disease severity in small-fiber neuropathy, which may not be detected by traditional physical, neurophysiologic, and neuropathologic tests [16]. In addition, serial skin punch biopsies have also been useful for monitoring disease progression.

It can easily be performed in the office under local anesthetic. A 3 mm sample of the skin is taken from any body site using sterile technique. The sample is specially prepared and immunohistochemically stained. The site of the biopsy easily heals within a week and can be performed multiple times [12].

MRI, fMRI, and MR Spectroscopy: Uses

The human brain processes pain signals and creates an interpretation of what people feel as pain. Different imaging modalities permit observation of these pain process in various areas of the brain, allowing clinicians and researchers to get a better understanding of signaling pathways.

Magnetic Resonance Imaging (MRI) operates on the principles of nuclear magnetic resonance, whereby in the presence of a magnetic field, different nuclei absorb and give off characteristic electromagnetic radiation, allowing visualization and identification of different structures. It can be used to identify areas of structural damage that can be causing pain. Functional magnetic resonance imaging (fMRI) uses similar principles; however it exploits the fact that there is an increase in blood flow to localized vasculature associated with neural activity in the brain [18]. The increased blood flow is associated with local reduction in deoxyhemoglobin (deoxyhemoglobin is paramagnetic, it alters the T2-weighted MRI signal) which functions as an endogenous contrast-enhancing agent and serves as the source of the signal for fMRI. fMRI can be used to obtain information about active signal processing occurring in real time and has permitted the discovery of various pain pathways and CNS pain signaling [12]. In clinical setting fMRI has been used to monitor disease progression and also to map the brain language centers in order to provide surgical planning for tumor resection.

Magnetic Resonance Spectroscopy (MRS) provides a measure of brain chemistry and can be used to monitor serial biochemical changes in patients with tumors, stroke, epilepsy, metabolic disorders, infections, and neurodegenerative diseases [12].

PET Scan: Uses

Positron Emission Tomography (PET) is a nuclear medicine imaging technique that produces a 3-dimensional image of functional processes in the body [12]. The patient is injected with a radioisotope tracer while performing a particular task. Brain areas participating in functional activation demand a higher level of oxygen and glucose energy, resulting in increased blood perfusion and subsequent tracer concentration, which is picked up by scanners. Computer analysis then uses complicated software algorithms for signal processing and analysis.

PET scan has a lower resolution and is considered to be more hazardous than fMRI due to involvement of radioactive tracers. However, it has utility in evaluating oncological involvement and spread in the body. Its use in pain management has been mainly limited to research and study of signaling pathways.

EEG and MEG: Uses

Electroencephalography (EEG) and Magnetoencephalography (MEG) are noninvasive techniques used to detect and measure electric potentials (EEG) and magnetic fields (MEG) generated by the neurons in the brain. EEG is recorded from the scalp by electrodes directly in contact with the skin. In contrast, MEG can be recorded directly from the array of SQUIDs (super quantum induction devices) placed above the head [17]. EEG characteristically shows alpha, beta, delta, and theta waves in varying frequencies and intensities. Varying levels of consciousness, seizures, and pain states show characteristic changes in these waves. MEG has the advantage of easy application without the lengthy preparation as in EEG and direct recording of current flow without interference from the different currents in the brain [17]. However, unlike EEG, it is not very sensitive to deep brain currents.

Clinically, EEG and MEG are used to detect and localize epileptiform spiking activity in patients with epilepsy. They are also used to localize brain areas important for speech, which should be avoided by the surgeon in planning for removal of brain tumors [12]. In chronic pain states, EEG and MEG have shown that chronic pain patients have characteristic signal patterns. Studies are being done to see whether EEG can be used to diagnose chronic pain states.

References

1. AANEM glossary of terms in neuromuscular &amp. Electrodiagnostic medicine. Muscle Nerve. 2015;52:145.
2. Ibrahim, A., et al., Analysis of electromyography (EMG) signal for human arm muscle: a review. 2016. p. 567.
3. Paganoni S, Amato A. Electrodiagnostic evaluation of myopathies. Phys Med Rehabil Clin North Am. 2013;24(1):193.
4. Feinberg J, et al. Electrodiagnostic medicine; 2006. p. 285.
5. Braddom RL, Chan L, et al., editors. Physical medicine and rehabilitation. Philadelphia: Saunders/Elsevier; 2011.
6. Thornton R, Michell A. Techniques and applications of EMG: measuring motor units from structure to function. J Neurol. 2012;259(3):585.
7. Mallik A, Weir A. Nerve conduction studies: Essentials and pitfalls in practice. Neurol Pract. 2005;76(2):ii23.
8. Guidelines in electrodiagnostic medicine. Somatosensory evoked potentials: clinical uses. Muscle Nerve Suppl. 1999;8:S111.
9. Palmieri RM, Ingersoll CD, Hoffman MA. The Hoffmann reflex: Methodologic considerations and applications for use in sports medicine and athletic training research. J Athl Train. 2004;39(3):268.
10. Oh SJ. In: Oh SJ, editor. Clinical electromyography: nerve conduction studies. Philadelphia: Lippincott Williams & Wilkins; 2003.
11. Preston DC. In: Preston DC, Shapiro BE, editors. Electromyography and neuromuscular disorders clinical-electrophysiological correlations. London/New York: Elsevier Saunders; 2013.
12. Gevirtz C. Review of clinical nerve function studies and imaging: part II. Top Pain Manag. 2011;26(12):1–7.
13. Valeriani M, Pazzaglia C, Cruccu G, Truini A. Clinical usefulness of laser evoked potentials. Neurophysiol Clin. 2012;42(5):345–53.
14. Treede RD, Lorenz J, Baumgärtner U. Clinical usefulness of laser-evoked potentials. Neurophysiol Clin. 2003;33(6):303–14.
15. Mücke M, Cuhls H, Radbruch L, et al. Quantitative sensory testing (QST). English version. Schmerz. 2016;
16. Gibbons CH, Griffin JW, Polydefkis M, et al. The utility of skin biopsy for prediction of progression in suspected small fiber neuropathy. Neurology. 2006;66(2):256–8.
17. Chen AC. New perspectives in EEG/MEG brain mapping and PET/fMRI neuroimaging of human pain. Int J Psychophysiol. 2001;42(2):147–59.
18. Cole LJ, Farrell MJ, Duff EP, Barber JB, Egan GF, Gibson SJ. Pain sensitivity and fMRI pain-related brain activity in Alzheimer's disease. Brain. 2006;129(Pt 11):2957–65.

Peripheral Nerve Blocks and Lesioning and Surgical Pain Management

19

Alan David Kaye, Elyse M. Cornett, Chris J. Cullom, Susan M. Mothersele, Yury Rapoport, Burton D. Beakley, Azem Chami, and Vibhav Reddy

Introduction

Peripheral nerve blocks are used to treat a variety of chronic pain conditions in the outpatient setting. In the perioperative setting, they have been shown to decrease hospital length of stay, provide better pain control, and have fewer side effects when compared to epidural anesthesia or patient-controlled opioid therapy [1]. The number of hospitals providing acute pain services is increasing, and peripheral nerve blocks are an important aspect of these services [2]. Blocks can be used as the sole modality for analgesia for a procedure or be used as an adjunct to general anesthesia or moderate/deep sedation to allow for improved pain control in the acute setting. Some contraindications to peripheral nerve blocks include infection of the skin over the area of needle insertion, neuropathy of the nerves to be blocked, and the presence of a coagulopathy. Risks of the procedure include, but are not limited to infection, nerve damage, bleeding, possible falls if the block is performed on a lower extremity and pneumothorax for brachial plexus and chest wall/thoracic spine procedures [3].

Peripheral nerve blocks are generally performed under ultrasound guidance to allow the practitioner to directly visualize the nerve and other relevant structures (i.e., blood vessels, pleura, etc.) in relation to the needle, as well as spread

of local anesthesia around the nerve. A nerve stimulator may also be used to locate the nerve, but has been shown to be less cost effective for hospitals and inferior to ultrasound techniques [3]. Nerves being viewed in a transverse plane appear as a honeycomb, while nerves visualized in a longitudinal plane appear as long, slender structures that consist of a mixture of hypoechoic and hyperechoic parallel lines [4]. The use of ultrasound has made it easier to perform distal nerve blocks in the upper extremity, which is beneficial in the event that a brachial plexus block provides incomplete analgesia [5].

Paresthesias are uncomfortable, shock-like sensations that can occur during the administration of a peripheral nerve block. The needle used in a block should be positioned close to the nerve, and if contact is made with the nerve, a paresthesia may be elicited. While this discomfort can help to indicate that the needle is in close proximity to the nerve, suggesting increased probability of a successful nerve block, anesthetic should not be injected if a paresthesia is persistent, as it could increase the chance of intraneural injection and potential nerve damage.

The use of peripheral nerve blocks for perioperative pain management has allowed for earlier mobilization and rehabilitation, leading to shorter hospital stays and improved satisfaction among patients [3]. Nerve blocks can either be single injection or continuous infusion with catheter placement [6]. Catheter-based pain management techniques allow for uninterrupted analgesia but are at increased risk for catheter displacement and infection [7].

Anatomical Considerations and Clinical Indications

Brachial Plexus Blocks: Upper Extremity

The brachial plexus innervates the upper extremity and is formed by the ventral rami of cervical nerve roots 5, 6, 7, and 8 and thoracic nerve root 1. Brachial plexus nerve roots

A. D. Kaye (✉)
Department of Anesthesiology, LSU School of Medicine, New Orleans, LA, USA

Louisiana State University Interim Hospital and Ochsner Hospital at Kenner, New Orleans, LA, USA

E. M. Cornett · C. J. Cullom · B. D. Beakley · A. Chami
Department of Anesthesiology, LSU School of Medicine, Shreveport, LA, USA

S. M. Mothersele
Department of Anesthesiology, LSU School of Medicine, New Orleans, LA, USA

Y. Rapoport · V. Reddy
Department of Anesthesiology, Tulane School of Medicine, New Orleans, LA, USA

© Springer Nature Switzerland AG 2019
Y. Khelemsky et al. (eds.), *Academic Pain Medicine*, https://doi.org/10.1007/978-3-030-18005-8_19

exit the spinal cord via the intervertebral foramina where they traverse between the anterior and middle scalene muscles and become trunks. The trunks then course between the first rib and clavicle where each of the trunks divides into an anterior and posterior division [9]. The divisions continue under the clavicle and then converge to form three cords. The lateral, posterior, and medial cords are named based on their relation to the axillary artery [8]. The cords divide again at the lateral border of the pectoralis minor muscle into the terminal nerves [10]. The lateral cord splits into the musculocutaneous nerve (with contributions from C5, 6, and 7) and into the median nerve (with contributions from C5, 6, 7, 8, and T1). The posterior cord divides into the axillary nerve (made up of C5, 6) and the radial nerve (with contributions from C5, 6, 7, 8, T1). The medial cord branches into the medial portion of the median nerve (with contributions from all the nerve roots of the brachial plexus, C5, 6, 7, 8, and T1) and the ulnar nerve (also made up of portions from C5, 6, 7, 8, and T1) [8]. Figure 19.1 depicts brachial plexus anatomy.

Commonly performed brachial plexus blocks include interscalene, supraclavicular, infraclavicular, and axillary. An interscalene block provides anesthesia for the shoulder and most of the upper extremity by targeting the trunks and roots of the brachial plexus, with the possibility of the inferior trunk, C8 and T1, being spared. This could lead to preservation of sensation on the ulnar side of the forearm and hand. Supraclavicular blocks block the trunks/divisions of the brachial plexus providing anesthesia from the shoulder to the hand. Colloquially known as "the spinal of the arm," this block tends to be the workhorse of upper extremity anesthesia. Infraclavicular block is performed at

Fig. 19.1 Brachial plexus anatomy (https://www.nysora.com/interscalene-brachial-plexus-block)

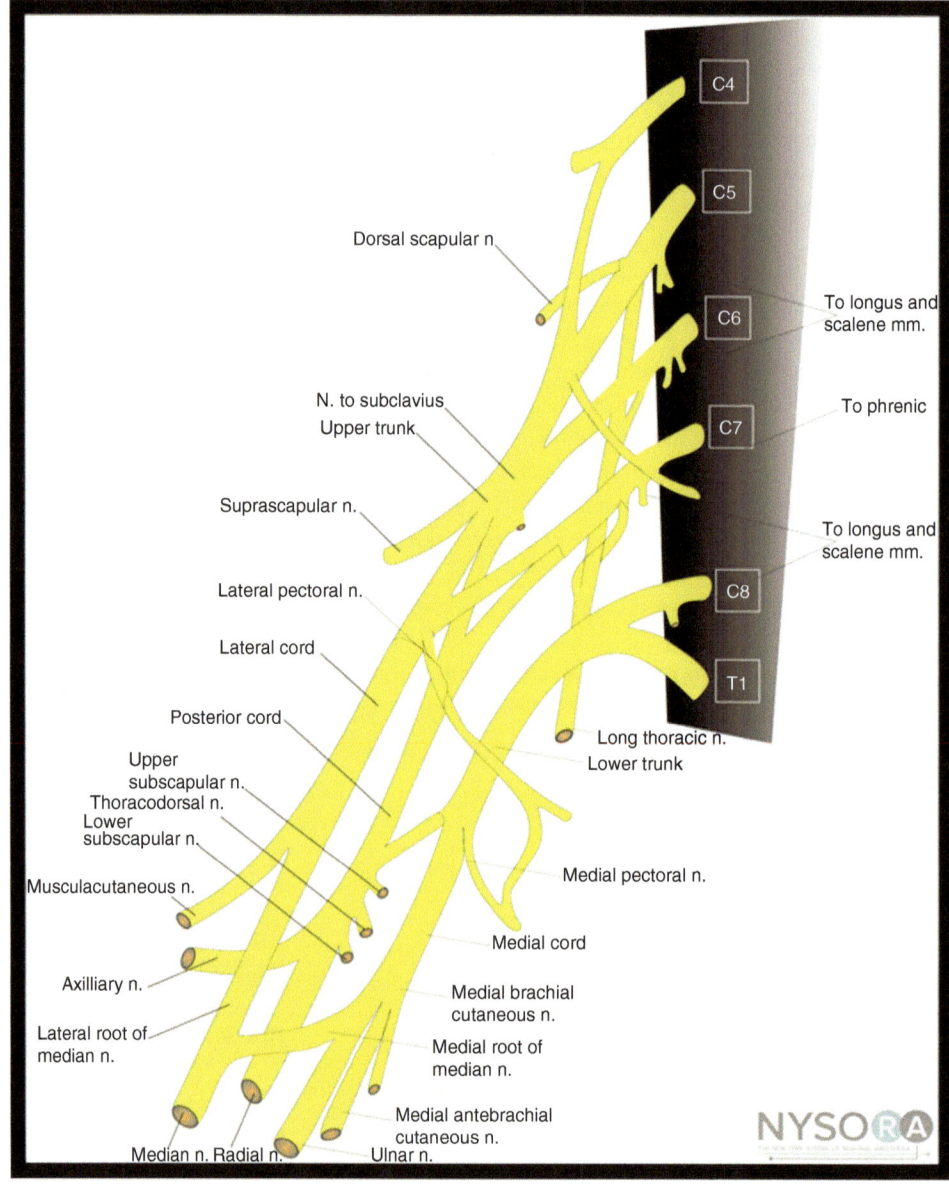

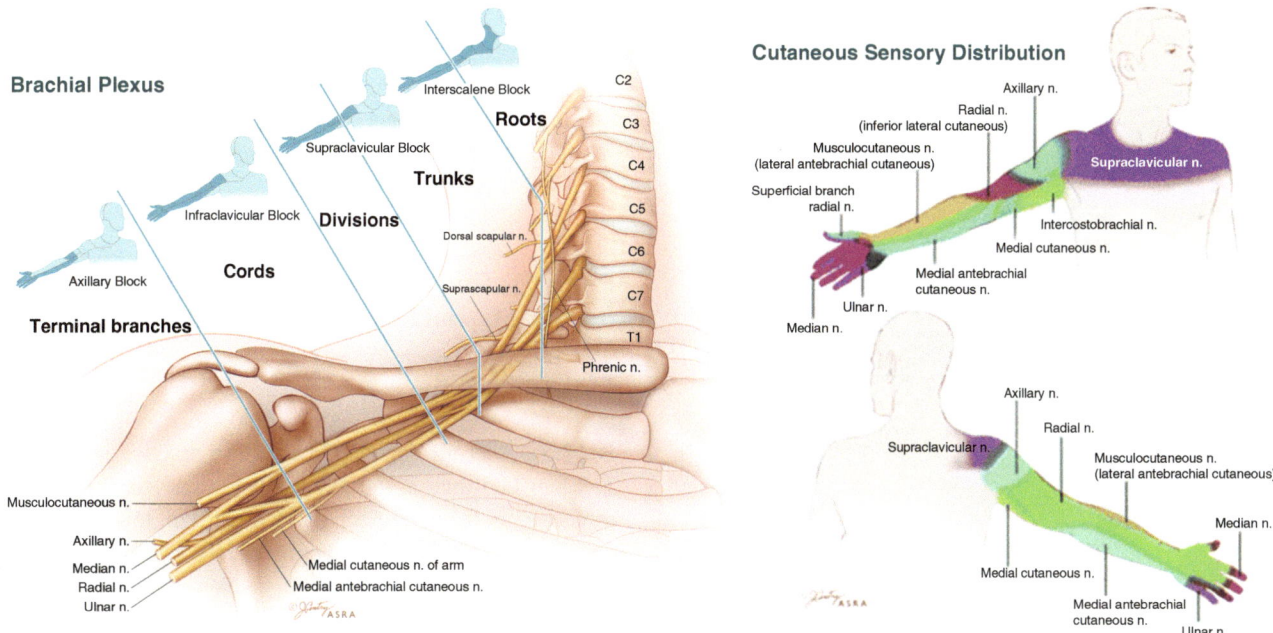

Fig. 19.2 Upper extremity blocks [10]

the level of the cords and provides coverage from the elbow down to the hand. Axillary block also provides anesthesia of the hand from the elbow down, but is performed at the level of the branches [10]. Deep and superficial cervical plexus blocks can be employed for carotid endarterectomy and superficial neck surgery such as excision of cervical lymph nodes. Figure 19.2 depicts the various types of brachial plexus blocks – including the areas expected to be anesthetized, as well as the cutaneous distribution of upper extremity nerves.

Truncal Blocks

Selective truncal blocks, best performed with the use of ultrasound, include the iliohypogastric nerve block, ilioinguinal nerve block, genitofemoral nerve block, penile nerve block, transversus abdominal plane block, lateral femoral cutaneous nerve block, and rectus sheath block. The iliohypogastric nerve, which is often blocked for hernia surgery, anatomically may have a small contribution from T12, but it primarily originates from L1. The genitofemoral nerve block, utilized as a treatment for chronic pain of the pelvis, the perineal area, and the upper thigh, can be combined with ilioinguinal/iliohypogastric nerve blocks for surgical procedures involving the groin area. The genitofemoral nerve originates from the L1 and L2 ventral rami and is formed within the psoas major. The nerve, primarily sensory in function, contains a small motor component and

descends obliquely, advancing through the psoas muscle to emerge at its abdominal surface near the medial border. There, the genitofemoral nerve divides into femoral and genital branches at varying distances from the inguinal ligament. The penile block has been widely used for circumcisions and other penile surgeries and is derived from the pudendal nerve (S2–S4). The penile nerve usually divides into the right and left dorsal nerves of the penis and courses under the pubis symphysis. It then travels under Buck's fascia to supply sensory innervations to the penis. The transversus abdominis plane (TAP) block is a local anesthetic injection into the fascial plane superficial to the transversus abdominis muscle and deep to the internal oblique muscle, which contains nerves responsible for the innervation of the anterior abdominal wall (arising from T6 to L1 levels) and is useful for providing analgesia for abdominal procedures (Fig. 19.3). Bilateral TAP blocks must be performed to provide analgesia to the entire abdominal wall. The rectus sheath block may be used to provide analgesia of the anterior abdominal wall. The lateral femoral cutaneous nerve, which is a pure sensory nerve, may be injected to treat meralgia paresthetica (lateral femoral cutaneous neuropathy). It arises from the dorsal divisions of L2–L3 and emerges from the lateral border of the psoas major muscle.

TAP and rectus sheath blocks can provide significant postoperative analgesia; however, it is important to note that they do not treat the visceral component of pain following intra-abdominal procedures.

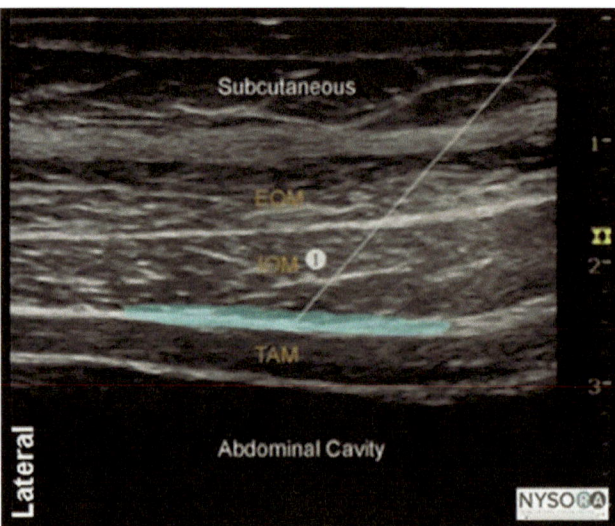

Fig. 19.3 Transversus abdominis plane (TAP) block, ultrasound guided. Shaded blue represents the area of desired local anesthetic spread. EOM, external oblique muscle; IOM, internal oblique muscle, TAM, transverse abdominal muscle (https://www.nysora.com/truncal-and-cutaneous-blocks)

Lower Extremity Blocks

Common nerve blocks of the lower extremity include the femoral, saphenous, sciatic, and popliteal. The ankle block, which is achieved by anesthetizing the five peripheral nerves that supply the foot, is also a commonly employed technique. The femoral nerve innervates the anterior aspect of the thigh and is formed from L2 to L3 to L4. It passes lateral to the femoral artery and vein below the inguinal ligament and is within the fascia iliaca of the iliopsoas muscle. This block is often used for total knee arthroplasty. The femoral nerve continues and gives off its terminal sensory branch, the saphenous nerve [9]. The saphenous nerve can be blocked just after it splits off the femoral nerve, located anterior to the femoral artery at mid-thigh level, beneath the sartorius muscle in the adductor canal [3]. The saphenous nerve provides sensation to the medial aspect of the lower leg, including the knee. The sciatic nerve is made up of nerves from the sacral plexus: L4, L5, S1, 2, and 3. This nerve can be located as it emerges deep to the piriformis muscle. It can be blocked to provide coverage for hip and knee surgery. A popliteal block targets the sciatic nerve in the popliteal fossa, just distal to where the nerve splits into the common peroneal and the tibial nerves. This block provides anesthesia for the foot and ankle and is often used in combination with a femoral or saphenous block. Figure 19.4 shows the innervation of the lower limb, as well as cutaneous coverage achieved with various types of blocks. An ankle block consists of blocking five separate nerves as they enter the foot [6]. These nerves are the posterior tibial, sural, saphenous, deep peroneal, and superficial peroneal.

Femoral and, more recently, saphenous blocks are used to provide analgesia after total knee arthroplasty. Popliteal blocks combined with saphenous blocks are typically employed to provide anesthesia/analgesia for surgery involving the leg and foot. Ankle blocks are commonly performed for procedures involving the foot.

Pharmacology of the Drugs Used During Interventional Pain Procedures

Corticosteroids

Neuraxial steroid injections came into practice in the early 1950s, when their epidural administration was shown to be effective in the treatment of sciatica and low back pain. Despite the fact that the exact mechanism of action was yet to be discovered, the effectiveness of initial attempts prompted utilization of the same approach for a variety of neuraxial, myofascial, and articular injections in the management of a multitude of chronic pain disorders. CS acts at ubiquitous cellular receptors and alters gene expression to modify cellular responses [11]. The direct effects include blockade of phospholipase A2, inhibition of pro-inflammatory mediators and cytokine expression, membrane stabilization, and suppression of both neuronal discharge and dorsal horn sensitization [12, 13]. A variety of corticosteroid drugs (i.e., triamcinolone, betamethasone, dexamethasone, etc.) have been developed, each with different biologic and chemical properties. Formulations prepared using particulates are anticipated to have a longer therapeutic effect, although evidence for this is mixed. When used for neuraxial injections, such as an epidural, depending on the type of agent, steroids impart both short (less than 6 weeks) and long (over 6 weeks) pain relief. CS knee injections for rheumatoid arthritis provided pain relief for 14–66 days after triamcinolone [14] and 8–56 days after administration of methylprednisolone [15].

Local Anesthetics

The use of local anesthetics (LA) as a sole therapeutic treatment in chronic pain is infrequent; however it is increasingly evident that these medications can provide analgesia that lasts far beyond their typical duration of anesthetic action. They are universally utilized for local anesthesia prior to procedures and are also commonly used as a part of multimodal interventional approaches and administered centrally or peripherally, in combination with corticosteroids or other agents. Traditionally, local anesthetics were known to physically block sodium (Na) voltage-gated channels; however, it has been recently suggested that local anesthetics exert their action through generating electrostatic forces that prevent

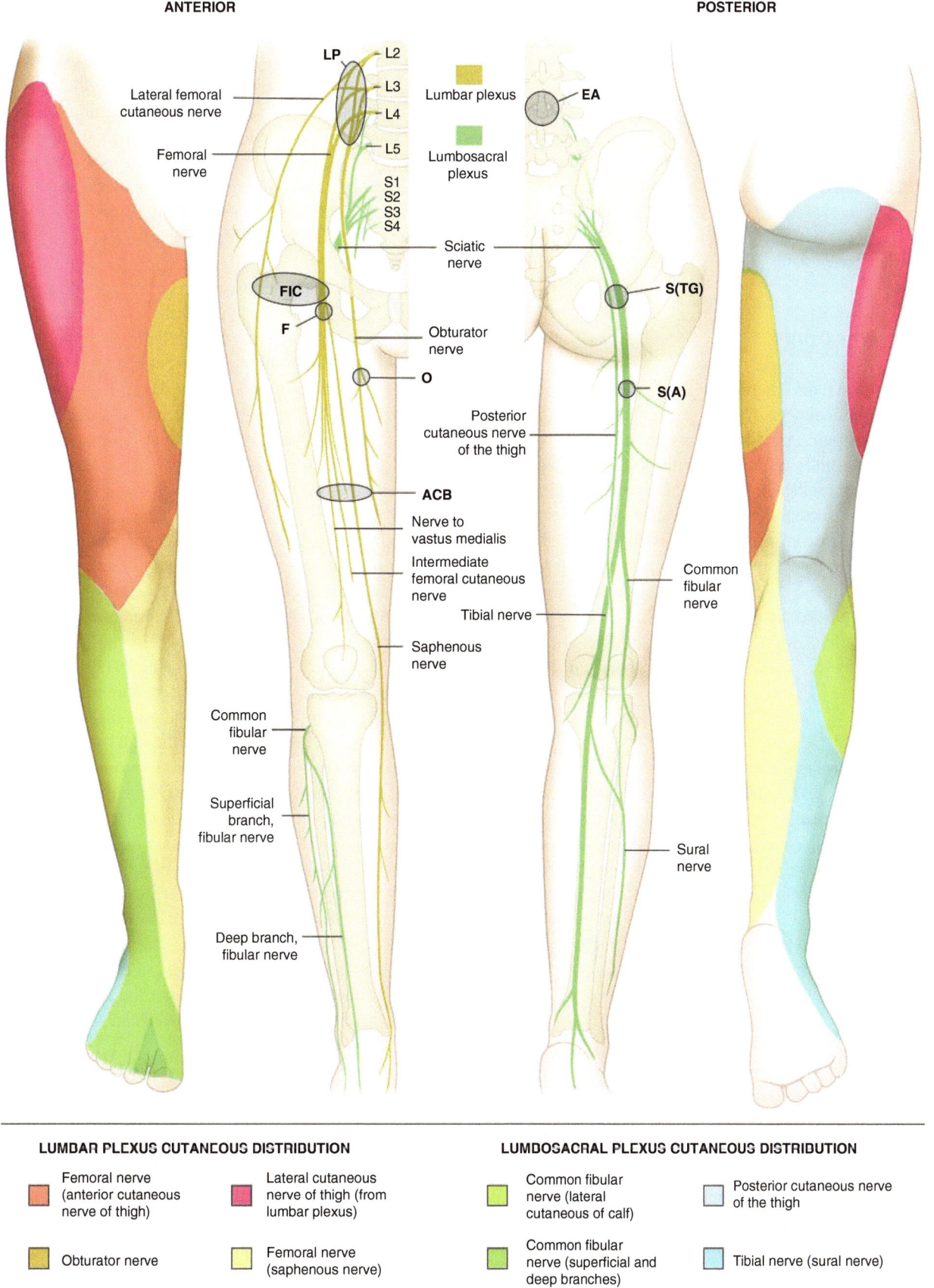

Fig. 19.4 Innervation of the lower limb and lower extremity blocks [49]

Na+ ions from binding and activating Na channels as opposed to direct occlusion [16]. Other potential mechanisms, including their action through non-Na+ ion channels and G-protein receptors, have also been described. Interruption of neuronal membrane depolarization leads to sustained dampening of C-fiber activity – decreasing nociceptive signal input. In addition, local anesthetics have anti-inflammatory properties.

Pka, protein binding, lipid solubility, thickness of perineurium, and vascularity of the specific anatomic location all determine the potency and duration of action of a particular LA drug.

Neurolytic Drugs

Neurolysis is the chemical/physical destruction of nerve fibers. Chemical neurolysis was a popular approach for management of pain in the past; however with the development of safer and more reliable techniques, the use of neurolytic agents has diminished. Nevertheless, neurolysis is a powerful tool in the arsenal of pain physician and has its place as a part of multimodal therapy in carefully selected patients, specifically in those with chronic intractable pain resistant to other modalities. There are several chemical preparations that are approved for injections including alcohol, phenol, and hypertonic saline. Physical neurolysis is typically achieved with radiofrequency (RF) lesioning or cryoablation.

Alcohol

Alcohol neurolysis is commonly utilized for destruction of the celiac plexus/splanchnic nerves [17]. Other uses such as intrathecal neurolysis (alcohol is hypobaric relative to the CSF) and hypophysectomy are increasingly rare. Alcohol is typically diluted with local anesthetics to a concentration of approximately 50% in order to attenuate the burning pain it creates after injection. Injection may be complicated by vasospasm. Full effect of neurolysis, mediated by lipid extraction and protein precipitation, may take several days to develop.

Phenol

While available as a sterile preparation at a concentration of 6.7%, glycerol and a contrast agent are often added to the mixture to lower the concentration. Addition of glycerol makes the solution more hyperbaric compared to CSF. Although the indications for phenol use are similar to those with alcohol, phenol appears to be a less effective neurolytic agent. Injection may precipitate arrhythmias, cardiovascular collapse, and seizures. In contrast to alcohol, there is no pain on injection of phenol. Full effect of neurolysis develops faster than with alcohol, within 24 hours, and is related to protein coagulation and necrosis.

Hypertonic Saline

The use of hypertonic saline was initially limited to intrathecal injection to treat intractable pain and was first described by Hitchcock in 1967. A 10% sodium chloride/water solution is available as a commercial preparation. Its effect is thought to be produced by C-fiber destruction while sparing sensory and motor function. The exact mechanism of its neurolytic action is not well elaborated; however it is hypothesized to be related to osmolality change with associated shift of free water. Similar to alcohol, it causes pain on injection, and thus pretreatment with local anesthetic is warranted. Side effects of intrathecal administration include an increase in intracranial pressure, hypertension, tachypnea, and temporary neurologic deficits. Gabor Racz pioneered the use of hypertonic saline in the management of spinal adhesions or scar tissue, known worldwide as the Racz procedure. The technique, well-described for over two decades, involves fluoroscopic placement of an epidural catheter with targeted instillation of hypertonic saline.

Botox

OnabotulinumtoxinA (Botox, BTX) injections are primarily used to treat disorders related to involuntary muscle contraction as found in focal dystonia and spasticity. Botox has also been effective in the treatment of chronic migraines and is FDA-approved for this indication. There are only two preparations that are FDA-approved for use: BTX-A and BTX-B. BTX-A has been successfully used in treatment of chronic low back pain, myofascial pain syndromes, and neuropathic pain. One mechanism of action is the blockade of acetylcholine release from synapses in the neuromuscular junction while sparing the sensory aspect of nerve conduction, which may produce analgesia via enhanced local blood flow, muscle relaxation, and subsequent release of muscular compression of nerve fibers. Other mechanisms of analgesia have also been proposed. For example, it appears that Botox is taken up in sensory afferents and transported to more central structures in the nervous system, cleaving certain proteins involved in nociception. It has been recently demonstrated that botulinum toxin interferes with the release of several neurotransmitters including glutamate and substance P [18].

Nerve Blocks and Neurolytic Techniques: Diagnostic and Treatment Purposes; Clinical Indications, Risks, and Associated Complications

Interscalene Block

The interscalene block is a brachial plexus block indicated for surgeries of the shoulder, humerus, and upper arm. Brachial plexus roots C5–C7 are anesthetized, but C8–T1 are spared. Risks include intravascular injection, hematoma, nerve injury, and pneumothorax. Ipsilateral Horner's syndrome is expected. Consideration is needed for patients with severe pulmonary disease as the ensuing blockade of the phrenic nerve (100% of the time) leads to paralysis of the hemidiaphragm, which may compromise respiratory effort. Bilateral blocks should be avoided for this reason, as well as the potential of pneumothorax. Caution should also be exercised if the patient has preexisting unilateral vocal cord paralysis, as recurrent laryngeal nerve blockade on the contralateral side could lead to complete airway obstruction. Vascular injury may result in pseudo-aneurysm formation [10, 19].

Supraclavicular Block

The block aims to anesthetize the trunks and divisions of the brachial plexus. The intercostobrachial nerve (T2) is not anesthetized; thus the skin of the inner arm is spared. There is a risk of pneumothorax, phrenic nerve paralysis (50% of the time), and recurrent laryngeal nerve paralysis. Similar to interscalene blocks, complications include intravascular injection, pneumothorax, phrenic nerve injury, and laryngeal nerve injury [10, 19, 20].

Infraclavicular Block

Infraclavicular block is another brachial plexus block indicated for procedures distal to the axilla. This approach is not indicated for procedures of the shoulder. The block targets the lateral, posterior, and medial cords of the brachial plexus from an infraclavicular approach. The block is ideal for continuous catheter placement as the pectoralis muscle holds the catheter in place. There is a risk of vascular puncture and pneumothorax although lower than the supraclavicular approach. Complications include hematoma formation and respiratory distress from the previously mentioned risks. Pacemakers or vascular access devices on the chest may obstruct needle placement [20, 21].

Axillary Block

The axillary block is the most distal brachial plexus block and is indicated for procedures distal to the elbow. The block targets the terminal branches of the brachial plexus; however the axillary, musculocutaneous, and medial brachial cutaneous nerves split proximally and are spared. There is no risk of pneumothorax or phrenic nerve paralysis. Hematoma is more likely with the trans-arterial approach [20–22].

Lumbar Plexus Block (Psoas Compartment Block)

Lumbar plexus blocks are indicated for procedures of the hip, anterior thigh, and knee. The lumbar plexus is made up of the ventral rami of L1–L4, which form the obturator, lateral femoral cutaneous, ilioinguinal, iliohypogastric, and genitofemoral nerves. Procedure-specific complications include peritoneal puncture, renal subcapsular hematoma, and psoas hematoma [23].

Femoral Nerve

Femoral nerve block is indicated for knee procedures. Additional blockade may be required as the posterior sensation provided by the sciatic nerve is unaffected. The femoral nerve innervates the hip flexors, knee extensors, and sensory fibers for the anterior thigh and hip. This block can anesthetize the femoral, lateral femoral cutaneous, and obturator nerves if there is spread of the local anesthetic. Risk of lower extremity weakness due to quadriceps motor blockade is possible. Complications include postoperative falls due to quadriceps weakness and hematoma formation from vascular injury [24, 25].

Obturator Nerve Block

Obturator nerve block is indicated for knee procedures or procedures involving the distal 2/3 of the thigh, but alone will not provide complete anesthesia for knee surgery. Full coverage requires combination with a sciatic nerve block. Obturator nerve block can also be used in urologic surgery to suppress the obturator reflex during transurethral resection of the bladder wall. The obturator nerve contributes sensory innervation to the medial thigh and medial aspect of the knee as well as motor control of the adductor compartment muscles. Lower extremity weakness due to adductor muscle block can result in falls, yet is unlikely due to sparing of much of the musculature in the thigh. If the needle is advanced too deep, the pelvic cavity can be punctured and the bladder, rectum, or spermatic cord can be damaged. The obturator vessels can be damaged by the needle as well [26].

Sciatic Nerve Block

Sciatic nerve block is useful for surgery involving the hip, thigh, knee, lower leg, and foot. However anesthesia is limited to the posterior portion of the thigh and knee. Sciatic nerve block is useful for knee arthroplasty in conjunction with femoral nerve block and lower leg surgery in conjunction with saphenous nerve block. The sciatic nerve originates from nerve roots L4–L5 and L5–S1. Anesthesia to the sciatic nerve blocks sensation to the posterior thigh, posterior knee, and most of the lower leg except the sensory domain of the saphenous nerve on the medial leg. Risks include vascular puncture with the anterior approach and direct nerve injection. Complications include falls due to hamstring weakness and foot drop, vascular injury, and neuropathy [27–29].

Popliteal Block

Popliteal fossa block is a distal sciatic nerve block indicated for procedures involving the knee, lower leg, and foot. Anesthesia excludes the anterior aspect of the knee as well as the medial aspect of the lower leg and ankle joint capsule. Addition of saphenous nerve block is required for complete anesthesia of the lower leg. Sciatic nerve block is performed at or slightly above the popliteal fossa, thus avoiding hamstring muscle weakness. Risks include vascular puncture and nerve injury. Complications include hematoma formation and falls due to foot drop [29, 30].

Adductor Canal Block

Adductor canal block is primarily indicated for knee surgery and procedures involving the thigh; however the posterior aspect of knee and thigh will be spared. Adductor canal block aims to anesthetize the saphenous nerve, obturator sensory branch, and nerve to the vastus medialis. The block provides anesthesia to the anterior portion of the knee and thigh. There is less involvement of the quadriceps muscles, thus less lower extremity weakness compared to other blocks. Risks include vascular puncture, local infection at the site, and minor quadriceps muscle weakness. Complications include bleeding and hematoma from vascular puncture and infection. Postoperative falls are possible; however they have been found to be significantly less common compared to femoral nerve blocks [24, 25, 31].

Ankle Block

Ankle block is indicated for surgeries of the ankle and foot; however a calf tourniquet will be proximal to the block, resulting in some degree of tourniquet-related pain. The block involves local anesthetic injection of the distal saphenous nerve, deep peroneal, superficial peroneal, posterior tibial, and sural nerves. Risks include vascular puncture, intravascular injection, infection, and nerve injury. Complications are very rare but include neuropathy, hema-

toma formation (most commonly with disruption of the saphenous vein medially), and local anesthetic toxicity [32].

Side Effects: Recognition and Treatment

As with all medical procedures, there are risks associated with the use of peripheral nerve blocks and lesioning. With all procedures involving the insertion of a needle or catheter, there is risk of bruising, bleeding, infection, and damage to surrounding structures. Bleeding disorders and pharmacological anti-coagulation increase the risk of hematoma formation. Vascular puncture during peripheral nerve catheter placement has an incidence of 5.7–6.6% [33]; however serious complications secondary to the puncture are rare. An understanding of the American Society of Regional Anesthesia's anticoagulation recommendations will help the physician with determination of bleeding risk. Infection at the site of injection is a contraindication [19]. While the benefits of peripheral nerve catheters are evident, the risk of infection is clearly greater than with single shot blocks [33]. The use of transparent dressing helps for early recognition of superficial infection, and strict aseptic technique can help reduce the incidence of infection, as well [34]. Bruising and soreness at the site of injection can occur with any injection, most being self-limited and managed conservatively. Up to 13% of patients receiving spinal anesthetics can develop a backache, thought to be secondary to local inflammatory response along with a degree of muscle spasm [35]. Intraneural injection, nerve laceration, vascular injury, or pneumothorax are also possible. With integration of ultrasound guidance into regional anesthesia practice, incidence of vascular injury, local anesthetic systemic toxicity, pneumothorax, and phrenic nerve block has decreased; however it is unclear if there has been a similar decline in the incidence of nerve injury [33]. Nerve injury can occur with peripheral blocks, and while rare, patients with underlying peripheral neuropathy or previous nerve injury can be at increased risk for these complications [19]. Studies suggest an incidence of 0.5–1.0%, with most cases presenting with transient mild mononeuropathies [33]. While post-peripheral nerve block neurologic deficits are rare and often transient, recognition and neurological follow-up until resolution and/or stabilization is necessary [33].

Local anesthetic toxicity (LAST) via accidental intravascular injection or systemic absorption can occur. LAST can be recognized early in the awake patient because of its initial CNS symptoms, including tinnitus, perioral numbness, dizziness, and tremors [8]. These CNS symptoms can progress to seizure. Treatment includes stopping administration of local anesthetic with signs of mild CNS symptoms, and in the case of seizures, small intravenous doses of a benzodiazepine often terminate the convulsions. LAST resulting in cardiotoxicity, while less common, and typically requiring higher doses of local anesthetic than needed to elicit CNS symptoms, can be fatal. It is important to note that the pharmacologic treatment of cardiac arrest secondary to LAST is different from other cardiac arrest scenarios – for example, epinephrine boluses should be limited to less than or equal to 1 mcg/kg, the nearest cardiopulmonary bypass team should be alerted, and intralipid (20% lipid emulsion) should be administered. The American Society of Regional Anesthesia (ASRA) has released a checklist that should be used in cases of LAST.

Surgical Pain Management

Introduction

Many surgical procedures have been attempted to treat intractable pain. These surgical interventions can be directed to target the peripheral nervous system, spinal cord, or the brain [36]. It is important to note that all the nonsurgical approaches of pain management should be exhausted before any surgical intervention is discussed [37]. The common surgical techniques used are ablative, augmentative, and decompressive approaches.

Ablative Procedures

Ablative techniques are not common in clinical practice and have been replaced by augmentative techniques such as the implantation of stimulating electrodes or chronic analgesic infusion pumps, among others [36]. Ablative methods are characterized by the destruction of the neural tissues in an attempt to modulate or modify the pain pathway or to prevent transmission of pain signals from an injured nerve to the central nervous system. However, ablation causes irreversible damage and may lead to the loss of function. In addition, some procedures like neurectomy and ganglionectomy are generally known for achieving only short-term benefits [38]. On the other hand, ablative procedures remain useful therapeutic options for appropriately selected cases. A definitive ablative procedure may be appropriate in patients with a terminal illness, such as a malignancy, because of a limited life span [36].

Ablative procedures are divided into three major categories:

1. Peripheral ablative procedures: Peripheral neurectomy, dorsal rhizotomy, ganglionectomy, and trigeminal nerve or glossopharyngeal nerve ablation. Trigeminal neuralgia is one of the most prevalent diseases successfully treated with ablation. Dorsal rhizotomy or sectioning of the dorsal root is generally effective. However, it is highly associated with sensory loss.
2. Spinal cord ablative procedures: Dorsal root entry zone lesioning, interrupting the ascending lateral spinothalamic tract by percutaneous or open anterolateral cordotomy, and commissural myelotomy.
3. Central ablative procedures: Postcentral gyrectomy, cingulotomy, and thalamotomy.

Augmentative Procedures

Augmentative procedures involve a variety of different techniques, ranging from implantation of electrical stimulating systems to the implantation of infusion pumps to provide spinal analgesia [39]. Choice of system depends on the type of pain being treated and the desired goal of therapy.

Electrical stimulating systems can be used for peripheral nerve, spinal cord, deep brain, and motor cortex stimulation [39]. The implantable infusion systems are intrathecal or epidural infusion catheters that allow infusion of opioids, local anesthetics, and other compounds. These technologist are discussed in greater detail in other chapters of this publication.

Decompressive Procedures

Decompressive surgical approaches are non-ablative procedures that may relieve pain caused by compression of nerves by adjacent connective tissue [38]. Commonly used decompressive procedures include laminectomy, trigeminal microvascular decompression, and decompression of median or ulnar entrapments [39].

Importance of General Health Status in Preoperative Evaluation

Surgical treatment is associated with variable degrees of risk of intraoperative and postoperative complications, and these generally increase with age and comorbidities. Thus, all patients should undergo a general preoperative assessment and evaluation to weigh the desirable benefits and outcomes against any potential risk and complications [40].

It is crucial to understand the general health issues that are relevant to successful surgery, particularly before considering any surgical procedure for pain management [41]. It is also important to exclude and treat any medical condition that might be the causative pathology of the pain before electing to proceed with an invasive management approach [36].

Distinguishing and differentiating the pathological cause of the pain, assessing the general health status, and life expectancy are important factors in the preoperative evaluation [41]. Decisions for selection of a specific technique may be based on the disease prognosis and life expectancy [42]. For patients with good prognosis, augmentative techniques or simple ablative techniques are used more frequently. Whereas patients with severe pain, poor prognosis and short life span are more appropriate candidates for destructive procedures [42].

In addition to physical health, psychological status is vital in the preoperative evaluation. Identification and assessment of psychological and environmental factors influencing pain behavior is important. Pre-surgical psychological assessment can improve patient selection, promote preparation for surgical interventions, and facilitate treatment of psychological and social issues related to pain [37].

Surgical Lesioning of the Brain, Brain Stem, Spinal Cord, Peripheral Nerves: Indications, Risks, and Associated Complications

Neurosurgical approaches to pain can be achieved at the level of brain, brainstem, spinal cord, or peripheral nerves. Although surgical approaches to achieving pain control have become less frequently used with advances in other forms of chronic pain treatment, it is still a viable option in certain situations.

Medial Thalamotomy

Nuclear targets for neuroablative medial thalamotomy are (1) centralis lateralis, (2) centrum medianum, and (3) parafascicularis. This procedure has been used to treat pain related to a variety of conditions including cancer pain, deafferentation pain (both central and peripheral), arthritis, and pain associated with Parkinson's disease [43].

Stereotactic Cingulotomy

A rarely used procedure, this surgery involves ablation of anterior cingulate gyrus and is used to alter emotional response to pain stimulation. Suitable indications for this procedure are for terminally ill patients with metastatic disease.

Spinal Neuroablation

These procedures were more common several decades ago and were most often used for nociceptive pain relief in patients with cancer pain. However, due to the risk involved with open spinal cord surgery as well as complications involved with the procedures in high-risk patients, this technique is used as last resort.

Anterolateral Cordotomy

This procedure consists of disruption of the lateral spinothalamic tract, located in the anterolateral quadrant of the spinal cord. This tract transmits pain and temperature from one side of the body, beginning approximately two to five segments below that level. Complications involved with the surgery are secondary to local disruption of other pathways in the area. The autonomic pathways for genitourinary as well ipsilateral automatic respiration are also in the anterolateral quadrant of the spinal cord and can lead to complications if transected. Other procedural complications include hypotension, dysesthesia, ataxia, and incontinence. In general, this procedure should be reserved for cancer patients with pain below the cervical levels [44].

Dorsal Root Entry Zone (DREZ) Ablation

The dorsal root entry zone is an area of nociceptive pain signaling found in the spinal cord. Indications for DREZ ablation include a variety of neuropathic pain syndromes of the peripheral nerves, but nerve root avulsion is considered the best indication. Main complications of the procedure include corticospinal tract injury and dorsal column injury due to close location to the DREZ [45].

Peripheral Neurectomy

Neurectomies ablate connection between peripheral nociceptors and the central nervous system.

Procedures aiming to destroy this connection are most used in disorders of peripheral joints or in treatment of peripheral nerve injuries, including post-traumatic neuromas. A significant complication of this procedure is creation neuromas, as well as issues related to the loss of motor function [46].

Radiofrequency Treatment

Radiofrequency ablation (RFA) is usually indicated in patients who are refractory to conservative pain management. RFA employs high-frequency current which runs through an insulated needle generating a localized electric field around the needle tip [47]. This results in generation of thermal energy which causes destruction of tissues (e.g., nerve) adjacent to the active electrode tip. The effect of pain relief is accomplished due to interruption of nociceptive signal propagation through lesioned nerve fibers and lasts until the nerve regenerates. The size of the lesion is determined by the length of the cannula tip, the diameter of the cannula tip, the lesion temperature, and duration of lesioning, as well as other factors such as the presence of heat sinks, such a nearby blood vessels [48]. The electrode tip should be placed alongside the target tissue (parallel). Figure 19.5 shows the factors influencing RF lesion size, and Fig. 19.6 displays the specific effects of increasing temperature and time on lesion size. Currently, the most common indication for the use of CRF is in the treatment of facet mediated pain. Unintended lesioning of surrounding structures is the most serious complication. Many patients may also experience a post-procedural neuralgia, which is typically self-limited, but may require treatments with analgesics.

Pulsed RF (PRF), a nondestructive technique, was later developed in an attempt to minimize unwanted destruction of neighboring structures. It is important to note that this is a completely different modality than CRF. In contrast to CRF, PRF utilizes radiofrequency current in short bursts (typically 20 ms) followed by a "silent" period which usually lasts 480 ms. This allows for extra heat to dissipate, keeping the target tissue at or below 42 °C. The mechanism by which PRF controls pain is unclear. The electric field density is greatest at the tip of the electrode; therefore it should be positioned perpendicular to the target (Fig. 19.7). The relative effectiveness of CRF vs PRF is likely dependent on the specific indication, as well as the allotment of adequate treatment time for PRF (longer than CRF).

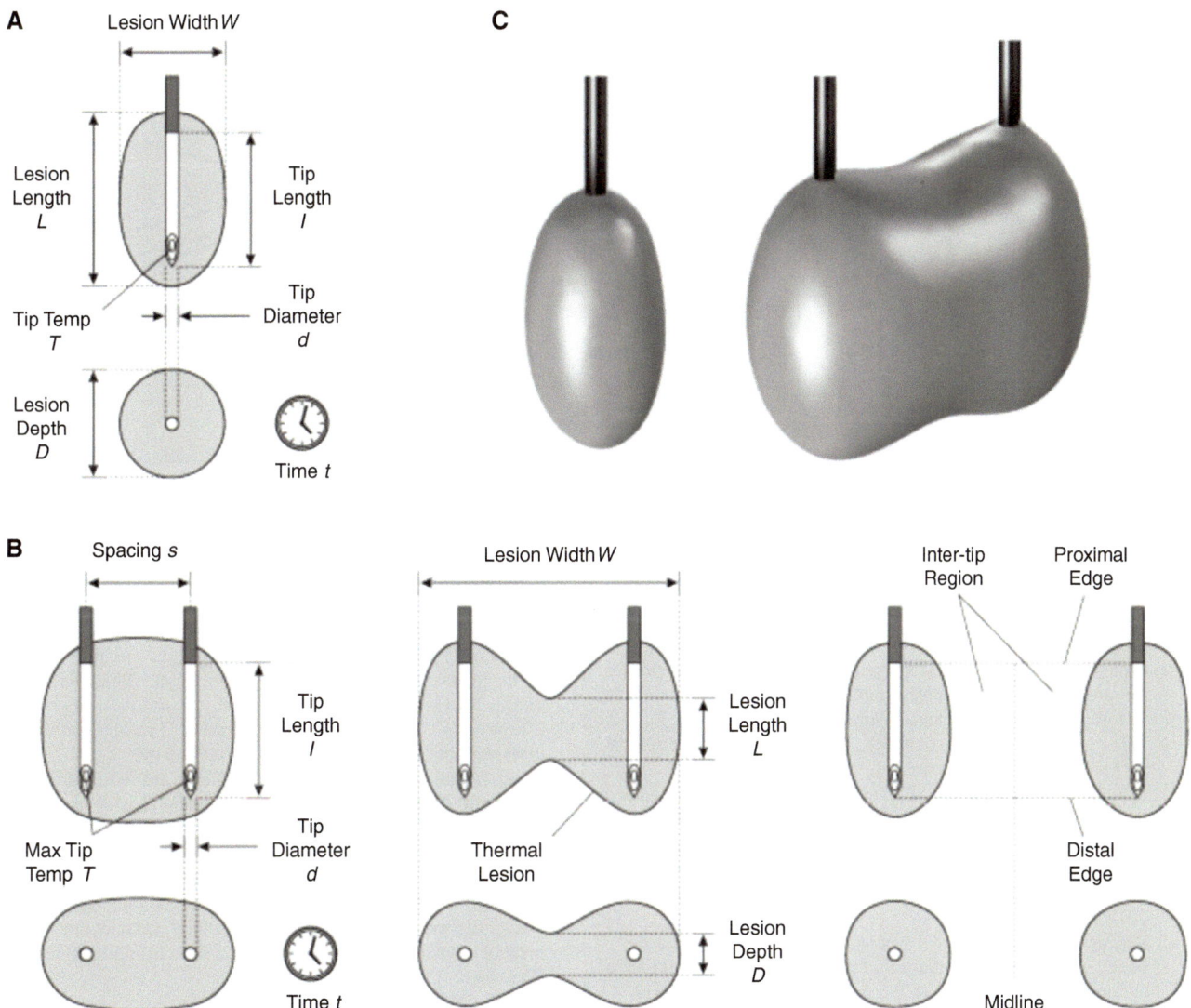

Fig. 19.5 Factors influencing RF lesion size. (From Ref. [48], Pain Med I © 2014 American Academy of Pain Medicine)

Temperature

20ga / 10mm 2:00min

60°C	70°C	80°C	90°C

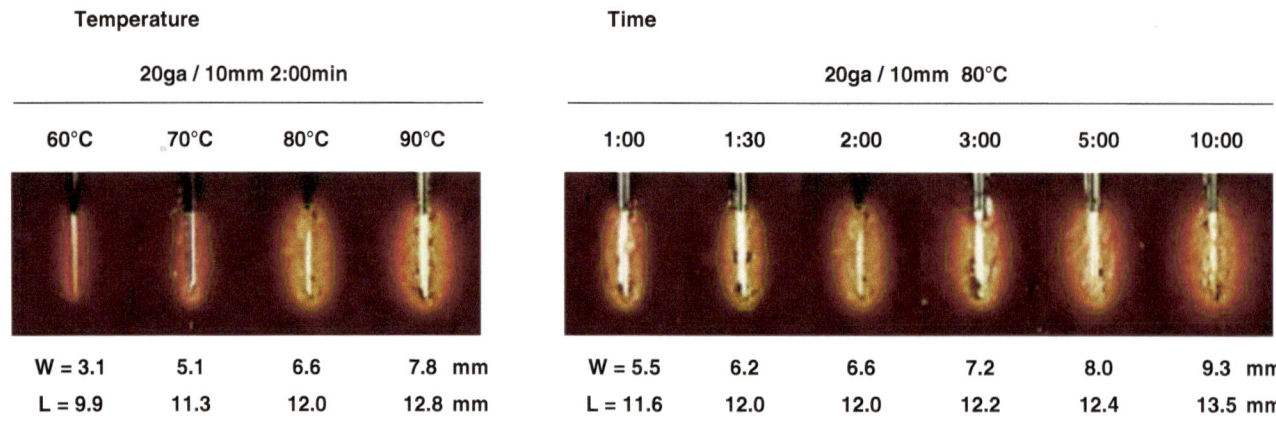

| W = 3.1 | 5.1 | 6.6 | 7.8 mm |
| L = 9.9 | 11.3 | 12.0 | 12.8 mm |

Time

20ga / 10mm 80°C

1:00	1:30	2:00	3:00	5:00	10:00

| W = 5.5 | 6.2 | 6.6 | 7.2 | 8.0 | 9.3 mm |
| L = 11.6 | 12.0 | 12.0 | 12.2 | 12.4 | 13.5 mm |

Fig. 19.6 Effect of temperature (*D*) and time (*E*) on lesion size. (From Ref. [48], Pain Med | © 2014 American Academy of Pain Medicine)

Fig. 19.7 Electric field in pulsed radiofrequency ablation. Density of field is strongest at the tip of the electrode

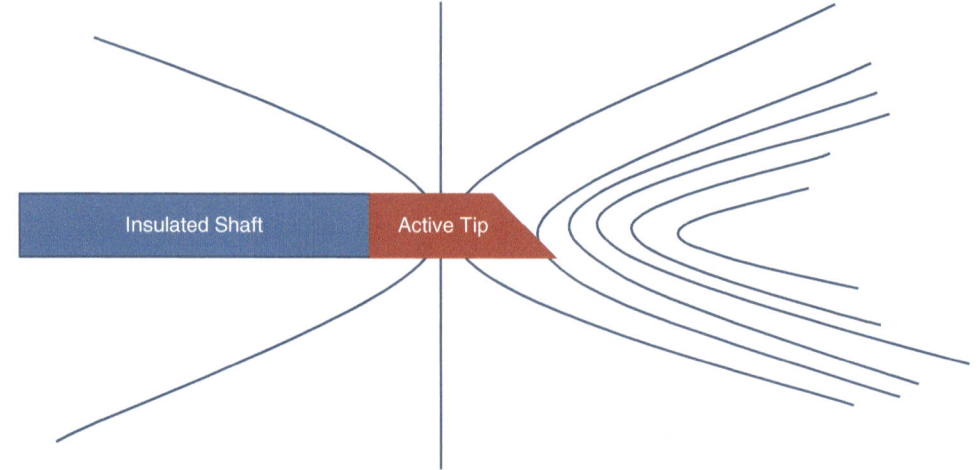

Insulated Shaft   Active Tip

References

1. Johnson RL, Kopp SL, Hebl JR, Erwin PJ, Mantilla CB. Falls and major orthopaedic surgery with peripheral nerve blockade: a systematic review and meta-analysis. Br J Anaesth. 2013;110(4):518–28.
2. Nasir D, Howard JE, Joshi GP, Hill GE. A survey of acute pain service structure and function in United States hospitals. Pain Res Treat. 2011;2011:934932.
3. Danninger T, Opperer M, Memtsoudis SG. Perioperative pain control after total knee arthroplasty: an evidence based review of the role of peripheral nerve blocks. World J Orthop. 2014;5(3):225–32.
4. Suk JI, Walker FO, Cartwright MS. Ultrasonography of peripheral nerves. Curr Neurol Neurosci Rep. 2013;13(2):328.
5. Sehmbi H, Madjdpour C, Shah UJ, Chin KJ. Ultrasound guided distal peripheral nerve block of the upper limb: a technical review. J Anaesthesiol Clin Pharmacol. 2015;31(3):296–307.
6. Aguirre J, Del Moral A, Cobo I, Borgeat A, Blumenthal S. The role of continuous peripheral nerve blocks. Anesthesiol Res Pract. 2012;2012:560879.
7. Kirksey MA, Haskins SC, Cheng J, Liu SS. Local anesthetic peripheral nerve block adjuvants for prolongation of analgesia: a systematic qualitative review. PLoS One. 2015;10(9):e0137312.
8. Butterworth J, Mackey J, Wasnick D. Morgan & Mikhail's clinical anesthesiology. 5th ed. New York: McGraw Hill; 2013.
9. Netter FH. Atlas of human anatomy. 5th ed. Philadelphia: Saunders/Elsevier; 2011.
10. Neal JM, Gerancher JC, Hebl JR, Ilfeld BM, McCartney CJL, Franco CD, Hogan QH. Upper extremity regional anesthesia: essentials of our current understanding. Reg Anesth Pain Med. 2008;34(2):134–70.
11. Im S-A, Gerelchuluun T, Lee C-K. Evidence for direct inhibition of MHC-restricted antigen processing by dexamethasone. Immune Netw. 2014;14(6):328–32.
12. McCarron RF, Wimpee MW, Hudkins PG, Laros GS. The inflammatory effect of nucleus pulposus. A possible element in the pathogenesis of low-back pain. Spine (Phila Pa 1976). 1987;12(8):760–4.
13. Murphy RW. Nerve roots and spinal nerves in degenerative disk disease. Clin Orthop Relat Res. 1977;(129):46–60.
14. Blyth T, Hunter JA, Stirling A. Pain relief in the rheumatoid knee after steroid injection. A single-blind comparison of hydrocortisone succinate, and triamcinolone acetonide or hexacetonide. Br J Rheumatol. 1994;33(5):461–3.
15. Ostergaard M, Stoltenberg M, Gideon P, Sørensen K, Henriksen O, Lorenzen I. Changes in synovial membrane and joint effusion volumes after intraarticular methylprednisolone. Quantitative assessment of inflammatory and destructive changes in arthritis by MRI. J Rheumatol. 1996;23(7):1151–61,. Jul.
16. Mcnulty MM, Edgerton GB, Shah RD, Hanck DA, Fozzard HA, Lipkind GM. Charge at the lidocaine binding site residue Phe-1759 affects permeation in human cardiac voltage-gated sodium channels. J Physiol. 2007;5812:741–55.

17. Chak A. What is the evidence for EUS-guided celiac plexus block/neurolysis? Gastrointest Endosc. 2009;69(2. Suppl):S172–3.
18. Sim WS. Application of botulinum toxin in pain management. Korean J Pain. 2011;24(1):1–6.
19. Madison S, Ilfeld B. Chapter 46. Peripheral nerve blocks. In: Morgan GE, Mikhail M, editors. Morgan & Mikhail's clinical anesthesiology. 4th ed. New York: Lange Medical Books; 2006.
20. Stav A, Reytman L, Stav M-Y, Portnoy I, Kantarovsky A, Galili O, Luboshitz S, Sevi R, Sternberg A. Comparison of the supraclavicular, infraclavicular and axillary approaches for ultrasound-guided brachial plexus block for surgical anesthesia. Rambam Maimonides Med J. 2016;7(2):e0013.
21. Gürkan Y, Hoşten T, Solak M, Toker K. Lateral sagittal infraclavicular block: clinical experience in 380 patients. Acta Anaesthesiol Scand. 2008;52(2):262–6.
22. Kang SB, Rumball KM, Ettinger RS. Continuous axillary brachial plexus analgesia in a patient with severe hemophilia. J Clin Anesth. 2003;15(1):38–40.
23. Bogoch ER, Henke M, Mackenzie T, Olschewski E, Mahomed NN. Lumbar paravertebral nerve block in the management of pain after total hip and knee arthroplasty: a randomized controlled clinical trial. J Arthroplast. 2002;17(4):398–401.
24. Kuang M-J, Xu L-Y, Ma J-X, Wang Y, Zhao J, Lu B, Ma X-L. Adductor canal block versus continuous femoral nerve block in primary total knee arthroplasty: a meta-analysis. Int J Surg. 2016;31:17–24.
25. Sharma S, Iorio R, Specht LM, Davies-Lepie S, Healy WL. Complications of femoral nerve block for total knee arthroplasty. Clin Orthop Relat Res. 2010;468(1):135–40.
26. Bolat D, Aydogdu O, Tekgul ZT, Polat S, Yonguc T, Bozkurt IH, Sen V, Okur O. Impact of nerve stimulator-guided obturator nerve block on the short-term outcomes and complications of transurethral resection of bladder tumour: a prospective randomized controlled study. Can Urol Assoc J. 2015;9(11–12):E780–4.
27. Shah S, Hadzic A, Vloka JD, Cafferty MS, Moucha CS, Santos AC. Neurologic complication after anterior sciatic nerve block. Anesth Analg. 2005;100(5):1515–7.
28. Levesque S, Delbos A. Sciatic nerve block for total-knee replacement: is it really necessary in all patients? Reg Anesth Pain Med. 2005;30(4):410–1.
29. Kinghorn K, Ellinas H, Barboi AC, Dolinski SY. Case scenario nerve injury after knee arthroplasty and sciatic nerve block. Anesthesiology. 2012;116(4):918–23.
30. Sinha SK, Abrams JH, Arumugam S, D'Alessio J, Freitas DG, Barnett JT, Weller RS. Femoral nerve block with selective tibial nerve block provides effective analgesia without foot drop after total knee arthroplasty: a prospective, randomized, observer-blinded study. Anesth Analg. 2012;115(1):202–6.
31. Lund J, Jenstrup MT, Jaeger P, Sørensen AM, Dahl JB. Continuous adductor-canal-blockade for adjuvant post-operative analgesia after major knee surgery: preliminary results. Acta Anaesthesiol Scand. 2011;55(1):14–9.
32. Shah S, Tsai T, Iwata T, Hadzic A. Outpatient regional anesthesia for foot and ankle surgery. Int Anesthesiol Clin. 2005;43(3):143–51.
33. Jeng CL, Torrillo TM, Rosenblatt MA. Complications of peripheral nerve blocks. Br J Anaesth. 2010;1:i97–107.
34. Gasparini JR, de Mello SS, Marques RS, Saraiva RA. Postoperative continuous plexular analgesia. A study on the side effects and risk factors of catheter infection. Rev Bras Anestesiol. 2008;58(6):602–13.
35. Rafique MK, Taqi A. The causes, prevention and management of post spinal backache: an overview. Anaesth Pain Intensive Care. 2011;15(1):65–9.
36. Ballantyne J, Fields HL, Massachusetts General Hospital. The Massachusetts General Hospital handbook of pain management. Bridgend: Seren; 2017.
37. Burchiel K. Surgical management of pain. New York: Thieme; 2015.
38. Fishman S, Ballantyne J, Rathmell JP, Bonica JJ. Bonica's management of pain. Baltimore: Lippincott, Williams & Wilkins; 2010.
39. Garcia J, Altman RD. Chronic pain states: invasive procedures. Semin Arthritis Rheum. 1997;27(3):156–60.
40. Mannion AF, Fekete TF, Porchet F, Haschtmann D, Jeszenszky D, Kleinstück FS. The influence of comorbidity on the risks and benefits of spine surgery for degenerative lumbar disorders. Eur Spine J. 2014;23(Suppl 1):S66–71.
41. J. E. Charlton and International Association for the Study of Pain. Committee on Education. Core curriculum for professional education in pain. Seattle: IASP Press; 2005.
42. Hassenbusch SJ. Surgical management of cancer pain. Neurosurg Clin N Am. 1995;6(1):127–34.
43. Shealy CN, Mortimer JT, Reswick JB. Electrical inhibition of pain by stimulation of the dorsal columns: preliminary clinical report. Anesth Analg. 1967;46(4):489–91.
44. Konrad P. Dorsal root entry zone lesion, midline myelotomy and anterolateral cordotomy. Neurosurg Clin N Am. 2014;25(4):699–722.
45. Denkers MR, Biagi HL, Ann O'Brien M, Jadad AR, Gauld ME. Dorsal root entry zone lesioning used to treat central neuropathic pain in patients with traumatic spinal cord injury: a systematic review. Spine (Phila Pa 1976). 2002;27(7):E177–84.
46. Agrawal SM, Kambalimath DH. Peripheral neurectomy: a minimally invasive treatment for trigeminal neuralgia. A retrospective study. J Maxillofac Oral Surg. 2011;10(3):195–8.
47. Shealy CN. Percutaneous radiofrequency denervation of spinal facets. Treatment for chronic back pain and sciatica. J Neurosurg. 1975;43(4):448–51.
48. Cosman ER, Dolensky JR, Hoffman RA. Factors that affect radiofrequency heat lesion size. Pain Med. 2014;15:2020–36. https://doi.org/10.1111/pme.12566.
49. Terkawi AS, et al. Pain management modalities after total knee arthroplasty: a network meta-analysis of 170 randomized clinical trials. Anesthesiology. 2017;126:923–37.

Matthew B. Novitch, Mark R. Jones, Cameran Vakassi,
Alexander Haroldson, and Robert Levy

Importance of General Health Status in Preoperative Evaluation

Overview

Surgical procedures for pain management can be efficacious treatment options for those experiencing chronic pain. Procedures can range from minimally invasive, such as single disc decompression, to complex, such as spinal reconstructive methods. Assessing a patient's general health status prior to indicating a surgical procedure is of the utmost importance. Properly identifying comorbidities and potential complications before procedures affords the opportunity to optimize perioperative management, effectively reducing the occurrence of adverse outcomes. Here we discuss the importance of properly evaluating a patient, identifying the most common comorbidities, and optimizing preoperative conditions to mitigate these comorbidities.

Preoperative Evaluation

Pulmonary

In procedures where general anesthesia is indicated, special emphasis should be placed on evaluation of the airways. Providers should obtain a complete history and physical exam focused on potential complications of anesthetic use. The goals of airway assessment are to predict the likelihood of airway obstruction and aspiration during the procedure. Patients may have unique respiratory anatomy or pathology that predisposes them to complications. Chronic obstructive pulmonary disease, for example, is a major risk factor for increased morbidity and mortality following surgical procedures [1]. Preoperative interventions for patients who require tracheal intubation and ventilation include early tracheal extubation, avoidance of high airway pressures, and positive end-expiratory pressure (PEEP) in patients with large bullae.

Cardiovascular

A proper cardiovascular evaluation should elicit information about angina, dyspnea, palpitations, syncope, and history of heart disease. Auscultation of the heart and an examination of the extremities for edema should be performed. Major clinical risk factors for increased perioperative morbidity and mortality include coronary artery disease, heart failure, cardiomyopathy, valvular disease, arrhythmias, and conduction problems [2].

Musculoskeletal

In chronic pain patients, often the underlying cause is musculoskeletal in nature. Preexisting musculoskeletal disorders can influence positioning or affect procedural decisions during surgery [3]. For example, cervical spine immobility could make airway management more difficult. Likewise, dental disease, such as loose teeth can complicate airway manipulation. Changes in the normal anatomy of the vertebral column can influence surgical technique.

Neurological

Of special importance in pain management is evaluation of the neurological system. A baseline should be established assessing both sensory and motor function for any deficits. Documentation of deficits will facilitate postoperative comparison and may guide site of anesthetic application and assessment. In especially invasive surgical pain management procedures such as targeted lesioning, this becomes an absolute necessity.

M. B. Novitch (✉)
Department of Anesthesiology and Critical Care Medicine,
University of Washington Medical Center, Seattle, WA, USA
e-mail: mnovitch@uw.edu

M. R. Jones · C. Vakassi
Department of Anesthesiology, Critical Care and Pain Medicine,
Beth Israel Deaconess Medical Center, Boston, MA, USA

A. Haroldson
Medical College of Wisconsin, Wausau, WI, USA

R. Levy
Institute for Neuromodulation, Boca Raton, FL, USA

© Springer Nature Switzerland AG 2019
Y. Khelemsky et al. (eds.), *Academic Pain Medicine*, https://doi.org/10.1007/978-3-030-18005-8_20

Metabolic

Underlying metabolic disorders and malnourishment increase the risk of perioperative complications. Diabetes mellitus, particularly, is an increasingly prevalent metabolic disorder that has been linked to adverse perioperative outcomes [4]. Perioperative stress and medications can worsen hyperglycemia and result in poor wound healing and/or increased risk of infection.

Immunological

Preoperative assessment should be broad and directed toward an individual's immunocompromised state. Particular attention should be given to HIV, cancer, recent transplant patients, and those on chronic immunosuppressant therapy. Immunocompromised individuals are at increased risk of infection, especially in procedures that necessitate the use of implanted devices.

Laboratory

The necessity for laboratory studies should be guided by the extent of the procedure; however special attention must be paid to the coagulation status of the patient.

Surgical Lesioning of Brain, Brainstem, Spinal Cord, and Peripheral Nerves

The surgical lesioning of pain pathways targets nociceptive transmission of afferent neurons. Interventions to interrupt these pain signals may be performed as distally as the peripheral nerve and extend to the cortex.

Peripheral Nerves

Surgical procedures targeting the peripheral nerves fall into two main categories: microvascular decompression and nerve transection. These procedures provide the possibility of permanent eradication of the pain signal. This is in contrast to radiofrequency nerve ablation, which is discussed in the next section.

Microvascular Decompression

Nerve decompression involves dissection of the affected nerve from surrounding tissue in order to relieve compression by adjacent structures [5]. Decompressive procedures provide the greatest benefit in neuropathic pain resulting from nerve entrapment syndromes. Pain results from anatomic impingement, leading to nerve ischemia and inflammation. The most common examples include carpal tunnel syndrome (median nerve entrapment), cubital tunnel syndrome (ulnar nerve entrapment), radial tunnel syndrome, thoracic outlet

syndrome, and meralgia paresthetica (lateral femoral cutaneous neuropathy). Surgery can provide relief to those who have failed conservative management with splinting, steroid injections, and NSAIDs [6]. Risks include wound infection, neuroma formation, incomplete decompression, re-entrapment due to fibrosis, and inadvertent transection of motor branches leading to weakness [7].

Neurectomy

A less common alternative to decompression is peripheral neurectomy. Surgical technique involves complete transection of the nerve at the site of injury with implantation of the ends in muscle or bone to prevent regrowth [8]. Given that surgery results in complete functional loss of the nerve, it is generally reserved for nerve pain resulting from neuroma formation or intractable trigeminal neuralgia [9]. It can, however, be used to treat neuropathic pain that has been successfully relieved with local anesthetic blockade and is not amenable to decompression. Examples include postamputation pain, post-thoracotomy pain due to intercostobrachial nerve injury, and pelvic pain due to trauma of the ilioinguinal, iliohypogastric, perineal, or genitofemoral nerves during hernia repair or pelvic surgery [10]. These procedures may be complicated by loss of sensation or motor function in the nerve distribution, resurgence of pain due to nerve regrowth, painful neuroma formation, and deafferentation pain [11].

Ganglia

The cell bodies of peripheral nerves reside in the dorsal root ganglia, making them a target for surgical lesioning of the pain pathway.

Dorsal Root Ganglionectomy

Resection of a whole ganglion is most commonly done for malignant pain due to tumors or at the C2 ganglion for refractory occipital neuralgia. It provides similar benefits and risks to neurectomy without the risk of nerve regrowth or neuroma formation [12].

DREZ Lesioning

A common approach for treating severe pain occurring in a specific dermatome is lesioning dorsal root entry zone (DREZ). The DREZ is an entry point of multiple sensory spinal rootlets to the spinal cord which transmits pain sensation from a specific region. DREZ lesioning provides the distinct advantage over full dorsal rhizotomy of preserving proprioception and light touch to the dermatome. It is typically performed via a laminectomy at the affected levels. Microvascular dissection is performed to expose the DREZ nerve rootlets at their entry to the spinal cord. Lesioning is done via multiple 2–3 mm deep incisions that extend from the dorsolateral sulcus to the dorsal rootlets. This maintains the viability of ventrally located sensory fibers. Less invasive lesioning can also be performed via radiofrequency ablation of the DREZ. Procedural indications include lesions localized to specific levels of spinal cord injury including cauda equina syndrome, spinal cord tumors, postherpetic neuralgia, and brachial plexus injuries. Complications include weakness from lesioning of ventral motor nerves, paresthesias, CSF leak, infection, stroke, and hemorrhage [13, 14].

Sympathectomy

Pain control for sympathetically mediated conditions, mainly CRPS, can be achieved with a sympathectomy. It may be appropriate for patients with CRPS whose symptoms are no longer relieved with sympathetic nerve blocks. Thoracic sympathectomy can be performed via open thoracotomy or thoracoscopy targeting the T2 and T3 ganglia. Potential complications include pneumothorax, compensatory hyperhidrosis, and Horner's syndrome. Lumbar sympathectomy occurs in the prone position with exposure via the flank. The lumbar sympathetic chain may also be lesioned. Major complications include damage to adjacent structures including major vessels and sexual dysfunction [15].

Spinal Cord

Spinal Cord Stimulation

Spinal Cord stimulation is an attractive choice for relief of chronic pain syndromes due to its wide array of indications. Analgesia is achieved by application of electrical energy via epidural leads that causes the patient to feel paresthesias in the region of pain. Newer modalities, such as high-frequency stimulation, offer the option of having the patient to not feel any paresthesias. There are multiple presumed mechanisms of relief including "masking" of the pain by sending alternate signals, release of inhibitory hormones such as GABA, inhibition of excitatory molecules such as glutamate and aspartate, and matching of oxygen supply and demand. FDA-approved indications include failed back surgery syndrome, CRPS, peripheral neuropathy, intractable angina, and visceral abdominal pain. The procedure involves a trial period with percutaneous lead placement via an epidural needle into the epidural space. If significant pain relief (>50%) is achieved during the trial, a permanent (that may be removed later) system, which includes the leads and an implantable pulse generator (IPG) may be implanted. Possible complications include lead migration (resulting in decrease of cessation of pain relief), lead fracture, infection, epidural hematoma, CSF leak, post-dural puncture headache, and nerve injury [22, 23].

Intrathecal Pump

Intrathecal instillation of pain medication via an implanted pump can be used to avoid high doses of systemic opioids and allow the use of other medications, such as ziconotide, clonidine, and local anesthetics. After an initial trial period, which typically entails an epidural or intrathecal infusion, a catheter is implanted into the subarachnoid space and then attached to a subcutaneous pump located in the abdominal wall. This pump contains a reservoir of medication that is infused at a programmed dosage. Complications include overdose, bleeding, infection, persistent CSF leak, catheter malfunction, and granuloma formation [14, 22].

Cordotomy

Less commonly used in the modern era, cordotomy disrupts the spinothalamic tract in the anterior spinal cord which contains nociceptive pain fibers. This procedure is performed percutaneously with fluoroscopic guidance via a small puncture site at the C1–C2 level. This procedure is reserved for intractable cancer pain, typically secondary to pleural and peritoneal mesothelioma [14, 19]. Profound unilateral relief may last for up to 2 years. Risks include dysesthesias, acquired central hypoventilation syndrome, and bowel/bladder dysfunction [14, 18].

Myelotomy

Similar to cordotomy, midline myelotomy is reserved for intractable severe abdominal or pelvic pain resulting from cancer. The goal is to percutaneously lesion the spinothalamic tract bilaterally via an incision at the midline of the posterior spinal cord, where the tracts decussate. Reports of 70% relief for up to 3 years have been shown without the adverse autonomic effects of cordotomy [20].

Brainstem

Mesencephalotomy

Surgical intervention at the midbrain enables alleviation of the emotional response to pain and suffering, rather than decreasing nociceptive transmission. The medial reticular formation is targeted, which lies between the spinothalamic tract and gray matter. Mesencephalotomy is indicated for palliative relief of refractory head and neck cancer pain. The main complication specific to this procedure is a persistent extraocular palsy [21].

Brain

Deep Brain Stimulation

While deep brain stimulation is generally known for its use in Parkinson's disease, other regions of the brain can be targeted to provide pain relief. The region of stimulation varies based on the pain condition. Most commonly, the electrodes are placed in the periaqueductal gray matter and thalamus. Indications include brachial plexus injuries, spinal cord injury, thalamic-mediated pain, and malignant pain. Intractable facial pain can be targeted at the ventral posterolateral nucleus. Stimulation is produced by a generator implanted in the chest. The electrical currents are hypothesized to prevent neuronal depolarization at the site of the electrodes. The highest success rate has been seen for failed back syndrome and cancer pain with reports of near-complete pain relief. Potential adverse effects include hemorrhage, infection, lead migration, and temporary postoperative brain swelling [16, 17].

Motor Cortex Stimulation (MCS)

MCS is a beneficial therapy in post-stroke neuropathic pain. These patients often have pain due to hyperactive neurons in the sensory cortex from disruption of the afferent spinothalamic pathway. The procedure is similar to DBS with electrode placement at the motor cortex, with a stimulation level that does not induce motor activity [14, 16, 17].

Cingulotomy

Similar to surgical lesioning of the midbrain, stereotactic radiofrequency lesioning of bilateral cingulate gyri targets the emotional response to pain rather than nociceptive pathways. This procedure is reserved for cancer pain refractory to all other forms of relief. It has also been described for relief of psychiatrically mediated pain. Potential complications include seizures, hemorrhage, gait disturbance, or bowel/bladder dysfunction [14, 24].

Radiofrequency Treatment: Indications, Risks, and Associated Complications

Indications

Radiofrequency ablation has been successfully used for the treatment of pain arising from the spine, major joints, and peripheral nerves. In the realm of peripheral nerve injury, the mechanism of radiofrequency ablation involves damage to the myelin, axon, and endoneurium. The fascicles, perineurium, and epineurium remain unharmed, but this is enough damage to compromise neural transmission of pain signals in most cases. Pulsed RF is not an ablative technique and does not depend on thermal injury to produce analgesia. It is an excellent option that may result in a shorter duration of pain relief, however, it has fewer side effects and negative outcomes when compared to thermal RF ablation. Pain recurrence after RF procedures is most likely due to Schwann cell proliferation, axonal sprouting, and increased trophic factors, ultimately leading to regrowth of the pain transmitting pathways [25].

Risks and Associated Complications

As with any interventional procedure, there are risks of bleeding, infection, and nerve injury. One study followed patients undergoing radiofrequency ablation of lumbar medial branches. Each patient underwent 2–8 individual neurotomies per operative procedure, for a total of over 600 procedures. A total of 10 complications were noted among 8 separate operative procedures, none being classified as major [26]. These included neuropathic pain lasting more than 2 weeks in 5 patients. Two patients reported prolonged localized pain and one presented with prolonged muscle spasm near the procedure site. There were no reports of infection, new sensory deficits, or new motor deficits. Therefore, the authors concluded that this procedure has a 6.5% minor complication rate and a negligible serious complication rate.

There is an additional side effect profile of this procedure of a neuropathic "sunburn" type of pain, which occurs in 3–5% of patients, but is usually not severe. This is thought to be due to a partially damaged, although not completely destroyed neural tissue [27].

References

1. Mills GH. Respiratory complications of anaesthesia. Anaesthesia. 2018;73(1):25–33.
2. Fleisher LA, et al. 2014 ACC/AHA guideline on perioperative cardiovascular evaluation and management of patients undergoing noncardiac surgery. J Am Coll Cardiol. 2014;64(22):77–137.
3. King MS. Preoperative evaluation. Am Fam Physician. 2000;62(2):387–96.
4. Leung V, Ragbir-Toolsie K. Perioperative management of patients with diabetes. Health Services Insights. 2017;10:1–5.
5. Learmonth J. The principle of decompression in the treatment of certain diseases of peripheral nerves. Surg Clin North Am. 1933;13:905–13.
6. Spinner M, Linscheid RL. Nerve entrapent syndromes. In: The elbow and its disorders, vol. 2. Philadelphia: Saunders; 1993. p. 813–32.
7. Louis DS, Greene TL, Noellert RC. Complications of carpal tunnel surgery. J Neurosurg. 1985;62(3):352–3563.
8. Downey MJ. Current concepts of peripheral neurectomy. In: Reconstructive surgery of the foot and leg: update. Tucker: Podiatry Institute; 1994. p. 219–23.
9. Agrawal SM, Kambalimath DH. Peripheral neurectomy: a minimally invasive treatment for trigeminal neuralgia. A retrospective study. J Maxillofac Oral Surg. 2011;10(3):195–8.
10. Hokkam E. The effect of ilioinguinal neurectomy in elective inguinal hernia repair on chronic postoperative pain. Egypt J Surg. 2009;4:156–62.
11. Hanakawa T. Neural mechanisms underlying deafferentation pain: a hypothesis from a neuroimaging perspective. J Orthop Sci. 2012;17(3):331–5. https://doi.org/10.1007/s00776-012-0209-9.

12. Pope JE, Deer TR, Kramer J. A systematic review: current and future directions of dorsal root ganglion therapeutics to treat chronic pain. Pain Med. 2013;14(10):1477–96.

13. Falci S, et al. Dorsal root entry zone microcoagulation for spinal cord injury—related central pain: operative intramedullary electrophysiological guidance and clinical outcome. J Neurosurg Spine. 2002;97(2):193–200.

14. Saab CY. Chronic pain and brain abnormalities. Amsterdam: Academic Press; 2013.

15. Mailis-Gagnon A, Furlan A. Sympathectomy for neuropathic pain. Cochrane Database Syst Rev. 2003;(2):CD002918.

16. Burchiel KJ, editor. Surgical management of pain. New York: Thieme; 2011.

17. Lozano AM, Gildenberg PL, Tasker RR, editors. Textbook of stereotactic and functional neurosurgery, vol. 1. Berlin Heidelberg: Springer Science & Business Media; 2009.

18. Rosomoff HL, et al. Percutaneous radiofrequency cervical cordotomy: technique. J Neurosurg. 1965;23(6):639–44.

19. Jackson MB, et al. Percutaneous cervical cordotomy for the control of pain in patients with pleural mesothelioma. Thorax. 1999;54(3):238–41.

20. Nauta HJW, et al. Punctate midline myelotomy for the relief of visceral cancer pain. J Neurosurg Spine. 2000;92(2):125–30.

21. Shieff C, Jr BSN. Stereotactic mesencephalotomy. Neurosurg Clin N Am. 1990;1(4):825–39.

22. Benzon HT, et al. Chronic pain management. In: Clinical anesthesia: seventh edition. Philadelphia: Wolters Kluwer Health; 2013.

23. Crapanzano JT, et al. High frequency spinal cord stimulation for complex regional pain syndrome: a case report. Pain Physician. 2017;20(1):E177–82.

24. Wilkinson HA, Davidson KM, Davidson RI. Bilateral anterior cingulotomy for chronic noncancer pain. Neurosurgery. 1999;45(5):1129–36.

25. Choi EJ, Choi YM, Jang EJ, Kim JY, Kim TK, Kim KH. Neural ablation and regeneration in pain practice. Korean J Pain. 2016;29(1):3–11. https://doi.org/10.3344/kjp.2016.29.1.3.

26. Oh WS, Shim JC. A randomized controlled trial of radiofrequency denervation of the ramus communicans nerve for chronic discogenic low back pain. Clin J Pain [Internet]. 2018;20(1):55–60.. Available from: http://www.ncbi.nlm.nih.gov/pubmed/14668658.

27. Kornick CA, et al. Complication rate associated with facet joint radiofrequency denervation procedures. Pain Med [Internet]. 2002;3(2):175–6.. Available from: https://academic.oup.com/painmedicine/article-lookup/doi/10.1046/j.1526-4637.2002.20249.x.

Spinal Cord Stimulation

Adeepa Singh and Jason Pope

Background

Spinal cord stimulation (SCS) was introduced nearly 40 years ago and has since rapidly evolved, with expanding indications and with high-quality evidence to support its safety and efficacy. Spinal cord stimulation and peripheral nerve stimulation (PNS) therapies have become instrumental in the treatment of pain and are becoming increasingly employed earlier in the treatment algorithms for many disease processes, often in lieu of surgery or chronic opioid therapy [1–3].

Mechanism of Action

There are many theories that describe mechanisms of action of spinal cord stimulation. The gate theory, proposed by Melzack and Wall, postulated that stimulation of large A-beta fibers of the dorsal column inhibits nociceptive input from the A-delta, C and wide dynamic range neurons (WDR) in the substantia gelatinosa. Essentially, the theory suggests that only one signal can pass through the "gate" at any given time, and stimulated larger fibers are able to "close the gate" to signals from the smaller pain fibers entering the dorsal horn. This helps to begin to explain the reason rubbing a hand over a painful site (preferential stimulation of A-beta fibers) helps to reduce nociceptive input from that location (mediated by C and A-delta fibers).

In neuropathic pain, multimodal WDR cells in the dorsal horn of the spinal cord express hyperexcitability which is secondary to release of glutamate and other excitatory amino acids. There is also a dysfunction of the GABA inhibitory system. Animal models of neuropathy demonstrate that SCS inhibits dorsal horn WDR hyperexcitability and induces release of GABA [11–15, 28].

The cholinergic neurotransmitter system also was recently found to play a major role in the effects of spinal cord stimulation (SCS). Release of acetylcholine in the dorsal horn with SCS was demonstrated and associated with activation of the muscarinic M4 receptor [16, 17]. The effect of cholinergic activation was first noted in a study of "enhanced spinal stimulation" [18] in which clonidine was administered intrathecally to rats which did not respond to SCS alone. Addition of an M4 agonist converted rats which did not respond to SCS to responders [18]. Additional studies also revealed that acetylcholine is released in the dorsal horn, and its effect is dependent on the muscarinic M4 receptor.

SCS-induced release of adenosine, serotonin, and noradrenaline in the dorsal horn may play a role in pain reduction [15, 19–21]. Earlier reports suggested that descending inhibition was also a mechanism of SCS [22, 23]. In neuropathic pain, 50% of the effects of SCS may be due to activation of supraspinal circuitry that involves serotonergic cells and the OFF cells in the rostroventral medial medulla [20, 25, 28]. There does not appear to be direct activation of noradrenergic neurons by SCS in the dorsal horn [21–23, 28].

The mechanism of action of different pulse trains continues to evolve. These include the Burst DR waveform [29], dorsal root ganglion stimulation [56], and HF10 stimulation [57].

Indications

Indications for SCS continue to evolve as new technologies come to market. As with any treatment, patient selection is a critical component of spinal cord stimulation, as are the medical indications. The most common indications that are best supported by literature include failed back surgery syndrome (FBSS) (also known as post-laminectomy syndrome), chronic radicular pain unresponsive to conservative treatments, ischemic pain, peripheral neuropathy, peripheral vascular disease, visceral pain, and Complex Regional Pain Syndrome (CRPS) types I and II. Other indications include visceral pain, multiple sclerosis-induced nerve pain, cancer

A. Singh
Montefiore Medical Center, New York, NY, USA

J. Pope (✉)
Evolve Restorative Center, Santa Rosa, CA, USA

© Springer Nature Switzerland AG 2019
Y. Khelemsky et al. (eds.), *Academic Pain Medicine*, https://doi.org/10.1007/978-3-030-18005-8_21

Table 21.1 Disease-specific indications for SCS

Failed back surgery syndrome in the absence of neurologic progression [4] (strongly recommended)

Consider high-frequency stimulation in patients with significant axial low back pain or in patients with low-frequency stimulation resistance [5] (recommended)

Complex regional pain syndrome (CRPS), type 1 and type II [6, 7] (strongly recommended)

Upper extremity neuropathic pain syndrome including, but not limited to, radiculopathy [8] (recommended)

Chronic refractory angina not controllable by a combination of maximal medical therapy, bypass surgery, and percutaneous angioplasty [9] (recommended)

Ischemic peripheral neuropathic pain from peripheral artery disease may respond better in patients with maintained microcirculation (i.e., local TcPO2 10–30 mmHg) [10]. SCS provides an improvement in limb survival rate compared with surgical sympathectomy in patients with nonreconstructable critical leg ischemia [11, 12] (recommended)

Painful diabetic peripheral neuropathy when conventional pharmacologic treatment has provided insufficient pain relief or intolerable side effects [13] (suggested)

Human immunodeficiency virus neuropathy [14] (suggested)

The success of SCS in postherpetic neuralgia is inversely correlated with the level of deafferentation [15–17] (suggested)

Raynaud's syndrome and other painful ischemic vascular disorders [18, 19] (suggested)

The evidence for SCS in patients with chronic abdominal pain (visceral hyperalgesia) is limited to case series [20]. SCS for visceral pain should be used on a case-by-case basis

Spinal cord injury patients with central neuropathic pain may respond to SCS if there is segmental pain at the level of injury as opposed to diffuse pain below the injury. A decision for using SCS should be made on a case-by-case basis

Postamputation pain may be secondary to neuroma, CRPS, somatic pain, and phantom limb pain. Evidence is limited to case series and suggests that phantom limb pain is more difficult to treat with traditional SCS, but may be more amenable to high-frequency SCS [21, 22].

In patients with chronic cancer-related pain, SCS should be reserved for those with expected long-term remission, slow disease progression, or resolution of disease [23]. Consider MRI-compatible SCS systems

Post-thoracotomy and post-mastectomy pain syndromes may respond less favorably to traditional SCS. Consider the use of dorsal root stimulation or high frequency stimulation therapies

Demyelinating central pain conditions such as multiple sclerosis may require repeated magnetic resonance imaging. Consider SCS with MRI compatible systems only if the potential benefits outweigh the risks [24]

From Deer et al. [63]

pain, and chemotherapy-induced neuropathy. Low likelihood of success is predicted when SCS is utilized for treatment of conditions such as deafferentation pain, spinal cord injury pain, central/post-stroke pain, cancer pain without neuropathy, nociceptive pain, and nerve root avulsion [58].

The most significant positive responses to SCS treatment have been noted with peripheral neuropathy (73%) and CRPS (100%) [8]. Historically, with traditional systems, FBSS had a 52% success rate secondary to its mixed neuropathic and nociceptive nature [58]. Patients who did not have surgical procedures prior to implantation of SCS had better responses and shorter implantation time after trial than those who had surgery in the past. Sympathetically mediated pain when treated with SCS has success rates that approach 70%. Disease-specific indications have been published by Neurostimulation Appropriateness Consensus Committee (NACC) and are detailed in Table 21.1.

Contraindications of SCS Therapy and Exclusion from Treatment Selection

Absolute contraindications include comorbidities that interfere with device placement, namely infection and coagulopathy. Infection poses a serious risk to the patient despite the minimally invasive nature of SCS implantation. Epidural

abscess formation can be a devastating complication resulting in severe neurological compromise, sepsis, and death. Recently, management safeguards intended to mitigate infectious and other risks of spinal cord stimulation were developed by the Neurostimulation Appropriateness Consensus Committee (NACC) (Table 21.2) [63]. It is imperative that careful attention is placed on sterilization of the skin near and around the entry points. It is important to note any history of methicillin-resistant *Staphylococcus aureus* (MRSA) infection and take additional precautions. Any systemic or localized infections should be treated prior to the procedure. Immunosuppression can affect the outcome of SCS trial and implantation resulting in delayed wound healing and infection. Immunosuppressed states include HIV, hepatitis, recent treatment with chemotherapy, malignancy, and high-dose steroid treatment.

Primary or secondary coagulopathy are major concerns, especially with neuraxial procedures. Epidural bleeding leading to the development of hematoma may result in permanent neurologic injury, even after emergent decompression. Detailed history, physical exam, and laboratory tests should be performed to assess for bleeding potential. The most recent version of the American Society of Regional Anesthesia's guidelines addressing the management of antiplatelet and anticoagulant medications in patients undergoing interventional spine and pain procedures should be reviewed.

Table 21.2 Recommended perioperative management safeguards

Preoperative

Use of a psychological assessment to address psychiatric comorbidities before proceeding with SCS [27]

Preoperative MRI to determine appropriateness of SCS prior to implant (i.e., neurologic compressive pathology) [25]

Consider, as clinically indicated, cervical and thoracic MRI to assess for critical stenosis or other anatomical abnormality that would compromise the SCS trial or permanent implant

Optimization of health management (diabetes, immunosuppression, and tobacco use) that would impact wound healing and increase infection risk [28]

Address recent systemic infection or local infection at surgical site. Patients in whom an infection cannot be cured should not undergo implantation [29, 31]

Address platelet counts of 100K or less, or abnormal clotting studies. Avoid implantation in patients with platelet counts less than 50K, unless managed in close collaboration with a hematologist [30]

Preoperative laboratory testing to include complete blood count, basic metabolic panel, coagulation profile, urinalysis, and urine culture if indicated [29–31]

Preoperative screening for carriers of *Staphylococcus aureus*. If the patient is *S. aureus* positive (methicillin-sensitive and methicillin-resistance), treat with mupirocin ointment twice daily and chlorhexidine washings daily for 5 days preoperatively [29, 31]

Intraoperative [29–31]

Use of weight-based preoperative antibiotics

Laminar-flow operating suites to minimize outside airborne pathogens

Chlorhexidine-alcohol or povidone-iodine-based preparations

Hair removal at surgical site by clipping immediately prior to surgery only if required

Minimize operating suite staff traffic

Minimize surgical time when possible

Use of careful hemostasis, gentle dissection, and minimizing tissue coagulation near skin edges

Multilayer closure to reduce postoperative wound dehiscence

Postoperative

Use of occlusive sterile dressing, including silver-impregnated antimicrobial barriers [29]

Postoperative wound inspection 7 to 10 days postoperatively

From Deer et al. [63]

This guideline is typically published in the journal *Regional Anesthesia and Pain Medicine* and a convenient App is also available for use on mobile devices.

Cardiac consultation should be considered in patients with cardiovascular implantable electronic devices (CIEDs), despite the fact that SCS is now cleared for concurrent use.

Relative contraindications may cause a physician to delay or modify the screening trial until the condition resolves or improves. These include:

- Unresolved major psychiatric morbidity
- Likelihood of secondary gain
- Untreated substance abuse disorder
- Occupational risk: responsibilities including climbing ladders, operating machinery

Conditions that require careful management and device selection and patient selection:

- Presence of a pacemaker, or defibrillator
- Need for future MRI
- Anticoagulation or antiplatelet therapy

Outcomes may be optimized with appropriate evaluation of the patient, and accurate identification of the type of pain, that is, nociceptive versus neuropathic pain. Traditional par-

esthesia inducing spinal cord stimulation is also less effective in patients with somatization or catastrophization, although this may be optimized by employing new pulse trains [59] or closed loop systems [60]. Other areas that may potentially result in increased failure rates include cauda equina syndrome, primary bone pain, pain from dystonia and paraplegia, arachnoiditis, and cancer pain [58]. Important patient selection considerations are listed in Table 21.3.

Spinal Cord Stimulator Trial and Implantation Process

Once spinal cord stimulation is selected as a treatment, a trial must be performed in order to determine efficacy and tolerability of the treatment. A pre-trial psychiatric evaluation is standard practice. A trial typically lasts 3–10 days. Percutaneous dorsal column leads are placed via an epidural needle, with the intent to remove them after the conclusion of the trial. Other trial strategies include the surgical staged trial, where leads (percutaneous or paddle) are placed surgically with the associated anchoring, as typically performed during permanent placement, with tunneling to an external battery source for the trial. There is little data supporting one methodology over another, although the infection risk for the latter strategy seems to be anecdotally higher. The NACC

Table 21.3 Patient selection considerations for SCS

Use SCS only when more conservative therapies (e.g., pharmacologic, psychologic, physical therapeutic, less invasive interventional pain therapies) have either failed or judged unsuitable

SCS trial within 2 years of chronic pain onset, when conventional therapies have proven ineffective (suggested)

Predominant pain source is neuropathic (e.g., failed back surgery syndrome, arachnoiditis, complex regional pain syndrome, causalgia, peripheral neuropathy, and chronic radiculopathy), as opposed to nociceptive (musculoskeletal irritation) or central neuropathic (poststroke)

No underlying untreated major psychiatric or drug habituation. Patients with inadequately controlled psychiatric/psychological comorbidity should not be implanted

Patients unable to cognitively participate in their care should not be implanted. In patients with partial cognitive impairment, consider a nonrechargeable SCS generator

Demonstration of at least 50% pain relief during temporarily implanted SCS of sufficient duration

The implanter must have access to the necessary facilities, equipment, and support personnel required for proper patient diagnosis, treatment, and follow-up

From Deer et al. [63]

has described risk mitigating strategies to avoid neurologic injury, with the hallmark being injury detection, either by patient feedback or neuro-monitoring [63].

After leads are positioned over the target areas, either with anatomic or paresthesia mapped placement, testing is performed, which varies based on the device employed. Programming variables that may be manipulated to evoke a desired response include pulse width, amplitude, pulse rate, and frequency. Once testing is complete, the leads are secured and further testing and optimization of stimulation is performed before discharge from the facility. The patient follows up in the office within several days for assessment of analgesia and removal of trial leads. If the patient reports greater than 50% pain relief, improvement in functional activities such as ambulation and activities of daily living, and reduction in pain medications, the trial is considered to be successful and the patient is deemed a candidate for implantation of a permanent device.

Permanent implantation typically involves either a percutaneous cylindrical lead placement similar to the trial after careful surgical dissection to the lumbodorsal fascia, or surgical placement of a paddle lead through a laminotomy. The leads are then secured and tunneled subcutaneously to the internal pulse generator (IPG) site. Careful tissue management intraoperatively and appropriate surgical technique is vital to ensure durable outcomes. The device is subsequently programmed and the patient is given a programmer for adjustment of program selection.

Table 21.4 Anatomic targets of SCS at specific spinal levels

Spinal level	Target
C2	Face, maxillary region
C2–C4	Neck, shoulder to hand
C4–C7	Forearm to hand
C7–T1	Anterior shoulder
T1–T2	Chest wall
T5–T6	Abdomen
T7–T9	Back and legs
T10–T12	Leg
L1	Pelvis
T12–L1	Foot
L5,S1	Foot, lower limb
S2–S4	Pelvis, rectum
Sacral hiatus	Coccyx

Adapted from Deer et al. [58]

the positive pole is used to shape the stimulation pattern. This is accomplished by using a variety of contact configurations. Amplitude of stimulation involves the intensity of the electrical field and strength of stimulation delivered to the patient. Increasing the amplitude may increase the spread of the impulse to additional areas beyond the target. Frequency of stimulation determines the number of impulses delivered over time. Pulse width is the period of time the nerve tissue is exposed to the current (duration). Increases in the pulse width can also increase the area of stimulation to areas beyond the target. Major stimulation patterns used in SCS are detailed in Table 21.5.

Programming of Spinal Cord Stimulation

If paresthesia-inducing systems are employed, precise positioning of the leads is crucial to achieving stimulation of the target structures (Table 21.4). Leads have multiple electrodes that may be programmed to stimulate the dorsal columns. A stimulating contact programmed as a negative pole is known as a cathode. Cathodal effects are predominant in SCS. An anode, or the stimulating contact programmed as

Risks and Associated Complications

Spinal Cord Stimulator trial and permanent implantation requires a procedure that although minimally invasive is not without risk or complications. Overall, neuromodulation of the spinal cord and periphery is safe; however hardware and biologic complications are reported in the literature. Complications can be divided into those that involve hardware, software, or biologic. Hardware complications are

Table 21.5 Stimulation patterns commonly used in SCS

Traditional	High frequency (HF)	Burst
40–50 Hz	Most common frequency used is 10 kHz	5 pulses of 500 Hz delivered with a 40 Hz frequency, charge balanced at the end of each burst.
Activates nucleus gracile in dorsal column	High frequency stimulation with low amplitude	Delivers closely spaced, high frequency stimulation
Tonic stimulation	Stimulation amplitude is subthreshold for sensory activation and thus free of paresthesias	No paresthesia experienced by the patient
Electrically stimulates A-beta fibers generating paresthesias		Lower amplitude, large pulse width allows for similar energy delivered during each pulse
Stimulation-induced paresthesias have to cover the painful area completely	Suppresses mechanical hypersensitivity while using half of the stimulation intensity	Amplitude can be increased to elicit paresthesia and decreased to below paresthesia thresholds.
Continuous individual pulses delivered at the same amplitude, duration (pulse width), and frequency	Onset of pain relief occurs in hours-days, not as rapid as tonic	Based on dual firing properties of the thalamic cells which fire in burst and tonic modes
Pain relief onset occurs immediately, quick onset of nociceptive transmission suppression in superficial and deep dorsal horn	May induce depolarization blockade of lower threshold, larger diameter fibers of the dorsal horn which carry vibration and pressure, thus there is less inhibition	Burst firing is similar to normal nerve activity
There is an abrupt decrease in dorsal horn sensitization		Activate cortical areas involved in pain perception → dorsal anterior cingulate and right dorsolateral prefrontal cortex
Activation of dorsal column blocks wind up of WDR neurons		Efficacy relates to electric charge per burst in animal models [37].
Hyperexcitability after neuronal injury can be normalized by traditional SCS		Effects do not rely on GABA-B receptors as with traditional SCS [37].
May induce postsynaptic potentials in dorsal horn and facilitate primary afferent depolarization to elicit presynaptic inhibition in the dorsal horn.		Burst DR SCS reduces connectivity between the dorsal anterior cingulate and parahippocampal cortices → modulates the medial pain pathway directly by actions on C fibers synapsing onto lamina 1 neurons with projections to the dorsomedial nucleus of the thalamus and from there to the dorsal anterior cingulum → thus burst stimulation disturbs the synchronous firing of high threshold fibers which results in halting the activation directly related to perception of pain [39–42]
Functional MRI reveals that lateral pain pathways are modulated by changes in oxygen levels in the somatosensory cortices [42]		Burst DR with low amplitude and sub-perception more effectively treats nociceptive back pain component of FBSS [30, 34, 35, 40, 41]
		Patients who respond to SCS may have further improvement with burst [30, 34, 35, 40, 41]

more frequent than biologic complications. Complications related to hardware involve lead migration, failure or fracture, disconnection of the device from internal leads, implantable pulse generator battery depletion, IPG flipping or recharging difficulties. Common biologic complications include infection, pain over implant, hematoma development over the device, post-dural puncture headache, and neurological damage secondary to spinal cord injury. Software complications involve a lack or reduced efficacy with programming and may represent tolerance and habituation.

Hardware

Lead migration is the most commonly reported complication of both spinal and peripheral nerve stimulation. Spinal cord stimulator leads have a lead migration rate of approximately 20% [44]. Some studies have demonstrated that migration rates are increased when leads are placed in the cervical spine compared with lower thoracic lead placements. This is likely related to high levels of mobility of the cervical compared to the thoracic, lumbar, and sacral spine. Lead migration rates between percutaneous and paddle leads are the same [63]. In peripheral nerve stimulation, lead migration occurs at a rate of 2–13%, although rates as high as 60% in 1 year and 100% in 3 years have been reported [29, 47, 48, 56, 57]. This wide range of outcomes may be explained by varied experience of the implanting physician, different definitions of migration, differing clinical context of therapy, and clinical practice differences [43, 49, 65]. Lead migration may lead to a loss of analgesia. Paresthesias may be recaptured by reprogramming, however the majority of instances of lead migration reported in the literature require re operation in order to correct lead positioning and most result in the utilization of a new lead.

Other common hardware complications include lead fracture and malfunction. These usually occur distal to the fixation point to the deep fascia where the lead enters the spinal canal. The incidence of lead fracture may be up to 10% [2, 43, 44, 50, 51]. In cases of lead fracture, revision surgery was needed in approximately 30% of cases.

Programming and Device Complications

The power generator for spinal cord stimulator can be either external or internal. IPGs may be either rechargeable or non-rechargeable. The durability of SCS is improved with the use of non-rechargeable devices (primary cells) [61]. Once depleted, replacement of the battery requires a repeat surgery. Battery failure is defined by a battery requiring replacement earlier than its expected date. Premature primary-celled battery depletion is rare, with expected life spans of 3–7 years. Primary celled therapies are usually employed for burst and traditional SCS, while rechargeable systems are used for higher consuming programming pulse trains, namely high frequency (HF) stimulation.

Rechargeable batteries limit quality of life by requiring daily or weekly recharging. The lifespan of such devices is 5–7 years or more when used properly and requires a higher level of patient understanding and awareness, as patients will need to maintain charge of their device. Patients may feel that recharging is an inconvenient or burdensome task [53, 54]. Should the battery become drained, most depleted rechargeable batteries can now be revived, however this may require the assistance of a trained technician.

Biological

Pain related to device components is often reported by patients with neuromodulation devices. This includes pain around the implanted pulse generator (IPG) site, the lead anchor sites, or lead extension junctions [2]. This can be related to the location of lead and IPG site, thus avoidance of prominent bony contact points along with highly mobile areas or areas of frequent contact or manipulation is critical.

Infection is a major complication and cause of explantation of SCS with an incidence of 4–8%. The majority of infection in SCS is caused by staphylococcus or pseudomonas. The most common site, accounting for over 50% of cases, is the IPG pocket site. Lead infections make up 17% of cases, mostly related to lumbar incision sites [55]. Risk factors for infection include diabetes, debilitated status, malnutrition, extremely thin body habitus, obesity, autoimmune disorders, corticosteroid use, decubitus ulcers, preexisting infection, poor hygiene, urinary or fecal incontinence, and malabsorption syndromes [63, 64]. Management SCS infection often involves removal of the device, treatment with appropriate antibiotics, and infectious disease consultation. Prevention of infection is key and is achieved by administration of prophylactic antibiotics, adequate skin preparation, sterile technique in the operating room and adequate wound hemostasis.

Dural puncture can occur with epidural needle placement during lead insertion. This may be lead to post-dural puncture headaches and a chronic CSF leak into the wound site. Risk factors for dural puncture include female gender, age 30–50, and a previous history of post-dural puncture headache [2, 43]. Due to the resulting intracranial hypotension, patients may experience diplopia, tinnitus, neck pain, nausea, and photophobia, which may cloud assessing the efficacy of an SCS trial.

Neurological injury is the most catastrophic complication of SCS; however it is uncommon, occurring in less than 1% of patients [63, 64]. Injury may occur secondary to needle puncture and percutaneous lead placement or during paddle lead placement. Delayed neurological injury can occur as a result of epidural hematoma or abscess development. Risk of neurological injury is higher in patients taking medications that impair coagulation. Additionally, risk is increased in patients who consume more than ten drinks weekly, have multilevel procedures, and have had previous spinal surgeries [43].

Conclusion

Spinal cord stimulation has evolved into one of the most durable and efficacious treatment strategies we can employ in the management of chronic pain. New technologies and techniques that result in improvements in outcomes and safety continue to be developed and position SCS and PNS as important analgesic methods in the armamentarium of pain physicians.

References

1. Kumar K, Taylor RS, Jacques L, Eldabe S, Meglio M, Molet J, Thomson S, O'Callaghan J, Eisenberg E, Milbouw G, Buchser E, Fortini G, Richardson J, North RB. Spinal cord stimulation versus conventional medical management for neuropathic pain: a multicentre randomized controlled trial in patients with failed back surgery syndrome. Pain. 2007;132:179–88.
2. Kumar K, Taylor RS, Jacques L, Eldabe S, Meglio M, Molet J, O'Callaghan J, Eisenberg E, Milbouw G, Buchser E, Fortini G, Richardson J, North RB. The effects of spinal cord stimulation in neuropathic pain are sustained: a 24-month follow-up of the prospective randomized controlled multicenter trial of the effectiveness of spinal cord stimulation. Neurosurgery. 2008;63:762–70.
3. Krames ES, Monis S, Poree L, Deer T, Levey R. Using the safe principles when evaluating electrical stimulation therapies for failed back surgery syndrome. Neuromodulation. 2011;14:299–311.
4. Kumar K, Taylor RS, Jacques L, Eldabe S, Meglio M, Molet J, O'Callaghan J, Eisenberg E, Milbouw G, Buchser E, Fortini G, Richardson J, North RB. Spinal cord stimulation versus conventional medical management for neuropathic pain: a multicentre randomized controlled trial in patients with failed back surgery syndrome. Pain. 2007;132:179–88.
5. Baysinger CL, Pope JE, Lockhart EM, Mercaldo ND. The management of accidental dural puncture and postdural puncture headache: a North American survey. J Clin Anesth. 2011;23(5):349–60. https://doi.org/10.1016/j.jclinane.2011.04.003. Epub 22 Jun 2011.

6. North RB, Kidd DH, Olin J, Sieraki JM, Farrokhi F, Petrucci L, Cutchis PN. Spinal cord stimulation for axial low back pain. A prospective, controlled trial comparing dual with single percutaneous electrodes. Spine. 2005;30:1412–8.
7. Melzack R, Wall PD. Pain mechanisms: a new theory. Science. 1965;150:971–9.
8. Kumar K, Toth C, Nath RK, Laing P. Epidural spinal cord stimulation for treatment of chronic pain some predictors of success: a 15-year experience. Surg Neurol. 1998;50:110–21.
9. Linderoth B, Meyerson BA. Spinal cord stimulation: exploration of the physiological basis of a widely used therapy. Anesthesiology. 2010;113:1265–7.
10. Guan Y, Wacnik PW, Yang F, et al. Spinal cord stimulation-induced analgesia: electrical stimulation of dorsal column and dorsal roots attenuates dorsal horn neuronal excitability in neuropathic rats. Anesthesiology. 2010;113:1392–405.
11. Stiller CO, Cui JG, O'Connor WT, Brodin E, Meyerson BA, Linderoth B. Release of GABA in the dorsal horn and suppression of tactile allodynia by spinal cord stimulation in mononeuropathic rats. Neurosurgery. 1996;39:367–75.
12. Cui JG, O'Connor WT, Ungerstedt U, Meyerson BA, Linderoth B. Spinal cord stimulation attenuates augmented dorsal horn release of excitatory amino acids in mononeuropathy via a GABAergic mechanism. Pain. 1997;73:87–95.
13. Ultenius C, Song Z, Lin P, Meyerson BA, Linderoth B. Spinal GABAergic mechanisms in the effects of spinal cord stimulation in a rodent model of neuropathic pain: is GABA synthesis involved? Neuromodulation. 2013;16:114–20.
14. Cui JG, Linderoth B, Meyerson BA. Effects of spinal cord stimulation on touch evoked allodynia involve GABAergic mechanisms. An experimental study in the mononeuropathic rat. Pain. 1996;66:287–95.
15. Cui JG, Meyerson BA, Sollevi A, Linderoth B. Effects of spinal cord stimulation on tactile hypersensitivity in mononeuropathic rats is potentiated by GABA-B and adenosine receptor activation. Neurosci Lett. 1998;247:183–6.
16. Schechtmann G, Wallin J, Meyerson BA, Linderoth B. Intrathecal clonidine potentiates suppression of tactile hypersensitivity by spinal cord stimulation in a model of neuropathy. Anesth Analg. 2004;99:135–9.
17. Schechtmann G, Song Z, Ultenius C, Meyerson BA, Linderoth B. Cholinergic mechanisms in the pain relieving effect of spinal cord stimulation in a model of neuropathy. Pain. 2008;139:136–14.
18. Song Z, Meyerson BA, Linderoth B. Muscarinic receptor activation potentiates the effect of spinal cord stimulation on pain related behaviour in rats with mononeuropathy. Neurosci Lett. 2008;436:7–12.
19. Linderoth B, Gazelius B, Franck J, Brodin E. Dorsal column stimulation induces release of serotonin and substance P in the cat dorsal horn. Neurosurgery. 1992;31:289–97.
20. Linderoth B, Foreman RD. Physiology of spinal cord stimulation. Review and update. Neuromodulation. 1999;2:150–64.
21. Linderoth B, Foreman RD. Mechanisms of spinal cord stimulation in painful syndromes: role of animal models. Pain Med. 2006;7:S14–26.
22. Saade NE, Tabet MS, Soueidan SA, Bitar M, Atweh SF, Jabbur SJ. Supraspinal modulation of nociception in awake rats by stimulation of the dorsal column nuclei. Brain Res. 1986;369:307–10.
23. Saade NE, Jabbur SJ. Nociceptive behavior in animal models for peripheral neuropathy: spinal and supraspinal mechanisms. Prog Neurobiol. 2008;86:22–47.
24. El-Khoury C, Hawwa C, Baliki M, Atweh SF, Jabbur SJ, Saade NE. Attenuation of neuropathic pain by segmental and supraspinal activation of the dorsal column system in awake rats. Neuroscience. 2002;112:541–53.
25. Yakhnitsa V, Linderoth B, Meyerson BA. Modulation of dorsal horn neuronal activity by spinal cord stimulation in a rat model of neuropathy: the role of the dorsal funicles. Neurophysiology. 1998;30:424–7.
26. Atkinson L, Sundaraj SR, Brooker V, Callaghan JO, Teddy P, Salmon J, Semple T, Majedi PM. Recommendations for patient selection in spinal cord stimulation. J Clin Neurosci. 2011;18(10):1295–302.
27. Deer T, Pope J. Atlas of implantable therapies for pain management. 2nd ed. New York: Springer; 2016. ISBN 978-1-4939-2109-6.
28. Linderoth B, Foreman R. Conventional and novel spinal stimulation algorithms: hypothetical mechanisms of action and comments on outcomes. Neuromodulation. 2017;20:535–3.
29. Deer T, Slavin KV, Amirdelfan K, North RB, Burton AW, Yearwood TL, Tavel E, Staats P, Falowski S, Pope J, Justiz R, Fabi AY, Taghva A, Paicius R, Houden T, Wilson D. Success using neuromodulation with BURST (SUNBURST) study: results from a prospective, randomized controlled trial using a novel burst waveform. Neuromodulation. 2017;21:56. https://doi.org/10.1111/ner.12698.
30. De Ridder D, Perera S, Vanneste S. Are 10kHz stimulation and burst stimulation fundamentally the same? Neuromodulation. 2017;20:650–3.
31. Chakravarthy K, Richter H, Christo PJ, Williams K, Guan Y. Spinal cord stimulation for treating chronic pain: reviewing preclinical and clinical data on paresthesia-free high-frequency therapy. Neuromodulation. 2017;21:10. https://doi.org/10.1111/ner.12721.
32. Hou S, Kemp K, Grabois M. A systematic evaluation of burst spinal cord stimulation for chronic Back and limb pain. Neuromodulation. 2016;19:398–405.
33. Kulkarni B, Bentley DE, Elliott R, Youell P, Watson A, Derbyshire SW, Frackowiak RS, Friston KJ, Jones AK. Attention to pain localization and unpleasantness discriminates the functions of the medial and lateral pain systems. Eur J Neurosci. 2005;21:3133–42.
34. DeRidder D, Plazier M, Kamerling N, Menovsky T, Vanneste S. Burst spinal cord stimulation for limb and back pain. World Neurosurg. 2013;80(5):642–9.
35. De Ridder D, Vanneste S, Plazier M, van der Loo E, Menovsky T. Burst spinal cord stimulation: toward paresthesia-free pain suppression. Neurosurgery. 2010;66:986–90.
36. Pope J, Falowski S, Deer TR. Advanced waveforms and frequency with spinal cord stimulation: burst and high-frequency delivery. Expert Rev Med. 2015;12:431–7.
37. Crosby ND, Goodman Keiser MD, Smith JR, Zeeman ME, Winkelstein BA. Stimulation parameters define the effectiveness of burst spinal cord stimulation in a rat model of neuropathic pain. Neuromodulation. 2015;18:1–8.
38. Crosby N, Weisshaar C, Smith J, Zeeman M, Goodman-Keiser M, Winkelstein B. Burst & tonic spinal cord stimulation differentially activate GABAergic mechanisms to attenuate pain in a rat model of cervical radiculopathy. IEEE Trans Biomed Eng. 2015;62:1604–13.
39. Slavin KV, North RB, Deer TR, Staats P, Davis K, Diaz R. Tonic and burst spinal cord stimulation waveforms for the treatment of chronic, intractable pain: study protocol for a randomized controlled trial. Trials. 2016;17:569. https://doi.org/10.1186/s13063-016-1706-5.
40. De Ridder D, Lenders MW, De Vos CC, et al. A two-center comparative study on tonic versus burst spinal cord stimulation: amount of responders and amount of pain suppression. Clin J Pain. 2015;3131:433–43.
41. De Ridder D, Vanneste S. Burst and tonic spinal cord stimulation: different and common brain mechanisms. Neuromodulation. 2016;19:47–59.
42. Stancak A, Kozak J, Vrba I, et al. Functional magnetic resonance imaging of cerebral activation during spinal cord stimulation in failed back surgery syndrome patients. Eur J Pain. 2008;12:137–48.
43. Eldabe S, Buchser E, Duarte RV. Complications of spinal cord stimulation and peripheral nerve stimulation techniques: a review of the literature. Pain Med. 2016;17(2):325–36.

44. Kumar K, Hunter G, Demeria D. Spinal cord stimulation in treatment of chronic benign pain: challenges in treatment planning and present status, a 22-year experience. Neurosurgery. 2006;58:481–96.

45. North RB, Kidd DH, Olin J, Sieracki JN, Petrucci L. Spinal cord stimulation for axial low back pain: a prospective controlled trial comparing 16-contact insulated electrodes with 4-contact percutaneous electrodes. Neuromodulation. 2006;9:56–67.

46. Levy R, Henderson J, Slavin K, Simpson BA, Barolat G, Shipley J, North R. Incidence and avoidance of neurologic complications with paddle type spinal cord stimulation leads. Neuromodulation. 2011;14:412–22. https://doi.org/10.1111/j.1525-1403.2011.00395.x.

47. Sator-Katzenshaclager S, Fiala K, Kress HG, Kofler A, Neuhold J, Kloimstein H, Ilias W, Mozes-Balla EM, Pinter M, Loining N, Fuchs W, Heinze G, Likar R. Subcutaneous target stimulation (STS) in chronic noncancer pain: a nationwide retrospective study. Pain Pract. 2010;10(4):279–86.

48. Verrills P, Vivian D, Mitchell B, Barnard A. Peripheral nerve field stimulation for chronic pain: 100 cases and review of the literature. Pain Med. 2011;12(9):1395–405.

49. Cameron T. Safety and efficacy of spinal cord stimulation for the treatment of chronic pain: a 20-year literature review. J Neurosurg. 2004;100:254–67.

50. Turner JA, Loeser JD, Deyo RA, Sanders SB. Spinal cord stimulation for patients with failed back surgery syndrome or complex regional pain syndrome: a systematic review of effectiveness and complications. Pain. 2004;108:137–47.

51. Mekhail NA, Mathews M, Nageeb F, Guirguis M, Mekhail MN, Cheng J. Retrospective review of 707 cases of spinal cord stimulation: indications and complications. Pain Pract. 2011;11:148–53. https://doi.org/10.1111/j.1533-2500.2010.00407.x.

52. Kumar K, Taylor RS, Jacques L, Eldabe S, Meglio M, Molet J, Thomson S, O'Callaghan J, Eisenberg E, Milbouw G, Buchser E, Fortini G, Richardson J, North RB. The effects of spinal cord stimulation in neuropathic pain are sustained: a 24-month follow up of the prospective randomized controlled multicenter trial of the effectiveness of spinal cord stimulation. Neurosurgery. 2008;63(4):762–70.

53. Taylor RJ, Taylor RS. Spinal cord stimulation for failed back surgery syndrome: a decision-analytic model and cost-effectiveness analysis. Int J Technol Assess Health Care. 2005;21:351–8.

54. Taylor RS, Ryan J, O'Donnell R, Eldabe S, Kumar K, North RB. The cost effectiveness of spinal cord stimulation in the treatment of failed Back surgery syndrome. Clin J Pain. 2010;26(6):463–9.

55. Follett KA, Boortz-Marx RL, Drake JM, Dupen S, Schneider SJ, Turner M, Coffey RJ. Prevention and management of intrathecal drug delivery and spinal cord stimulation system infections. Anesthesiology. 2004;100:1582–94.

56. Deer TR, Levy RM, Kramer J, Poree L, Amirdelfan K, Grigsby E, Staats P, Burton AW, Burgher AH, Obray J, Scowcroft J, Golovac S, Kapural L, Paicius R, Kim C, Pope J, Yearwood T, Samuel S, McRoberts WP, Cassim H, Netherton M, Miller N, Schaufele M, Tavel E, Davis T, Davis K, Johnson L, Mekhail N. Dorsal root ganglion stimulation yielded higher treatment success rate for complex regional pain syndrome and causalgia at 3 and 12 months: a randomized comparative trial. Pain. 2017 Apr;158(4):669–81. https://doi.org/10.1097/j.pain.0000000000000814.

57. Kapural L, Yu C, Doust MW, Gliner BE, Vallejo R. Novel 10-kHz high-frequency therapy (HF10 therapy) is superior to traditional low-frequency spinal cord stimulation for the treatment of chronic back and leg pain: the SENZA-RCT randomized controlled trial. Anesthesiology. 2015;123:851–60. https://doi.org/10.1097/ALN.0000000000000774.

58. Deer T, Pope J. Disease indications. In: Atlas of implantable therapies. New York: Springer; 2016. p. 11–4.

59. Schu S, Slotty PJ, Bara G, Von Knop M, Edgar D, Vesper J. A prospective, randomised, double-blind, placebo-controlled study to examine the effectiveness of burst spinal cord stimulation patterns for the treatment of failed back surgery syndrome. Neuromodulation. 2014;17(5):443–50. https://doi.org/10.1111/ner.12197. Epub 19 Jun 2014.

60. Russo M, Cousins MJ, Brooker C, Taylor N, Boesel T, Sullivan R, Poree L, Shariati NH, Hanson E, Parker J. Effective relief of pain and associated symptoms with closed-loop spinal cord stimulation system: preliminary results of the Avalon study. Neuromodulation. 2017; https://doi.org/10.1111/ner.12684. [Epub ahead of print].

61. Pope JE, Deer TR, Falowski S, et al. Multicenter retrospective study of neurostimulation with exit of therapy by explant. Neuromodulation. 2017;20(6):543–52.

62. Van Buyten JP, Wille F, Smet I, et al. Therapy-related explants after spinal cord stimulation: results of an international retrospective chart review study. Neuromodulation. 2017;20(7):642–9. https://doi.org/10.1111/ner.12642. Epub 18 Aug 2017.

63. Deer TR, Provenzano DA, Hanes M, Pope JE, Thomson SJ, Russo MA, McJunkin T, Saulino M, Raso LJ, Lad SP, Narouze S, Falowski SM, Levy RM, Baranidharan G, Golovac S, Demesmin D, Witt WO, Simpson B, Krames E, Mehkail N. The Neurostimulation Appropriateness Consensus Committee (NACC) recommendations for infection prevention and management. Neuromodulation. 2017;20(1):31–50. https://doi.org/10.1111/ner.12565. Epub 2 Jan 2017.

64. Deer TR, Mekhail N, Provenzano D, Pope J, Krames E, Thomson S, Raso L, Burton A, DeAndres J, Buchser E, Buvanendran A, Liem L, Kumar K, Rizvi S, Feler C, Abejon D, Anderson J, Eldabe S, Kim P, Leong M, Hayek S, McDowell G, Poree L, Brooks ES, McJunkin T, Lynch P, Kapural L, Foreman RD, Caraway D, Alo K, Narouze S, Levy RM, North R. The appropriate use of neurostimulation: avoidance and treatment of complications of neurostimulation therapies for the treatment of chronic pain. Neuromodulation. 2014;17:571–98. https://doi.org/10.1111/ner.12206.

65. Kumar K, Buchser E, Linderoth B, Meglio M, Van Buyten JP. Avoiding complications from spinal cord stimulation: practical recommendations from an international panel of experts. Neuromodulation. 2007;10:24–33.

Intrathecal Drug Delivery: Indications, Risks, and Complications

22

Mark N. Malinowski, Nicholas Bremer, Chong H. Kim, and Timothy R. Deer

Introduction

Neuromodulation through the use of implantable drug delivery (IDD) has been shown to be effective in treating chronic pain [1]. Physicians must determine the optimal point at which this therapy is most appropriate. The pain care continuum can provide an algorithmic approach to the use of interventional pain techniques, as well as a framework in the decision-making process [2]. However, a uniform, stepwise approach should not supplant a well-tailored, fluid plan of care for the individual patient's needs. The SAFE principles include "safety," "appropriateness," "fiscal neutrality," and "efficacy" and should be employed when considering the appropriateness of IDD as a treatment option [3].

Indications

The use of IDD is indicated in the treatment of refractory trunk and limb pain of malignant and nonmalignant origin [4, 5]. Intractable pain that exists in spite of appropriate interventions is considered "refractory." Recently, refractory pain has been suggested to be pain that persists when multiple evidence-based treatments have been attempted and desired end points of pain reduction, return to acceptable function, and absence of intolerable effects of pain have not been achieved [6]. Success of IDD is predicated on the accurate diagnosis of the underlying disease state and underlying

M. N. Malinowski (✉)
Adena Regional Medical Center, Adena Spine Center, Chillicothe, OH, USA

N. Bremer
Department of Anesthesiology and Pain Medicine, Columbia University Medical Center, New York, NY, USA

C. H. Kim
PM&R and Anesthesiology, Case Western Reserve University, Cleveland, OH, USA

T. R. Deer
The Spine and Nerve Centers of Virginia, Charleston, WV, USA

pathophysiology of symptoms, and the proper evaluation of the clinical scenario as elucidated by a thorough history and physical [7].

Refractory pain disease states of malignant and nonmalignant origin can be categorized into nociceptive, neuropathic, and mixed pain syndromes and often subcategorized into visceral and somatic pain [8]. Examples of nociceptive pain include post-laminectomy syndrome (also known as failed back surgery syndrome – FBSS), gastrointestinal malignancies, or bone tumors. Examples of neuropathic pain include diabetic peripheral neuropathies and plexopathies. Mixed pain syndromes include complex regional pain syndrome or burst fractures with associated myelomalacia. While IDD itself is a uniform option for treating this variety of conditions, successful treatment is heavily reliant upon the ability to deliver the appropriate drug to the appropriate receptors responsible for mediating the disease state by strategic catheter placement in the neuraxis [5, 9–11].

Patient Selection

Proper patient selection is paramount. The selection of candidates involves a complex evaluation of the clinical scenario which includes, but is not limited to, the patient diagnosis, prognosis, previous therapies, current medications, medication allergies and associated intolerances, and comorbid conditions [4, 12, 13]. Subsequent to accurate diagnosis, patients who are candidates for IDD are those who have tried and failed less aggressive measures. These patients demonstrate minimal or no benefit with both opioids and non opioid therapies. However, current best practice guidelines suggest a trend away from failure of high-dose opioids as a prerequisite to IDD [14]. Furthermore, clinical presentation should demonstrate failure to thrive (i.e., reduction of activities of daily living, decreased appetite, mood and sleep disturbance, socioeconomic effects, etc.) with worsening scores through pain assessment tools [8].

Patients considered for IDD should have proper prescreening to identify comorbid conditions that could be maximized prior to implantation. Strong consideration should be given to the surgical candidacy of the patient. In patients with non-malignant pain, comorbidities that may negatively respond to IDD (i.e., cardiopulmonary disease, morbid obesity, etc.) or patients who demonstrate conditions that impair wound healing (i.e., diabetes, morbid obesity, smoking etc.) warrant special attention and pre-surgical optimization [14, 15]. Psychiatric assessment is also critical, as patient perceptions, expectations, and suboptimal coping skills may negatively impact outcomes. Furthermore, the presence or history of psychosis may contraindicate the use of certain medications (e.g., ziconotide) [14, 15].

Patients with pain of malignant origin warrant special consideration. No clear consensus exists in managing this population. Ongoing chemotherapy or radiation and the presence of metastatic disease may impact not only the surgical candidacy of the patient but also the timing of instituting IDD in the care plan [16].

Trial of Therapy

While there is no clear consensus, some physicians use intrathecal (IT) or epidural trialing as a part of the pre-implantation screening process [4]. Trialing may provide measurable data of improvement as compared to the patient's pre-procedural presentation, as well as provide a reference point for initiating continuous IT drug delivery after implantation [14].

Intrathecal Therapy

Risks and Complications

Complications of IDD can be organized into several categories: procedural, pharmacologic, mechanical, refill-related, and patient-specific comorbidities. Since 2000, PolyAnalgesic Consensus Conference (PACC) guidelines have been published to improve efficacy and safety, and to provide recommendations for IDD. In the most recent update in 2016, 15 key safety-related aspects of IT therapy were delineated. These included patient management, medications, procedural and biologic challenges of trialing, implantation, maintenance and explanation, and device-related complications and failures [14].

Procedural or surgical complications include bleeding, infection, cerebrospinal fluid (CSF) leakage, seroma formation, neurologic injury, shredded catheters, and malpositioned subcutaneous pockets [17]. For patients on systemic anticoagulation therapy, the joint society guidelines on neuraxial pain procedures should be followed [18]. Although

bleeding is common, it is rarely clinically significant. However, undiagnosed and untreated epidural hematoma can be catastrophic. In any patient where an epidural hematoma is suspected, immediate imaging and surgical evaluation is warranted.

Some patients experience pain at the reservoir site due to tissue irritation, formation of a neuroma, seroma, or infection. Patient may present with fever, chills, tenderness, edema, warmth, erythema, discharge, or induration along the incision or at the pump site. Laboratory studies, including white blood cell count, erythrocyte sedimentation rate (ESR), or C-reactive protein (CRP) levels should guide clinical decision-making. Sampling and culturing pocket fluid can help distinguish infection from seroma. Infection rates range from 2% to 5%, with most infections being superficial [19–21]. Given the direct conduit to the central nervous system, any degree of infection can result in neurologic sequelae. Although most infections do not require removal of the device, deep infections including epidural abscess, discitis, and meningitis require immediate removal and intravenous antibiotics. While the most common organism is staphylococcus, culture and sensitivity testing should guide antimicrobial therapy after the explanation [22]. Fortunately, the rates of infection have decreased with improved training, strict sterile technique, preoperative antibiotics, and postoperative monitoring.

During the placement of the catheter into the IT space, persistent CSF leak can occur in as many as 20% of the patients, resulting in post-dural puncture headache [23]. Most resolve without treatment, but severe symptoms may require an epidural blood patch or even surgical closure of the dural tear. Peri-catheter CSF leaks have been described and can lead to persistent intracranial hypotension. Even in the absence of a classic positional headache, the presence of clear fluid within the pocket can indicate peri-catheter leaks. For recalcitrant cases, epidural blood/fibrin glue patching or complete system explanation may be required [24].

Pharmacologic adverse effects are the most common complication associated with IDD [25]. Serious pharmacologic complications of IDD include anaphylaxis, respiratory arrest, and meningitis from a contaminated infusion. Specifically, IT opioids may cause centrally mediated respiratory depression, nausea, vomiting, sedation, pruritus, constipation, urinary retention, cognitive impairment, and headache [17]. IT ziconotide may cause nausea, vomiting, dizziness, urinary retention, gait imbalance, nystagmus, and confusion. Psychosis, suicide, and rhabdomyolysis have also been seen with ziconotide, particularly at high doses. IT baclofen has been shown to potentially cause nausea, vomiting, dizziness, urinary retention, constipation, headaches, fatigue, hypotonia, and paresthesias. In cases of sudden discontinuation of baclofen, prompt oral supplementation, resumption of IT infusion with supportive care is required as life-threatening withdrawal can occur. IT clonidine can cause hypotension, bradycardia, and sedation. Paradoxical hypertension may be seen with sudden discontinuation. IT local anesthetics can cause autonomic dysfunction (i.e., hypotension, bradycardia, etc.), motor impairment, and sensory deficits and, at higher doses, neurotoxicity, weakness, fatigue, somnolence, paresthesias, and urinary retention.

Mechanical complications can arise at any point from the catheter to the pump. The catheter can become displaced or migrate, kink, fracture, or disconnect from the pump. The most common catheter-related malfunction is catheter migration [26]. Catheter displacement, disconnection, and fracture can cause CSF leakage and leakage of the drug agent outside of the IT space and potentially cause a hygroma formation. Fractures are frequently seen at points of high stress, such as at the anchoring site and at the reservoir. Kinking can cause altered rate of drug delivery, typically under-infusion or even a motor stall. The pump can flip 180 degrees within the abdomen, preventing access to the reservoir. In addition, complications from the pump device malfunction have been reported, particularly with off label IT drug uses [27]. The annual rate for mechanical complications requiring surgical intervention is approximately 10%, with majority being catheter-related [28]. Recent advances in the design of catheters and devices may reduce mechanical-related complications.

Refill-related complications can occur during pump refill or reprogramming. Incorrect medications or concentrations can be refilled, or the medication can be deposited outside of the pump reservoir. Erroneous programming can result in inappropriate dosing of medications. Systematic and standardized practices should be employed to minimize refill-related complications.

Patient-specific complications can be varied in IDD. Hormonal fluctuations have been seen with opioid use. Levels of testosterone and other hormones have been found to decrease with IT opioid use, as sole agents or in combination with other agents [29]. In patients with symptoms of fatigue, reduced libido, and sexual dysfunction, screening should be considered. Though titration off the opioid is an option, hormone replacement therapy may be more appropriate [4].

Finally, one of the most serious potential complications of IDD is an inflammatory mass. Also known as a granuloma, this inflammatory mass is a noninfectious collection of inflammatory cells located at the catheter tip. The major risk factor is high dose or concentration of opioid, especially morphine. No inflammatory masses have been reported with fentanyl or ziconotide. The etiology of this collection is unknown, but it can cause devastating consequences [30]. Fortunately, mass formation is rare, 0.04% incidence at 1 year, 1.2% after 6 years [31]. Mass formation has been consistently associated with opioids in the IT space, either alone or in combination. Signs of inflammatory masses include loss of analgesia, increasing pain, and development of neuro-

logic dysfunction (i.e., numbness, weakness, bowel or bladder dysfunction, etc.). In suspected cases, prompt evaluation with contrast-enhanced MRI (alternatively CT myelogram of MRI is unavailable) is the gold standard. In confirmed cases without neurologic deficits, revision of the catheter inferiorly, reduction of the drug concentration or dose, or switching to another agent can be considered as majority of granulomas regress when the offending agent is removed [32]. Neurosurgical evaluation is warranted in cases of significant or progressive neurologic deficits.

Conclusion

Neuromodulation through the use of implantable IDD is an effective treatment option for chronic intractable pain. However, understanding of appropriate patient selection, risks, and potential complications is critical for optimal patient outcomes.

References

1. Wang J, Nauss L, Thomas J. Pain relief by intrathecally applied morphine in man. Anesthesiology. 1979;50(2):149–51.
2. Deer T, Winkelmuller W, Erdine S, Bedder M, Burchiel K. Intrathecal therapy for cancer and nonmalignant pain: patient selection and patient management. Neuromodulation. 1999;2(2):55–66.
3. Krames E, Poree L, Deer T, Levy R. Implementing SAFE principles for the development of pain medicine therapeutic algorithms that include neuromodulation techniques. Neuromodulation. 2009;12(2):104–13.
4. Deer T, Prager J, Levy R, Rathmell J, Buchser E, Burton A, Caraway D, Cousins M, De Andres J, Diwan S, Erdek M, Grisby E, Huntoon M, Jacobs M, Kim P, Kumar K, Leong M, Liem L, McDowell G, Panchal S, Rauk R, Saulino M, Sitzman T, Staats P, Stanton-Hicks M, Stearns L, Wallace M, Willis KD, Witt W, Taksh T, Mekhail N. Polyanalgesic consensus conference 2012: Polyanalgesic consensus conference −2012: recommendations for the management of pain by IT (intraspinal) drug delivery: report of an interdisciplinary expert panel. Neuromodulation. 2012;15:436–66.
5. Hayek S, Deer T, Pope J, Panchal S, Patel V. Intrathecal therapy for cancer and non-cancer pain. Pain Physician. 2011;14:219–48.
6. Deer T, Caraway D, Wallace M. A definition of refractory pain to help determine suitability for device implantation. Neuromodulation. 2014;17:711–5.
7. Smyth C, Ahmadzai N, Wentzell J, Pardoe A, Tse A, Nguyen T, Goddard Y, Nair S, Poulin P, Skidmore B, Ansari M. Intrathecal analgesia for chronic refractory pain: current and future prospects. Drugs. 2015;75:1957–80.
8. Deer T, Smith H, Cousins M, Doleys D, Levy R, Rathmell J, Staats P, Wallace M, Webster L. Consensus guidelines for the selection and implantation of patients with noncancer pain for intrathecal drug delivery. Pain Physician. 2010;13:E175–213.
9. Dougherty P, Staats P. Intrathecal drug delivery for chronic pain. Anesthesiology. 1999;91:1891–918.
10. Krames E, Buchser E, Hassenbusch S, Levy R. Future trends in the development of local drug delivery systems: intraspinal, intracerebral and intraparenchymal therapies. Neuromodulation. 1999;2(2):133–48.

11. Pope J, Deer T, Bruel B, Falowski S. Clinical uses of intrathecal therapy and its placement in the pain care algorithm. Pain Pract. 2016;16(8):1092–196.

12. Deer T, Pope J. Factors to consider in the choice of intrathecal drug in the treatment of neuropathic pain. Expert Rev Clin Pharmacol. 2015;8(5):507–10.

13. Deer T, Smith H, Burton A, Pope J, Doleys D, Levy R, Staats P, Wallace M, Webster L, Rauck R, Cousins M. Comprehensive consensus based guidelines on intrathecal drug delivery systems in the treatment of pain caused by cancer pain. Pain Physician. 2011;14:E283–312.

14. Deer TR, Pope JE, Hayek S, et al. The polyanalgesic consensus conference (PACC): recommendations on intrathecal drug infusion systems best practices and guidelines. Neuromodulation. 2017;20(2):96–132.

15. Deer TR, Pope JE, Hayek S, et al. The polyanalgesic consensus conference recommendations on intrathecal drug delivery: guidance for improving safety and mitigating risks. Neuromodulation. 2017;20(2):155–76.

16. Bruel B, Burton A. Intrathecal therapy for cancer-related pain. Pain Med. 2016;17:2404–21.

17. Upadhay SP, Mallick PN. Intrathecal drug delivery system (IDDS) for cancer pain management: a review and updates. Am J Hops Palliat Care. 2012;29:388–98.

18. Narouze S, Benzon H, Provenzano D, et al. Interventional spine and pain procedures in patients on antiplatelet and anticoagulant medications: guidelines from the American Society of Regional Anesthesia and Pain Medicine, the European Society of Regional Anaesthesia and Pain Therapy, the American Academy of Pain Medicine, the International Neuromodulation Society, the North American Neuromodulation Society, and the World Institute of Pain. Reg Anesth Pain Med. 2015;40(3):182–212.

19. Kumar K, Nath R, Wyant GM. Treatment of chronic pain by epidural spinal cord stimulation: a 10 year experience. J Neurosurg. 1991;111:881–91.

20. Lang P. The treatment of chronic pain by epidural spinal cord stimulation-15 year follow up; present status. Axon. 1997;18:71–3.

21. Meglio M, Coini B, Rossi GF. Spinal cord stimulation in management of chronic pain. A 9 year review. J Neurosurg. 1989;70:519–24.

22. Follett K, Boortz-Marx R, Drake J, et al. Prevention and management of intrathecal drug delivery and spinal cord stimulation system infections. Anesthesiology. 2004;100:1582–94.

23. Knight KH, Brand FM, Mchaourab AS, Veneziano G. Implantable intrathecal pumps for chronic pain: highlights and updates. Croat Med J. 2007;48:22–34.

24. Kari M, Jaycox M, Lubenow T. Complications associated with intrathecal drug delivery systems. In: Deer T, editor. Intrathecal drug delivery for pain and spasticity. Philadelphia: Saunders Elsevier; 2012. p. 102–8.

25. Bhatia G, Lau ME, Gulur P, Koury KM. Intrathecal drug delivery (ITDD) systems for cancer pain. Version 3. F1000Res. 2013;2(96):1–13.

26. Follett K, Naumann C. A prospective study of catheter-related complications of intrathecal drug delivery systems. J Pain Symptom Manag. 2000;19:209–15.

27. Galica R, Hayek S, Veizi IE, Lawrence M, Khalil AA, McEwan M. Sudden intrathecal drug delivery device motor stalls: a case series. Reg Anesth Pain Med. 2016;41(2):135–9.

28. Stearns L, Boortz-Marx R, Du Pen S, Friehs G, Gordon M, Halyard M, Herbst L, Kiser J. Intrathecal drug delivery for the management of cancer pain: a multidisciplinary consensus of best clinical practices. J Support Oncol. 2005;3:399–408.

29. Kim CH, Garcia R, Stover J, Ritchie K, Whealton T, Ata M. Androgen deficiency with long term intrathecal opioid administration. Pain Physician. 2014;17:E543–8.

30. Deer T, Prager J, Levy R, Rathmell J, Buchser E, Burton A, Caraway D, Cousins M, De Andres J, Diwan S, Erdek M, Grisby E, Huntoon M, Jacobs M, Kim P, Kumar K, Leong M, Liem L, McDowell G, Panchal S, Rauk R, Saulino M, Sitzman T, Staats P, Stanton-Hicks M, Stearns L, Wallace M, Willis KD, Witt W, Taksh T, Mekhail N. Polyanalgesic consensus conference 2012: Polyanalgesic consensus conference −2012: consensus on diagnosis, detection, and treatment of catheter-tip granulomas (inflammatory masses). Neuromodulation. 2012;15:483–96.

31. Yaksh TL, Hassenbusch S, Burchiel K, Hildebrand KR, Page LM, Coffey RJ. Inflammatory masses associated with intrathecal drug infusion: a review of preclinical evidence and human data. Pain Med. 2002;3:299–312.

32. Jourdain V, Cantin L, Prud'Homme M, Fournier-Gosselin M. Intrathecal morphine therapy-related granulomas: faster to grow than thought. Neuromodulation. 2009;12:164–8.

Physical Medicine and Rehabilitation

23

Sumeet Arora, Samantha Erosa, and Houman Danesh

Introduction

Strategies discussed in this chapter include, but are not limited to, temperature modalities, manipulation and traction, casting/splinting, and exercise therapy. These techniques should be used liberally to either augment analgesic plans or to provide the first line of analgesia for acute injuries.

Temperature Modalities

Cold

Cold therapy, also known as cryotherapy, is defined as therapeutic lowering of localized tissue temperature. It is implemented with the goals of decreasing cellular metabolism, inflammation, transmission of painful stimuli, and muscle spasm. Application of cold stimulus induces localized vasoconstriction, reaching maximal narrowing at a temperature of 50 °F (10 °C).

Initial vasoconstriction decreases the release of inflammatory mediators and cytokines that increase nociceptive input from the site of insult. Of note, paradoxical vasodilation occurs when temperatures begin to decrease below 50 °F, usually after 15 minutes of application. Vasculature is maximally dilated at 32 °F (0 °C). This phenomenon is hypothesized to occur due to spinal cord reflexes in an attempt to maintain thermoregulation along with direct paralysis of the vessel musculature from nerve conduction inhibition.

Localized analgesia is attained through decreased conduction velocity in peripheral pain fibers, as cryotherapy decreases excitability in free nerve endings. This effect is also seen in fibers supplying the muscle spindle and golgi tendon resulting in alleviation of muscle spasm. Depth penetration of cryotherapy, maximally approximately 5 cm, is dependent on duration and magnitude of treatment. Therapeutic efficacy is inversely related to depth of the tissue requiring treatment [1, 2].

Indications for cryotherapy include acute soft tissue injury, acute postsurgical pain, and certain chronic pain syndromes. Tissue injury, whether traumatic or postsurgical, is attenuated with utilization of cold therapy. As adipose acts as an insulator to resist heat transfer, deeper tissues require longer application times in order to lower the temperature. Decreased temperature results in decreased metabolic rates and production of inflammatory mediators in injured tissue and protects against further damage from relative hypoxia. Edema and hemorrhage are reduced as a result of vasoconstriction, while recovery of muscular activity is accelerated. Chronic pain states also display benefit from cryotherapy. Acute flares of chronic inflammatory conditions such as osteoarthritis and rheumatoid arthritis are managed with application of cold therapy for its anti-inflammatory effects. Trigger points associated with myofascial pain syndrome are responsive to cryotherapy, as desensitization of peripheral free nerve endings and alleviation of spasm in the localized nodule provides symptomatic relief. Other conditions responsive to cryotherapy include tenosynovitis, bursitis, tendinitis, ligament/muscle strain, and contusion. Contraindications include hypersensitivity to cold, disease states causing impaired circulation, open wounds, or infection [3, 4].

Various methods exist for the delivery of cryotherapy. Ice packs and chemical sprays are most commonly utilized with ice massage, cold whirlpool, and contrast baths also being options. Ice packs and ice massage employ penetration to subcutaneous and muscular layers, generally requiring 20 minutes of application to achieve effect. Contrast baths

S. Arora
Metro Pain & Vein, Clifton, NJ, USA

S. Erosa
Department of Physical Medicine and Rehabilitation,
Montefiore Medical Center, Bronx, NY, USA

H. Danesh (✉)
Department of Anesthesiology, Perioperative and Pain Medicine,
Mount Sinai Hospital, New York, NY, USA
e-mail: houman.danesh@mountsinai.org

involve alternating application of hot and cold immersions to reduce swelling via fluctuating vasodilation-vasoconstriction responses. Chemical cold sprays act on superficial skin layers by stimulating A-beta fibers [4].

Superficial Heat

Superficial thermotherapy acts on cutaneous tissue with less than 1 cm in depth penetration. Primary effects include vasodilation, direct analgesia, and muscle relaxation. Localized vasodilation aids in reducing inflammation by removing noxious mediators. Analgesia is explained by gate theory, as heat receptors reach peak recruitment and discharge between 99 °F and 104 °F. Temperatures exceeding this range result in further stimulation of pain receptors. The increase in temperature decreases the gamma fiber firing rate in muscle spindles thereby causing skeletal muscles to relax [5].

Subacute and chronic conditions respond favorably to superficial heat therapy. Examples include osteoarthritis, ligament sprain, contusion, muscle strain, spasm, and myofascial pain syndrome. In contrast to deep heating modalities, superficial thermotherapy spares the deep tissues, including the muscles, as hypodermal fat insulates and prevents heat transfer. The maximum degree of temperature elevation occurs in the skin and subcutaneous tissues within 0.5 cm of the skin surface. Acute pain syndromes, open wounds, active infections, and conditions involving impairment of circulation are instances in which heat treatment is contraindicated.

Manipulation, Traction, and Massage

Introduction

Manipulation, massage, and traction incorporate hands-on techniques that are both relatively new and have been utilized in medicine for thousands of years. These techniques focus on using the practitioner's hands as a diagnostic and therapeutic tool and can be applied to a wide variety of disorders, particularly musculoskeletal conditions of the neck, back, and joints.

Manipulation

Manipulation, or manual medicine, is the application of passive mechanical forces to vertebral segments, joints, muscles, and fascia. The primary goal of manipulation is to improve or restore range of motion where an area of restriction is encountered. Restoration of musculoskeletal function can also lead to decreased pain, increased circulation, and improved lymphatic drainage. A variety of musculoskeletal conditions, particularly those involving the back, neck, pelvis, ribs, and thorax have been treated with manipulation techniques [6].

The main principles of manipulation medicine are the barrier concept and somatic dysfunction. The barrier concept states that the normal range of motion of a joint is relatively free in one direction and restricted in the other direction. A restrictive barrier refers to a restriction that is functional in nature and occurs within the normal range of motion of the joint. These barriers are typically due to abnormal muscle contraction or the development of ligamentous or capsular shortening in one direction that prevents normal range of motion. This impaired musculoskeletal function is termed somatic dysfunction. Somatic dysfunction can be detected on physical exam based on tenderness, asymmetry, range of motion abnormalities, and tissue texture changes. In the technique of manipulation, the practitioner applies an additional force in an attempt to correct somatic dysfunction and restore normal range of motion [7].

Manipulation techniques are typically categorized into soft tissue techniques, articulatory techniques, or specific joint mobilization. Furthermore, these techniques can be applied either directly or indirectly. In the direct technique, the practitioner moves the body part in the direction of the restrictive barrier, which is known as engaging the restrictive barrier. Indirect techniques involve directing the body part away from the restrictive barrier.

Examples of direct techniques are thrust, articulation, muscle energy, and direct myofascial release, while indirect techniques include strain-counterstrain, indirect balancing, indirect myofascial release, and craniosacral.

Thrust technique is a high velocity, low amplitude approach. First, the restriction barrier is assessed through flexion-extension, rotation, and side bending of the vertebra. Once diagnosed, the identified joint is moved to its limit of motion, and a brief, controlled thrust is applied.

Articulation involves mobilizing a joint repeatedly in a back and forth motion to increase range of motion. It is a low velocity, high amplitude approach. In soft tissue technique, the goal is to mechanically stretch skin, muscle, and fascia to relieve tension, encouraging circulation and lymphatic flow.

Muscle energy is a direct non-thrusting technique that requires the patient to exert an isometric force and contract against the resistance offered by the practitioner.

Direct myofascial release targets tissue restriction by applying a constant force, allowing fascial release to occur through inherent mechanisms. Myofascial release can also be applied using an indirect technique [8].

Strain-counterstrain utilizes positioning and tender points to relieve pain. A tender point associated with an area is first identified. A palpating finger is then applied to the tender point, and the patient's position is adjusted until the tenderness is eliminated or reduced significantly. While the patient is held in this position of ease, the restricting muscle is shortened (counterstrained), and its antagonist muscle is overstretched (strained). Neurophysiologically, strain-counterstrain resets the restricted muscles and normalizes their proprioceptive input to the spinal cord.

Indirect balancing, also known as functional technique, is similar to strain-counterstrain in its goal of finding the position of ease in order to reset inappropriate afferent signals to the spinal cord. However, in indirect balancing, the position of ease is found entirely by the practitioner, who must be experienced enough to detect increased or decreased tissue tension during the positioning process.

In craniosacral manipulation, pressure is applied to the cranial and sacral areas to restore normal rhythmic wave motion. The wave motion is thought by some to represent the state of fluidity in the cerebrospinal fluid [8].

Generally, low-velocity techniques are considered safer than high-velocity thrust techniques. Contraindications include vertebral malignancy, inflammatory arthropathy, acute spondyloarthropathy, ligamentous instability, infection, fracture or dislocation, severe osteoporosis, coagulopathy, tumor, and cauda equina syndrome. The most feared complication during cervical manipulation is stroke due to vertebrobasilar artery dissection [9].

Traction

Traction involves application of pulling forces to cause stretch in a certain part of the body. Different types of traction delivery include mechanical, hydraulic or motorized, manual, gravity, and autotraction. Mechanical traction involves use of a weighted pulley system, along with a harness or sling that is attached to the patient. Manual traction utilizes the body weight of the practitioner to provide the traction. Gravity can also be utilized to provide traction. In autotraction, a specially designed device allows the patient to self-administer traction [10].

Physically, traction stretches the muscles and ligaments, enlarges the intervertebral space and intervertebral foramen, and separates the apophyseal (e.g., facet) joints. Traction use is typically limited to the cervical and lumbar spine for conditions such as radiculopathy, pain, muscle spasm, and facet spondylosis. For cervical traction, 25 pounds of force is needed to begin noticing distraction of the cervical vertebral segments. For lumbar traction, the force necessary is a much greater, typically reported to range from 70 to 150 pounds. Positioning is an important consideration in traction [11]. There are no clear indications as to what types of neck of back pain may benefit from traction. Generally, scientific literature supporting the efficacy of traction is scant and its use has declined over the years.

Absolute contraindications to traction include the conditions that might predispose to cervical ligamentous instability, such as previous trauma, Down's syndrome, Marfan syndrome, and rheumatoid arthritis. The presence of vertebrobasilar insufficiency could predispose to dissection if manipulation is performed. A positive history of spinal cord tumor or malignancy, osteopenia, infection, and pregnancy are also contraindicated. Advanced age is a relative contraindication due to degenerative changes of the spine [10].

Massage

Massage therapy involves utilizing a variety of techniques of pressure, compression, and stretching on the soft tissues to produce reflexive, mechanical, neurologic, and psychological effects. The goals are relaxation, relief of tension, decreased pain, increased circulation, and improved mobility. Massage leads to an improvement in circulation secondary to reflex vasodilation. Release of endogenous endorphins, as well as gate control are likely responsible for analgesia. Mechanically, the compressive, shearing, and vibratory forces cause fluid shifts within tissues. Massage assists in increased venous return from the periphery, as well as lymphatic drainage. Muscle tightness is decreased, adhesions and scars in the muscles, tendons and ligaments are broken down or softened [12].

Types of massage can be categorized based on geographic origin – Western versus Eastern. Forms of Western massage include effleurage, pétrissage, tapotement, and friction massage. Effleurage is performed by gliding the hands and/or fingers across the skin in a rhythmic fashion. It promotes blood flow and relaxation and is usually employed as an initial maneuver prior to more aggressive massage techniques. Pétrissage is a kneading, rhythmic motion that compresses soft tissue between the hands and fingers, leading to soft tissue release and increased blood flow. Pétrissage can be superficial, which causes relaxation, and deep, which increases blood flow, decreases adhesions, and mobilizes tissue deposits. Tapotement is the act of repetitive percussion of soft tissue with varying degrees of pressure, which loosen and clear secretions. Friction massage is the forceful application of an increasing amount of pressure when moving from superficial to deep, with the goal of loosening adhesions [8]. Eastern forms of massage include acupressure, shiatsu, and reflexology. In Chinese philosophy, energy, or qi, circulates through the body along 12 meridians. Acupressure points are situated along the course of these meridians. In acupressure, digital pressure is applied to acupuncture points with the goal of restoring qi. Shiatsu is a Japanese system also based on the Chinese meridian theory. In reflexology, it is believed that a homuncular representation of the body exists on the extremities, including the soles of the feet. Dysfunctional areas of the body can be treated by applying digital pressure to the corresponding areas of the feet [8].

Massage therapy should not be utilized when there is potential exacerbation of an existing condition, tissue destruction, or spread of disease. Therefore, it should not be used over areas of known deep venous thrombosis or atherosclerosis, infection, malignancy, or lymphangitis. Traumatic areas with recent bleeding or patients with coagulopathies should also be treated with caution [13].

Casting and Splinting

Basic Principles

Prior to determining if a patient requires a cast or splint, a thorough physical exam should be performed to assess for neurovascular damage or other findings that necessitate prompt orthopedic surgeon referral. Casting and splinting are both methods of immobilization in musculoskeletal injuries. Immobilization is the foundation of fracture healing by maintaining alignment of the associated bones, protecting the site of injury, and promoting recovery. Although splints and casts both provide immobilization, they differ in their structure, indications, benefits, and risks. It is important to utilize proper casting and splinting techniques as improper application will not be beneficial and can result in harm to the patient [14, 15].

Splints are often used in the acute orthopedic setting for a variety of conditions, including simple or stable fractures, sprains, post-laceration repairs, and severe soft tissue injuries. Splints typically require less time to perform than casts and are also more easily removed, which allows for more frequent inspection of the site of injury. However, due to easy removal, splints tend to have lower compliance rates. Splints may be static to prevent motion and further injury or dynamic to assist with motion. As splints are non-circumferential, they are more permissive of swelling that occurs during the acute inflammatory phase, which, if severe enough with a circumferential cast, could lead to neurovascular compromise [14, 15].

Casts provide more effective immobilization than splints and are therefore utilized for definitive management of simple, complex, unstable, or potentially unstable fractures. Splinting is inappropriate for definitive management of such cases, but may be used in the acute setting to accommodate for swelling and provide some stability while awaiting more definitive care such as casting or orthopedic intervention. Casts are more technically difficult to apply, and as mentioned before, improper application of splints or casts can lead to complications related to tissue compression [14].

Materials

The two most commonly used materials for splinting or casting are Plaster of Paris and fiberglass. Plaster of Paris, a powdered form of gypsum, recrystallizes and hardens in an exothermic reaction with the presence of water. Plaster is more pliable and has a slower setting time than synthetic fiberglass, allowing more time for application and molding before setting. However, plaster is heavier, messier, and more prone to breaking down. Due to a slower setting time, plaster produces less heat and reduces discomfort and the risk of burns. Fiberglass sets faster and is lighter, stronger and more breathable than plaster, but is more expensive [16].

Water temperature is a significant factor in determining setting time. Warmer water temperature leads to a shorter setting time. However, shorter setting times produce more heat, increasing the risk of thermal injury. Generally, room temperature water is recommended for plaster and cool water for fiberglass. The amount of material or layers used is proportional to the amount of heat generated. Thus, it is ideal to use only the amount of material required to stabilize the injury [16].

Application of Splints and Casts

The general principles for applying a splint or cast are similar. Again, prior to applying a splint or cast, the full extent of injury should be ascertained. Emergent orthopedic referral is indicated for open, angulated or displaced fractures, dislocations that are unable to be reduced, and injuries with positive neurovascular findings. The proximal and distal joints to the fracture site should be included for maximal immobilization (not possible for distal fractures below the elbow or knee). For dislocations, the bone above and below the reduced joint should be immobilized. Joints should be casted or splinted while in their position of function (for the hands and fingers, position of safety is preferred) to prevent stiffness and loss of function [14].

The first layer of a splint or cast begins with stockinette application in order to provide skin protection. An appropriate stockinette size is selected and applied, covering about 10 cm beyond the proximal and distal ends of the destined splint or cast site. Afterwards, layers of cotton padding are added over the stockinette (extending 2–3 cm beyond intended splint or cast site) to prevent maceration and to accommodate for swelling. The padding is wrapped circumferentially, with each new layer overlapping the previous layer by 50%. Wrinkles should be avoided as they are potential sources of pressure points. Bony prominences and high pressure areas should receive extra padding. Prominences at high risk include the olecranon, malleoli, heel, and ulnar styloid. Excess padding should also be avoided, as this can lead to a loose fit and inadequate immobilization [15].

Finally, the splinting or casting tape (plaster or fiberglass material) should be moistened, applied over padding, molded, and allowed to set. The difference between splitting and casting is that the casting material is applied circumferentially, similar to the application of the padding. Care should be taken during molding as to not cause any unevenness or indentations that could lead to pressure sores or ulcers. Beginners should use the palms and heels of the hands rather than the fingers to avoid improper, uneven molding. After application of the splint or cast material, excess stockinette and padding material should be folded back to create a smooth edge. Neurovascular status should always be reassessed after application, and the patient should also be reexamined 24–48 hours after application. A follow-up exam is indicated 7–10 days after injury, at which time most of the swelling has subsided. At this time, a splint may be exchanged for a cast if deemed necessary [15].

Complications of Splinting and Casting

While immobilization is the overall goal in splinting and casting, this can lead to stiffness, atrophy, and disuse syndromes. Splints or casts that are applied too tightly can lead to skin breakdown and neurovascular compromise, including compartment syndrome (more likely with casts). A patient who experiences increasing pain, tingling, burning, or numbness should undergo immediate evaluation for potentially severe complications [48].

The most common complication is skin breakdown from sores or abrasions. This can be due to pressure from an unpadded, wrinkled, or uneven area of the splint or cast that overlies the tissue or bone. Confirming that there is smooth and sufficient padding helps to minimize skin breakdown. Thermal injuries can also occur during the splinting or casting process due to heat generation. Infectious complications are more likely to occur with open wounds but can also occur from the moist, warm environment of a splint or cast. Prolonged immobilization after fracture is also a risk factor for complex regional pain syndrome (CRPS).

Therapeutic Exercise

An important part of a healthy lifestyle, regular physical activity has been shown to reduce the mortality risk from all causes. There has been increasing evidence that moderate-intensity physical activity is associated with health benefits, even in the face of unchanged overall fitness. In order to benefit from the many health-related benefits associated with exercise, the Centers for Disease Control and Prevention (CDC) and the American College of Sports Medicine (ACSM) recommend that all adults achieve 30 minutes or more of moderate-intensity activity on preferably all days of the week [17].

The goals of therapeutic exercise include enhancement of physical fitness, correction of an impairment, and maintenance of a state of well-being. Exercise prescriptions should be individualized with attention to the patient's overall health condition, risk factors, behavioral propensities, goals, and medications [18]. The major components of any exercise therapy program consist of intensity, duration, frequency, and progression. Mode refers to the specific type of exercise (i.e., running, swimming, cycling, etc.). Duration is the length of an exercise session. Frequency is how often each exercise session occurs. Progression is the improvement in activity over time with continual training [18, 19].

The major categories of therapeutic exercise are endurance training, strength training, and flexibility training. An exercise prescription is targeted towards improving one of these components of overall fitness. Before a patient embarks on a therapeutic exercise regimen, he or she should undergo a comprehensive medical evaluation. Patients with cardiac conditions or other significant comorbidities should have relevant testing performed, such as an electrocardiogram and exercise stress test.

Endurance Training

The ACSM recommendations for endurance training are listed in Table 23.1 [8].

Table 23.1 ACSM recommendations for endurance training [8]

Mode	Frequency	Duration	Intensity	Progression
Aerobic exercise[a]	3–5 days per week	20–60 minutes[b]	About 60–90% of maximum heart rate, or 50–85% of V_{O2max} or heart rate reserve (HRR)	5 to 10 minute increase in activity every 1–2 weeks over the first 4–6 weeks[c]

[a]Exercises that engage large muscle groups and are rhythmic in nature
[b]May be one continuous session or several intermittent sessions each lasting greater than 10 minutes
[c]Depends on current physical status, goals, and compliance

Strength Training

Muscle fibers are classified into two main categories (slow or fast) based on their speed of contraction. Type I muscle fibers are slow twitch fibers and contain a high amount of oxidative enzymes due to the large amounts of mitochondria. They have a rich capillary supply and are suited for low-intensity, endurance activities. Type I fibers have low glycogen content, low glycolytic activity, and are small in diameter.

Type II fibers are fast-twitch fibers and are suited for high-intensity, short-duration activities. They can achieve rapid peak tension and relaxation, but have a higher rate of fatigue compared to Type I fibers. Type II fibers generally have high ATPase activity, high levels of glycogen content, high levels of glycolytic activity, and large fiber diameters.

Type II fibers are further subdivided into Type IIA and Type IIB fibers. Type IIA fibers, known as fast oxidative glycolytic or fatigue resistant fibers, have more oxidative enzymes and a richer capillary supply compared to Type IIB fibers. Type IIB fibers are known as fast glycolytic or fast fatigable fibers.

There are generally three categories of strengthening exercises: isotonic, isometric, and isokinetic.

Isotonic Exercise

Isotonic contractions occur when muscles contract against a fixed external resistance. As the external resistance is overcome, limb motion is produced at a variable speed. Resistance training with free weights and machines is an example of isotonic exercise.

The DeLorme technique utilizes isotonic contractions and is an example of a progressive resistance exercise. In this regimen, the patient determines a 10 repetition maximum, or 10 RM, which is the maximum weight able to be lifted 10 times with correct technique. Starting at 50% of the 10 RM, the patient would perform a set of 10 repetitions. The second and third set are performed using 75% and 100% of the 10 RM, respectively. The individual gradually increases the percentage of the 10 RM as strength increases. The Oxford technique is the reverse of the DeLorme technique (regressive resistance exercise) in that the patient begins with 10 repetitions at 100% of the 10 RM, then 10 repetitions at 75% of the 10 RM, and finally 10 repetitions at 50% of the 10 RM. Both the DeLorme and Oxford techniques are effective in strengthening, since reaching the RM means that progressive recruitment of muscle fibers has occurred and the muscle is operating at a high intensity [20, 21].

With isotonic contractions, muscle fibers can contract eccentrically or concentrically. In eccentric contraction, as muscle resists a stretching force as it lengthens. Eccentric contractions occur during the lowering phases of resistance exercise. Though eccentric contractions generate the largest amount of force, it tends to cause a greater amount of muscle injury. With concentric contractions, muscle develops tension as it shortens to overcome resistance. Concentric contractions occur during the lifting phase of the resistance exercise.

Isometric Exercise

Isometric contractions are a form of static exercise and simple to perform. Muscle contracts against a fixed load, but since the resistance is not overcome, no limb motion occurs. An example of this would be exertion against an immovable object.

Isokinetic Exercise

During isokinetic contraction, muscle contracts against a variable load at a constant velocity. The same velocity is maintained throughout the contraction cycle. Isokinetic exercises are usually performed with specialized equipment, such as a Cybex™ or Nautilus™.

Flexibility

Flexibility describes the amount of excursion attainable by a part of the body through its range of motion. The goal of flexibility training is to improve and maintain the range of motion of specific joints by lengthening tendons and muscles. Flexibility exercises should be executed in a slow, controlled manner and gradually progressed to achieve greater ranges of motion. The three main types of flexibility exercises are static, passive, ballistic or dynamic, and proprioceptive neuromuscular facilitation (PNF) [22].

Static stretching involves the steady stretching of a muscle to a position where one begins to feel mild discomfort and then holding that position for a period of time. Static stretching is easy and safe to perform with little assistance required, and good efficacy with little time investment.

Passive stretching is performed with assistance from a partner, who applies a slow force to a relaxed extremity to create stretch.

Ballistic or dynamic stretching utilizes repetitive rapid bouncing and jerking motions to create momentum. Muscles are stretched as the generated momentum carries the specific body part through its range of motion. The risk of muscle tear and injury is higher with this type of stretching.

Proprioceptive neuromuscular facilitation (PNF) usually requires assistance from a therapist or trainer. With this technique muscles alternate between contraction and relaxation. The muscle first undergoes an isometric or concentric contraction, followed by a passive stretch. A rest or relaxation period follows before the next contraction and stretch phase takes places. PNF produces the largest improvements in flexibility, but is more likely to cause muscle soreness.

Exercises for Common Pain Conditions

Before prescribing an exercise plan, all pain conditions should undergo a complete evaluation of the affected joint in addition to the joint above and below. Patients should be instructed to pay close attention to proper technique when performing all exercises and to be monitored by trained professionals to decrease risk of injury secondary to incorrect exercise technique.

Hip Osteoarthritis: [23–25]

1. Nordic Walking
2. Strength training exercises:
   • Leg press
   • Leg raise
   • Leaping squat
3. Home-based exercises:
   • Flexibility exercises
     (i) Hip ROM
     (ii) Psoas release
   • Chair-stand exercise
   • Pelvic-lift
   • Isometric hip flexion in standing position
   • Side-lying leg lift
4. Aquatic exercise program
   • Swimming (Table 23.2)

Knee Osteoarthritis: [26–29]

1. Resistance exercise:
   • Seated leg presses (or a variation of squats)
   • Knee extensions
   • Hamstring curls

Table 23.2 ACSM guidelines for arthritis [19]

Exercise	Duration	Description

Aerobic exercise	3–5 days per week	Activities with low joint stress:
		  Walking
		  Cycling
		  Swimming

Resistance exercise	2–3 days per week	Begin with maximum voluntary isometric contractions around affected joint with progression to dynamic training.
Flexibility exercise	Daily	ROM exercises to include all major muscle groups

• Hip adduction (with machine or resistance bands)
• Hip abduction (with machine or resistance bands)
• Calf/toe presses
2. Flexibility exercises
   • Quadricep release
   • IT band release
3. Aquatic exercise program
   • Swimming

Lumbar Radiculopathy: [30, 31]

1. Core strengthening exercises:
   • "Bird dog" pose
   • Side plank
   • Tri-ped exercise with balance ball
   • Tri-planar exercise with weights using forward lunge and rotation
   • "Lawn mower" exercise (weight free)
2. Flexibility exercises:
   • "Cat and Camel" exercise
   • Knee to chest stretch
   • Ankle over knee stretch
   • Kneeling lunge

Cervical Radiculopathy: [32–34]

1. Stretching exercises:
   • Cervical flexion/extension
   • Contralateral rotation
   • Side flexion
2. Strengthening exercises:
   • Cervical strengthening:
     (i) Supine craniocervical flexion
     (ii) Prone craniocervical extension
     (iii) Seated craniocervical flexion
   • Scapular strengthening:
     (i) Scapular retraction with resistance bands or pulleys
     (ii) Prone horizontal abduction
     (iii) Side-lying forward flexion
     (iv) Prone extension of each shoulder
     (v) Prone push-ups with emphasis on shoulder protraction

Myofascial Pain Syndrome: [35, 36]

1. Post-isometric relaxation
2. Spray and stretch technique

Cervical Spondylosis: [37, 38]

1. Cervical retraction (McKenzie exercise)
2. Supine cervical flexion

3. Scapular retraction
4. Pectoralis stretching (hands placed behind head, abduction, external rotation)

Lumbar Spondylosis: [39–41]

1. Stretching exercises:
   - Piriformis stretch
   - Erector spinae stretch
2. Strengthening exercises:
   - Supine: contraction of transversus abdominis in supine position
   - Supine: pelvic lift with contraction of transversus abdominis
   - Prone: head and shoulder lift on elbows
   - Prone: bilateral leg lift
   - Postural correction with sitting
   - Leg extensions while on knees and hands (add assistive weight via pulleys)
   - Single leg reverse lunges
   - Trunk lifting

Fibromyalgia: [42–47]

1. Resistance exercises:
   - Leg press
   - Knee flexion/extension with weight machine
   - Bicep curls and hand grip with free weights
   - Heel raise/core stability using body weight
2. Aerobic exercise:
   - Land-based or water-based
     (i) Walking (indoor, outdoor, treadmill)
     (ii) Running
     (iii) Low-impact aerobics
     (iv) Cycle ergometer
     (v) Aerobic dance
     (vi) Swimming
3. Flexibility exercises:
   - Tailored stretching programs targeting major muscle groups
   - ROM exercises (especially in shoulders, hips, knees, and ankles)

References

1. Olson J, Stravino V. A review of cryotherapy. Phys Ther. 1972;52:840–53.
2. Galvan H, Tritsch AJ, Tandy R, Rubley MD. Pain perception during repeated ice-bath immersion of the ankle at varied temperatures. J Sports Rehabil. 2006;15(2):105–15.
3. Bleakley C, McDonough S, MacAuley D. The use of ice in the treatment of acute soft-tissue injury: a systematic review of randomized controlled trials. Am J Sports Med. 2004;32:251–61.
4. Lehmann J. Therapeutic heat and cold. 4th ed. Baltimore: Williams & Wilkins; 1990.
5. Fischer E, Solomon S. Physiologic responses to heat and cold. In: Licht S, editor. Therapeutic heat and cold. New Haven: Elizabeth Licht; 1965. p. 126–9.
6. DeStefano L. Greenman's principles of manual medicine. 4th ed. Philadelphia: Lippincott Williams & Wilkins; 2011.
7. Korr I. Proprioceptors and somatic dysfunction. J Am Osteopath Assoc. 1975;74(7):634–50.
8. Cifu DX. Braddom's physical medicine & rehabilitation. 5th ed. Philadelphia: Elsevier; 2016.
9. Assendelft W, LM B, PG K, LM B, PG K. Complications of spinal manipulation: a comprehensive review of the literature. J Fam Pract. 1996;42(5):475–80.
10. Hinterbuchner C. Traction. In: Basmajian J, editor. Manipulation, traction and massage. Baltimore: Williams & Wilkins; 1985.
11. Colachis S Jr, Strohm BR. A study of tractive forces and angle of pull on vertebral interspaces in the cervical spine. Arch Phys Med Rehabil. 1965;46(12):820–30.
12. Beard G. Massage: principles and techniques. Philadelphia: WB Saunders; 1964.
13. Knapp M. Massage. In: Kottke F, Lahman J, editors. Krusen's handbook of physical medicine and rehabilitation. Philadelphia: Saunders; 1990.
14. Boyd A, Benjamin H, Asplund C. Principles of casting and splinting. Am Fam Physician. 2009;79(1):16–22.
15. Chudnofsky C, Byers S. Splinting techniques. In: Roberts J, Hedges J, Chanmugam A, editors. Clinical procedures in emergency medicine. 4th ed. Philadelphia: Saunders; 2004.
16. Wehbé M. Plaster uses and misuses. Clin Orthop Relat Res. 1982;(167):242–9.
17. Franklin B, Whaley M, Howley E, Balady G. General principles of exercise prescription. In: Franklin BA, Whaley MH, Howley ET, editors. ACSM's guidelines for exercise testing and prescription. 6th ed. Philadelphia: Lippincott Williams & Wilkins; 2000.
18. Seto C. Basic principles of exercise training. In: O'Connor F, Sallis R, Wilder R, et al., editors. Sports medicine: just the facts. New York: McGraw-Hill; 2005. p. 75–83.
19. Thompson WR, Gordon NF, Pescatello LS. ACSM's guidelines for exercise testing and prescription. 8th ed. Philadelphia: Wolters Kluwer/Lippincott Williams & Wilkins; 2010.
20. DeLorme T, Watkins A. Progressive resistance exercise. New York: Appleton-Century-Crofts; 1951.
21. Zinovieff A. Heavy-resistance exercises the "Oxford technique". Br J Phys Med. 1951;14(6):129–32.
22. Saal J. Flexibility training. In: Kibler W, editor. Functional rehabilitation of sports and musculoskeletal injuries. Gaithersburg; 1998.
23. Bieler T, Siersma V, Magnusson S, Kjaer M, Beyer N. Exercise induced effects on muscle function and range of motion in patients with hip osteoarthritis. Physiother Res Int. 2017;23(1) https://doi.org/10.1002/pri.1697.
24. Bieler T, Siersma V, Magnusson S, Kjaer M, Christensen H, Beyer N. In hip osteoarthritis, Nordic Walking is superior to strength training and home-based exercise for improving function. Scand J Med Sci Sports. 2016;27(8):873–86.
25. Tak E, Staats P, Van Hespen A, Hopman-Rock M. The effects of an exercise program for older adults with osteoarthritis of the hip. J Rheumatol. 2005;32(6):1106–13.
26. Vincent KR, Vincent H. Resistance exercise for knee osteoarthritis. PM&R. 2012;4(5):S45.
27. Baker K, Nelson M, Felson D, Layne J, Sarno R, Roubenoff R. The efficacy of home based progressive strength training in older adults with knee osteoarthritis: a randomized controlled trial. J Rheumatol. 2001;28(7):1655–65.

28. Lu M, Su Y, Zhang Y, Zhang Z, Wang W, He Z, et al. Effectiveness of aquatic exercise for treatment of knee osteoarthritis. Z Rheumatol. 2015;75(6):543–52.

29. Ottawa panel evidence-based clinical practice guidelines for therapeutic exercises and manual therapy in the management of osteoarthritis. Phys Ther. 2005;85(9):907–71.

30. Kennedy DJ, Noh MY. The role of core stabilization in lumbosacral radiculopathy. Phys Med Rehabil Clin N Am. 2011;22(1):91–103.

31. Durstine L. ACSM's exercise management for persons with chronic diseases and disabilities. Champaign: Human Kinetics; 2009.

32. Fritz J, Thackeray A, Brennan G, Childs J. Exercise only, exercise with mechanical traction, or exercise with over-door traction for patients with cervical radiculopathy, with or without consideration of status on a previously described subgrouping rule: a randomized clinical trial. J Orthop Sports Phys Ther. 2014;44(2):45–57.

33. Langevin P, Desmeules F, Lamothe M, Robitaille S, Roy J. Comparison of 2 manual therapy and exercise protocols for cervical radiculopathy: a randomized clinical trial evaluating short-term effects. J Orthop Sports Phys Ther. 2015;45(1):4–17.

34. Falla D, Lindstrøm R, Rechter L, Boudreau S, Petzke F. Effectiveness of an 8-week exercise programme on pain and specificity of neck muscle activity in patients with chronic neck pain: a randomized controlled study. Eur J Pain. 2013;17(10):1517–28.

35. Bron C, de Gast A, Dommerholt J, Stegenga B, Wensing M, Oostendorp R. Treatment of myofascial trigger points in patients with chronic shoulder pain: a randomized, controlled trial. BMC Med. 2011;9(1)

36. Lewit K, Simons D. Myofascial pain: relief by post-isometric relaxation. Arch Phys Med Rehabil. 1984;65(8):452–6.

37. Wani S, Raka N, Jethwa J, Mohammed R. Comparative efficacy of cervical retraction exercises (McKenzie) with and without using pressure biofeedback in cervical spondylosis. Int J Ther Rehabil. 2013;20(10):501–8.

38. Diab AA, Moustafa IM. The efficacy of forward head correction on nerve root function and pain in cervical spondylotic radiculopathy: a randomized trial. Clin Rehabil. 2011;26(4):351–61.

39. van Middlekoop M, Rubinstein S, Verhagen A, Ostelo R, Koes B, van Tulder M. Exercise therapy for chronic nonspecific low-back pain. Best Pract Res Clin Rheumatol. 2010;24(2):193–204.

40. Pardo GB, Lluch Girbés E, Roussel N, Gallego Izquierdo T, Jiménez Penick V, Pecos Martín D. Pain neurophysiology education and therapeutic exercise for patients with chronic low back pain: a single-blind randomized controlled trial. Arch Phys Med Rehabil. 2018;99(2):338–47.

41. Smeets RJ, Vlaeyen JW, Hidding A, Kester AD, van der Heijden GJ, van Geel AC, et al. Active rehabilitation for chronic low back pain: cognitive-behavioral, physical, or both? first direct post-treatment results from a randomized controlled trial [ISRCTN22714229]. BMC Musculoskelet Disord. 2006;7(1)

42. Larsson A, Palstam A, Löfgren M, Ernberg M, Bjersing J, Bileviciute-Ljungar I, et al. Resistance exercise improves muscle strength, health status and pain intensity in fibromyalgia--a randomized controlled trial. Arthritis Res Ther. 2015;17(1):161.

43. AJ AB, Webber S, Brachaniec M, Bidonde J, Bello-Haas V, Danyliw A, et al. Exercise therapy for fibromyalgia. Curr Pain Headache Rep. 2011;15

44. Häuser W, Klose P, Langhorst J, Moradi B, Steinbach M, Schiltenwolf M, Busch A. Efficacy of different types of aerobic exercise in fibromyalgia syndrome: a systematic review and meta-analysis of randomised controlled trials. Arthritis Res Ther. 2010;12(3):R79.

45. Brosseau L, Wells G, Tugwell P, Egan M, Wilson K, Dubouloz C, et al. Ottawa panel evidence-based clinical practice guidelines for aerobic fitness exercises in the management of fibromyalgia: part 1. Phys Ther. 2008;88(7):857–71.

46. Busch AJ, Overend TJ, Schachter CL. Fibromyalgia treatment: the role of exercise and physical activity. Int J Clin Rheumatol. 2009;4(3):343–80.

47. Cazzola M, Atzeni F, Salaffi F, Stisi S, Cassisi G, Sarzi-Puttini P. Which kind of exercise is best in fibromyalgia therapeutic programmes? A practical review. Clin Exp Rheumatol. 2010;28:S117–24.

48. Pons T, Shipton EA, Williman J, Mulder RT. Potential risk factors for the onset of complex regional pain syndrome type 1: a systematic literature review. Anesthesiol Res Pract. 2015;2015:956539. https://doi.org/10.1155/2015/956539. https://www.ncbi.nlm.nih.gov/pubmed/25688265

Stimulation-Produced Analgesia (TENS and Acupuncture)

Max Snyder and Naum Shaparin

Introduction

The concept of utilizing electrical stimulation to relieve pain dates back to at least the first century of the Common Era. In his book *De Materia Medica* ("On Medical Matters"), the Greek scholar Pedanius Dioscorides noted that "the sea torpedo [fish], when applied for chronic pain about the head, lightens the severity of the pain" [1]. In the eighteenth century, Benjamin Franklin experimented with capacitors and utilized electrical discharges to treat various pain conditions [2]. Despite these and many other historical anecdotes regarding the ability of electrical stimulation to relieve pain, it was not until the twentieth century that theories regarding the mechanism underlying this type of analgesia were espoused.

The Gate Control Theory of Pain was proposed by Ronald Melzack and Charles Patrick Wall in 1965. This theory recognized the concept of descending modulation of painful stimuli, but proposed a more complex system than previously thought. Melzack and Wall proposed that signals from nociceptors and touch receptors in the skin are transmitted to synapses in the dorsal horn of the spinal cord [3]. They proposed that a "gate" exists in this area of synapse which modulates the transmission of sensory information from peripheral nociceptors to central pain centers in the spinal cord and brain. The idea that sensory information from peripheral receptors could be modulated, transformed, or attenuated by the action of competing peripheral sensory input prior to reaching the central nervous system, forms the theoretical basis for modern stimulation-produced analgesic techniques.

In the late 1960s, it was reported that electrical stimulation of the periaqueductal gray (PAG) region in the midbrain of rats triggers profound analgesia [4]. Following several confirmatory experiments, the term "stimulation-produced analgesia" was coined to describe this phenomenon [5].

Today, stimulation-produced analgesia is a term that describes many techniques used to relieve acute or chronic pain via electrical stimulation of the peripheral or central nervous system. Methods used to produce analgesia by nerve stimulation include noninvasive or minimally invasive techniques such as acupuncture/acupressure, electroacupuncture, vibration, and transcutaneous electrical nerve stimulation (TENS). These techniques are typically used as a supplementary analgesic option for many acute and chronic pain conditions. More invasive options which produce analgesia by a similar mechanism include electronic stimulators which can be implanted adjacently to peripheral nerves, in the epidural space, or in the brain. These more invasive techniques are usually reserved for pain conditions refractory to more conventional treatments.

Peripheral Stimulation Techniques

TENS

The modern TENS device was initially developed by neurosurgeon Dr. C. Norman Shealy and the first commercial patent in the US was filed by Medtronic in 1974 [6]. Initially, TENS was used to predict success prior to dorsal column stimulator implantation. However, patients and physicians quickly realized that TENS could be used as an independent analgesic modality.

A TENS unit is a noninvasive device that generates and transmits electrical impulses to electrodes placed directly onto the skin. These electrical impulses then traverse the skin to stimulate the underlying nerves or muscles. A TENS unit consists of three basic components: a computer chip which can be used to adjust the characteristics of the stimulus, a battery source, and gel pad electrodes.

The electrical pulse waveform created by a TENS unit consists of three parts: pulse rate, pulse duration, and

M. Snyder · N. Shaparin (✉)
Department of Anesthesiology, Montefiore Medical Center, Bronx, NY, USA
e-mail: NSHAPARI@montefiore.org

© Springer Nature Switzerland AG 2019
Y. Khelemsky et al. (eds.), *Academic Pain Medicine*, https://doi.org/10.1007/978-3-030-18005-8_24

intensity. The pulse rate, also commonly referred to as frequency or pulses per second, is measured in hertz (Hz). Commonly used pulse rates may range from approximately 1 to 250 Hz. The pulse duration, also known as pulse width, is measured in microseconds (μS). This parameter determines the time interval during which each pulse is delivered. Typically, pulse duration may range from 1 to 250 μS. Increasing the pulse duration will cause the stimulation to feel more powerful and if increased sufficiently can elicit muscle contraction. The intensity, commonly referred to as amplitude, is measured in milliamps (mA). The intensity determines how strongly the stimulation will be felt by the patient. TENS units typically offer intensity in the range of 1–100 mA and it may be adjusted to patient comfort. Different pulse rates, pulse durations, and intensities may be used to maximize analgesia and depending on the patient's preference or underlying pain condition.

There are three main classifications of stimulation modes based on the pulse rate: high frequency (~50–250 Hz), low frequency (~10 Hz), or burst TENS. Different frequency settings are thought to elicit analgesia by different mechanisms. High-frequency stimulation is thought to excite large diameter peripheral afferents which in turn inhibit input from smaller diameter afferents in the substantia gelatinosa of the spinal cord (e.g., gate theory) [7]. Alternatively, low-frequency/high-intensity TENS is thought to work by activating an endogenous opioid pathway [7]. This is supported by evidence that the analgesia produced by low-frequency/high-intensity TENS can be reversed by administering naloxone [8].

Conventional TENS involves placing the electrodes directly over the painful dermatome and delivering high-frequency (10–250 Hz), low-amplitude currents for 30 minutes at a time several times a day. This mode elicits a comfortable tingling sensation without causing any motor excitation. Analgesia is produced by selective activation of large diameter non-noxious afferents which block afferent activity originating from nociceptors. Several studies suggest that this mode may also involve the neurotransmitters GABA and/or glutamate rather than endogenous opioids [9–11]. This is the most commonly used TENS mode and is the most reliable method for producing rapid, but short acting analgesia in the majority of patients.

Acupuncture-like TENS describes a low-frequency, high-amplitude mode often used in patients with pain refractory to conventional TENS. This mode uses a stimulus with a higher amplitude and pulse width but delivered at a frequency less than 10 Hz. With this mode, electrodes are placed over muscles, acupuncture points, or trigger points and a comfortable muscle contraction is elicited. As mentioned previously, this mode is thought to work by releasing endogenous opioids and is often considered to provide longer lasting analgesia

than high-frequency TENS [7]. Low-frequency TENS often does not produce analgesia in opioid-tolerant patients due to its mechanism of action. Interestingly, repeated TENS treatments utilizing this mode has also been shown to induce opioid tolerance in rats [12].

Several other modes of TENS exist including burst TENS, intense TENS, and modulation TENS. Each mode has its own postulated mechanism of action and benefits. Despite many studies explaining TENS mechanisms of action, some authors still believe that a significant part of its analgesic action is due to placebo effect [13]. Alternatively, some practitioners suggest that patients may report improved analgesia when using TENS simply due to an enhanced feeling of control over their pain [14].

MENS

A concept similar to TENS is microcurrent electrical neuromuscular stimulation (MENS). This modality delivers a stimulus one thousand times less intense than a typical TENS unit and well below a typical sensory level. Proponents of MENS believe that it can be beneficial for treatment of neuropathic pain and to accelerate healing [15]. However, rigorous studies demonstrating efficacy are lacking and many insurance companies consider this an experimental/investigational treatment [16].

TENS Indications

TENS devices have been considered for treatment of various pain conditions including relief of acute postsurgical pain, musculoskeletal pain, neurologic pain, phantom limb pain, arthritis, angina, labor pain, and dysmenorrhea [7, 17].

TENS Complications/Contraindications

Reported complications associated with TENS therapy are rare, but include mild electrical burns (typically caused by inappropriate use), minor skin irritation beneath electrodes, and mild autonomic responses [18, 19]. TENS should not be placed close to transdermal drug patches as there is a possibility that electrical stimulation can increase drug delivery to the patient. Device manufacturers consider cardiac pacemakers, pregnancy, epilepsy, and bleeding disorders to be contraindications [19]. However, some specialists believe that TENS may be used with care in these patient groups, as long as electrodes are not applied directly over the implanted device, pregnant abdomen, or head/neck (in epileptic patients) [19–22]. TENS electrodes should not be applied over the anterior neck, over the eyes, over areas of active malignancy, on open wounds or damaged skin, or to skin with diminished sensation caused by nerve damage [19].

Acupuncture

Acupuncture is an ancient alternative medicine technique used all over the world to treat various pain conditions as well as other non-painful ailments. Although the exact origins are unknown, acupuncture has its strongest ties to Traditional Chinese Medicine and is believed to have been developed in China around 100 BCE [23]. During the seventeenth century, acupuncture spread to Europe and by the nineteenth century was ubiquitous throughout the world.

The word acupuncture (derived from the latin word "acus" meaning "needle" or "pin") means "to puncture with a needle." Acupuncture treatment involves the insertion of multiple thin gauge needles along special pathways [24]. Once inserted, practitioners may periodically twist, heat, or apply mild electrical currents to the needles (e.g., electroacupuncture) to produce an enhanced effect. Needles are often left in place for 10 to 20 minutes at a time.

Traditionally, acupuncture is thought to work by correcting disruptions in the flow of energy (qi) along invisible pathways (meridians) throughout the body and restoring a natural balance [23]. In recent years, many studies have been performed in an attempt to discover a more scientific explanation for the pain relieving effects of acupuncture. Currently, the most widely accepted scientific theory asserts that acupuncture stimulates small diameter afferents that activate spinal cord, brainstem, and hypothalamic neurons which release endogenous opioids to dull pain. This endorphin theory is supported by the fact that the analgesic action of acupuncture seems to be reversed by naloxone in experiments with mice, but studies in humans are conflicting [25, 26]. Despite many theoretical mechanisms of action, a definitive scientific explanation for its observed effects has not been elucidated [23]. Other proposed mechanisms of action include modulation of immune function, inhibition of inflammatory responses, regulation of neuropeptide gene expression, alteration of hormone levels, and placebo effect [23].

Innumerable studies have been performed over many years in an attempt to prove the efficacy of acupuncture for the treatment of various pain conditions, but to date, the data is conflicting. Studies comparing acupuncture to sham needling typically show no difference in effect [27–29]. Studies comparing acupuncture to no treatment often show that acupuncture does work to reduce pain [29–31]. However, most physicians agree that this effect is largely due to a placebo effect [23]. According to the NIH, expectation and belief may play important roles in the beneficial effects of acupuncture on pain [32]. Various authors have similarly concluded that patient expectations may influence outcomes independent of the actual treatment effects [30, 33].

Despite the continued controversy regarding its efficacy, acupuncture continues to be widely used for the treatment of pain. In 1998, an National Institutes of Health consensus panel concluded that acupuncture was acceptable as "an adjunct treatment or acceptable alternative or may be included in a comprehensive management program" for the treatment of headache, tennis elbow, fibromyalgia, myofascial pain, low back pain, and osteoarthritis [34]. Similarly, a World Health Organization (WHO) publication summarizing the findings from an expert panel convened in 1996 concluded that "in developing countries, where medical personnel and medicines are still lacking, the need for acupuncture maybe considerable [and that] proper use of this simple and economic therapy could benefit a large number of patients" [35].

Acupuncture is considered relatively safe if performed by a trained practitioner. Unfortunately, rare but serious adverse outcomes caused by acupuncture are well documented. The following adverse events have been described: epidural hematoma, subarachnoid hemorrhage, pneumothorax, right ventricular puncture, cardiac tamponade, aortic rupture, intestinal perforation, tracheal injury, peritonitis, subcutaneous emphysema, tetanus, abscess formation, and other bacterial/viral infections [36].

Acupressure

Acupressure is a technique similar to acupuncture wherein the practitioner applies physical pressure to acupuncture points instead of inserting needles. Pressure can be applied manually or with various instruments. The basic mechanism of action and indications are considered to be the same for acupressure as for traditional acupuncture.

Vibration

The application of vibration to reduce pain has been used for many years. Historically vibration was produced manually; however, more recently it is produced by electronic devices. The proposed mechanisms by which vibration induces analgesia are similar to TENS. Vibration stimulates cutaneous A-β nerve fibers which activate inhibitory interneurons in the spinal cord that act to decrease the transmission of nociceptive information from A-δ and C fibers up the spinal cord to the brain (gate control theory). Additionally, part of the analgesia produced by vibration is likely due to placebo effect [37]. Vibration does not seem to be associated with the release of endogenous opioids and therefore cannot be reversed with naloxone [38].

Vibration therapy has been used to treat acute and chronic musculoskeletal type pains, thermal pain, sinus pain, pressure pain, as well as pain from local anesthetic infiltration or Botox injection [39]. Typically, the stimulation is applied with moderate pressure directly on the painful area, along the affected muscle or tendon, or along the antagonist muscle. Treatment sessions are 20–45 minutes in duration. Patients often describe an initial period of increased discomfort which is followed by numbness and analgesia which can last for several hours. A Lancet editorial from 1992 concludes that the use of vibration is "simple, safe, and highly effective and has the added advantage of being cheap to establish and maintain" [40].

Summary

Stimulation-produced analgesia techniques continue to be a popular choice for many acute and chronic pain conditions. Despite a dearth of randomized controlled trials clearly demonstrating effectiveness, many practitioners continue to tout its benefits based on their own professional experiences and patient feedback. Due to the relatively benign nature of most of these techniques and the possibility of modest benefit, stimulation-produced analgesia may be considered as an adjunctive analgesic modality.

References

1. Finger S, Piccolino M. Torpedoes in the Greco-Roman world: Pt. 2. From therapeutic shocks to theories of the discharge. In: The shocking history of electric fishes: from ancient epochs to the birth of modern neurophysiology. 1st ed. New York: Oxford University Press; 2011. p. 47–58.
2. Deer TR, Mali J. History of neurostimulation. In: Atlas of implantable therapies for pain management. 2nd ed. New York: Springer; 2016. p. 3–6.
3. Melzack R, Wall PD. Pain mechanisms: a new theory. Science. 1965;150(3699):971–9.
4. Reynolds DV. Surgery in the rat during electrical analgesia induced by focal brain stimulation. Science. 1969;164(3878):444–5.
5. Mayer DJ, Wolfle TL, Akil H, Carder B, Liebeskind JC. Analgesia from electrical stimulation in the brainstem of the rat. Science. 1971;174(4016):1351–4.
6. Maurer D, inventor; Medtronic Inc, assignee. Transcutaneous stimulator and stimulation method. United States patent US 3,817,254. 1974.
7. Sluka KA, Walsh D. Transcutaneous electrical nerve stimulation: basic science mechanisms and clinical effectiveness. J Pain. 2003;4(3):109–21.
8. Sluka KA, Deacon M, Stibal A, Strissel S, Terpstra A. Spinal blockade of opioid receptors prevents the analgesia produced by TENS in arthritic rats. J Pharmacol Exp Ther. 1999;289(2):840–6.
9. Duggan AW, Foong FW. Bicuculline and spinal inhibition produced by dorsal column stimulation in the cat. Pain. 1985;22(3):249–59.
10. Maeda Y, Lisi TL, Vance CG, Sluka KA. Release of GABA and activation of GABAA in the spinal cord mediates the effects of TENS in rats. Brain Res. 2007;1136:43–50.
11. Sluka KA, Vance CG, Lisi TL. High-frequency, but not low-frequency, transcutaneous electrical nerve stimulation reduces aspartate and glutamate release in the spinal cord dorsal horn. J Neurochem. 2005;95(6):1794–801.
12. Chandran P, Sluka KA. Development of opioid tolerance with repeated transcutaneous electrical nerve stimulation administration. Pain. 2003;102(1–2):195–201.
13. Carroll D, Tramer M, McQuay H, Nye B, Moore A. Randomization is important in studies with pain outcomes: systematic review of transcutaneous electrical nerve stimulation in acute postoperative pain. Br J Anaesth. 1996;77(6):798–803.
14. Köke AJ, Schouten JS, Lamerichs-Geelen MJ, Lipsch JS, Waltje EM, van Kleef M, Patijn J. Pain reducing effect of three types of transcutaneous electrical nerve stimulation in patients with chronic pain: a randomized crossover trial. Pain. 2004;108(1–2):36–42.
15. Mercola JM, Kirsch DL. The basis for microcurrent electrical therapy in conventional medical practice. J Adv Med. 1995;8(2):107–20.
16. Electrical stimulation for pain – Medical Clinical Policy Bulletins | Aetna [Internet]. Aetna.com. 2018 [cited 17 Mar 2018]. Available from: http://www.aetna.com/cpb/medical/data/1_99/0011.html.
17. Mannheimer C, Carlsson CA, Vedin A, Wilhelmsson C. Transcutaneous electrical nerve stimulation (TENS) in angina pectoris. Pain. 1986;26(3):291–300.
18. Carroll D, Moore RA, McQuay HJ, Fairman F, Tramer M, Leijon G. Transcutaneous electrical nerve stimulation (TENS) for chronic pain. Cochrane Database Syst Rev. 2001;3(3):CD003222.
19. Jones I, Johnson MI. Transcutaneous electrical nerve stimulation. Contin Educ Anaesth Crit Care Pain. 2009;9(4):130–5.
20. Chen D, Philip M, Philip PA, Monga TN. Cardiac pacemaker inhibition by transcutaneous electrical nerve stimulation. Arch Phys Med Rehabil. 1990;71(1):27–30.
21. Keskin EA, Onur O, Keskin HL, Gumus II, Kafali H, Turhan N. Transcutaneous electrical nerve stimulation improves low back pain during pregnancy. Gynecol Obstet Investig. 2012;74(1):76–83.
22. Rathmell JP, Viscomi CM, Ashburn MA. Management of non-obstetric pain during pregnancy and lactation. Anesth Analg. 1997;85(5):1074–87.
23. Ernst E. Acupuncture–a critical analysis. J Intern Med. 2006;259(2):125–37.
24. Rosenquist RW, Vrooman BM. Chronic pain management. In: Morgan and Mikhail's clinical anesthesiology. New York: McGraw Hill Professional; 2013. p. 1.
25. Pomeranz B, Chiu D. Naloxone blockade of acupuncture analgesia: endorphin implicated. Life Sci. 1976;19(11):1757–62.
26. Chapman CR, Benedetti C, Colpitts YH, Gerlach R. Naloxone fails to reverse pain thresholds elevated by acupuncture: acupuncture analgesia reconsidered. Pain. 1983;16(1):13–31.
27. Lembo AJ, Conboy L, Kelley JM, Schnyer RS, McManus CA, Quilty MT, Kerr CE, Drossman D, Jacobson EE, Davis RB, Kaptchuk TJ. A treatment trial of acupuncture in IBS patients. Am J Gastroenterol. 2009;104(6):1489.
28. Manheimer E, Linde K, Lao L, Bouter LM, Berman BM. Meta-analysis: acupuncture for osteoarthritis of the knee. Ann Intern Med. 2007;146(12):868–77.
29. Park J, White A, Stevinson C, Ernst E, James M. Validating a new non-penetrating sham acupuncture device: two randomised controlled trials. Acupunct Med. 2002;20(4):168–74.
30. Kalauokalani D, Cherkin DC, Sherman KJ, Koepsell TD, Deyo RA. Lessons from a trial of acupuncture and massage for low back pain: patient expectations and treatment effects. Spine. 2001;26(13):1418–24.
31. Madsen MV, Gøtzsche PC, Hróbjartsson A. Acupuncture treatment for pain: systematic review of randomised clinical trials with acupuncture, placebo acupuncture, and no acupuncture groups. BMJ. 2009;338:a3115.

32. NCCIH. Acupuncture: in depth. 2018 [online]. Available at: https://nccih.nih.gov/health/acupuncture/introduction [Accessed 17 Mar 2018].

33. Linde K, Witt CM, Streng A, Weidenhammer W, Wagenpfeil S, Brinkhaus B, Willich SN, Melchart D. The impact of patient expectations on outcomes in four randomized controlled trials of acupuncture in patients with chronic pain. Pain. 2007;128(3):264–71.

34. Acupuncture. NIH Consens Statement. 1997;15(5):1–34.

35. World Health Organization. Acupuncture: review and analysis of reports on controlled clinical trials. Geneva: World Health Organization; 2002.

36. White A. A cumulative review of the range and incidence of significant adverse events associated with acupuncture. Acupunct Med. 2004;22(3):122–33.

37. Ekblom A, Hansson P. Extrasegmental transcutaneous electrical nerve stimulation and mechanical vibratory stimulation as compared to placebo for the relief of acute oro-facial pain. Pain. 1985;23(3):223–9.

38. Lundeberg T. Naloxone does not reverse the pain-reducing effect of vibratory stimulation. Acta Anaesthesiol Scand. 1985;29(2):212–6.

39. Smith KC, Comite SL, Balasubramanian S, Carver A, Liu JF. Vibration anesthesia: a noninvasive method of reducing discomfort prior to dermatologic procedures. Dermatol Online J. 2004;10(2)

40. Vibration therapy for pain. Lancet. 1992;339(8808):1513–4.

Work Rehabilitation

Andrew Gitkind and Adeepa Singh

Importance of Early Intervention and Early Return to Work in Reducing Absence

Injury and resulting disability have become an increasing cause of missed work. Musculoskeletal injuries have been shown to be the most likely cause of time lost from work, and of these low back pain is the most prevalent subgroup [1, 2]. Rapid return to work is of benefit to the individual, employer, and society for a variety of socioeconomic reasons. Typically, the longer it takes for one to return to the work force, the lower the probability of return [3].

By 1995 it was estimated that the total cost due to time spent out of work due to injury exceeded $95 billion in the United States, and this number has continued to rise over the last two decades [4]. The three main contributing factors to this sum include lost wages, lost revenue and healthcare costs. In addition to the economic impact of being out of work, there exists extensive research which has examined the effect of being out of work on the worker. Being an active participant of the work force has beneficial effects on overall mental and physical health [5]. The ability to rejoin the work force has multiple positive psychological effects. These include reduced incidence of depression, increased feelings of improved self-worth, a sense of societal contribution and feelings of increased productivity. Remaining out of work can result in feelings of worthlessness and dependence, particularly in an individual who has spent the majority of his/her life as part of the work force. Additionally, there is a clearly demonstrated increase in the incidence of family-related stress issues when a worker has been out for an extended period of time as a result of chronic pain [6].

Psychosocial Factors and Socioeconomic Determinants as Predictors of Prolonged Work Absence

There are many psychosocial factors which can be examined when attempting to differentiate an injured worker who will return to work in a timely fashion, and one who will remain out of work for an extended period. While some of these factors are debated in the literature, most have been shown to have consistent correlations with return to work rates even when accounting for gender, age, and race.

Psychosocial factors that may predict return to work rates can be divided into two main categories: personal and work-related. This can be further subdivided into modifiable and non-modifiable groups. Personal psychosocial factors have strong correlations with poor or delayed return to work rates. Personal psychosocial factors may be either modifiable or non-modifiable. Non-modifiable factors such as gender, age, and race have been closely studied. While there is no correlation with one's race and likelihood of return to work, both gender and age may be predictive. Women have been found to have a worse recovery at 1 year than their male counterparts [7]. This may be due to a difference in responses from their respective support groups, as well as inherent experience of the underlying illness. On the other hand, women return to work more rapidly than their male counterparts after total joint replacement as a cause of disability [8]. Thus, the cause of injury is a factor in gender-related return to work. It should be noted that there are significant disparities in the existing literature, suggesting a lack of consistent evidence to demonstrate the impact of gender on return to work rates. With respect to age and return to work, older groups of workers tend to have lower rates of returning to work, especially after the age of 25 [7].

Many modifiable psychosocial factors have also proven to have a direct impact on the likelihood of return to work following injury. These include one's individualized concerns and expectations, those pertaining to

A. Gitkind (✉)
Department of Rehabilitation Medicine, Montefiore Medical Center, Bronx, NY, USA
e-mail: agitkind@montefiore.org

A. Singh
Montefiore Medical Center, New York, NY, USA

© Springer Nature Switzerland AG 2019
Y. Khelemsky et al. (eds.), *Academic Pain Medicine*, https://doi.org/10.1007/978-3-030-18005-8_25

their employment, as well as interpersonal and familial relationships. An individual's pre-injury job satisfaction is a major indicator of the likelihood of return to work independent of ethnicity or age. The more dissatisfied a worker was prior to injury, the less likely they are to return to work.

Factors that may contribute to increased job dissatisfaction may include poor interpersonal relationships with peers or supervisors, one's perception of being treated fairly or unfairly and the degree of hard or intensive manual labor involved in one's vocation. Those from a lower socioeconomic class typically have more labor-intensive jobs. It can therefore be extrapolated that those with a lower socioeconomic status, who have jobs with increased physical demands and responsibilities, are likely to have lower job satisfaction rates and are therefore less likely to return to work following injury. Conversely, those with higher levels of education and jobs with lower physical demands have a higher rates of returning to work [7, 9].

Familial relationships directly influence the probability of returning to work. Individuals who are the main earners in a family have significantly higher rates of return to work at more rapid rates, as the well-being of their family is directly dependent on their continued wage earning. On the other hand, employees who do not have a strong support network, or those who do not feel they receive the support of their family during the course of their injury and recovery period, have a lower likelihood of returning to work [4, 10].

Finally, one's own health status and interpretation of such also have a direct impact on return to work. In further examining the psychosocial aspects of how one's health relates to the likelihood of returning to work, health-related issues which preexisted the injury as well as health-related concerns directly related to the injury are considered. Individuals who are overweight and in poor overall health have a significantly decreased frequency of returning to work. Similarly, those individuals who have a negative perception of their overall health prior to injury or those perceive a negative change to their well-being occurred as a result of the injury also have a lower likelihood and frequency of returning to work [4, 10, 11].

Patients who seek early intervention and help for the ailment which has caused them to be out of work have shown a higher incidence of an early return to work. On the other hand, those who delay treatment, or who fear pain related to increased activity or treatment of their condition have been shown to have a lower prospect of returning to work. Those who catastrophize pain or other health issues take longer to return to work [9].

Identification and Management of Obstacles to Recovery

Rehabilitative measures such as physical or occupational therapy may be hindered by obstacles that result in diminished patient motivation. Such factors may be related to patient's fear of re-injury and persistent pain after recovery from injury. Pain during rehabilitation can also amplify this fear and result in more guarded attitudes toward therapy.

Depressed mood or anxiety related to rehabilitation tasks or time expected for recovery can also deter one from participation in rehabilitation therapies and ultimately delay recovery. This may be the result of a prolonged duration of disability or inability to perform at a pre-injury level. Anxiety as a result of pain or functional limitation can further decrease motivation and ultimate return to work.

Patients and families play a role in rehabilitation participation and recovery. Unrealistic expectations that arise from patients or their support systems can result in mistrust of medical advice and result in poor clinical outcomes. These include expected return to baseline function prior to injury or complete resolution of pain or disability. Resulting mistrust of therapy can significantly delay time required for recovery and return to work. It has been demonstrated that significant others and spouses that expect substantial or complete resolution of pain after injury contribute to skepticism of treatment and delay return to work [12]. Thus, clear communication regarding anticipated outcomes and possible complications must occur between patient, families and providers.

Components of Successful Comprehensive Rehabilitation Program

The definition of a successful rehabilitation program can vary greatly. When the employer examines a rehabilitation program, success is typically defined by the ability of the employee to return to work at pre-injury work capacity. Loved ones typically consider a program successful when their family member is no longer in pain, happy, and returning to a pre-injury level of function. In the setting where the injured individual was also the breadwinner for the family, success of rehabilitation may be determined by a return to a wage-earning position. The definition of a successful rehabilitation program as it pertains to the patient and their rehabilitation team may often have a predetermined set of goals. At the beginning of a comprehensive program, a reasonable outcome should be agreed upon by the patient and healthcare team. These should include short-, intermediate-, and long-term goals [4, 10, 13].

Multidisciplinary Approaches for Those Who Do Not Return to Work Within a Few Weeks

Work instability or disability is influenced by several factors that include physical limitations, psychosocial factors, and workplace environment. Acknowledging this multidimensional nature of delayed return to work is necessary in developing a program that is effective in reducing disability and promoting return to work.

A multidisciplinary biopsychosocial approach to the treatment of injuries, such as lower back pain, which targets physical, psychological, and social influences on disability and recovery has been noted to result in decreased pain and faster recovery times [14]. Care approaches involving work assessment and adjustment followed by graded activity for patients who have not returned to work after 8 weeks is effective in reducing disability and increasing likelihood to return to work [15].

Disability duration is reduced by employers allowing for accommodations at work, open communication between providers and employers, ergonomic interventions, and the presence and participation of return to work coordinators or case managers. Accommodations, such as work restrictions determined by functional capacity evaluation, may be provided in order to promote return to work. An industrial therapist at the work site may address ergonomic issues, job-specific therapeutic tasks, strengthening, work hardening, pacing, safe work methods, and job modification training.

The transitional work therapy model describes a method of evaluation of the injured worker and work environment and implementation of a plan for return to employment. This starts with job analysis to identify the purpose of the job position and expectations, current environmental conditions, scheduling, safety issues, and work methods. Then, a functional analysis of the worker is performed; this evaluation is described in detail in the next section. Data from a functional capacity evaluation is used to assign job tasks that the worker is able to perform safely. These tasks are also therapeutic and contribute to work hardening for the individual. Accommodation at the place of employment is required when work tasks exceed the worker's capabilities after an injury or illness [16].

Functional Capacity Evaluation

A functional capacity evaluation, also known as a functional assessment, is essential in determining the ability to return to work [17]. It allows for determination of a person's capacity to perform work-related tasks and is an important aspect of the rehabilitation process. It consists of several items related to performance including weight handling and strength, posture and mobility, locomotion, balance and hand coordination [16]. It is an essential part of pre-employment and post-offer screening, determinations based on level of disability, performing goal setting treatment planning for industrial rehabilitation and monitoring progress.

Functional assessments which directly measure work-related functional activities are often utilized for determination of level of disability in individuals with chronic pain or musculoskeletal injuries. These can determine and quantify specific restrictions or tolerances related to work environments and tasks when return to work is being considered.

Key components of a well-conducted and designed job-specific functional assessment include comprehensive medical history, as well as details of the injury. A review of the worker's lifestyle, job demands, and limitations after injury is necessary in order to determine current and expected levels of function. Additionally, diagnostic testing records, physical examination, including active range of motion limitations and functional test results that relate to job specific functions are required. Finally, the worker is monitored during real or simulated job tasks and a summary describing his/her performance is generated (Job Matching) [16].

Limitations to functional assessment include high cost, which is related to lengthy multi-item assessments performed by highly trained professions. Complicating matters further is that these evaluations are often not covered by insurance or reimbursed. Physicians often estimate functional capacity based on a comprehensive evaluation and their experience with chronic pain and musculoskeletal injury [17, 18]. These estimations of functional capacity are valid as long as very specific limitations are not needed. Patient effort is also a limiting factor in these assessments, as maximal effort is required on behalf of the patient in order to be certain that functional capacity evaluations are objective quantifications of function. In order to maintain objectivity, many methods have been applied to eliminate bias including Waddell's signs (Table 25.1), coefficients of variation, and the relationship between heart rate and pain intensity [17, 19–23]. Overall functional capacity evaluations can objectively quantify a patient's function and determine his or her limitations provided that participants provide a conscientious effort.

Table 25.1 Waddell's signs

Tests	Signs
Tenderness	Superficial skin tenderness to light touch over a wide area
	Non-anatomic deep tenderness not localized to one area, is felt over a wide area and extends to the thoracic spine, sacrum or pelvis
Simulation tests	Axial loading pressure on the skull induces lower back pain
	Rotation of the shoulders and pelvis in the same plane induces pain
Distraction	A positive physical finding is demonstrated in the routine manner, this exam is repeated while the patient's attention is distracted. A non-organic component may be present if the finding disappears with distraction.
	Straight leg raise: examiner lifts the patient's foot as when testing plantar reflexes in the seated position, a non-organic component may be present if the leg is lifted higher without pain than when tested in supine position.
Regional disturbances	Dysfunction of motor or sensory functions involving a widespread region of the body in a manner not explained neurologically or anatomically
	Sensory disturbance: diminished sensation fitting a "stocking" distribution rather than a dermatomal pattern
	Weakness: demonstrated by a partial cogwheel "giving away" of muscle groups that cannot be explained on a neurological basis
Overreaction	Disproportionate verbalization, facial expression, muscle tension and tremor, collapsing, or sweating

References

1. Opsahl J, Eriksen HR, Tveito TH. Do expectancies of return to work and Job satisfaction predict actual return to work in workers with long lasting LBP? BMC Musculoskelet Disord. 2016;17(1):481.
2. Hoy D, March L, Brooks P, Blyth F, Woolf A, Bain C, et al. The global burden of low back pain: estimates from the Global Burden of Disease 2010 study. Ann Rheum Dis. 2014;73(6):968–74.
3. Luk KD, Wan TW, Wong YW, Cheung KM, Chan KY, Cheng AC, et al. A multidisciplinary rehabilitation programme for patients with chronic low back pain: a prospective study. J Orthop Surg (Hong Kong). 2010;18(2):131–8.
4. MacKenzie EJ, Morris JA Jr, Jurkovich GJ, Yasui Y, Cushing BM, Burgess AR, et al. Return to work following injury: the role of economic, social, and job-related factors. Am J Public Health. 1998;88(11):1630–7.
5. Plomb-Holmes C, Luthi F, Vuistiner P, Leger B, Hilfiker R. A return-to-work prognostic model for orthopaedic trauma patients (WORRK) updated for use at 3, 12 and 24 months. J Occup Rehabil. 2017;27(4):568–75.
6. Hamer H, Gandhi R, Wong S, Mahomed NN. Predicting return to work following treatment of chronic pain disorder. Occup Med (Lond). 2013;63(4):253–9.
7. Schultz IZ, Law AK, Cruikshank LC. Prediction of occupational disability from psychological and neuropsychological evidence in forensic context. Int J Law Psychiatry. 2016;49(Pt B):183–96.
8. Sankar A, Davis AM, Palaganas MP, Beaton DE, Badley EM, Gignac MA. Return to work and workplace activity limitations following total hip or knee replacement. Osteoarthr Cartil. 2013;21(10):1485–93.
9. Steenstra IA, Munhall C, Irvin E, Oranye N, Passmore S, Van Eerd D, et al. Systematic review of prognostic factors for return to work in workers with sub acute and chronic low back pain. J Occup Rehabil. 2017;27(3):369–81.
10. MacKenzie EJ, Shapiro S, Smith RT, Siegel JH, Moody M, Pitt A. Factors influencing return to work following hospitalization for traumatic injury. Am J Public Health. 1987;77(3):329–34.
11. Bültmann U, Franche R-L, Hogg-Johnson S, Côté P, Lee H, Severin C, et al. Health status, work limitations, and return-to-work trajectories in injured workers with musculoskeletal disorders. Qual Life Res. 2007;16(7):1167–78.
12. McCluskey S, Brooks J, King N, Burton K. Are the treatment expectations of "significant others" psychosocial obstacles to work participation for those with persistent low back pain? Work. 2014;48(3):391–8.
13. Meijer EM, Sluiter JK, Frings-Dresen MHW. Evaluation of effective return-to-work treatment programs for sick-listed patients with non-specific musculoskeletal complaints: a systematic review. Int Arch Occup Environ Health. 2005;78(7):523–32.
14. Marin TJ, Van Eerd D, Irvin E, Couban R, Koes BW, Malmivaara A, et al. Multidisciplinary biopsychosocial rehabilitation for subacute low back pain. Cochrane Database Syst Rev. 2017;6:CD002193.
15. Bieniek S, Bethge M. The reliability of WorkWell Systems Functional Capacity Evaluation: a systematic review. BMC Musculoskelet Disord. 2014;15:106.
16. Basich M, Driscoll T, Wickstrom R. Transitional work therapy on site: work is therapy! Prof Case Manag. 2007;12(6):351–5.
17. Walker WC, Cifu DX, Gardner M, Keyser-Marcus L. Functional assessment in patients with chronic pain: can physicians predict performance? Am J Phys Med Rehabil. 2001;80(3):162–8.
18. Lee GK, Chan CC, Hui-Chan CW. Consistency of performance on the functional capacity assessment: static strength and dynamic endurance. Am J Phys Med Rehabil. 2001;80(3):189–95.
19. Claar RL, Walker LS. Functional assessment of pediatric pain patients: psychometric properties of the functional disability inventory. Pain. 2006;121(1–2):77–84.
20. Cheng AS, Cheng SW. Use of job-specific functional capacity evaluation to predict the return to work of patients with a distal radius fracture. Am J Occup Ther. 2011;65(4):445–52.
21. Fishbain DA, Cole B, Cutler RB, Lewis J, Rosomoff HL, Rosomoff RS. A structured evidence-based review on the meaning of nonorganic physical signs: Waddell signs. Pain Med. 2003;4(2):141–81.
22. Waddell G, McCulloch JA, Kummel E, Venner RM. Nonorganic physical signs in low-back pain. Spine (Phila Pa 1976). 1980;5(2):117–25.
23. Wygant DB, Arbisi PA, Bianchini KJ, Umlauf RL. Waddell nonorganic signs: new evidence suggests somatic amplification among outpatient chronic pain patients. Spine J. 2017;17(4):505–10.

Complementary and Alternative Medicine

Rehan Ali, Jeffrey Ciccone, and Pavan Dalal

Introduction

Complementary and alternative medicine (CAM) generally consists of healthcare practices and products not considered to be conventional medicine. According to The National Cancer Institute, complementary medicine consists of treatments that are used along with standard medical treatments but are not considered to be standard treatments. Alternative medicine consists of treatments that are used in lieu of standard medical treatments. One example of the latter is using a special diet to treat cancer instead of anticancer drugs that are prescribed by an oncologist.

CAM has become an increasingly popular mode of therapy for patients, especially among those who suffer from chronic illness such as malignancy or chronic pain. Often, it's the patient's spiritual, religious, cultural, and other personal beliefs that drive interest in CAM. Despite continued controversy, medical practitioners have become more accepting of treatment regimens that incorporate conventional therapies alongside CAM treatments.

CAM and Pain

While CAM therapies are poorly understood and often dismissed by many clinicians, CAM use is widespread among many patient populations. For example, during the first year of treatment up to 90% of cancer patients integrate CAM into their care plans. Chronic pain, specifically back pain, is the most common reason for complementary and alternative medicine (CAM) use in the United States, and patients with back pain have more office visits to CAM practitioners than to primary care physicians. Little is known about the pattern of CAM use, the reasons for its usage, and the perceived benefit of CAM nationally among patients with back pain.

CAM Therapies and Evidence

There are several categories of therapies sought by patients that fall under the CAM designation. These include alternative medical systems (i.e., traditional Chinese medicine, homeopathy, mind–body interventions, etc.), biologically based therapies (i.e., herbs, foods, vitamins, etc.), and manipulative methods (e.g., osteopathy), to name a few.

Acupuncture

The practice of acupuncture originated in China approximately 2000 years ago. Since then, it has grown to include a wide variety of techniques and practices. The cornerstone of acupuncture practice is to stimulate discreet anatomical points with not just needles, but also pressure (including negative pressure "cupping"), heat, lasers, ultrasonic waves, and electrical stimulation. The purported goal is to harmonize an imbalance in an internal life force energy known as Qi (pronounced "Chee") [1]. Qi energy flows through the body along channels known as meridians which consist of 14 major foci [2]. These are representative of 6 yin and 6 yang organs that organize bilaterally in addition to two more midline meridians, one anterior (conception) and the other posterior (governing). These 14 channels are associated with organs though their location is not related to the anatomic location of said organ (Fig. 26.1).

Along these meridians there are hundreds of points (traditionally 361) where needle insertion can regulate the flow of Qi, thereby treating a designated ailment. Each acupoint is

R. Ali
Icahn School of Medicine, Mount Sinai Department
of Anesthesiology, Division of Pain Medicine, New York, NY, USA

J. Ciccone (✉)
Department of Anesthesiology, Perioperative and Pain Medicine,
Icahn School of Medicine at Mount Sinai Health System,
New York, NY, USA
e-mail: jeffrey.ciccone@mountsinai.org

P. Dalal
Department of Anesthesiology, Perioperative and Pain Medicine,
Mount Sinai Hospital, New York, NY, USA

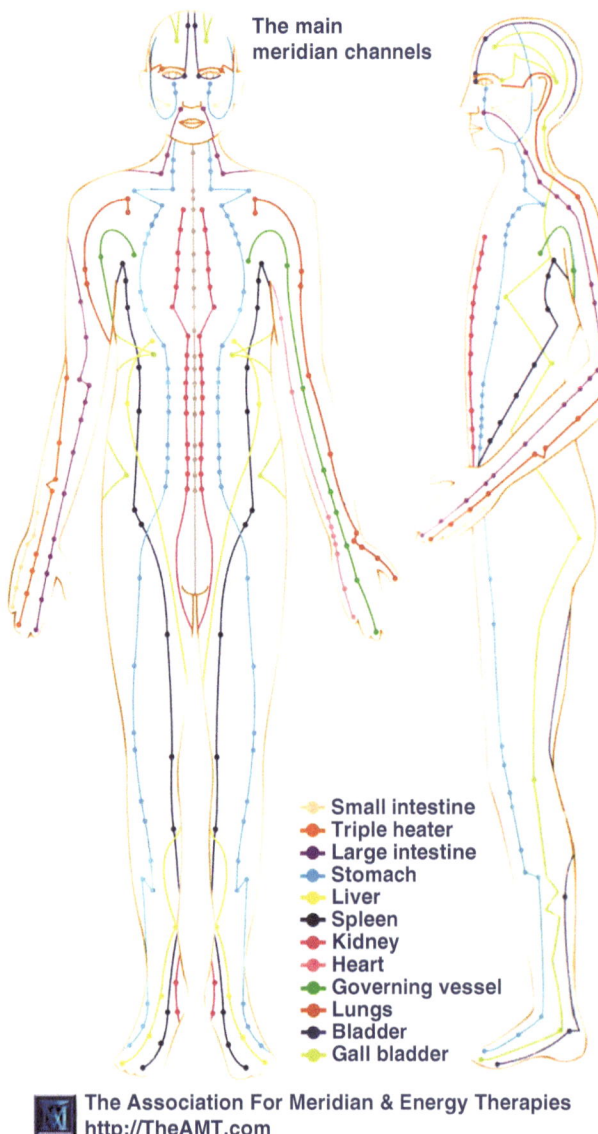

The main
meridian channels

- Small intestine
- Triple heater
- Large intestine
- Stomach
- Liver
- Spleen
- Kidney
- Heart
- Governing vessel
- Lungs
- Bladder
- Gall bladder

The Association For Meridian & Energy Therapies
http://TheAMT.com

Fig. 26.1 The main meridians

designated via its organ designated meridian and an identifying number (i.e., "Liver 43," "Heart 17," etc.).

Since its inception, many more meridians and thousands more acupoints have been added to the practice of acupuncture [3].

Acupuncture has been studied extensively since the 1970s. Since then, thousands of studies have yet to demonstrate definitive conclusions regarding the efficacy of this therapy. There have been almost 500 randomized controlled trials (RCTs), about half of these having a placebo control. Studies with positive results have been for the treatment of nausea and vomiting, dental pain, and fibromyalgia. Meanwhile, studies involving conditions such as lower back pain, general back pain, chronic pain, osteoarthritis, and headache have yielded contradictory and inconclusive results [4]. Despite decades of research, the fact that definitive

evidence regarding the efficacy of acupuncture for a variety of indications remains elusive is in no small part due to the nature of acupuncture practice itself. Difficulties in ascertaining objective outcomes of acupuncture include projection by practitioners of positive treatment outcomes (leading to bias), a significant placebo effect, and heterogeneity of acupuncture practice among practitioners [5].

Despite these limitations, surveys show that acupuncture has the strongest credibility in the medical community of all the complementary medical therapies. Members of the medical community are encouraged by basic science research that supports physiologic mechanisms of therapeutic action.

Many mechanistic theories behind acupuncture have been proposed, including the mediation of inflammatory factors, afferent modulatory neural pathways, endogenous opioid pathways, antinociceptive networks, and higher level cortical modulation of pain perception.

Studies in the 1980s suggested that acupuncture stimulated small diameter nerves that led to spinal cord, brainstem, and hypothalamic triggering of endogenous opioid pathways that led to changes in concentration of these opioids and stress hormones in plasma or CSF [6]. It has been shown that naloxone, a mu receptor antagonist, can reverse acupuncture-mediated analgesia in a dose-dependent manner [7].

Acupuncture has many documented adverse effects. Needle use in acupuncture can result in disease transmission, foreign body entrapment, infection, hematoma, nerve injury, pneumothorax, pneumoperitoneum, and viscus perforation. Acupuncture can also be associated with pain and paresthesia development at the site [8]. Despite the wide range of possible side effects, their rare occurrence makes acupuncture an overwhelmingly safe modality.

Herbal Remedies

Herbal therapies are often sought by patients with chronic pain, particularly back pain, arthritis, headache, and abdominal pain. Many widely used "conventional drugs" today trace their origin to botanical (herbal) usage that predated their chemical isolation. Opium was used in ancient Mediterranean civilizations thousands of years before the isolation of morphine in 1804, and willow and other salicin-rich plants were also used thousands of years before the first NSAIDs were developed in the late nineteenth century. However, unlike the eliminative process of chemical isolation that leads to conventional drug development, the intake of botanical remedies containing various ingredients leads to the activation of an array of pharmacological pathways, thereby compounding the difficulty in studying these therapies. In 2014, a systematic review of randomized trials of herbal therapies in lower back pain found that compared to placebo, topical *Capsicum frutescens* (cayenne) had the

Table 26.1 Examples of botanical/herbal treatment of pain

Herbal remedy	Review/ article	Route	Control arm	Efficacy evidence
Capsicum frutescens (*Cayenne*)	[9]	Topical	Placebo or plaster, homeopathic gel	Strongly positive
Harpagophytum procumbens (*Devil's claw*)	[9]	Oral	Placebo or rofecoxib	Supportive evidence
Salix alba (*White willow bark*)	[9]	Oral	Placebo or rofecoxib	Supportive evidence
Symphytum officinale (*Comfrey root extract*)	[9]	Topical	Placebo or plaster, homeopathic gel	Supportive evidence
Lavender essential oil	[9]	Topical	No treatment	Supportive evidence
Boswellia serrata (*Indian frankincense*)	[10–13]			Equivocal, some studies support OA use

strongest evidence for effectiveness. Other therapies such as oral devil's claw and white willow bark along with topical comfrey root extract and lavender essential oil had some supportive evidence (Table 26.1) [9]. Risks of herbal therapies include lack of stringent monitoring during manufacturing, absence of dose standardization in many preparations, and unforeseen interactions with other supplements or pharmaceuticals.

With regard to pain management, curcumin, commonly known as turmeric, is widely believed to hold anti-inflammatory properties and has been shown to exhibit antioxidant properties [17]. Employed as a supplement, it has been utilized in pain control for various osteoarthritic and other inflammatory disorders of the musculoskeletal system, and for inflammatory bowel disease. Overall quality of evidence is poor, but remains suggestive of a benefit for pain control in these conditions [18]. Common side effects of use include gastrointestinal upset, increased risk of bleeding, increased liver function tests, hypotension, and uterine contraction in pregnancy. Toxicity, and efficacy, is limited due to its poor bioavailability and absorption [19].

St. John's wort, or *hypericum perforatum*, is another commonly used supplement in various pain states and related diseases, specifically mild-to-moderate depression, musculoskeletal pain, dermatologic conditions and gastrointestinal upset. Evidence is limited for these indications. Neuropathic pain states are being considered as potential targets from animal studies [20] and neuraxial-related painful conditions [21]. Reported side effects include gastrointestinal upset, headaches, sensitivity to sunlight, fatigue, dizziness, and sexual dysfunction. Concerning its metabolism, patients should be counseled on its use due to its significant induction of the hepatic P450 system, specifically the CYP3A4 system [22]. Therefore patients maintained on digoxin, warfarin, some oral contraceptives, some HIV inhibitors, immunosuppressants and selective serotonin reuptake inhibitors (SSRIs) must be educated on the potential for reduced efficacy of the medication, or the increased risk of serotonin syndrome with the use of SSRIs [23].

Saw palmetto, also plant derived, has been popularized in benefitting symptoms of benign prostatic hypertrophy and in androgenic alopecia (male and female pattern baldness). Side effects are typically mild and include dizziness, nausea, and headache. Currently the NIH does not support its use for any medical condition based on high quality evidence [24]. Because it may decrease the effects of estrogen in the body, it may reduce the effects of estrogen-containing oral contraceptives. Saw palmetto has also been implicated in increased postoperative bleeding, as a solitary supplement, and with concomitant use of anticoagulation agents [25].

With the advent of increased use of herbal supplements, the interventional pain physician must take appropriate precaution when performing neuraxial procedures. Particularly, increased supplemental use of garlic, ginseng, and gingko biloba has been implicated in higher risk of increased bleeding due to inhibition of platelet aggregation and increased prothrombin time [26]. Garlic, in supplemental doses, may inhibit platelet aggregation irreversibly, and caution is advised with other antiplatelet agents, with up to 7 days before normal platelet function resumes [26]. Ginseng and gingko biloba do not appear to increase surgical or neuraxial bleeding independently, but may pose a possible increased risk when taken in conjunction with other antiplatelet agents, with 36 and 24 hours, respectively, required before return of normal platelet function after discontinuation [26].

Mind–Body and Chronic Pain

Mindfulness meditation is a technique based on ancient Eastern meditation and spiritual practices during which one pays attention to the present moment with openness, curiosity, and acceptance. These techniques have use in managing substance abuse, tobacco cessation, stress reduction, and treatment of chronic pain [14]. The most commonly used mindfulness-based intervention is mindfulness-based stress reduction (MBSR). Key components of the program are sitting meditation, walking meditation, yoga, and a mindfulness practice in which attention is focused on different parts of the body [15].

Spinal Manipulation and Osteopathy

Osteopathic medicine is one of the registered professions legally allowed to practice spinal manipulative therapy (SMT). Spinal manipulative therapy (manual therapy) combines moving joints, massage, exercise, and physical therapy. It is designed to relieve pressure on joints, reduce inflammation, and improve nerve function. In spinal *manipulation*, the practitioner rapidly applies a controlled force, while in spinal *mobilization*, a practitioner uses less force and more stretching. There is a lack of quality clinical trials testing osteopathic/manipulative intervention in adult patients with chronic low back pain, and more data is required. A Cochrane review of SMT in low back pain concluded that despite over 800 publications addressing this issue, evidence for the effect on low back pain is equivocal [16]. Certain types of manipulation of the cervical spine may carry a risk of stroke. Further clinical trials into this subject are required in order to validate the long-term benefit of spinal manipulation for chronic low back pain.

References

1. Birch S, Felt R. Understanding acupuncture. London: Churchill Livingstone; 1999.
2. Kaptchuk TT. Acupuncture: theory, efficacy, and practice. Ann Intern Med. 2002–03;136:374–83.
3. http://www.acos.org/images/meridian-channels.gif.
4. Nahin Richard L, Straus Stephen E. Research into complementary and alternative medicine: problems and potential. BMJ. 2001;322:161.
5. Astin JA, Marie A, Pelletier KR, Hansen E, Haskell WL. A review of the incorporation of complementary and alternative medicine by mainstream physicians. Arch Intern Med. 1998;158(21):2303–10. https://doi.org/10.1001/archinte.158.21.2303.
6. Pomerantz S. Scientific basis of acupuncture. Berlin: Springer-Verlag; 1989.
7. Cheng RSS, Pomeranz BH. Electroacupuncture analgesia is mediated by stereospecific opiate receptors and is reversed by antagonists of type I receptors. Life Sci. 1980;26(8):631–8.
8. Lao L, Hamilton GR, Fu J, Berman BM. Is acupuncture safe? A systematic review of case reports. Altern Ther Health Med. 2003;9(1):72.
9. Oltean H, Robbins C, van Tulder MW, Berman BM, Bombardier C, Gagnier JJ. Herbal medicine for low-back pain. Cochrane Database Syst Rev. 2014;(12):CD004504. https://doi.org/10.1002/14651858. CD004504.pub4.
10. Kimmatkar N, Thawani V, Hingorani L, Khiyani R. Efficacy and tolerability of *Boswellia serrata* extract in treatment of osteoarthritis of knee – a randomized double blind placebo controlled trial. Phytomedicine. 2003;10(1):3–7. https://doi.org/10.1078/094471103321648593.
11. Etzel R. Special extract of *Boswellia serrata* (H 15) in the treatment of rheumatoid arthritis. Phytomedicine. 1996;3:91–4.
12. Sander O, Herborn G, Rau R. Is H15 (resin extract of *Boswellia serrata*, "incense") a useful supplement to established drug therapy of chronic polyarthritis? Results of a double-blind pilot study [in German, English abstract]. Z Rheumatol. 1998;57:11–6.
13. Chopra A, Lavin P, Patwardhan B, Chitre D. Randomized double blind trial of an ayurvedic plant derived formulation for treatment of rheumatoid arthritis. J Rheumatol. 2000;27:1365–72.
14. Hilton L, Hempel S, Ewing B, Apaydin E, et al. Mindfulness meditation for chronic pain: systematic review and meta-analysis. Ann Behav Med. 2017;51:199–213.
15. Bishop SR, Lau M, Shapiro S, Carlson L, Anderson ND, Carmody J, Segal ZV, Abbey S, Speca M, Velting D, Devins G. Mindfulness: a proposed operational definition. Clin Psychol Sci Pract. 2004;11:230–41.
16. Assendelft WJJ, Morton SC, Yu EI, Suttorp MJ, Shekelle PG. Spinal manipulation for low-back pain. Cochrane Database Syst Rev. 2004;(1):CD000447.
17. Srivastava S, Saksena AK, Khattri S, Kumar S, Dagur RS. *Curcuma longa* extract reduces inflammatory and oxidative stress biomarkers in osteoarthritis of knee: a four-month, double-blind, randomized, placebo-controlled trial. Inflammopharmacology. 2016;24(6):377–88.
18. Pagano E, Romano B, Izzo AA, Borrelli F. The clinical efficacy of curcumin-containing nutraceuticals: an overview of systematic reviews. Pharmacol Res. 2018;134:79–91.
19. Prasad S, Tyagi A, Aggarwal B. Recent developments in delivery, bioavailability, absorption and metabolism of curcumin: the golden pigment from golden spice. Cancer Res Treat. 2014;46(1):2–18.
20. Uslusoy F, Nazıroğlu M, Çiğ B. Inhibition of the TRPM2 and TRPV1 channels through *Hypericum perforatum* in sciatic nerve injury-induced rats demonstrates their key role in apoptosis and mitochondrial oxidative stress of sciatic nerve and dorsal root ganglion. Front Physiol. 2017;8:335.
21. Raak C, Scharbrodt W, Berger B, Büssing A, Geißen R, Ostermann T. *Hypericum perforatum* to improve post-operative pain outcome after monosegmental spinal microdiscectomy (HYPOS): a study protocol for a randomised, double-blind, placebo-controlled trial. Trials. 2018;19(1):253.
22. Moore LB, Goodwin B, Jones SA, Wisely GB, Serabjit-Singh CJ, Willson TM, Collins JL, Kliewer SA. St. John's wort induces hepatic drug metabolism through activation of the pregnane X receptor. Proc Natl Acad Sci U S A. 2000;97(13):7500–2.
23. Mannel M. Drug interactions with St John's wort: mechanisms and clinical implications. Drug Saf. 2004;27(11):773–97.
24. https://nccih.nih.gov/health/palmetto/ataglance.htm. Accessed 16 Dec 2017.
25. Wang CZ, Moss J, Yuan CS. Commonly used dietary supplements on coagulation function during surgery. Medicines (Basel). 2015;2(3):157–85.
26. Horlocker TT, Wedel DJ, Rowlingson JC, Kayser Enneking F, Kopp SL, Benzon HT, Brown DL, Heit JA, Mulroy MF, Rosenquist RW, Michael L. Regional anesthesia in the patient receiving antithromboticor thrombolytic therapy American Society of Regional Anesthesia and Pain Medicine evidence-based guidelines (third edition). Reg Anesth Pain Med. 2010;35:64–101.

Acute Pain

Erica B. John, Marc W. Kaufmann, Richard A. Barnhart, Jaime L. Baratta, and Eric S. Schwenk

Introduction

Acute perioperative pain is a complex physiologic response to tissue injury that has significant physical and psychological manifestations. Recent surveys show that in the estimated 51 million surgeries occurring annually in the United States [1], 80% of patients report experiencing acute pain with the majority rating that pain as moderate, severe, or extreme [2]. A better understanding of the epidemiology and pathophysiology of acute pain in recent years has resulted in a focus on multimodal analgesia as a way to improve pain management, speed recovery, and reduce the significant morbidity and mortality that can result from poorly controlled postsurgical pain.

Uncontrolled pain can have many deleterious effects for patients, including the development of deep vein thrombosis, pulmonary embolism, coronary ischemia, myocardial infarction, pneumonia, poor wound healing, insomnia, functional impairments, development of postoperative delirium and the progression to chronic persistent postsurgical pain (CPSP) [3, 4]. Recognizing and treating acute pain is critically important, as up to 50% of patients may develop CPSP [4]. For example, women undergoing breast cancer surgery suffer from chronic persistent postsurgical pain between 20% and 50% of the time [5]. Furthermore, in a study of patients undergoing total knee arthroplasty, up to 42% met criteria for the diagnosis of complex regional pain syndrome at 4 weeks and then 3 months postoperatively [6].

E. B. John
Department of Anesthesiology and Acute Pain Management, Thomas Jefferson University, Philadelphia, PA, USA

M. W. Kaufmann · R. A. Barnhart
Department of Anesthesiology, Thomas Jefferson University Hospital, Philadelphia, PA, USA

J. L. Baratta · E. S. Schwenk (✉)
Sidney Kimmel Medical College, Thomas Jefferson University, Philadelphia, PA, USA
e-mail: Eric.Schwenk@jefferson.edu

Poorly controlled acute pain has multiple effects on a person's well-being, both physiologically and psychologically. Although there is a physiologic role for pain, it triggers a cascade of events involving sympathetic nervous system activation that can be detrimental, particularly in the perioperative setting (Fig. 27.1). Tachycardia and hypertension can lead to myocardial ischemia in susceptible patients with coronary artery disease. Activation of the stress response can cause immunosuppression [7]. This can lead to wound breakdown and increased risk of infection. Additionally, there is a strong mind–body interaction of pain where pain can elicit anxiety, which can then contribute to the conversion of acute to chronic pain [8]. Uncontrolled acute pain is the most common cause of delay in discharge from the Post Anesthesia Care Unit and unanticipated readmissions [9]. Inadequate acute pain management may result in significant increases in health-care costs, decreases in patient satisfaction, and thus hospital reimbursement.

Pharmacologic Approach to Acute Pain

Depending on the type of surgery, acute perioperative pain may manifest as nociceptive, inflammatory, neuropathic pain, or a combination of these types of pain. Nociceptive pain is generally aching, sharp or throbbing, while inflammatory pain may be dull and aching, and neuropathic pain is often burning, tingling, or stabbing. Pain is complex and successful treatment requires targeting multiple levels along the pain pathway in both the peripheral and central nervous systems. Various classes of medications target these receptors and pathways and it is important to fully understand the mechanism of action and type of pain best treated by each type of medication (Table 27.1). For example, one of the most commonly used analgesics, acetaminophen, is thought to act on the central nervous system and possibly prostaglandin synthesis. Nonsteroidal anti-inflammatory medications inhibit cyclooxygenase enzymes 1 and 2 (COX 1 and COX 2), which then inhibit prostaglandin synthesis and ultimately

Fig. 27.1 Depiction of the sympathetic response to uncontrolled acute pain. (Adapted from [71])

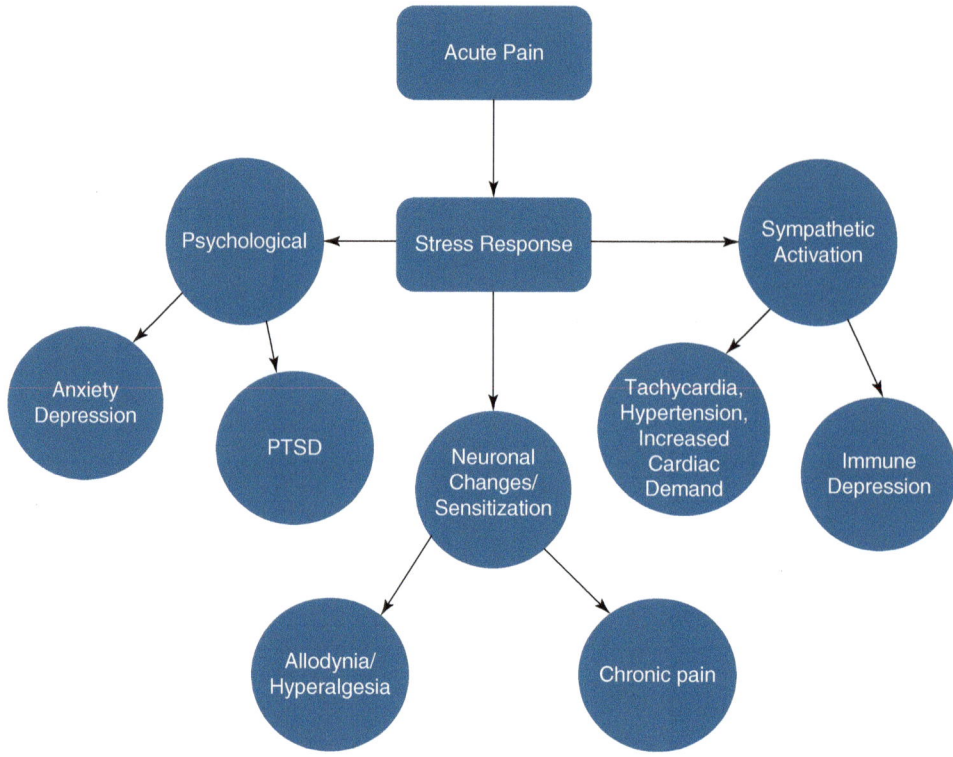

Table 27.1 Summary of medications utilized in the treatment of pain

Drug name or class	Mechanism of action	Routes of administration	Contraindications	Comments
Acetaminophen	Centrally acting analgesic; may inhibit prostaglandin synthesis	IV/PO/PR	Absolute: Hepatic failure Relative: Hepatic insufficiency	Exert caution when combining multiple analgesics containing acetaminophen and keep total daily dose to under 4 g for adults ≥50 kg
Nonsteroidal anti-inflammatory drugs (NSAIDS) (e.g., ibuprofen)	Reversibly inhibits COX 1 and 2, reducing prostaglandin formation; may also decrease neutrophil activity	IM/IV/PO/PR	Absolute: Severe renal disease, peptic ulcer disease Relative: Asthma	Exert caution when combining with other agents that affect coagulation
Local anesthetics (e.g., lidocaine)	Blocks initiation and propagation of nerve impulses by inhibiting sodium channels	IV, perineural, SQ, topical	Absolute: Allergy to local anesthetics (esters much more likely; amides extremely rare)	Cumulative local anesthetic doses should be monitored
NMDA antagonists (e.g., ketamine)	Inhibits NMDA glutamate receptors; may modulate central sensitization	IM, intranasal, IV	Relative: Increased ICP or intraocular pressure, psychiatric disorders	Patients must be monitored for psychomimetic side effects
Mu-opioid agonists (e.g., morphine)	Binds to mu opioid receptors in brain, spinal cord, and peripheral nervous system	IM, IV, PO, transdermal	None	Reduce dose and exert extreme caution in the elderly and patients with obstructive sleep apnea
Gabapentinoids (e.g., gabapentin)	Modulates presynaptic calcium channels	PO	Relative: Suicidal ideation	Can cause sedation in the elderly
Tricyclic antidepressants (e.g., amitriptyline)	Increases synaptic concentration of serotonin and/or norepinephrine by blocking re-uptake	PO	Absolute: Suicidal ideation, seizure disorder, prolonged QT syndrome	Anticholinergic side effects (dry mouth, fatigue, nausea), orthostatic hypotension
Alpha-2-receptor agonists (e.g., clonidine)	Decreases sympathetic outflow; disrupts the transmission of pain signals in spinal cord	IV, PO, transdermal	Absolute: Avoid in pregnancy Relative: Cardiac or cerebrovascular disease, AV block, depression	Watch for bradycardia and administer slowly; rebound hypertension is possible after suddenly stopping
Benzodiazepines (e.g., lorazepam)	Potentiates action of GABA on the GABA1A receptor	IM, IV, PO	Absolute: Narrow-angle glaucoma	Sedation is synergistic with opioids

Adapted from Ref. [72]

Legend: *COX* cyclooxygenase, *GABA* gamma aminobutyric acid, *IM* Intramuscular, *IV* intravenous, *NMDA* N-methyl-D-aspartate, *PO* by mouth, *PR* by rectum, *SQ* subcutaneous

reduce inflammation. Local anesthetics target sodium channels along axons and neurons, inhibiting pain signal propagation. They can be used locally at the site of tissue trauma, along the neuraxis, and at peripheral nerves to target pain perception. Ketamine is an NMDA-receptor antagonist that can be a useful adjunct in managing acute postsurgical pain in the opioid-tolerant patient and has also been used recently to help relieve intractable migraines [10]. Ketamine has been implicated in reducing opioid requirements and resetting opiate receptor sensitivity [74]. Opioids, some of the oldest pain relievers in use, primarily target the mu-opioid receptors and exert their effects both peripherally and centrally. Other medications, such as gabapentinoids, tricyclic antidepressants, alpha 2 agonists, and benzodiazepines, can be used as adjunctive pain relievers with other analgesics to target multiple sites along the pain pathway (Table 27.1).

Perioperative Approach to Acute Pain Management

Perioperative pain management involves taking steps before, during, and after a procedure to reduce or eliminate postoperative pain [11]. The type and cause of acute pain in the perioperative setting can vary widely, and several patient-specific factors can influence the pain management plan including type of surgery, severity of postoperative pain, and pre-existing medical conditions (i.e., significant cardiac or pulmonary disease, psychiatric conditions, allergies, etc.) [11]. In addition to these factors, patient preference and available expertise and resources influence the perioperative pain management plan.

Preoperative Evaluation

Optimal perioperative pain management begins with a preoperative evaluation, which should include a pain history, physical examination, and a preoperative pain control plan [11] Current and past analgesic use including opioids and non-opioids, as well as the character of the pain being treated should be addressed in the preoperative evaluation (Table 27.2). Exact medications taken and their dosages, frequencies, and durations of use should be established. It is important to determine the level of pain experienced following previous surgeries, and which medications or analgesic methods proved successful in the past [12]. Patients taking preoperative opioids should generally continue their opioid regimen up to the time of surgery, and can often maintain this regimen with minimal alterations for most operations [13]. There are situations in which tapering opioids may be appropriate if begun early enough prior to surgery and with consultation with a pain management specialist. Tapering regimens are beyond the scope of this chapter. If patients are taking high doses of opioids, such as greater than 100-mg equivalents of oral morphine daily, adjustments

Table 27.2 Types of pain, characteristics, and treatment

Category	Characteristics	Treatment(s)
Somatic (nociceptive)	Localized Sharp, stabbing, and/or aching Superficial	Opioids Regional anesthesia Acetaminophen NSAIDs Ketamine
Visceral (nociceptive)	Diffuse Deep, dull Often referred to superficial structures	Opioids Regional anesthesia Acetaminophen NSAIDs Ketamine
Neuropathic	Paresthesia (tingling, numbness, burning) Dysesthesia Allodynia	Gabapentinoids (gabapentin, pregabalin) Serotonin-norepinephrine reuptake inhibitors Tricyclic antidepressants Ketamine

should be made through consultation with a pain physician. Non-opioid analgesics should be continued throughout the perioperative period. Some surgeons may request the discontinuation of NSAIDs due to concern for bleeding, although evidence for this practice is questionable [14]. In general, patients should continue analgesics and return to their regular medication regimen following surgery as soon as possible [13]. If the anesthesia provider performing the preoperative evaluation differs from the intraoperative anesthesia team, early communication between these providers is paramount in formulating a plan and identifying potential problems prior to the day of surgery [15].

Multimodal Analgesia

Traditionally, perioperative analgesia has relied heavily on opioids. However, their unfavorable side-effect profile, which ranges from nuisance (pruritus) to potentially fatal (respiratory depression), can increase hospital length of stay and health-care costs [16]. In addition, the opioid epidemic has prompted anesthesiology and pain providers to carefully consider use of these medications during the perioperative period and seek alternatives whenever possible.

Multimodal analgesia is the utilization of several classes of medications (Table 27.1) [11, 12, 21] often via several routes of administration (e.g., enteral, parenteral, regional), to improve analgesia and minimize the side effects of any one class of medication, especially opioids [12]. The technique or combination of techniques chosen for any multimodal plan should take into consideration the type of surgery/procedure and the patient-specific risk-benefit profile. Epidural and/or peripheral nerve blockade should be incorporated into the multimodal analgesic plan whenever possible. Both forms of regional anesthesia provide excellent analgesia and can reduce the amount of systemic analgesics necessary to achieve adequate pain relief.

Epidural Analgesia

Epidural analgesia provides better postoperative pain control [17] and is superior in reducing the surgical stress response to pain compared to opioids [18]. By reducing pain and the physiologic stress response to pain, epidural analgesia can speed recovery, decrease postoperative complications such as pulmonary embolism, deep vein thrombosis, and myocardial infarction, and improve patient satisfaction [17]. The benefits from epidural blockade depend on appropriate placement of the epidural catheter to provide anesthesia to the dermatomes affected by the surgical site [12]. Thoracic epidurals are appropriate for thoracic and upper abdominal surgeries, while lumbar epidurals are better suited for low abdominal, pelvic, and lower extremity surgeries. Epidural anesthesia has been shown to provide superior analgesia compared to parenteral opioids following thoracic surgery [19, 20], intra-abdominal surgery [20, 22, 23], and breast surgery with tissue flap reconstruction [24].

Peripheral Nerve Blocks

Similar to epidural analgesia, peripheral nerve blocks provide superior pain relief compared to systemic opioids [25], improve rehabilitation, and can reduce surgical stress [12]. Superficial peripheral nerve blocks are an optimal choice for patients undergoing surgery on the extremities, and are a viable option for patients who cannot receive neuraxial anesthesia due to anticoagulation. Peripheral nerve blockade can be the sole anesthetic or can be combined with monitored anesthesia care for less-invasive procedures (i.e., arteriovenous fistula surgery, minor foot or hand surgery, etc.). For more invasive procedures (i.e., surgery on major joints, repair of fractured long bones, etc.), peripheral nerve blocks can be an adjunct to general or neuraxial anesthesia with the goal of improving postoperative analgesia. Peripheral nerve blocks for orthopedic procedures have been shown to hasten same-day recovery and decrease hospital readmission compared to general anesthesia [26]. Furthermore, continuous peripheral nerve blocks provide superior analgesia, and reduce both opioid consumption and opioid-related adverse effects [27]. The management of continuous peripheral nerve blocks both in the hospital and ambulatory settings should include verbal and written instructions regarding infusion pump details, analgesic expectations, catheter site care, limb and fall precautions, breakthrough pain instructions, and signs of local anesthetic toxicity. Furthermore, patients should have 24-hour contact information for an anesthesia provider for emergencies and questions [15].

The perioperative pain management team, which may include both an intraoperative anesthesia team as well as an acute pain service, should educate both the patient and family on the expected level of postoperative pain, methods of evaluating pain, and the proper use of the designated analgesic method(s) (i.e., patient-controlled analgesia (PCA), patient-controlled epidural analgesia (PCEA), etc.) [11]. Patients provided with information regarding expected level and duration of pain often report less pain, require fewer analgesics, and have a shortened length of hospital stay [21].

Non-pharmacologic Treatment

The goal of any pain management plan should be to provide the most effective analgesia with as few risks and side effects as possible [12]. Adding non-pharmacologic techniques to a multimodal analgesic regimen can further reduce the total pharmacologic burden and associated side effects. Non-pharmacologic treatment of pain can be divided into cognitive-behavioral interventions or physical interventions (Table 27.3) [11, 12].

Cognitive-Behavioral Interventions

The goal of cognitive-behavioral interventions is to change patients' perception of pain, influence the reaction to pain, and create a sense of situational control [28]. Before the advent of pharmacologic-based anesthesia, hypnosis, mental imagery, and relaxation techniques were utilized to assist in surgical procedures [12]. Relaxation techniques can decrease anxiety prior to surgery, improve patient comfort, and decrease pharmacologic analgesic requirements [28]. Hypnosis has been shown to reduce the amount of pharmacologic analgesics needed during radiologic procedures [28]. In a three-day postoperative period after orthopedic hand surgery, patients receiving hypnosis experienced improved analgesia [29]. Relaxation strategies and guided imagery are simple techniques that can be taught in minutes by almost any provider, while others like hypnosis and biofeedback may require professional involvement. Therefore, utilization of these techniques may be limited by availability of resources.

Table 27.3 Non-pharmacologic treatment of pain

Cognitive behavioral interventions	Physical interventions
Imagery	Topical (heat/cold)
Preparatory information	Exercise
Relaxation training	Electroanalgesia (TENS and PENS therapy)
Distraction	
Hypnosis	Acupuncture
Biofeedback	

Physical Interventions

Physical interventions are designed to affect the transmission of pain signals and pathways, positively alter the physiologic response to pain, and decrease anxiety surrounding pain-related physical limitations or disabilities [21]. Acupuncture gained popularity in Western countries in the mid-twentieth century and has since been endorsed by the Food and Drug Administration, National Institutes of Health, and World Health Organization as a treatment for many medical problems, including the treatment of acute and chronic pain [12]. Acupuncture is based on the principle that energy flows through the human body via pathways called meridians. Needles are inserted at various points between these meridians creating an afferent stimulus, which in turn restores energy flow and alleviates symptoms [12]. Several studies investigating acupuncture's effectiveness in postoperative analgesia have found that while patient-reported pain scores are no different, analgesic medication consumption is significantly reduced in the acupuncture group compared to controls [30, 31]. Transcutaneous electrical nerve stimulation (TENS) and percutaneous electrical nerve stimulation (PENS) work similarly to acupuncture; however, with these modalities, the stimulus is an electrical current [12]. Many studies have shown decreased pharmacologic analgesic requirements [32, 33], as well as increased time to analgesic request in the postoperative setting, with the use of TENS [34]. TENS and PENS are used widely in treating chronic pain, but have not yet been used widely in the treatment of postoperative pain.

Given the relatively safe side-effect profile of these modalities, they may be tried with relatively low risk. The availability of experienced personnel and resources limits their use. Future efforts may provide additional data regarding the efficacy of these techniques, especially compared to established pharmacologic techniques.

Tools for Assessment and Measurement of Pain

In order to effectively devise an analgesic regimen for acute perioperative pain, it is imperative to accurately identify the type and assess the level of pain. Although no ideal tool exists to measure pain, a thorough history combined with existing, validated tools can help guide the treatment plan. Pain is multifactorial and in order to treat it effectively it not only has to be quantified, but its quality must also be assessed (e.g., nociceptive, neuropathic, visceral). Other important details include location, intensity, character, aggravating or relieving factors, response to current therapy, pre-existing level of chronic pain, and prior opioid and non-opioid usage. In order to properly assess the level of postoperative pain,

several validated tools of measurement can be used to measure pain intensity. The following is a brief review of some commonly used pain scales, but is by no means an exhaustive list, as many other instruments exist for evaluation of pain.

The visual analogue scale (VAS) is a simple method used to measure variations in pain intensity [35]. Patients are instructed to place a mark along a 100-mm line labeled with no pain on one end and worst pain possible on the other. This scale is easy to understand for patients and is useful for comparing pain scores during a hospital stay and before and after therapy. It can, however, be more difficult for patients to use with cognitive impairments, children, and in the immediate postoperative period while patients are sedated and still recovering from anesthesia.

The 11-point numeric rating scale (NRS) is equally sensitive to the VAS [36]. This scale involves patients rating their pain on a scale of 0–10, with 10 being the worst possible pain. This scale is perhaps the easiest to use and understand for both patients and providers and is the most commonly used pain scale in clinical practice. This scale does not need clear vision, dexterity, or paper and pen.

The four-point verbal categorical scale (VRS) uses a scale of 0–3 with 0 indicating no pain, 1 mild pain, 2 moderate pain, and 3 severe pain. This scale is less accurate and underestimates pain compared to the VAS. Thus, it should only be used as a coarse screening tool [37].

The Wong-Baker FACES Scale consists of pain scores 0–5 that each correspond to a facial expression drawing. This scale allows patients who cannot express their pain as a number to quantify it as an emotion and is the preferred pain scale in patients ages 3–18 [38].

Due to their subjective nature, these tools cannot be used alone to guide adjustments to analgesic regimens. Along with a thorough history and physical to determine the quality and intensity of the current pain, these validated assessment tools combined with hemodynamic parameters, functional status, physical therapy milestones, and ability to eat, sleep, and perform activities of daily living can help you make a reliable assessment of patient's pain and further guide treatment (Table 27.4).

Role of Patient and Family Education

Postoperative pain that is poorly controlled is a significant source of patient dissatisfaction with economic implications, such as extended lengths of stay and readmissions [39, 40]. Postoperative pain is an individual experience, with multiple factors playing a role. Besides the physical aspect of the surgery, patient's emotional, psychological, and behavioral states can play a role in postoperative pain management. Several studies examining pre-surgical pain scores found

Table 27.4 Commonly used pain scales

Pain scale	Description				Strengths	Weaknesses
VAS [35]	No pain ——————— Worst pain				Allows comparison of pain scores during hospital stay and before and after treatment. Validated for research.	Difficult to understand in the cognitively impaired, children, and immediately postop.
NRS [36]	0- Pain: No	1-2-3- Mild	-4-5-6- Moderate	-7-8-9-10 Severe	Easy to use, understand, and perform.	Difficult to use in pediatrics and cognitively impaired.
VRS [37]	0 No pain	1 Mild pain	2 Moderate pain	3 Severe pain	Coarse screening tool.	Less accurate, underestimates pain compared to VAS.
Wong-Baker FACES [75]	0 1 2 3 4 5				Good for children and non-verbal patients.	Tendency to select faces at extremes of scale [73].

that higher expectations of pain prior to surgery predicted higher pain scores and lower functional status postoperatively [41, 42]. Patients with more positive expectations for pain control and outcome following total knee arthroplasty (TKA) experienced greater pain relief and functional status compared to those with more negative expectations [43, 44]. It is therefore imperative during pre-anesthetic evaluation to ascertain patient expectations, especially in those with a history of chronic pain who are at risk for more significant challenges in the postoperative period. It is also important to prepare patients for the pain that they will experience and educate them regarding which analgesic modalities will be available. Equally important is educating patients and their families regarding their roles in achieving comfort, reporting pain, and the proper usage of patient-controlled analgesics [11]. For example, if a patient receives a continuous nerve block, the patient as well as the family should be aware that the density of the primary block will wane and some pain is to be expected with primary block resolution. This can prevent unnecessary concern and help prepare the patient and family to address and treat postoperative pain in a timely manner.

Treatment of Acute Nonsurgical Pain

The role of acute pain specialists expands beyond the prevention and management of acute postsurgical pain. Several patient populations may present with acute episodes of pain that can be very challenging for primary care teams to handle, such as sickle cell crises, burn victims requiring multiple dressing changes, migraine headaches, and phantom limb pain. These patient populations are challenging due to

baseline chronic pain and ongoing opioid therapy. During acute flares of nonsurgical pain, these patients must first be evaluated for a medical cause of the pain before concluding the cause is an acute on chronic flare.

Sickle cell anemia is an autosomal recessive disease characterized by large amounts of hemoglobin S, resulting in the sickling of red blood cells [45]. Due to the decreased ability to conform to the small diameter of the microcirculation, sickled red blood cells cause occlusion and resulting ischemic necrosis [46]. This occlusion is thought to be responsible for the vaso-occlusive crisis (VOC) that leads to significant pain experienced by these patients. VOCs can be precipitated by certain conditions such as infections, cold, hypovolemia, hypoxia, and stress. The pain is thought to be the result of both the infarction secondary to the occlusion, as well as the inflammatory mediators released in response [47, 48]. Due to the recurrent nature of these painful episodes and the development of chronic pain, many of these patients are maintained on chronic opioid therapy, which makes controlling acute exacerbations more difficult.

Management of these patients should begin with addressing the factors inciting the VOC, including optimization of oxygenation and hydration. Similar to the initial management of pain from most etiologies, treatment should begin with utilizing a comprehensive multimodal analgesic regimen when appropriate. Severe VOC pain can be managed with opioids via several routes. Patient-controlled analgesia (PCA) allows patients to administer their own analgesic, giving them a sense of control and providing relief when needed. This may decrease the overall opioid requirements, as well [49]. The majority of sickle cell patients experiencing a VOC require larger doses of opioids compared to the general population. This is due not only to the extreme pain experienced by these patients, but increased renal clearance, hepatic metabolism, as well as opioid tolerance [50]. In addition, regional techniques can be employed in this population. Epidural analgesia has been used with success, reducing pain, as well as improving oxygenation in pediatric patients presenting with acute chest syndrome [51]. Ketamine, an NMDA-receptor antagonist, has been shown to modulate opioid tolerance and opioid-induced hyperalgesia [52]. At low doses, ketamine serves as a safe adjunct to opioid analgesia in patients with sickle cell disease. Several case series have shown an improvement in pain and a significant reduction in opioid consumption in this group of patients [53–55].

Burn victims present with pain due to the injury, typically consisting of both nociceptive and neuropathic components, as well as the pain experienced with frequent dressing changes [56]. Pain from burns is primarily treated with acetaminophen, NSAIDs, opioids, and ketamine. Morphine via intravenous patient-controlled analgesia pumps, IV-PCA, has been shown to be effective in the adult, as well as pediatric burn population, with its pharmacokinetics remaining unchanged [57–59]. Gabapentinoids are effective at treating neuropathic pain and can reduce pain ratings and opioid consumption [60, 61]. Ketamine is a useful adjunct that provides analgesia, reduces opioid consumption, and may prevent hyperalgesia. Ketamine also serves as an effective adjunct during dressing changes [62]. Regional anesthesia is beneficial in providing intraoperative anesthesia, improving postoperative analgesia, and facilitating rehabilitation [63]. Techniques such as fascia iliaca and saphenous nerve blocks have been shown to reduce pain at graft donor sites, reduce late post-burn primary and secondary hyperalgesia. Indwelling catheters are effective when bolused during dressing changes [64, 65].

Phantom limb pain occurs in the area of a missing body part after amputation. It affects up to 80% of people who undergo limb amputation and is due to a combination of CNS, PNS, and psychological mechanisms [66]. Epidural analgesia started 48 hours prior to surgery and continued 48 hours postoperatively has been shown to reduce phantom pain intensity, prevalence, and frequency 6 months after amputation [67]. Morphine, gabapentin, and ketamine have demonstrated favorable short-term analgesic efficacy for treatment of phantom pain [68]. Peripheral nerve blockade, though effective for postoperative pain, has shown inconsistent results in preventing phantom pain [69, 70].

Conclusion

Acute pain is a complex process that if left untreated can have detrimental effects resulting in significant morbidity and mortality. A thorough understanding of the different types of pain, the tools for assessment, available pharmacologic and non-pharmacologic methods of treatment are necessary in order to develop a multimodal analgesic regimen and effectively treat acute pain whether in the perioperative setting or resulting from nonsurgical causes.

References

1. Fast stats. National Center for Health Statistics, Atlanta. 2010. http://www.cdc.gov/nchs/data/nhds/4procedures/2010pro4_numberprocedureage.pdf. Accessed 20 Dec 2016.
2. Apfelbaum JL, Chen C, Mehta SS, Gan TJ. Postoperative pain experience: results from a national survey suggest postoperative pain continues to be undermanaged. Anesth Analg. 2003;97(2):534–40.
3. Breivik H. Postoperative pain management: why is it difficult to show that it improves outcome? Eur J Anaesthesiol. 1998;15:748–51.
4. Kehlet H, Jensen TS, Woolf CJ. Persistent postsurgical pain: risk factors and prevention. Lancet. 2006;367:1618–25.
5. Wallace MS, Wallace AM, Lee J, Dobke MK. Pain after breast surgery: a survey of 282 women. Pain. 1996;66:195–205.
6. Stanos SP, Harden RH, Wagner-Raphael R, et al. A prospective clinical model for the development of CRPS. In: Harden RN, Baron R, Jianig W, editors. Complex regional pain syndrome, progress in pain research and management. Seattle: IASP Press; 2001. p. 151–64.
7. Weissman C. The metabolic response to stress: an overview and update. Anesthesiology. 1990;73:308–27.
8. Theunissen M, Peters ML, Bruce J, et al. Preoperative anxiety and catastrophizing: a systemic review and meta-analysis of the association with chronic postsurgical pain. Clin J Pain. 2012;28:819–41.
9. Pavlin DJ, Chen C, Penaloza DA, et al. Pain as a factor complicating recovery and discharge after ambulatory surgery. Anesth Analg. 2002;95:627–34.
10. Pomeroy JL, Marmura MJ, Nahas SJ, Viscusi ER. Ketamine infusions for treatment refractory headache. Headache. 2016;57(2):276–82.
11. Carr DB. Practice guidelines for acute pain management in the perioperative setting. Anesthesiology. 2012;116(2):248–73.
12. Sinatra RS, De Leon-Casasola OA, Ginsberg B, Viscusi E. Acute pain management. Cambridge: Cambridge University Press; 2009.
13. Viscusi ER, Pappagallo M. A review of opioids for in-hospital pain management. Hosp Pract. 2012;40:149–59.
14. White PF, Recart A, Issioui T, et al. The efficacy of celecoxib premedication on postoperative pain and recovery times after ambulatory surgery: a dose ranging study. Anesth Analg. 2003;96:1631–5.
15. Schwenk ES, Baratta JL, Gandhi K, Viscusi ER. Setting up an acute pain management service. Anesthesiol Clin. 2014;32(4):893–910.
16. Wheeler M, Oderda GM, Ashburn MA, Lipman AG. Adverse events associated with postoperative analgesia: a systematic review. Clin J Pain. 2002;3:159–80.
17. Block BM, Liu SS, Rowlington AJ, Cowan AR, Cowan JA, Wu CL. Efficacy of postoperative epidural analgesia: a meta-analysis. JAMA. 2003;290:2455–63.
18. Adams HA, Saatweber P, Schmitz CS, Hecker H. Postoperative pain management in orthopedic patients: no differences in pain score, but improved stress control by epidural anaesthesia. Eur J Anaesthesiol. 2002;19:658–65.
19. Flisberg P, Tornebrandt K, Walther B, Lundberg J. Pain relief after esophagectomy: thoracic epidural analgesia is better than parenteral opioids. J Cardiothorac Vasc Anesth. 2001;15(3):282–7.
20. Wu CL, Cohen SR, Richman JM, et al. Efficacy of postoperative patient-controlled and continuous infusion epidural analge-

sia versus intravenous patient-controlled analgesia with opioids. Anesthesiology. 2005;103:1079–88.

21. Carr DB, Jacox AD. Acute pain management: operative or medical procedures and trauma. Rockville: U.S. Dept. of Health and Human Services, Public Health Service, Agency for Health Care Policy and Research; 1992.

22. Carlie F, Trudel JL, Belliveau P. The effect of intraoperative thoracic epidural anesthesia and postoperative analgesia on bowel function after colorectal surgery. Dis Colon Rectum. 2001;44:1083–9.

23. Werawatganon T, Charuluxananan S. Patient controlled intravenous opioid analgesia versus continuous epidural analgesia for pain after intra-abdominal surgery. Cochrane Database Syst Rev. 2005;(1):CD004088.

24. Correll DJ, Viscusi ER, Grunwald Z, Moore JH. Epidural analgesia compared with intravenous morphine patient-controlled analgesia: postoperative outcome measures after mastectomy with immediate TRAM flap breast reconstruction. Reg Anesth Pain Med. 2001;26(5):444–9.

25. Capdevilla X, Barthelet Y, Biboulet P, et al. Effects of perioperative analgesic technique on the surgical outcome and duration of rehabilitation after major knee surgery. Anesthesiology. 1999;91:8–15.

26. Chelly JE, Ben-David B, Williams BA, Kentor ML. Anesthesia and postoperative analgesia: outcomes following orthopedic surgery. Orthopedics. 2003;26:S865–71.

27. Richman JM, Liu SS, Courpas G, et al. Does continuous peripheral nerve block provide superior pain control to opioids? A meta-analysis. Anesth Analg. 2006;102:248–57.

28. Lang EV, Benotsch EG, Fick LJ, et al. Adjunctive non-pharmacological analgesia for invasive medical procedures: a randomised trial. Lancet. 2000;355:1486–90.

29. Mauer MH, Burnett KF, Oullette EA, Ironson GH, Dandes HM. Medical hypnosis and orthopedic hand surgery: pain perception, postoperative recovery, and therapeutic comfort. Int J Clin Exp Hypn. 1999;47:144–61.

30. Lao L, Bergman S, Hamilton GR, Langebnberg P, Berman B. Evaluation of acupuncture for pain control after oral surgery: a placebo-controlled trial. Arch Otolaryngol Head Neck Surg. 1999;125:567–72.

31. Usichenko TI, Lysenyuk VP, Groth MH, Pavlovic D. Detection of ear acupuncture points by measuring the electrical skin resistance in patients before, during and after orthopedic surgery performed under general anesthesia. Acupunct Electrother Res. 2003;28:167–73.

32. Lin JG, Lo MW, Wen YR, et al. The effect of high and low frequency electroacupuncture in pain after lower abdominal surgery. Pain. 2002;99:509–14.

33. Hamza MA, White PF, Ahmed HE, Ghoname EA. Effect of the frequency of transcutaneous electrical nerve stimulation on the postoperative opioid analgesic requirement and recovery profile. Anesthesiology. 1999;91:1232–8.

34. Benedetti F, Amanzio M, Casadio C, et al. Control of postoperative pain by transcutaneous electrical nerve stimulation after thoracic operations. Ann Thorac Surg. 1997;63:773–6.

35. Chapman CR, Case KL, Dubner R, et al. Pain measurement: an overview. Pain. 1985;22:1–31.

36. Breivik EK, Bjornsson GA, Skovlund E. A comparison of pain rating scales by sampling from clinical trial data. Clin J Pain. 2000;16:22–8.

37. Breivik EK, Borchgrevink PC, Allen SM, et al. Assessment of pain. Br J Anaesth. 2008;101(1):17–24.

38. Wong D, Baker C. Pain in children: comparison of assessment scales. Pediatr Nurs. 1988;14(1):9–17.

39. Gan TJ, Habib AS, Miller TE, White W, Apfelbaum JL. Incidence, patient satisfaction, and perceptions of post-surgical pain: results from a US national survey. Curr Med Res Opin. 2014;30:49–160.

40. Twersky R, Fishman D, Homel P. What happens after discharge? return hospital visits after ambulatory surgery. Anesth Analg. 1997;84:319–24.

41. Brander V, Gondek S, Martin E, Stulberg SD. Pain and depression influence outcome 5 years after knee replacement surgery. Clin Orthop Relat Res. 2007;464:21–6.

42. Brander VA, Stulberg SD, Adams AD, et al. Predicting total knee replacement pain: a prospective, observational study. Clin Orthop Relat Res. 2003;416:27–36.

43. Gandhi R, Davey JR, Mahomed N. Patient expectations predict greater pain relief with joint arthroplasty. J Arthroplast. 2009;24:716–21.

44. Mahomed NN, Liang MH, Cook EF, et al. The importance of patient expectations in predicting functional outcomes after total joint arthroplasty. J Rheumatol. 2002;29:1273–9.

45. Kato GJ, Gladwin MT, Steinberg MH. Deconstructing sickle cell disease: reappraisal of the role of hemolysis in the development of clinical subphenotypes. Blood Rev. 2007;21:37–47.

46. Nagel RL, Fabry ME, Billett HH, et al. Sickle cell painful crisis: a multifactorial event. Prog Clin Biol Res. 1987;240:361–80.

47. Chiang EY, Frenette PS. Sickle cell vasco-occlusion. Hematol Oncol Clin North Am. 2005;19:771–884.

48. Kim SK, Miller JH. Natural history and distribution of bone and bone marrow infarction in sickle cell hemoglobinopathies. J Nucl Med. 2002;43:896–900.

49. Shapiro BS, Cohen DE, Howe CJ. Patient-controlled analgesia for sickle cell related pain. J Pain Symptom Manag. 1993;8:22–8.

50. Dunlop RJ, Bennet KC. Pain management for sickle cell disease. Cochrane Database Syst Rev. 2006;2:CD003350.

51. Yaster M, Tobin JR, Billett C, Casella JF, Dover G. Epidural analgesia in the management of severe vaso-occlusive sickle cell crisis. Pediatrics. 1994;93:310–5.

52. Visser E, Schug SA. The role of ketamine in pain management. Biomed Pharmacother. 2006;60(7):341–8.

53. Jennings CA, Bobb BT, Noreika DM, Coyne PJ. Oral ketamine for sickle cell crisis pain refractory to opioids. J Pain Palliat Care Pharmacother. 2013;27(2):150–4.

54. Meals CG, Mullican BD, Shaffer CM, Dangerfield PF, Ramirez RP. Ketamine infusion for sickle cell crisis pain in an adult. J Pain Symptom Manag. 2011;42(3):e7–9.

55. Tawfic QA, Faris AS, Kausalya R. The role of a low-dose ketamine-midazolam regimen in the management of severe painful crisis in patients with sickle cell disease. J Pain Symptom Manag. 2014;47(2):334–40.

56. Gray P. Acute neuropathic pain: diagnosis and treatment. Curr Opin Anaesthesiol. 2008;21(5):590–5.

57. Choiniere M, Grenier R, Paquette C. Patient-controlled analgesia: a double-blind study in burn patients. Anaesthesia. 1992;47(6):467–72.

58. Gaukroger PB, Chapman MJ, Davey RB. Pain control in paediatric burns—the use of patient-controlled analgesia. Burns. 1991;17(5):396–9.

59. Perreault S, Choiniere M, du Souich PB, et al. Pharmacokinetics of morphine and its glucuronidated metabolites in burn injuries. Ann Pharmacother. 2001;35(12):1588–92.

60. Cuignet O, Pirson J, Soudon O, et al. Effects of gabapentin on morphine consumption and pain in severely burned patients. Burns. 2007;33(1):81–6.

61. Wong L, Turner L. Treatment of post-burn neuropathic pain: evaluation of pregablin. Burns. 2010;36(6):769–72.

62. McGuinness SK, Wasiak J, Cleland H, et al. A systematic review of ketamine as an analgesic agent in adult burn injuries. Pain Med. 2011;12(10):1551–8.

63. Bittner EA, Shank E, Woodson L, Martyn JA. Acute and perioperative care of the burn-injured patient. Anesthesiology. 2015;122:448–64.

64. Cuignet O, Mbuyamba J, Pirson J. The long-term analgesic efficacy of a single-shot fascia iliaca compartment block in burn patients undergoing skin-grafting procedures. J Burn Care Rehabil. 2005;26(5):409–15.

65. Pedersen JL, Crawford ME, Dahl JB, et al. Effect of preemptive nerve block on inflammation and hyperalgesia after human thermal injury. Anesthesiology. 1996;84(5):1020–6.

66. Flor H. Phantom-limb pain: characteristics, causes, and treatment. Lancet Neurol. 2002;1:182–9.

67. Karanikolas M, Aretha D, Tsolakis I, et al. Optimized perioperative analgesia reduces chronic phantom limb pain intensity, prevalence, and frequency: a prospective, randomized, clinical trial. Anesthesiology. 2011;114(5):1144–54.

68. Alviar MJM, Hale T, Dungca M. Pharmacologic interventions for treating phantom limb pain. Cochrane Database Syst Rev. 2016;10:CD006380.

69. Borghi B, D'Addabbo M, White PF, et al. The use of prolonged peripheral neural blockade after lower extremity amputation: the effect on symptoms associated with phantom limb syndrome. Anesth Analg. 2010;111(5):1308–15.

70. Halbert J, Crotty M, Cameron ID. Evidence for the optimal management of acute and chronic phantom pain: a systematic review. Clin J Pain. 2002;18(2):84–92.

71. Roberts D, Aldington D. Why pain relief is important: the physiologic response. In: Combat anesthesia: the first 24 hours. Washington DC: Department of the Army; 2015. p. 201.

72. Lexicomp Online®, Lexi-Drugs®. Hudson: Lexi-Comp, Inc.; cited December 27, 2016. Available from: http://online.lexi.com.

73. Stein P. Indices of pain intensity: construct validity among preschoolers. Pediatr Nurs. 1995;21(2):119–23.

74. Subramaniam K, Subramanium B, Steinbrook R. Ketamine as adjuvant analgesic to opioids: a quantitative and qualitative systemic review. Anesth Analg. 2004;99:482–95.

75. Wong DL, Hockenberry MJ, Wilson D. Wong's nursing care of infants and children. St. Louis: Mosby/Elsevier; 2011.

Cancer Pain

Jonathan Silverman and Amitabh Gulati

Introduction

Cancer pain is thought to affect 17 million people worldwide [1]. Frequently the presenting symptom of malignancy, pain can affect patients at all stages of disease and typically gets worse with disease progression. Moderate-to-severe pain is estimated to affect as many as 90% of patients with metastatic or advanced disease [2]. Therapies aimed at decreasing tumor burden can be effective but are associated with significant morbidity. Moreover, one third of patients report ongoing pain following curative treatment [3]. Pain is inadequately controlled in 43% of cancer patients, a statistic which has remained stable over the last four decades despite increased attention being paid to cancer pain management [4].

This highlights the multiple barriers that exist to providing effective cancer pain palliation. With cancer treatments becoming more accessible, oncologic care is moving out of large regional centers into smaller, local hospital systems with limited resources to dedicate to robust multidisciplinary pain management teams. The increasing cost of oncologic care, combined with the adoption of value-based healthcare reimbursement models, ensures ongoing emphasis on resource allocation [5]. Traditional management approaches have come under increased scrutiny and regulation due, in large part, to data derived from non-oncologic populations. Ongoing research efforts are required to overcome these barriers. Until new treatment paradigms can be elucidated, management approaches must be extrapolated from existing literature. The prolonged life expectancy afforded by improved cancer treatment has also added the challenge of sustainability to the development of cancer pain treatment algorithms. To meet these challenges, creation and implementation of cost-effective, evidence-based pain management strategies is necessary.

Palliative Care

The term palliative care was coined in the 1970s to subjugate negative connotations of the word "hospice" in French culture, but also highlighted efforts to make available these services to patients at all stages of terminal illness. Through the 1990s, palliative care further integrated into mainstream medicine and the American Board of Medical Specialties first recognized it as a subspecialty in 2006 [6]. Today, palliative care practitioners not only serve as experts in symptom management at all stages of life-limiting illness but also have an integral role in the management of cancer pain.

Comprehensive Evaluation of Patients with Cancer Pain

Evaluation of the patient seeking relief of pain is similar regardless of etiology, but special considerations need to be made for a patient presenting with pain of known or suspected oncologic origin.

History

The goal of obtaining a history of present illness (HPI) is to characterize the patient's pain such that it fits within a broad contextual framework; for example, nociceptive versus neuropathic versus mixed pain. This will later be used to apply treatment algorithms, but first needs to be more precisely defined. The PQRST method, which seeks details regarding provocation, palliation (successful or unsuccessful), quality, radiation, severity, and timing of pain, is a handy memory tool which can

J. Silverman (✉)
Department of Anesthesiology, Weill-Cornell Medical Center, New York, NY, USA

A. Gulati
Department of Anesthesiology and Critical Care Medicine, Memorial Sloan Kettering Cancer Center, New York, NY, USA

© Springer Nature Switzerland AG 2019
Y. Khelemsky et al. (eds.), *Academic Pain Medicine*, https://doi.org/10.1007/978-3-030-18005-8_28

be utilized quickly and effectively to gather the necessary information. Acute versus chronic, somatic versus visceral, and iatrogenic versus organic are all subdivisions within the framework that help to narrow down potential etiologies.

Ancillary Studies

Ancillary studies, especially imaging modalities, play a much greater role in the management of cancer pain than in that of noncancer pain. Unlike degenerative back pain, in which strong evidence exists that expensive imaging modalities should be utilized only after failure of first-line treatments, diagnostic imaging is often available at the time of referral for a patient seeking specialist care for cancer-related pain [7]. MRI provides excellent tissue contrast and is used when high anatomical definition is required. It can detect bony metastases before disruption of the bony matrix can be detected on CT and is without the risk of ionizing radiation. CT offers superior spatial resolution compared to MRI and is rapid, making it the workhorse of diagnostic evaluation in the cancer pain population. The development of more efficient CT detector technology has allowed an increase in the spatial resolution of CT images and has decreased the radiation dose needed to generate detailed images [8]. Given its ability to obtain high-quality images rapidly, CT is also utilized in many advanced interventional pain management techniques to reduce procedural morbidity. The use of intravenous contrast significantly improves the ability of computed tomography to identify neoplastic lesions. PET scanning highlights metabolically active tissue and has become the test of choice for detection and monitoring of neoplastic lesions. It is important to review any available imaging prior to evaluation, as this can help significantly narrow the differential diagnosis and guide subsequent physical examination and treatment.

Physical Examination

Examination of a patient presenting for evaluation of cancer pain should be focused but thorough and guided by knowledge of the sensitivity and specificity of the available diagnostic maneuvers. It is important to approach the physical examination with a well-formulated differential diagnosis. It is often prudent to personally review relevant imaging prior to performing a physical examination, as pain-provoking maneuvers may be unnecessary for diagnosis and cause undue distress to the patient. In the absence of such radiographic evidence, or to confirm a degenerative etiology of pain, an algorithmic approach to physical diagnosis is recommended. Often in the cancer pain population, distinguish-

ing between a degenerative and disease-related cause of pain is difficult based on history and physical examination alone. In these instances, diagnostic interventions may be pursued. This approach is especially useful prior to neuroablative procedures or higher-risk advanced interventional pain management techniques.

Principles of Treatment

Once a target for treatment has been identified through history, physical examination, and review of ancillary tests, several treatment principles must be applied. Chief among them is that all pain management is palliative. It therefore stands that any treatment approach offering the potential for cure should take precedence. Chemotherapy, surgical resection, immunomodulation, radiation therapy, and others can provide such advantages, and referral to the appropriate specialists should be offered, if appropriate. It is for this reason that many of the top institutions hold regular meetings of interested parties that go by the name of "tumor board," "spine conference," or the like. Here, specialists from pain medicine, palliative care, medical and surgical oncology, diagnostic and interventional radiology, rehabilitation medicine, radiation oncology, and others discuss cases, disseminate ideas, and work cooperatively toward the common goal of optimizing patient care. Recent data show that the care delivered by a multidisciplinary team was more likely to meet quality and utilization benchmarks such as early, accurate preoperative staging, guideline-concordant treatment, and appropriate surveillance [9–11]. Compliance with guidelines is associated with improved patient outcomes, including survival [11].

While definitive treatment should not be delayed, neither should pain control be forsaken while awaiting response to potentially curative treatment. The two ought not to be mutually exclusive. Just as disease-modifying treatments may hold the promise of pain control, pain management can help promote disease-modifying efforts by improving tolerability or restoring performance status, thereby reestablishing eligibility for further treatment [12].

Functional modalities, such as physical therapy and tai chi, can be particularly beneficial for patients recovering from prolonged treatment courses whose pain and dysfunction limit further treatment options. Psychological modalities, such as CBT, biofeedback, and mindfulness meditation, are safe, effective ways in which patients can be trained to contribute positively to their own healing. Modalities such as acupuncture, massage, and osteopathy, provided through institutional integrative medicine departments or other community resources, can offer analgesia for appropriately selected patients. Pharmacotherapy is a staple of analgesia offered by nearly all members of an oncologic treatment team, regardless of specialization.

Interventional pain management strategies provide targeted therapies in an effort to reduce the burden of pharmacotherapeutics. The role of each modality will be discussed in greater detail below, because the adroit pain medicine specialist must understand how and when each may be implemented to best manage the complex condition of cancer pain.

Analgesic Ladder Approach

Forty-five years ago, Marks and Sachar revealed that 73% of cancer patients being treated in preeminent hospitals in New York City reported moderate-to-severe pain despite analgesic optimization [13]. Their findings inspired investigations into the adequacy of analgesia in cancer patients worldwide and, in 1982, a meeting of the World Health Organization (WHO) in Milan, Italy, in order to review the data and generate recommendations. This group of experts from the fields of anesthesiology, neurosurgery, oncology, surgery, neurology, pharmacology, psychology, and nursing evaluated the data from 32 publications as a basis for their recommendations. Born of this collaboration was a document which would be finalized in 1984 at the WHO Meeting on the Comprehensive Management of Cancer Pain in Geneva, Switzerland, and published in 1986 [14]. This document served as a call to action, not only for practitioners managing cancer pain but also for policymakers of national and international legislation concerning the regulation of opioid drugs, for experts in healthcare delivery and education, and for decision makers in pharmaceutical research and manufacturing. Among the guidance provided, the authors proposed a simple 3-step ladder approach to medication management of cancer pain.

The first step of the analgesic ladder calls for maximization of non-opioid analgesics, including aspirin, other non-steroidal anti-inflammatory medication, and acetaminophen. These, the panel felt, would be adequate to control mild pain when used routinely. If optimized non-opioid pharmacotherapy is unable to provide adequate relief or if pain is moderate at onset, the second step of the WHO ladder calls for the addition of a weak opioid. If uncontrolled by tier-1 and tier-2 pharmacotherapy, or if severe at onset, the panel recommended advancing to the third step of the ladder, which involves the addition of a strong opioid. At each step, co-administration of adjuvant medications, including antidepressants, antispasmodics, opioid receptor antagonists, NMDA receptor antagonists, corticosteroids, anticonvulsants, and sodium channel blockers, is advised. Their guidelines also included a series of recommendations emphasizing use of oral analgesics, individual dose-finding strategies, and systematic management of associated side effects.

Early field testing of the analgesic ladder approach suggested that stepwise escalation of pharmacotherapy was capable of controlling pain in up to 87% of cancer patients [15]. Ten-year data evaluating the approach, likewise, remained encouraging [16]. More recently, however, support for the analgesic ladder approach has waned, with newer studies scrutinizing the approach as ineffective and outdated [17–19]. This mounting dissent has contributed to widespread noncompliance with the WHO's recommendations [20].

Nonsteroidal Anti-inflammatory Medications

NSAIDs act peripherally by blocking cyclooxygenase (COX) to prevent conversion of arachidonic acid to thromboxane and prostaglandins in the inflammatory cascade. Traditional NSAIDs (i.e., ibuprofen, diclofenac, aspirin, naproxen, etc.) block, to varying degrees, both the constitutively active COX-1 isoform and the inducible COX-2 isoform [21]. Upon discovery of the COX-2 isoform, which is believed to be primarily responsible for the initiation and maintenance of inflammation, COX-1 became more closely associated with the gastrointestinal and renal side effects seen clinically [22–24]. Newer data, however, suggest that COX-2 inhibition contributes to these side effects as well [25]. Initially brought to market in the 1990s, commercially available selective COX-2 antagonists included celecoxib, rofecoxib, valdecoxib, parecoxib, lumiracoxib, and etoricoxib. While early data suggested equipotent anti-inflammatory activity with an anticipated reduction in gastrointestinal side effects compared to their nonselective predecessors, post-marketing data revealed an alarmingly high rate of cardiovascular events, prompting most members of the class to be pulled from the market [26–28]. Today, although rofecoxib is attempting to return to market, only celecoxib remains in widespread clinical use [29]. While its persistence was proposed to be due to its relative nonselectivity, it is now accepted that that the risk of adverse cardiovascular outcomes depends more on the extent of COX-2 inhibition than on the selectivity of inhibition [30].

Despite their potential risks, NSAIDs remain widely used in the management of malignant pain on the strength of primarily mechanistic and retrospective data [1, 31, 32]. While a 2005 Cochrane review found limited data suggesting that NSAIDs were more effective than placebo for the management of cancer pain, recent systematic reviews looking at various populations, including the update to the 2005 Cochrane review, found little evidence supporting this claim [33–36]. While data regarding the anti-tumor properties of NSAIDs seem promising, the role of anti-inflammatory medication in malignant pain control is inadequately supported by the current body of evidence [37–40].

Acetaminophen

While the mechanism of acetaminophen remains incompletely understood, it appears to be quite complex, involving all levels of pain stimulus generation, conduction, and processing [41]. Data support a role of acetaminophen in the modulation of descending serotonergic pain inhibition pathways, L-arginine/nitrous oxide free radical scavenging mechanisms, and the endogenous cannabinoid system, where it may work by activating transient receptor potential cation channel, subfamily V, member 1 (TRPV1) receptors [42–44]. Acetaminophen has also been shown to, like NSAIDs, reduce prostaglandin production via inhibition of cyclooxygenase, particularly COX-2 [45, 46]. Unlike NSAIDs, however, acetaminophen's effects are most pronounced in the central nervous system (CNS), where its effects appear to be determined by the local oxidation/reduction microenvironment [45, 47]. Other mechanisms have been proposed, but as of now, remain unproven.

Like NSAIDs, data supporting the use of acetaminophen in the management of cancer-related pain outside of the acute postoperative setting is suboptimal. A 2017 Cochrane review found only three small (122 total participants) studies which evaluated the use of acetaminophen for management of malignant pain [48]. Follow-up was 1 week in two studies and 5 days in the third. While each study investigated the addition of acetaminophen to a standing regimen of opioid analgesics, there was significant disparity in the average opioid doses between studies, with patients in one study receiving, on average, greater than three times the dose of patients in the other studies [49]. There was also significant heterogeneity in outcome measures, limiting comparison. All studies were associated with a high risk of bias. Overall, the data produced no convincing evidence that acetaminophen, when added to a standing regimen of opioid analgesics, improved pain control, quality of life, need for rescue analgesia, or participant satisfaction in patients with cancer pain. Unfortunately, the included studies did not permit comment on the use of acetaminophen in the role recommended by the WHO analgesic ladder – prior to initiation of opioid analgesia.

The only study published more recently than those considered for inclusion in the Cochrane review was a retrospective review of hospitalized cancer patients receiving chronic opioid analgesia who were administered intravenous acetaminophen for breakthrough analgesia [48]. Seventy-six percent of patients experienced pain relief, defined as a 1+ point improvement on a 4-point scale, following administration. A cut-off above which relief would not be expected was determined to be 45 morphine milligram equivalents per day.

Unlike that for management of chronic pain, the evidence supporting acetaminophen's use in acute cancer treatment-related pain is more robust. Several recent, high-quality studies investigating the use of acetaminophen following operative intervention for colorectal, gastric, brain, and esophageal cancers have been published [50–53]. Results of these studies indicate that acetaminophen may help enhance pain control, reduce opioid requirements, diminish side effects, and increase overall satisfaction compared to usual care or placebo. Another series of recent randomized, double-blind clinical trials found that acetaminophen, as part of a single-dose, multidrug cocktail including pregabalin and naproxen with or without dextromethorphan, effectively reduced postoperative pain and morphine consumption in patients undergoing radical neck dissection or laparotomy for cancer debulking [54, 55].

Acetaminophen is an exceptionally safe drug when used appropriately but can have important renal and hepatic effects when consumed at supratherapeutic doses or by patients whose baseline hepatic function is impaired by alcoholism, malnutrition, hepatitis, concomitant use of cytochrome P450 inducers such as omeprazole, and others. Its inclusion in myriad over-the-counter and prescription combinations contributes significantly to the risk of unintentional overdose [56, 57]. Although public education efforts were undertaken, the upper limit of safe use in the general public (e.g., over the counter dosing) was decreased from 4 to 3 grams daily, and new FDA regulations require clear labeling of all acetaminophen-containing compounds, acetaminophen toxicity remains the foremost cause of acute liver failure in the developed world [58].

Weak Opioids

The WHO panel's prototype drug in this class is codeine, but tramadol and hydrocodone were common substitutes at the time of publication. Hydrocodone has since been reclassified as a strong opioid, but codeine and tramadol, in addition to tapentadol, are weak opioids that remain widely used. Codeine is a classic mu-opioid receptor agonist. Both tramadol and tapentadol exhibit dual modes of action [59]. They act as agonists of the mu-opioid receptor in addition to inhibitors of central norepinephrine reuptake. Tramadol also adds weak serotonin reuptake inhibition, which tapentadol lacks [60].

Wiffen et al., in one of a series of 2017 Cochrane reviews investigating various pharmacologic interventions for cancer pain, found limited, low-quality evidence that use of tramadol effectively relieved cancer pain [61]. Likewise, most trials fail to show that other weak opioids have superior analgesic efficacy compared with paracetamol or NSAIDs [62, 63]. The role of weak opioids within the WHO analgesic ladder was further questioned by the results of a well-designed randomized controlled trial showing that low-dose morphine reduced pain significantly more effectively than weak opioids, with similar tolerability and a more rapid effect [19].

All weak opioids are associated with the same dose-dependent adverse effects as morphine, including nausea, vomiting, constipation, dizziness, drowsiness, pruritus, and respiratory depression. Additionally, tramadol can reduce the seizure threshold, contribute to the development of serotonin syndrome, cause hyponatremia, and increase intracranial pressure [64]. Liver or kidney disease, as well as genetic cytochrome P450 polymorphisms, can dramatically alter metabolism and excretion of these compounds (e.g., codeine), increasing the risk of inadvertent overdose [65]. There is also no evidence that weak opioids carry a lower risk of addiction than equianalgesic doses of morphine [66].

Strong Opioids

The prototype, morphine, is an opioid receptor agonist isolated from the opium poppy (*Papaver somniferum*). Along with codeine and thebaine, these substances make up the "opiates" or natural opioids. Semisynthetic opioids are derived from morphine or codeine and include hydrocodone, hydromorphone, oxycodone, and oxymorphone. Synthetic opioids include fentanyl and methadone. Buprenorphine, a derivative of thebaine, is a partial opioid agonist with an analgesic potency 50 times greater than that of morphine [67]. These substances bind G protein–coupled opioid receptors centrally and peripherally, initiating downstream effects which limit the release of neurotransmitters necessary for pain signal propagation, such as glutamate and substance P [68].

All opioids share a side effect profile that includes, to varying degrees, nausea, vomiting, constipation, dizziness, drowsiness, pruritus, respiratory depression, hypogonadism, hyperalgesia, and immune system dysfunction. Extensive preclinical and clinical data suggest that opioids may play a role in cancer recurrence and metastasis by promoting immune suppression and angiogenesis, among other mechanisms [69–71]. The data do not yet permit clinically meaningful conclusions, but rather provide additional impetus for maximizing a multimodal approach to analgesia that limits reliance on this class of medication. Tolerance, defined as requiring an increased dose of medication to achieve the same analgesic effect; dependence, defined as the presence of withdrawal symptoms with abrupt discontinuation of treatment; and addiction, defined as continued use despite physical, emotional, occupational, or social harm have proven equally problematic in populations of cancer pain patients as in those with chronic pain of noncancer origin [72]. Buprenorphine may be associated with reduced risk of respiratory depression, pruritus, addiction, and dependence, garnering it increased attention for the management of chronic pain, including that of oncologic origin [73, 74].

Given the significant safety risks, the question of opioids' clinical value turns to efficacy. A recent review of Cochrane reviews evaluated 152 studies, comprising over 13,500 patients and found the quality of the evidence for the use of opioids in the management of cancer pain to be "disappointingly low" [75]. Their findings did indicate efficacy, however, in that approximately 95% of cancer patients with moderate-to-severe pain who can tolerate opioids can expect their pain to be significantly reduced within 14 days. The ability to tolerate treatment is a significant caveat to their conclusion, as in the studies they reviewed, as many as 77% of participants experienced at least one adverse event and cessation of therapy due to adverse reactions was reported at rates of up to 19%. A retrospective study found that patients suffering adverse opioid-related drug events had a 36% higher risk of 30-day readmission, a 55% longer hospital stay, a 3.4-fold increased risk of inpatient mortality, and 47% more costly care when compared to patients who did not report an opioid-related adverse drug event [76]. Long-term efficacy of these medications has also yet to be proven [77]. This risk-benefit imbalance has led some authors to call into question the validity of the opioid-heavy WHO analgesic ladder approach [16–19].

Antidepressants

In 1956, Henry Beecher studied wounded soldiers and concluded that the significance of an injury, not the degree of tissue damage, was the primary determinant of analgesic requirement [78]. His conclusion spawned decades of research into the affective component of pain, which is now well established [79]. Cancer, likewise, is strongly associated with mood disorders [80]. Depression is known to worsen treatment outcomes in both pain and cancer populations [81, 82]. It is therefore no surprise that antidepressants are widely used in patients with cancer-related pain. While numerous antidepressant classes exist, including selective serotonin reuptake inhibitors, monoamine oxidase inhibitors, serotonin and norepinephrine reuptake inhibitors, and tricyclic antidepressants, the latter two classes are most often used in the management of pain. The mechanism by which these medications help ameliorate pain is unclear, but the finding that pain relief is achieved well before improvement in mood and that mood alterations are not necessary for analgesic effects suggests that they work differently for each indication. Modulation of norepinephrine appears to play a key role in the analgesic properties of these drugs [83–85]. This is consistent with the finding that serotonin-selective medications provide almost no pain relief [86]. Norepinephrine-induced activation of α2-adrenergic receptors in the dorsal horn of the spinal cord has been shown in animal models to reduce allodynia and hyperalgesia associated with neuropathic pain [87]. Additionally, descending noradrenergic neurons from the locus coeruleus play an important role in endogenous analgesia [88]. Other systems are likely to be involved as well. Various antidepressants have been shown to affect sodium channels, NMDA receptors, α1-adrenergic receptors, calcium channels, potassium channels, the adenosine system, GABA-B receptors, and opioid receptors [89–96]. The way antidepressants act upon each of these systems in an effort to reduce pain remains imprecisely elucidated.

Many antidepressants can be used to manage the significant affective component of chronic pain, but some, such as duloxetine, have evidence of efficacy in treating cancer-related nociceptive and neuropathic pain [97–101]. Venlafaxine and milnacipran also have proven superiority over placebo in the treatment of chemotherapy-induced peripheral neuropathy [100–102]. Tricyclic antidepressants, while effective for neuropathic pain in the setting of fibromyalgia and diabetes, do not appear to provide statistically significantly better control of chemotherapy-induced neuropathies than placebo [103–107].

While typically well tolerated, antidepressants have important class-related side effects. In a large survey-based study of patients on antidepressants, greater than 5% of patients taking SNRIs reported dizziness, hot flushes, GI upset, changes in appetite, weight gain, headaches, tremors, restless legs, abnormal dreams, anxiety, confusion, emotional numbing, somnolence, insomnia, sexual dysfunction, and sweating [108]. Venlafaxine, which requires relatively larger doses to achieve significant norepinephrine reuptake inhibition, is uniquely associated with an increased risk of elevated blood pressure at higher doses [109]. Tricyclic antidepressants have the most side effects, which include anticholinergic, antihistaminergic, and antiadrenergic effects in addition to those of other norepinephrine-modulating antidepressants mentioned above. While sedation and dry mouth are the most common clinical manifestations, urinary retention and orthostasis are the most clinically worrisome and can limit their use in many patients. All antidepressants carry a black box warning of increased suicidal thinking, feeling and behavior in young people; an adverse effect reported by almost 6% of the over 3000 patients surveyed by Hughes et al. [108]. Use of these medications is also limited by the potential for drug-drug interactions, including precipitation of serotonin syndrome when used alongside tramadol, among other medications. Ultimately, most patients are able to find a member of the class which they tolerate. Often, a medication's side effects can be exploited for the benefit of the patient. TCAs, for example, are often dosed at night to take advantage of their sedating properties.

Antispasmodics

This heterogeneous class of medications includes, among others, tizanidine, cyclobenzaprine, methocarbamol, baclofen, valium, chlorzoxazone, and carisoprodol. Given their disparate mechanisms, these drugs can be used in the management of a variety of painful conditions, but are most frequently used for management of myofascial pain. These medications have been shown to act synergistically with opioids and anti-inflammatory medications to improve their pain-relieving efficacy and reduce their risk of side effects [110, 111]. The centrally acting alpha-2 adrenergic agonist tizanidine has evidence supporting its efficacy in managing neuropathic and postoperative pain [112, 113]. Clonidine, another central alpha-2 adrenergic agonist, is a common additive to intrathecal admixtures, where it potentiates the effect of local anesthetics to improve management of neuropathic cancer pain [114]. Baclofen, a central GABA-B receptor agonist, has been used to manage pain and spasticity due to spinal cord injuries, multiple sclerosis, cerebral palsy, and a number of other neuropathic pain conditions [115–118]. Valium, a GABA-A receptor agonist, and carisoprodol, which shares structural similarity with barbiturates, have antispasmodic properties, but also carry with them the potential for significant side effects, including addiction and respiratory depression (especially when combined with opioids). Use of other members of this class of medications is limited mostly by cognitive side effects and sedation. The latter can be beneficial in patients with disordered sleep.

NMDA Receptor Antagonists

Ketamine, an N-methyl-D-aspartate (NMDA) receptor antagonist, was synthesized from phencyclidine in the 1960s for use as a battlefield anesthetic in Vietnam before being introduced to the general public in the 1970s [119]. It has since been replaced by less hallucinogenic anesthetics but retains a role in the management of refractory neuropathic (specifically sympathetically mediated) pain, nociceptive pain in opioid-tolerant patients, burn victims, and nonpainful conditions such as depression. There is evidence of its efficacy in the management of refractory cancer pain, although a recent Cochrane review found the data to be of insufficient quality to accurately assess the role of ketamine for this indication [120, 121]. A more recent well-designed, randomized, controlled trial found that ketamine was no better than placebo at treating cancer-related neuropathic pain while associated with significantly greater risk [122].

Although it is predominantly used intravenously, topical and intranasal formulations have been gaining in popularity [123–125]. Once in the bloodstream, ketamine's lipophilic properties allow it to easily cross the blood-brain barrier into the central nervous system, where it acts primarily by binding NMDA receptors, ultimately reducing release of the excitatory neurotransmitter glutamate [126]. Additionally, ketamine has been shown to interact with mu- and kappa-opioid receptors and to modulate central monoaminergic, muscarinic, and nicotinic processes. At high doses, ketamine exhibits local anesthetic properties, indicating an ability to inhibit neuronal sodium channels [119].

The most prominent side effects of ketamine are neurological or psychological in nature and include dissociation, agitation, confusion, dizziness, sedation, nystagmus, catatonia, and frank psychosis. Emergence from ketamine-induced analgesia can feature alterations in mood, panic attacks, sensations of weightlessness, vivid dreams, audiovisual hallucinations, and delirium [119]. These effects usually disappear once fully awake, but re-experiencing of the illusions (e.g., "flashbacks") has been reported [127]. Ketamine has a direct myocardial depressant effect, which is typically counteracted by increased sympathetic tone, creating the clinical picture of tachycardia, hypertension, and increased cardiac output [128]. In patients with a limited cardiac reserve, ketamine may cause hemodynamic decompensation. Hypersalivation is another common side effect that may be attenuated by co-administration of anti-cholinergic medications. Additionally, ketamine has been shown to cause adverse GI effects – most commonly nausea/vomiting and, rarely, hepatotoxicity. Benzodiazepine co-administration may help reduce the risk of adverse psychologic and cardiovascular events [129].

The opioid receptor antagonist naltrexone, when used at doses 10–100 times smaller than those used to manage opioid addiction (e.g., low-dose naltrexone), may also work by modulating activity at the NMDA receptor. Unlike ketamine, its effects upon the receptor are likely indirect, via inhibition of glial cell activation through toll-like receptor 4 pathways [130, 131]. Other mechanisms of action may include enhancement of endogenous opioid production, modulation of the cannabinoid system and suppressed production of inflammatory mediators from peripheral macrophages, but our understanding remains incomplete [132–136].

Data evaluating low-dose naltrexone in the management of cancer pain is sparse, but there is some evidence that it may have an opioid-sparing effect [137, 138]. The mechanism of this effect is unclear and may simply be due to prescriber's warnings of potential opioid withdrawal with concomitant use versus improved analgesia. There is, however, some evidence of its ability to reduce self-reported pain in other conditions, such as multiple sclerosis, Crohn's disease, and fibromyalgia [139]. In addition to its analgesic and anti-inflammatory potential, studies suggest it may help improve chemotherapeutic response or even exhibit direct anticancer properties through modulation of opioid growth factor pathways across multiple cancer subtypes [140, 141].

Orally administered low-dose naltrexone is typically very well tolerated [139]. Its side effects include anxiety, nausea, drowsiness, headache, dizziness, sleep disturbances, vivid dreams, muscle pain, and anorexia, but these tended to be short-lived and did not require discontinuation of treatment at a rate any greater than that of placebo [142, 143]. Although full-dose naltrexone carries a black box warning regarding the risk of hepatotoxicity, this does not seem to be an issue at lower doses [144–146]. Its use can, however, be limited by its delayed onset of efficacy. Its potential to interact with concomitantly prescribed opioids remains unknown as many available studies excluded patients receiving opioid analgesics.

Corticosteroids

Corticosteroids have a multitude of uses in the patient with pain of oncologic origin. Their mechanism of action is complex but includes transcriptional suppression of several cytokines and chemokines involved in the regulation of the inflammatory reaction as well as downstream suppression of cytokine-induced COX-2 expression [147]. In so doing, they have been used effectively for pain from bony metastasis and to reduce the radiation "flare" following radiation therapy to a bony lesion [148]. For the management of headaches due to tumor-associated cerebral edema or pain following ablation of metastatic liver lesions, administration of corticosteroids has been shown to produce rapid pain relief [149, 150]. In a 2015 Cochrane review, Haywood and colleagues performed a meta-analysis of six randomized, controlled trials and found that corticosteroids, primarily dexamethasone, provided better short-term relief of cancer-related pain than controls [151]. Overall, they found the evidence supporting the use of corticosteroids for pain control in cancer patients to be weak, but that significant pain relief was possible. In addition to pain, corticosteroids are commonly used in the management of primary or metastatic central nervous system tumors to reduce edema and improve neurologic function [149, 152–154]. Additionally, they have been proven useful in the relief of ureteral obstruction, can help reduce the risk of encephalopathy in patients undergoing whole-brain radiation therapy, and reduce nausea, vomiting, and anorexia caused by cancer or its treatments [149, 155, 156].

Corticosteroid use is associated with multiple, potentially serious side effects, including hirsutism, impaired wound healing, capillary fragility leading to easy bruising/bleeding, CNS excitation (i.e., jitteriness, euphoria, psychosis, etc.), immunosuppression, hypertension, glucose intolerance, insomnia, fluid retention, avascular necrosis, growth retardation, cataracts, and blurry vision [157]. These side effects tend to be dose and duration dependent, with the risk of side effects following brief, low-dose corticosteroid regimens in various populations of cancer patients proving no greater than that of placebo controls [158–160]. A systematic review investigating the safety of short courses of corticosteroids, albeit at highly variable doses, found the most common adverse drug reaction to be vomiting, which occurred in just over 5% of patients [161]. Chronic or high-dose use, however, can result in suppression of endogenous steroid production and the emergence of more worrisome side effects, such as myopathy, bone demineralization, HPA axis dysregulation, and gastrointestinal bleeding [162].

Anticonvulsants

Anticonvulsants, especially gabapentin and pregabalin, have become first-line agents for patients suffering neuropathic pain of a variety of etiologies. Structurally similar to gamma-aminobutyric acid (GABA), these medications' mechanisms of action are not entirely clear, but likely have to do with their affinity for voltage-gated calcium channels, where they may decrease neural firing by reducing calcium currents [163, 164]. Despite an unclear mechanism, both gabapentin and pregabalin have evidence of efficacy in reducing chemotherapy- or radiation-induced neuropathic pain [98, 165–167]. A recent systematic review found that both gabapentin (in 5 of 6 studies) and pregabalin (in 6 of 8 studies) were associated with significant reductions in tumor-related pain [168]. Both can also be used preoperatively to reduce postoperative pain and opioid requirements, or in combination with neuraxial procedures to improve pain relief [169, 170]. These medications are typically well tolerated, but can be limited by sedation, dizziness, GI side effects, peripheral edema, or weight gain. Pregabalin is associated with euphoria in 5% of patients, which earned it a schedule V designation on the FDA's list of controlled substances [171]. Gabapentin, uniquely, carries a black box warning regarding increased suicidality when initiating treatment – a risk validated by a 2010 meta-analysis [172].

Valproate, whose mechanism is unclear but may involve modulation of the GABAergic system, voltage-gated sodium channel blockade, or inhibition of histone deacetylases, may have protective effects against the development of chemotherapy-induced peripheral neuropathy [173, 174]. While data from animal and small human studies suggest that this may be the case, robust data in support of this theory do not exist [175, 176]. Valproic acid has a well-established safety profile, including nausea, vomiting, dry mouth, cardiac arrhythmias, central nervous toxicities, pancreatitis, and hepatotoxicity, but the more serious of these tend to be associated with doses significantly higher than those used in the aforementioned studies. This medication has also been associated with teratogenicity, so should be avoided by women of childbearing age.

Sodium Channel Blockers

Local anesthetics prevent the opening of transmembrane voltage-gated sodium channels, thereby inhibiting depolarization of the neural membrane, halting subsequent action potential propagation. They have been utilized in a variety of ways for the management of cancer-related pain, most commonly in interventional applications which will be discussed in detail later in the chapter. Topical lidocaine also has evidence supporting its efficacy in the management of myofascial pain or rib pain, such as from pathologic fractures or bony metastases [177, 178]. Intravenous lidocaine infusions have proven effective in treating refractory chemotherapy-induced peripheral neuropathy [179] and for reducing opioid requirements following colorectal surgery [180]. Mexiletine, an oral, nonselective, voltage-gated sodium channel blocker which also serves as a class IB antiarrhythmic agent, has some animal evidence of efficacy in relieving chemotherapy-induced neuropathic pain, but human data are lacking [181, 182]. Carbamazepine and its structurally related counterpart, oxcarbazepine, are anticonvulsants that work by blocking voltage-gated sodium channels. In a clinical trial of patients with colon cancer and chemotherapy-induced peripheral neuropathy, oxcarbazepine produced a significantly greater improvement in symptoms compared with no treatment [183]. In a similar population, carbamazepine proved more effective than controls at preventing peripheral neuropathy in patients treated with oxaliplatin-based chemotherapy, although the study was underpowered for their primary outcome [184].

Although topical formulations are typically quite safe and interventional procedures are more commonly limited by procedural risks than they are by local anesthetic pharmacodynamics, there is a risk of local anesthetic systemic toxicity (LAST) following any procedure in which local anesthetics are used. The risk is increased following high-volume blocks or intravenous infusions.

Oral administration of sodium channel antagonists is also associated with potentially significant side effects. Nausea and dizziness, experienced by 40% and 26% of patients, respectively, were the most common side effects reported in a study of mexiletine [185]. Discontinuation of mexiletine therapy in this group was significant, with 50% of patients stopping treatment within 6 weeks and fewer than 20% continuing treatment beyond 1 year. An important concern with the use of carbamazepine and oxcarbazepine is the development of hyponatremia. Oxcarbazepine is associated with fewer side effects and drug-drug interactions than carbamazepine and does not require routine monitoring for hematologic or hepatic toxicities [186].

Interventional Approaches

Once considered the fourth step of the WHO analgesic ladder, interventional approaches have assumed an earlier and more prominent role in the management of cancer pain as evidence regarding the risk-benefit ratio of chronic opioid use has been elucidated [14]. The 1986 WHO publication admits that "neurolytic and neurosurgical blocks may be necessary as a supplementary approach in a small number of cases," but more recent data suggest that conservative management may leave greater unmet need than previously estimated [14, 187].

Pain signals can be interrupted at the site of signal generation, along the afferent nerve, at the level of the sympathetic chain, or in the neuraxis. Interruption of nociceptive signaling with local anesthetic can provide valuable diagnostic information in addition to temporary relief. Sustained relief can be achieved with the addition of corticosteroid or through neurolysis with cryoablation, chemical, or radiofrequency ablation. The choice of where and how to intervene is dependent on myriad variables, including pathoanatomic considerations, anticipated progression of disease, and practitioner experience. While evidence-based treatment algorithms have been proposed, novel approaches continue to emerge, obligating practitioners to remain up-to-date in order to provide the highest quality care [188, 189].

Peripheral Nerves

Precise targeting of nerves within muscular or fascial planes demands an intimate knowledge of neuromuscular anatomy, but accuracy may be improved with ultrasound guidance [190, 191]. Common targets for peripheral nerve blockade include the trigeminal, suprascapular, intercostal, intercostobrachial, ilioinguinal/iliohypogastric, pudendal, and saphenous nerves, among others [192–198]. Approaches to targeting multiple intercostal nerve branches with a single injection have also been described. These traditionally involve the paravertebral space or fascial planes surrounding the serratus anterior, transversus abdominis, or pectoralis muscles, but new targets touting improved safety and efficacy routinely emerge [199–204]. Perineural injection of local anesthetic produces a diagnostic blockade, but may also be therapeutic, especially with the addition of corticosteroid. More permanent neurolysis can be achieved with chemical such as alcohol or phenol and thermal or cryoablation. Anesthesia dolorosa, or deafferentation pain, is a condition characterized by persistent, painful anesthesia or hyperesthesia in a denervated region. It is estimated to occur in as many as 1.5% of patients following chemical neurolysis and 3% of patients following thermocoagulation [205, 206]. The resulting pain is often described as being worse than the pain initially being treated. Treatment of this devastating consequence is often suboptimal, even with the use of advanced neurosurgical approaches.

Sympathetic Chain

Like peripheral nerves, sympathetic ganglia have been targeted for decades in the management of a variety of neuropathic and visceral pain states. The most common targets for neural blockade along the sympathetic axis include the stellate ganglion, celiac plexus, superior hypogastric plexus, lumbar plexus, and ganglion impar. Proposed mechanisms for the effects of sympatholysis include inhibition of adrenergic hypersensitivity, interruption of positive nociceptive feedback circuits, and reduction of central hyperexcitability [207]. Given the frequency of mixed pain states, sympathetic blocks rarely eliminate cancer pain. They have, though, been shown to provide significant pain relief, improve quality of life, and reduce the need for analgesic medication.

Stellate Ganglion

The stellate ganglion is most typically formed by the fusion of the inferior cervical ganglion with the first thoracic sympathetic ganglion [208]. It is located anterior to the transverse process of the seventh cervical vertebra, between the scalene and longus coli muscles. It provides sympathetic input to the upper extremity, chest, face, and head. Blockade is typically achieved by injecting local anesthetic with or without corticosteroid along the plane of the longus coli muscle at the level of the sixth cervical vertebra, where the adjacent vertebral artery is protected by the bony Chassaignac tubercle. This is commonly done using ultrasound guidance but can also be accomplished with the use of fluoroscopy, computed tomography, or palpation alone. A successful block is indicated by temperature changes in the upper extremity. Although most commonly used in the management of upper extremity CRPS, stellate ganglion blocks can be used successfully in the management of pain and other sequelae from cancers of the head and neck, esophagus and breast, or their treatment [209–211]. Risks include needle trauma to the many important structures surrounding the ganglion in the neck, including the carotid artery, vertebral artery, inferior thyroid artery, recurrent laryngeal nerve, vagus nerve, brachial plexus, thyroid, and trachea. Pneumothorax is a known complication but can be avoided by choosing a target cephalad to the first thoracic vertebra. Spinal or epidural blockade is possible if the needle is advanced or medication spreads into the neural foramen.

Celiac Plexus

The celiac plexus is located at approximately the twelfth thoracic or first lumbar vertebral level in the retroperitoneal space, just anterior and caudad to the crura of the diaphragm. It surrounds the anterior and lateral aspects of the aorta and celiac and superior mesenteric trunks as they divide from the aorta. The plexus receives sympathetic fibers from the greater (T9-T10), lesser (T10-T11), and least (T12) splanchnic nerves, parasympathetic fibers from the vagus nerve, and sensory fibers from the phrenic and vagus nerves [212]. The primary indication for celiac plexus blockade is visceral pain in the setting of pancreatic cancer, although pain from malignancies involving any of the upper abdominal viscera can be treated with this technique [213].

There are several approaches to the block. Most commonly, a posterior percutaneous approach utilizing fluoroscopic or computed tomography guidance is employed. The target of this approach can vary, based on patient characteristics and extent of disease. The retrocrural approach uses bilateral needles to place medication along the anterior border of the first lumbar vertebral body. While more appropriately referred to as a splanchnic nerve block, this method is effective, avoids penetration of the aorta, and may be preferred when the celiac plexus anatomy is distorted by lymphadenopathy [214]. It does, however, carry the potential for neurologic injury if the drug spreads to involve the somatic nerve roots or epidural and subarachnoid spaces. The transcrural approach starts with a single-needle approach from the left with a target of the lower one third of the first lumbar vertebral body. The needle is advanced through the diaphragmatic crux. If the aorta is penetrated, the needle is advanced through the anterior wall of the aorta until the tip lies on the anterior surface of the aorta near the midline, within the celiac plexus. Penetration of the muscular wall of the aorta is often of no significant consequence given the small gauge of the needles used. If an antecrural needle tip position is achieved without penetration of the aorta and contrast spread is unilateral, a needle is placed through the diaphragm from the right to block the remaining fibers. This approach reduces the risk of paravertebral spread. Anterior approaches have also been described. This approach uses palpation or ultrasound guidance and, although it necessitates traversing abdominal structures such as intestines and liver, is ordinarily inconsequential, is well tolerated, and can be performed quickly [215]. An approach gaining popularity in the literature utilizes endoscopic ultrasound to access the celiac plexus through the posterior gastric wall [216]. The advantages of this approach are the fine control of needle placement, the ability to visualize needle movement in real time, and the ability to perform the procedure in the same session as staging or sampling of an inoperable pancreatic tumor. No approach has proven superior to another regarding safety or efficacy.

Regardless the approach, high-quality data support the use of celiac plexus blockade in the management of upper abdominal cancer-related pain. Superior pain relief, improved quality of life, and diminished analgesic requirements were noted when celiac plexus blockade was compared to baseline, placebo, or active control groups [217]. Some studies have even provided evidence that, through improved nutrition and reduction in oral analgesic side effects, celiac plexus neurolysis can contribute to prolonged survival in patients with advanced pancreatic cancer, although newer data refute this [218–220].

Complications of celiac plexus blockade differ based on approach, but imaging-guided approaches are considered relatively safe. Injection site pain, orthostatic hypotension due to dilation of the splanchnic vasculature following loss of sympathetic tone, and transient diarrhea from unopposed parasympathetic activity are the most commonly described complications. Severe complications include pneumothorax, vascular injury, transient hematuria, sexual dysfunction, pleuritis, pericarditis, and retroperitoneal abscess [212]. There are several reports of spinal cord injury after celiac plexus block, thought to be the result of occlusion or spasm of radicular arteries, including the artery of Adamkiewicz [221, 222].

Lumbar Sympathetics

The lumbar sympathetic plexus is located anterolateral to the second, third, and fourth lumbar vertebral bodies. Blockade of the plexus, or the splanchnic nerves along which visceral afferent signals are transmitted from the plexus to the sympathetic trunk, is typically approached posteriorly using fluoroscopic guidance. Computed tomography and magnetic resonance-guided approaches have been described [223, 224]. Commonly, a single, high-volume injection at the level of the third lumbar vertebra is performed. While this is typically adequate, a multilevel approach may be more effective [225]. Lumbar sympathetic blocks have been used in the management of many painful conditions of the lower abdomen, pelvis, and lower extremity, but high-quality evidence supporting the use of the technique is sparse and comes primarily from studies of patients with CRPS affecting the lower extremities [226]. In this population, radiofrequency denervation and injections of local anesthetic with and without clonidine, saline, phenol, and botulinum toxin have all been shown to provide relief, with only botulinum toxin proving more effective than the others in comparative studies. Time to analgesic failure was also significantly longer in the group receiving botulinum toxin [227]. Adverse effects include pain at the injection site, motor or sensory deficits secondary to spread of medication into the intrathecal or epidural space, visceral perforation, genitofemoral nerve injury, and priapism [228–230].

Superior Hypogastric Plexus

The superior hypogastric plexus is located ventral to the bifurcation of the abdominal aorta, extending from the lower third of the fifth lumbar vertebra to the upper third of the first sacral vertebra. It contains sympathetic, parasympathetic, and visceral afferent fibers [231]. It has been targeted in the management of pelvic pain secondary to genitourinary, gynecologic, and colorectal cancers. Traditionally, bilateral needles are inserted inferior and lateral to the transverse process of the fifth lumbar vertebra. Fluoroscopic guidance is used to guide the needle tip to a position alongside the anterolateral vertebral body [232]. Injections of local anesthetic, alcohol, and phenol can be employed. Computed tomography is used for guidance in some centers, and, more recently, transdiscal and ultrasound-guided approaches have been described [233–235]. Pain relief on the order of 70% has been demonstrated in several studies, which can be improved to greater than 90% when used as part of multimodal therapy [232, 236].

Ganglion Impar

The ganglion impar is found in the midline on the ventral surface of the coccyx, where it forms the caudal termination of the bilateral sympathetic chain. It supplies nociceptive and sympathetic fibers to the perineum, rectum, distal urethra, vulva, scrotum, and distal one third of the vagina [237]. Neurolysis of this structure was initially described in 1990 by Plancarte for management of pelvic malignancies but is now also commonly used in the management of nonmalignant coccygodynia [207, 232, 238]. Initially accessed through the anococcygeal ligament, the transsacrococcygeal approach is now preferred because it requires less expertise and allows a more direct needle path [238]. In some patients, the sacrococcygeal joint or intercoccygeal joints are fused, necessitating a paracoccygeal approach [239]. Fluoroscopy is the primary means of image guidance, but computed tomography, ultrasound, and magnetic resonance-based techniques have been described [240–242]. Evidence of the block's efficacy in the cancer pain population is limited to case studies and small case series. The largest studies are in patients with nonmalignant pain and show success rates above 80% [243, 244]. Complications are rare but can include motor, sexual, or bowel/bladder dysfunction, rectal perforation, and sciatic nerve impingement.

Neuroaxial Procedures

Neuroaxial procedures include epidural injections or infusions; pulsed radiofrequency ablation or chemical neurolysis of the nerve root within the epidural space; electrical stimulation of the dorsal columns or dorsal root ganglion; intrathecal drug delivery; and stereotactic neurosurgical procedures such as cordotomy and myelotomy. Here, we will introduce treatment strategies involving the epidural space. Advanced central neuroablative approaches will be discussed in more detail later in the chapter.

Epidural Injection

Epidural injections are the most commonly performed procedure in the management of nonmalignant chronic pain, but their role in the care of patients with malignant pain is increasing as improved disease-management strategies have created chronic diseases of cancers that were once imminently terminal. The extensive body of literature discussing the most appropriate approach (e.g., caudal, transforaminal, or interlaminar) and injectate (e.g., local anesthetic with or without steroid, saline) does not yield any definitive conclusions [245–249]. Likewise, the efficacy of this commonly performed procedure has been questioned in light of its risks, which include epidural abscesses and hematomas, dural tears resulting in spinal headaches, and transient or permanent neurologic deficits related to inadvertent involvement of the radiculomedullary arterial system [250]. A thorough discussion of these considerations is, however, beyond the scope of this chapter.

Although less commonly utilized since the emergence of intrathecal drug delivery systems, epidural infusion via an external pump remains an effective alternative for the management of pain at the end of life [251]. In patients too debilitated to undergo the surgery or whose limited life expectancy brings the cost-effectiveness of IT therapy into question, epidural anesthesia should be considered. A catheter can be placed to provide days to weeks of relief or tunneled for longer use. With the option of patient-controlled boluses, epidural analgesia has advantages over intravenous patient-controlled analgesia or high-dose systemic opioids, including improved pain control and reduced risk of side effects [252]. Limitations include a high rate of catheter migration which is only modestly mitigated by tunneling or the use of commercial anchoring devices, effects on motor and bowel/bladder function, risk of infection, and concerns regarding monitoring and maintenance of the system outside of the healthcare setting.

Intrathecal Neurolysis

Intrathecal dorsal rhizolysis via delivery of alcohol or phenol into the dorsal subarachnoid space preferentially destroys the small sensory nerve rootlets which occupy the area between the dorsal root ganglion (DRG) and the dorsal horn of the spinal cord. Their greater surface area increases susceptibility to neurolysis when compared with the DRG or nerve root proper [253]. Owing to the anatomic separation of motor and sensory fibers within the intrathecal space, destruction of sensory fibers without harm to motor function is possible, although not typically seen in clinical practice, where absolute sensory selectivity is rarely achieved. The procedure has fallen out of favor given its potential for significant side effects and the boon of implanted intrathecal drug delivery systems. Ideal candidates for the procedure have a life expectancy less than 12 months and severe, well-localized pain covering three or fewer dermatomes which remains resistant to maximal tolerated doses of analgesics and adjuvants [253]. Response to a diagnostic local anesthetic block may also be considered a prerequisite for moving forward with subarachnoid neurolysis.

There is little data supporting the choice of neurolytic agent. The duration of relief following the use of both alcohol and phenol vary widely, but alcohol may have the potential to provide prolonged benefits [254]. Phenol has a shorter onset of action, requires less volume (allowing greater dermatomal specificity) and, due to its local anesthetic properties, does not cause the intense burning discomfort upon injection that is typical of alcohol [253]. At concentrations of 5–6%, phenol destroys nociceptive fibers with minimal motor side effects. At concentrations greater than 6%, however, it can cause axonal degradation, nerve root damage, spinal cord infarcts, arachnoiditis, and meningitis [255]. At higher doses, phenol is neurotoxic, causing central nervous system depression and cardiovascular collapse, similar to local anesthetic toxicity [256]. Additionally, phenol can damage the neural tube, destroying the pathway along which neuronal regeneration would otherwise follow, increasing the risk of aberrant re-innervation and resultant neuropathic pain [257]. Regardless of agent used, side effects can include sensory, motor, and autonomic system derangements (i.e., dysesthesias, paralysis, loss of sphincter control, nausea, etc.), postdural puncture headache, incomplete nociceptive blockade, and brief duration of relief. It is these safety concerns that have relegated this potentially effective technique to use in only the most refractory cases.

Surgical and Interventional Radiologic Approaches

When pharmacologic, percutaneous, and other conservative treatment options fail, multiple surgical options exist with evidence for efficacy in managing refractory oncologic pain. While some of these techniques fall under the purview of an adequately trained interventionalist, collaboration with surgical oncology, neurosurgery, and interventional radiology is vital to provide additional treatment options for the hardest-to-manage patients.

Intrathecal Drug Delivery

Intrathecal drug delivery (IDD) is one such approach that has been used effectively in the most refractory cancer pain

patients. The primary indication for use of an implanted IDD system is pain uncontrolled by an oral medication regimen whose further titration is limited by the development of intolerable side effects. Unlike oral medication, IDD provides direct access to receptor sites in the dorsal horn of the spinal cord and reduces drug delivery to the brain (when compared to systemic medications) via the blood–brain barrier [258]. IDD also allows rapid medication titration at initiation of therapy or following disease progression. While cases of drug abuse using implanted intrathecal systems have been described, IDD is associated with less risk of medication misuse than oral regimens [259]. Follow-up appointments for pump refills and reprogramming are generally less frequent and more streamlined than those required during chronic oral opioid management. Implanted IDD systems do not interfere with the ability to obtain an MRI or receive other oncologic care, although cases of pump failure following exposure of the device to a radiation therapy field have been reported [260]. Medication delivery can be programmed based on the patient's varying needs throughout the day; for example, increased rate at meal time for patients whose appetite is limited by abdominal pain. Furthermore, these pumps allow for administration of patient-delivered rescue medication within parameters set by the managing physician. There is even some evidence that IDD can contribute to prolonged survival by reducing the burden of medication side effects and restoring eligibility for disease-modifying treatment by improving nutritional and functional parameters [261].

Morphine was the first and remains the most commonly used medication in IDD systems. As one of three medications, along with baclofen and ziconotide, approved by the FDA for intrathecal use, morphine is recommended as a first-line pump medication by the Polyanalgesic Consensus Conference [262]. Other opioids such as fentanyl, sufentanil, hydromorphone, and methadone are also commonly used, alone or in combination with bupivacaine, clonidine, baclofen, midazolam, ketamine, octreotide, and other adjuvants. Ziconotide deserves special mention as the only medication that requires intrathecal administration to maximize its anti-nociceptive effectiveness and minimize sympatholysis [263]. A selective N-type voltage-sensitive calcium channel blocker isolated from the venom of the marine snail *Conus magus,* ziconotide, can be highly effective in the management of neuropathic pain [264]. While it has been studied in various admixtures, ziconotide is most commonly utilized as monotherapy, for which it carries an FDA indication [265–268]. Use of this medication is limited by substantial cost and a slow titration schedule necessitated by significant neurologic, cognitive, and psychological side effects common with rapid dose escalation [264, 269].

The choice of IDD regimen is multifactorial and includes consideration of patient age, disease stage, prognosis, life expectancy, previous opioid exposure, pain type, and location of pain, among other variables. Unlike for the management of nonmalignant pain, the Polyanalgesic Consensus Conference supports the use of opioid-bupivacaine combinations as first-line IDD therapy for the management of cancer pain [262]. When multiple medications are used in combination, however, stability of the admixture, priming bolus errors, and permeability of medications into the pump rotor resulting in corrosion and premature pump failure become concerns [267–269]. Once the decision to pursue IDD has been made and a medication or admixture has been chosen, catheter tip location and drug concentration need to be decided upon.

The catheter tip is ideally placed at the spinal level corresponding to the area of greatest pain. Studies of CSF fluid dynamics demonstrate little laminar flow within the spinal canal, contrary to what was previously theorized [270]. Instead, CSF flow is pulsatile, with oscillatory displacements creating eddy micro-currents but minimal net bulk flow [271]. Essentially, CSF radiates away from a source of disruption, much like water in a pond rippling away from an invading pebble. Physiologically, the source of disruption is a change in intrathoracic pressure (with heart rate, stroke volume, or respiratory cycle), intra-abdominal pressure (Valsalva), or spinal motion. In the presence of an IDD catheter, flow of medication produces ripples of CSF in all directions away from the tip, creating a concentration gradient across relatively few spinal levels. Factors influencing the degree of medication distribution within the CSF remain incompletely understood, but include anatomic variation (including pathoanatomic changes, such as in spinal stenosis or scoliosis), postural changes, drug solution density, binding characteristics of drugs at the dorsal horn, CSF volume, and variations in physiologic CSF flow [272–274].

Dose can be estimated based on the patient's current opioid requirement and level of pain control. Choosing an appropriate concentration will allow rapid dose titration without creating the need for unnecessarily frequent refill appointments. Concentration is limited by drug solubility, as precipitation has been shown to damage to the pump tubing, eventually resulting in corrosion of the pump mechanism and early malfunction of the device [275]. A medication's solubility changes based on the presence of other molecules in solution, which explains the previously mentioned risk of hardware corrosion seen in pumps containing medication admixtures. Additionally, delivery of highly concentrated intrathecal opioids, especially morphine, at a slow rate increases the risk of catheter tip granuloma [276]. These noninflammatory masses obstruct the delivery of medication, rendering the IDD system ineffective, and can cause mass effect on the nearby neural structures. The risk of catheter tip granuloma formation also plays into determination of the level at which the catheter tip should be placed, as some advocate placement of the tip below the conus medullaris to reduce the risk of adhesion to the spinal cord parenchyma, which can require an extensive, complicated resection [277].

Along with the benefits offered by IDD come substantial risks that must be reconciled when choosing this approach to symptom management. Risks of IDD can be broken down into three categories: procedural risks, device complications, and patient risks. Procedural risks include those related to general anesthesia, those related to holding anticoagulation, pocket infections, catheter infections, bleeding, neurologic injury, and persistent CSF leaks. Device-related complications include any number of causes of premature pump failure but, overwhelmingly, involve the catheter. Catheters can migrate out of the subarachnoid space, kink, tear, become entangled with the nerve roots, or develop tip granulomas. Patient risks include noncompliance with pump refill appointments resulting in withdrawal from medication and potential damage to the pump. Consequences of withdrawal range from harmless (ziconotide) to unpleasant (opioids) to life-threatening (clonidine and baclofen) [278–280]. Education regarding the early signs of withdrawal should be discussed at each visit. When intrathecal baclofen is utilized, it is important to provide oral baclofen to be taken at the first signs of withdrawal. It is also beneficial to periodically activate both the critical and noncritical alarms for the patient while in the clinic, so they are aware of what to listen for if something is amiss. Fortunately, patient-related risks can be minimized through appropriate patient selection and is one reason why psychological clearance is mandatory prior to implant.

Vertebral Augmentation

Vertebroplasty and kyphoplasty are image-guided percutaneous techniques used in the treatment of insufficiency and pathologic fractures of the vertebral body. They differ in that kyphoplasty uses a balloon tamponade to create a void in the bone prior to injection of the bone cement poly methyl methacrylate (PMMA). Spinal metastases occur in up to 40% of patients with cancer, most commonly from a primary lesion in the breast, lung, prostate or kidney, or multiple myeloma [281]. Each year, 5% of cancer patients will develop spinal metastases. These patients are commonly in the advanced stages of their disease with a median survival of less than a year, so conservative treatment options are limited and, unfortunately, often provide suboptimal results [282, 283]. Therefore, the goals of vertebral augmentation are primarily palliative and include pain reduction, functional optimization, mechanical fracture stabilization, and, to whatever extent possible, restoration of vertebral body height. The latter helps minimize the development of central or foraminal stenosis and their associated neurologic deficits, including paraplegia. Added benefits of these procedures are that, once access to the vertebral body is achieved, spine biopsies can be taken to confirm the primary diagnosis and cooled radiofrequency ablation of the tumor can be performed for additional pain management.

While surgical options can improve pain and stabilize vertebral compression fractures, many patients with end-stage disease are reluctant to pursue extensive surgery. Vertebral augmentation with or without radiofrequency ablation offers these patients safe and effective alternatives to surgery [284–288]. Complications are infrequent and often minor, but major complications occur at a rate of 1–2% [289]. Most complications result from cement extravasation. Published rates of cement extravasation vary widely, but the risk has been shown to increase with injection of cement volumes greater than 4 mL [283, 290]. Although most cement leaks are clinically insignificant, the potential for severe neurologic and cardiorespiratory compromise exists with extravasation of PMMA into the central canal, neural foramen, vasculature, or pleural cavity. Kyphoplasty theoretically reduces the risk of cement extravasation by establishing a cavity into which PMMA can be injected under relatively low pressure, but there is no evidence that kyphoplasty provides a superior safety or efficacy profile versus vertebroplasty in the management of pathologic vertebral compression fractures. Other procedural risks include bleeding, infection, fracture, fat emboli, radiculopathy, and hypotension [291]. An increased incidence of both remote and adjacent level fractures has been noted after cement augmentation of an index lesion [292]. Alterations in spine biomechanics are the most likely explanation for this finding, but a definitive causal relationship has not been established.

Tumor Ablation and Sacroplasty

Tumor ablation is an alternative to surgical resection that uses computed tomography or magnetic resonance guidance for percutaneous radiofrequency, microwave, and cryo- or chemical ablation of tumor cells. It is most effective for primary or secondary tumors involving the lung, thyroid, bone, liver, and kidney [293–297]. The risks are procedure- and site-specific but also include risks from procedural sedation, often general anesthesia. These techniques offer the possibility for complete destruction of the tumor, however, making them viable alternatives in properly selected patients. Sacroplasty is a procedure quite similar to vertebral augmentation in which PMMA is used to stabilize insufficiency or pathologic fractures of the sacrum. This technique has been incorporated into evidence-based treatment algorithms for sacroiliac tumors [189]. Unlike the evidence supporting the use of kyphoplasty for pathologic vertebral fractures, however, the evidence for the role of sacroplasty for pathologic sacral fractures is of low quality, including only case reports and small case series to date [189, 298–303]. Despite the lack of high-quality evidence, the safety of the procedure warrants its consideration for treatment-refractory cases.

Cordotomy

Percutaneous cordotomy involves CT-guided radiofrequency thermocoagulation of the lateral spinothalamic tract, which carries pain and temperature sensation from the contralateral extremities and trunk, in the upper cervical spinal cord. The lateral spinothalamic tract is organized such that selective lesioning of fibers from a single extremity is possible when using appropriate myelographic confirmation, impedance measurements, and sensory-motor dissociation testing. The procedure can provide complete resolution of pain in the affected extremity [304]. The most common complication is a headache in a C2 dermatomal distribution [305]. Other complications include transient motor weakness or dysesthesias, bleeding, infection, sensorimotor changes from inadvertent injury to neighboring spinal tracts, bowel or bladder dysfunction, hypotension, and Horner's syndrome. Bilateral procedures, especially those done using an open surgical approach without sensory testing, are not recommended as accidental involvement of the neighboring reticulospinal tract can disrupt their role in sustaining subconscious respiratory drive, resulting in sleep-induced respiratory arrest (Ondine's curse) and death [306]. Overall, however, cordotomy is felt to be a safe procedure, with the risk of major complications being less than 1% [307].

Destruction of Trigeminal Pathways

Trigeminal tractotomy/nucleotomy involves destruction of descending trigeminal nerve fibers in the medulla (tractotomy) or nucleus caudalis (nucleotomy) at the occipitocervical level. Alternatively, nucleus caudalis dorsal root entry zone (DREZ) lesioning involves destruction of the entire substantia gelatinosa along the rostral-caudal extent of the nucleus caudalis [308, 309]. Pain fibers from cranial nerves VII, IX, and X descend with the spinal tract of the trigeminal nerve into the upper cervical cord. Reliable topographic localization of cranial nerve nociceptive fibers in this region makes it an attractive target for intervention. Destruction of these tracts can be used to relieve dysesthetic, neurogenic, or deafferentation types of craniofacial pain, including pain from cancers of the head and neck; glossopharyngeal, vagal, and geniculate neuralgias; postherpetic neuralgias; and atypical forms of trigeminal neuralgia, including anesthesia dolorosa following neurolysis [309]. The first description of these procedures appeared in the 1930s and stereotactic radiofrequency denervation was first described in the early 1970s [310–312]. In large case series, as many as 85% of patients with pain from craniofacial malignancies responded favorably to one or more of these procedures [306, 309, 313, 314]. The most important complication is ataxia, which is caused by lesioning of the adjacent dorsal spinocerebellar tract and is most often transient [313]. The authors of the largest case series to date opined that, in light of its efficacy and safety, CT-guided trigeminal tractotomy, nucleotomy, and nucleus caudalis DREZ lesioning should be considered early in the treatment of refractory facial pain [314].

Myelotomy

Extralemniscal myelotomy involves stereotactic lesioning of the central canal at the occiput-C1 level. Experience with this procedure dating back to 1968 suggests efficacy in relieving pain in the upper extremities, lower extremities, and trunk, including visceral pain, pain in the anatomic midline, and even central pain [306]. Schvarcz is credited for coining the term in 1977 [315]. His stated goal with the approach was interruption of a nonspecific, extralemniscal, polysynaptic ascending system. Al-Chaer posited that interruption of dorsal column fibers may "tip the balance" away from pain perception [316]. This explanation accounted for what was seen clinically – pain relief without significant sensory loss. Another theory claims that a pathway responsible for transmitting visceral pain exists in the dorsal funiculus and that destruction of this pathway disrupts "extensive cross-connections within the propriospinal system" therein [317]. The true mechanism remains unclear. Following success of the procedure when performed in the upper cervical cord, others reported lesioning of the central cord at various thoracic levels, with good results [318, 319]. Given the unclear mechanism of pain relief and the low methodological quality of available data, only procedures in the upper cervical cord can be recommended currently. The ideal candidates for the procedure are patients with intractable visceral pain due to pelvic or abdominal malignancies, including gastric, pancreatic, renal, colon, and rectal carcinomas. Reported efficacy in the available case studies and case series is significantly less than with previously discussed procedures, but complications were rare and included transient hypoesthesia [306].

Neurostimulatory Approaches

Clinically relevant since antiquity, neuromodulation is now the most rapidly evolving field within the entire subspecialty of pain management. Despite significant growth of the field, however, evidence of these techniques for the management of oncologic pain is sparse.

Transcutaneous Stimulation

The most common approach to neuromodulation, transcutaneous electrical nerve stimulation (TENS), is inexpensive, noninvasive, safe, and simple to use. Although the efficacy of TENS for the management of cancer pain has been challenged, there is some evidence that TENS can be an effective nonpharmacologic adjunct in properly selected patients with pain of oncologic origin [320–323]. Cancer-related fatigue and lymphedema as well as chemotherapy-induced myelosuppression, peripheral neuropathy, and nausea/vomiting also have some evidence of improvement with the use of transcutaneous stimulation [324–328]. Studies of Calmare scrambler therapy found treatment to be associated with significantly decreased NRS pain scores, as well as reduced rescue opioid requirements in patients with chemotherapy-induced peripheral neuropathy, metastatic bone pain, and postsurgical neuropathic pain [329–331]. A phase 2 study of acupuncture-like TENS for chemotherapy-induced peripheral neuropathy revealed significant improvement in neuropathy scores at 6 months, although a subsequent study revealed worse outcomes than with sham acupuncture-like TENS at 12 weeks [327, 332].

Relative contraindications to the use of transcutaneous electrical therapy include use over broken or dysesthetic skin, use over implantable devices such as pacemakers, and the theoretical risk of worsening lymphedema, although the latter has been challenged [325]. While the application of transcutaneous stimulation has changed little over time, interest in waveform manipulation has grown across the field, resulting in the recent emergence of devices capable of producing kilohertz frequency stimulation. Preclinical data investigating the use of these devices suggest efficacy in managing neuropathic pain of non-oncologic origin, but clinical trials are lacking [333].

Dorsal Column Stimulation

Dr. C. Norman Shealy, a neurosurgeon in Wisconsin, is credited with implanting the first dorsal column stimulator when he sutured a vitallium electrode to the dura of a man with terminal metastatic bronchogenic carcinoma in 1967 [334]. Trial stimulation abolished pain for 36 hours following implant, spawning intense interest in the technology across all areas of pain management. Although high-quality data supporting its use in malignant pain are lacking, case series- and case report-level data support its use in various malignant pain states [335, 336]. Recent mitigation of MRI compatibility issues removes a significant barrier to the use of this technology in the cancer population. Emergence of paresthesia-free stimulation paradigms has made possible conduction of studies with more rigorous study designs, including blinded, randomized, placebo-controlled trials.

Charging requirements, as well as device and implantation-related complications including infection, bleeding, dural puncture/tear, lead migration, and positional changes in stimulation, limits the use of dorsal column stimulation. These issues, too, are improving as device technology and implantation techniques are refined. Obligatory cessation of anticoagulation for the duration of the trial can be especially problematic in the cancer population. No data exist to guide trial duration, but clinical experience suggests the risk of a false-positive response to stimulation after a 48- to 72-hour trial is probably low, so an abbreviated trial may be considered.

Dorsal Root Ganglion Stimulation

Similar in application to dorsal column stimulation, dorsal root ganglion (DRG) stimulation has been introduced as a more targeted neuromodulation technique. While improved target specificity is intriguing, no evidence exists of its successful application in the cancer population. Currently, DRG stimulation is limited by the same concerns for MRI compatibility and device- and procedure-related complications that early dorsal column stimulation systems were.

Peripheral Nerve Stimulation

Introduced prior to dorsal column stimulation in the mid-1960s, early application of this technology required highly invasive, risky surgical implantation of electrodes on or around the target nerve and quickly fell out of vogue as percutaneous or minimally invasive dorsal column stimulation techniques grew in popularity [337, 338]. It experienced resurgence when spinal cord stimulation hardware was applied peripherally in the management of refractory neuropathies of the head and neck [339, 340]. More recently, dedicated peripheral nerve stimulators have been introduced and are credited with renewed interest in this approach to neuromodulation [341, 342].

These newer systems feature small, percutaneously implantable electrodes designed with features to reduce the risk of migration and infection. They are powered percutaneously or transcutaneously by small, efficient energy sources that can be worn inconspicuously under clothing for all-day use. Associated with less morbidity than surgically implanted devices, these devices can be utilized earlier in the treatment algorithm and may be more appropriate for medically complex cancer pain patients. Required time off anticoagulation is minimal. They are less costly than devices utilizing implanted pulse generators and are not limited by cutaneous pain receptor activation as are inexpensive transcutaneous stimulation systems. While fully implanted options must contend with issues of MRI compatibility, temporary percutaneous devices can be quickly and safely removed if the need for imaging arises. Despite these theoretical benefits, high-quality data supporting the use of this technology in the management of malignant pain are lacking.

Peripheral Nerve Field Stimulation

Introduced following the success of craniofacial peripheral nerve stimulation, this technology was designed to overcome the electrical diffusion barrier provided by the skin and superficial soft tissues. Clinically, it has been used in the treatment of axial low-back pain, which tonic dorsal column stimulation often fails to adequately treat, and abdominal/pelvic pain that is not confined to an identifiable peripheral nerve distribution [343, 344]. The evidence supporting application of this technology in the management of malignant pain consists of a single case study [345]. In their report, the authors present a case in which a patient with intractable radiation-induced neuropathic pain following treatment for laryngeal cancer achieved complete resolution of pain following implantation of bilateral subcutaneous facial electrodes. Given the paucity of evidence supporting its use and the emergence and refinement of DRG stimulation, peripheral nerve field stimulation is unlikely to gain significant popularity in the management of malignant pain.

Physical Modalities

Cancer and its treatments are physically, mentally, emotionally, and socially disabling. Physical activity, whether freelance, as part of a regimented exercise prescription or performed under the direct supervision of a physical therapist or personal trainer, is unique in its potential to improve all aspects of a patient's life.

Exercise

In the most recent edition of *Physical Activity Guidelines for Americans*, the US Department of Health and Human Services recommends healthy adults participate in 150 minutes of moderate or 75 minutes of vigorous aerobic activity weekly, as well as muscle-strengthening exercises on two or more days per week [346]. Similarly, recommendations for physical activity in cancer survivors include both aerobic activity and strength training [347]. Evidence supports the physical, mental, and social health benefits of exercise in mitigating the negative effects of treatment for many types of cancer [348–357]. Strength training, specifically, has been linked to improvements in treatment-related side effects, lymphedema, and muscle wasting in patients with breast and prostate cancers and may even be associated with reduced cancer mortality [353–355, 357–359]. A series of Cochrane reviews further support the benefits of regular activity in patients at various stages of multiple types of cancer [350–352, 360, 361]. Compliance with exercise guideline recommendations, however, has been shown to be low in cancer patients of both sexes, with the odds of female cancer survivors meeting activity guideline minimums lower than that of their peers without a history of cancer [362]. A 2013 Cochrane review investigated various interventions aimed at promoting exercise in sedentary cancer patients [363]. The authors found that interventions which resulted in greater levels of adherence utilized one or more common behavior-modifying techniques, including goal setting, prompting practice, self-monitoring, and encouraging participants to apply behaviors learned in supervised exercise environments to unsupervised contexts. Ultimately, however, the authors conceded that expecting most sedentary cancer patients to achieve 150 minutes per week of aerobic exercise is unrealistic. As in the general population, reasons for cancer patients' noncompliance with an exercise prescription are innumerable. Fear of exacerbating disease- or treatment-related pain and concern over causing structural damage are some of the most common. These fears, however, are unfounded and must be overcome before patients suffering with malignant pain can reap the full benefits of physical activity [364, 365].

Physical Therapy

The role of physical therapy in the management of patients with malignant pain is broad and can include development and oversight of a strengthening and stretching program, functional training, manual therapies, lymphedema therapy, vestibular therapy, wound care, orthotic management, gait and balance training, proprioceptive neuromuscular facilitation, assistive device evaluation and maintenance, caregiver education, and application of modalities such as ultrasound, electrical stimulation, kinesiotaping, dry needling, and phono- or iontophoresis, among others. While there is a great deal of data supporting the benefits of various therapeutic modalities on quality of life in patients with cancer, the evidence supporting its role in pain reduction is less robust [366–375].

Myofascial therapy was recently shown to be effective at decreasing arm pain in breast cancer survivors, but previous data published by the same group were less optimistic [376, 377]. A systematic review investigating the use of photobiomodulation (laser therapy) for lymphedema in breast cancer patients found strong evidence of its benefit in reducing limb circumference, but only moderate evidence for pain relief [378]. A small but well-designed study of breast cancer survivors with shoulder and arm pain found that VAS scores decreased after a single session of myofascial induction therapy to a significantly greater degree than after placebo electrotherapy [379]. Kinesiotaping was found to be associated with reduced levels of thoracic wall pain in the immediate postoperative period following lung lobectomy [380]. NRS pain scores were also significantly reduced after 4 weeks of physical therapy, with or without manual lymphatic drainage, in a cohort of breast cancer patients with axillary web syndrome [369]. Despite these potential benefits, over two thirds of patients with late-stage cancer associated with high levels of disability and related distress reported no interest in receiving rehabilitation services [370]. The authors concluded that patient misconceptions regarding the role of rehabilitation may be a barrier to improved pain control, function, and quality of life in this cohort.

Psychological Approaches

In women with early breast cancer, the prevalence of a diagnosable mood disorder in the year following diagnosis approaches double that of the general female population [381]. At each stage of disease, emotional distress negatively affects quality of life and comorbid depression has even been associated with decreased survival in multiple studies [82, 382–385]. The influence of psychological factors in the development, persistence, and treatment of chronic pain has also been established [386–388]. Although there is evidence that appropriate management of depression might be associated with improved cancer treatment outcomes, recent data has questioned this finding [389–393]. Regardless of the survival benefits, given the impact of comorbid psychiatric disease on the quality of life and experience of pain in cancer patients, the importance of understanding the role of psychological interventions cannot be understated.

Cognitive Behavioral Therapy

A class of short-term, multidimensional approaches to managing emotional and physical issues, cognitive behavioral therapy focuses on changing the cognitive precursors of a behavior [394–396]. When used in the management of pain, cognitive behavioral therapy focuses on changing the way a person thinks about and interprets pain to re-structure its perceived cause, meaning, and effects of treatment [394]. Cognitive behavioral therapy has proven valuable in relieving pain in various cancer populations, including multiple myeloma, lymphoma, and solid tumors of the breast, ovaries, prostate, colon, cervix, and lung [397–399]. It is theorized to work by altering the conceptualization of pain, increasing tolerance to pain, regulating the emotional response to pain, and diverting attention from pain [396]. Techniques with evidence of efficacy in the management of cancer pain include activity pacing, contingency management, behavioral activation, cognitive/attentional distraction, cognitive restructuring, goal setting, imagery, pleasant activity scheduling, hypnosis, meditation, role playing, modeling, problem solving, biofeedback, systematic, relaxation training, visualization, desensitization, and assertiveness/communication training [400]. High-quality efficacy data, however, is lacking. Current practice guidelines suggest that cognitive behavioral methods might help to lower opioid requirements in the cancer population, so given its safety, it should have a role in the multidisciplinary approach to cancer pain management [398].

Mindfulness-Based Techniques

Mindfulness-based intervention, likewise, can be used safely and effectively in the management of pain. Mindfulness-based stress reduction and mindfulness-based cognitive therapy have proven effective in diverse pain populations, including women undergoing treatment for breast cancer [401–403]. Mindfulness-based intervention is proposed to improve the experience of pain by multiple mechanisms. First, by fostering openness and acceptance, patients are taught to uncouple the sensation of pain from the affective and cognitive experience of pain [404]. By encouraging self-compassion, mindfulness-based interventions help patients respond to painful thoughts and feelings with self-kindness, acknowledging distressing situations without avoidance or overidentification [405]. Finally, pain catastrophizing, which has been shown to be predictive of the pain experience [406], can be effectively reduced with mindfulness-based techniques [407]. While traditionally assumed to target the negative impact of pain rather than the painful sensation itself, a recent randomized controlled trial revealed a statistically significant effect of mindfulness-based intervention on pain intensity [408]. Moreover, the beneficial effects of mindfulness-based techniques were sustained for several weeks after completion of training [409].

Complementary and Alternative Therapies

Complementary and alternative therapy is defined as a medical system, practice, or product that is not part of conventional medical care and encompasses "complementary medicine" or therapies used alongside conventional medicine, "alternative medicine," or therapies used in place of conventional medicine and "integrative medicine" which refers to coordinated use of evidence-based complementary practices and conventional care [410]. Integrative medicine is the approach employed by leading multidisciplinary cancer pain management centers worldwide to enhance wellness, improve quality of life, and relieve symptoms of disease or side effects of conventional treatment [411]. The number of integrative oncology programs at top institutions has grown exponentially as data has emerged regarding the clinical utility of such services [412]. The Society for Integrative Oncology published clinical practice guidelines in 2014, which were recently updated, to inform patients and providers about the appropriate use of integrative therapies during cancer treatment [411, 413]. Using United States Preventive Services Task Force methods, they sought to provide graded recommendations on the use of specific integrative therapies for defined clinical indications based on the strength of available evidence [414]. Unfortunately, the data remained insufficient to make recommendations for or against the use of specific modalities in most cases [411].

Acupuncture

Acupuncture involves the placement of fine-gauge solid metallic needles at specific points, with or without mechanical or electrical stimulation, to stimulate the flow of a form of energy called "qi" [415]. In the oncology population, acupuncture is a popular modality for the treatment of chemotherapy-induced nausea and vomiting, musculoskeletal complaints, hot flashes, fatigue, stress, anxiety, and sleep disorders in addition to pain [411, 415]. One trial assessed acupuncture for pain after tumor resection surgery and found a small positive effect [416]. Five trials have evaluated the use of acupuncture for musculoskeletal pain related to the use of aromatase inhibitors, but all were small, and their results were conflicting [417–421]. Similarly, a 2015 Cochrane review found conflicting evidence and a high risk of bias in their evaluation of five trials which enrolled a total of 285 participants with cancer-associated pain [422]. The authors were, ultimately, unable to judge whether acupuncture is effective in treating cancer pain. A 2016 systematic review and meta-analysis looking at data from 20 randomized controlled trials enrolling patient with malignant pain found that acupuncture plus pharmacologic therapy resulted in greater immediate pain relief, longer pain remission, and improved quality of life than pharmacologic therapy alone, but the risk of bias in the included studies was high and the quality of the data was low [423]. The 2017 Society for Integrative Oncology practice guidelines found the data supporting the use of acupuncture to treat a variety of cancer-related pain states to be of low quality (grade C, indicating that the evidence is equivocal or that there is at least moderate certainty that the net benefit is small) [411].

Though questionably effective, acupuncture is safe. Two large studies including over 300,000 patients revealed the most common side effects to be local pain, bruising, minor bleeding, and orthostatic hypotension [424, 425]. Serious side effects, or those requiring intervention, are rare [425]. Use in the oncology population presents unique challenges, however, and is best performed with knowledge of the patient's underlying disease state and most recent blood counts. Despite the risks, acupuncture is contraindicated only for patients with cutaneous lesions (infectious or malignant) overlying the anticipated site of needle insertion, thrombocytopenia, or neutropenia [412]. Placement of needles through lymphedematous areas, in theory, increases risk for infection, but no data exist to compel avoidance of this modality in patients with lymphedema. Given its long track record of safety, potential for efficacy, and proven utility treating other symptoms associated with cancer and its treatment, acupuncture remains one of the most commonly utilized integrative medicine approaches for the management of malignant pain.

Manual Therapies

Healing touch is a therapeutic modality based on the presence of a vital energy, which practitioners attempt to influence with the goal of restoring balance and harmony in the patient's energy system to promote self-healing. Practitioners use touch in a manner that is "heart-centered and intentional" to clear, energize, and balance the human and environmental energy fields in an attempt to improve physical, mental, emotional, and spiritual health" [426]. A single large clinical trial assessed, as a secondary outcome, the effects of healing touch on pain after chemotherapy and found a small positive effect of the therapy [427].

More traditional forms of massage include Swedish, Shiatsu, and deep-tissue, among others. Each is intended to meet slightly different goals but, in general, massage aims to relieve pain by promoting relaxation, increasing blood and lymph flow, aiding muscle relaxation, and soothing nerves [428]. Massage techniques utilizing light to medium pressure are often most appropriate in the oncology setting, where bony or soft tissue metastases, radiation-induced dermatitis, and chemotherapy-induced peripheral neuropathy can interfere with the therapeutic benefits of touch. In appropriately selected patients, however, massage therapy may help mitigate pain, anxiety, depression, constipation, and high blood pressure [429]. There is even some data suggesting that massage may promote immune system function, making it especially beneficial during periods of profound immune suppression, when other treatment modalities are contraindicated [430].

Efficacy data on the use of massage for the management of pain in patients with cancer is conflicting. A 2015 systematic review and meta-analysis by Lee et al. reviewed data from 12 studies including 559 participants [431]. Nine of the included studies were considered to be of high-quality based on the PEDro scale [432]. From this data, the authors observed that massage therapy significantly reduced cancer pain compared with conventional care. Among the various massage techniques, reflexology appeared to be more effective than body massage with or without aromatherapy. A 2016 Cochrane review found 19 studies investigating massage with or without aromatherapy for the management of cancer-associated pain [433]. Their data suggested that massage was beneficial for short-term pain relief, but, unlike Lee et al., these authors found the data to be of very low quality. While statistically significant, data regarding relief of medium- to long-term pain was not felt to be clinically significant and was similarly limited by poor methodologic quality. Recommendations regarding clinical applicability, therefore, could not be made, and the authors concluded a lack of evidence regarding the clinical effectiveness of massage for pain relief in people with cancer. A more recent pilot study suggests that massage, in combination with aromather-apy, significantly reduces the incidence of peripheral neuropathy in patients undergoing oxaliplatin-based chemotherapy regimens [434]. In another recent study, massage therapy was associated with statistically and clinically significant improvements in pain as well as fatigue, anxiety, well-being, and sleep in patients undergoing active cancer treatment [435].

Like many of the complementary and alternative treatment approaches discussed herein, manual therapies are felt to be quite safe. Although data regarding the risks of these modalities is sparse, the two studies featured in the Cochrane review which reported side effects listed only physical distress, rash, and general malaise as adverse reactions of treatment [436, 437].

Yoga/Qigong

Yoga is a mind-body practice derived from ancient South Asian philosophy, the objective of which is to unite the individual with the entirety of the universe [438]. It can be offered as a group class or delivered in a focused one-on-one program with a yoga therapist. Programs are made available to all patients through modification of postures to meet an individual's limitations. Qigong, a form of traditional Chinese medicine, integrates movement, meditation, and controlled breathing to enhance vital energy and balance a patient's mental, physical, spiritual, and emotional well-being [411]. Each can be practiced in a variety of forms and are often used in the oncology setting to reduce stress, anxiety, and fatigue; improve physical, emotional, and spiritual balance; enhance quality of life; improve treatment efficacy and compliance; and restore social function [439–446].

Data supporting these modalities in the management of cancer-related pain, however, are sparse. A single large, randomized, controlled trial examining the efficacy of yoga for treating musculoskeletal complaints among breast cancer survivors was identified [447]. Participants in this study randomized to the yoga intervention demonstrated greater reductions in general pain, muscle aches, and total physical discomfort than participants in the wait-list control group. A smaller feasibility and preliminary efficacy study in patients having been treated for head and neck cancer found that those participating in yoga had a significantly greater decrease in pain and pain interference than wait-list controls [448].

The safety of these interventions has been well established. Multiple studies investigating the benefits of yoga for nonpainful cancer-related symptoms reported safety data [449–453]. Reported side effects include only transient arthralgias and myalgias. All adverse events were minor and, in studies employing active controls, occurred at similar rates between groups. Similarly, the feasibility study mentioned previously reported no adverse events in any of their study subjects [448]. Given the safety, availability, wide applicability, and potential efficacy, it is reasonable to incorporate yoga and qigong into a multimodal cancer pain treatment program.

Hypnosis

The use of hypnosis in cancer treatment dates back to the 1800s, at which time it was referred to as "magnetic sleep" [454]. The modality is characterized by a trance-like state which facilitates awareness and focus while allowing a patient to be more open to suggestion by functionally disconnecting the decision-making centers of the prefrontal cortex from the attentional/motivational centers of the anterior cingulate gyrus [455, 456]. Functional neuroimaging suggests that hypnosis modulates pain perception by altering activity within multiple brain regions involved in pain processing, including the somatosensory cortex [457]. There is evidence supporting its use in several chronic pain conditions, and hypnosis has been shown to help relieve stress, anxiety, fatigue, generalized suffering, and pain in patients with cancer [458–462]. A common approach for patients with cancer involves confronting disease-related stressors while dissociating the experience from somatic arousal [463].

Early trials assessing hypnosis for pain after tumor resection surgery showed small positive effects favoring the therapy [461, 464]. More recent data further support its use in a variety of malignant pain states, including pancreatic, colonic, breast, brain, and GYN cancers, soft tissue sarcomas, leukemia, and lymphoma [459, 465–467]. A small randomized, controlled, clinical trial comparing hypnosis plus cognitive behavioral therapy with education controls in the domains of pain intensity, pain interference, pain catastrophizing, depression, and cancer treatment distress reported significantly greater improvement in all outcomes following treatment relative to controls [466]. Benefits of treatment were maintained at 3-month follow-up. A recent clinical trial assessing early integration of hypnosis in palliative care enrolled 13 end-stage oncology patients [467]. The authors found hypnosis to be associated with a statistically significant decrease in pain and anxiety, as well as the need to escalate pharmacologic analgesia, compared to controls. They concluded that hypnosis is an effective adjuvant therapy for pain control in cancer patients receiving palliative care. Another study compared breast cancer patients undergoing breast surgery under general anesthesia versus hypnosis sedation and found significantly reduced lengths of hospital stay, anxiety, nausea, vomiting, arthralgias, and myalgias in the hypnosis group [468]. Of patients who then went on to receive adjuvant therapy, those in the hypnosis group experienced fewer treatment-related side effects, including asthenia during chemotherapy, radiodermatitis, post-radiotherapy

asthenia, and hot flashes. The authors concluded that hypnosis provides beneficial effects on nearly all modalities of breast cancer treatment.

Medical Marijuana

Use of medical marijuana is gaining popularity, especially within the oncologic population, based on anecdotal evidence of effect in managing a host of cancer- and treatment-related symptoms. As political attitudes shift toward greater acceptance and jurisdictions pass regulations allowing medicinal or recreational cannabis use, access and availability continues to increase. Although synthetic analogues of the main active component of marijuana, delta(Δ)9-tetrahydrocannabinol (THC), have been commercially available for quite some time, the use of unregulated inhaled, sublingual, or edible versions has become increasingly prevalent [469]. In the 2014–15 National Survey on Drug Use and Health, 9.8% of respondents reported using illicit marijuana in the past month for medical reasons [470]. A study of adult cancer patients utilizing survey data with urine test verification suggests that use in the adult oncology population is significantly greater [471].

Evidence exists regarding the potential benefits of marijuana in the management of cancer-related pain, nausea/vomiting, anorexia, weight loss, and insomnia, but the strength of the evidence is poor [472–474]. A 2016 retrospective study supported marijuana's ability to decrease opioid use and medication side effects as well as improve quality of life in patients with chronic pain [475]. A meta-analysis of five RCTs suggested that cannabis use results in short-term reductions in chronic neuropathic pain with a number needed to treat rivaling that of gabapentin [476]. Neither of these studies included oncology patients. A review of five studies investigating the use of various doses and formulations of THC with or without cannabidiol (CBD) in cancer pain concluded that medical cannabis has a potential role in cancer pain management but that the data supporting this conclusion is of "limited" quality [474]. Nabiximols (THC/CBD oromucosal spray) has been studied extensively in the cancer pain population, with varying results. An early multicenter, double-blinded, randomized, placebo-controlled trial showed that subjects given nabiximols were statistically more likely to achieve 30% reduction in their pain than controls or patients using THC alone after 2 weeks [477]. This result was disputed by the results of a series of methodologically rigorous trials, which showed no statistical difference in pain relief between trial and control patients [478, 479]. In all studies, the incidence of adverse effects, including nausea, vomiting, somnolence, and dizziness, was greater in patients receiving the study drug [477–479].

Although the short-term adverse effects of inhaled marijuana have been well described, insufficient data exist to adequately inform cancer patients of the potential long-term risks of medical marijuana use [480]. Each of the studies included in Blake et al.'s recent review reported side effects of medical cannabis use, although statistical evaluation of the prevalence of these effects was inconsistent [474]. The most common side effects included nausea, drowsiness, dizziness, slurred speech, blurred vision, dry mouth, and mental clouding. These seemed to occur in a dose-dependent manner [477, 478, 481, 482]. The reviewers noted, however, that side effects did not lead to discontinuation of any study participants [474].

Physical and psychological effects of chronic use, drug-drug and drug-disease interactions, quality control uncertainties, and the potential for conflict with federal regulations remain barriers to widespread study and use of this potential treatment modality. Research efforts continue, but for now, evidence is insufficient to guide clinical practice.

Conclusion

Pain is a common experience among patients with cancer and contributes significantly to the suffering and poor quality of life reported in this population. Effective management requires accurate diagnosis, application of a multimodal treatment plan inclusive of complementary/integrative therapies, timely application of interventional modalities, and prompt subspecialist consultation when required. This is best accomplished by a multidisciplinary care team composed of practitioners skilled and experienced in applying their craft to the care of patients with cancer pain. While safety is paramount, the time-sensitive nature of the diagnosis often requires rapid escalation of treatment should initial measures prove ineffective. An aggressive approach, however, must be balanced with concerns for sustainability, as advanced disease management options will continue to create chronic conditions of diagnoses which were previously imminently terminal. Through a team-based, patient-centric approach, pain becomes a manageable symptom of cancer and its treatment.

References

1. Vendrell I, Macedo D, Alho I, Dionísio MR, Costa L. Treatment of cancer pain by targeting cytokines. Mediat Inflamm. 2015;2015:984570.
2. Mantyh PW, Clohisy DR, Koltzenburg M, Hunt SP. Molecular mechanisms of cancer pain. Nat Rev Cancer. 2002;2(3):201–9.
3. Portenoy RK. Treatment of cancer pain. Lancet. 2011;377(9784):2236–47.
4. Haumann J, Joosten EBA, Everdingen MHJVDB. Pain prevalence in cancer patients: status quo or opportunities for improvement? Curr Opin Support Palliat Care. 2017;11(2):99–104.
5. Centers for Medicare & Medicaid Services: Oncology Care Model; 2016. https://innovation.cms.gov/initiatives/oncology-care.
6. Loscalzo MJ. Palliative care: an historical perspective. Hematology Am Soc Hematol Educ Program. 2008;1:465.
7. Chou R, Deyo RA, Jarvik JG. Appropriate use of lumbar imaging for evaluation of low back pain. Radiol Clin N Am. 2012;50(4):569–85.
8. Cuevas C, Shibata D. Medical imaging in the diagnosis and management of cancer pain. Curr Pain Headache Rep. 2009;13(4):261–70.
9. Pillay B, Wootten AC, Crowe H, Corcoran N, Tran B, Bowden P, Crowe J, Costello AJ. The impact of multidisciplinary team meetings on patient assessment, management and outcomes in oncology settings: a systematic review of the literature. Cancer Treat Rev. 2016;42:56–72.
10. Trogdon JG, Chang Y, Shai S, Mucha PJ, Kuo TM, Meyer AM, Stitzenberg KB. Care coordination and multispecialty teams in the care of colorectal cancer patients. Med Care. 2018;56(5):430–5.
11. Licitra L, Keilholz U, Tahara M, Lin JC, Chomette P, Ceruse P, Harrington K, Mesia R. Evaluation of the benefit and use of multidisciplinary teams in the treatment of head and neck cancer. Oral Oncol. 2016;59:73–9.
12. Schnipper LE, Smith TJ, Raghavan D, et al. American Society of Clinical Oncology identifies five key opportunities to improve care and reduce costs: the top five list for oncology. J Clin Oncol. 2012;30:1715–24.
13. Marks RM, Sachar EJ. Undertreatment of medical inpatients with narcotic analgesics. Ann Intern Med. 1973;78(2):173–81.
14. World Health Organization. Cancer pain relief. Geneva: World Health Press; 1986.
15. Takeda F. The development of use of oral morphine within the last 10 years in Japan. Eur J Pain. 2001;5(Suppl A):79–82.
16. Zech DF, Grond S, Lynch J, Hertel D, Lehmann KA. Validation of World Health Organization Guidelines for cancer pain relief: a 10-year prospective study. Pain. 1995;63(1):65–76.
17. Vargas-Schaffer G. Is the WHO analgesic ladder still valid? Twenty-four years of experience. Can Fam Physician. 2010;56(6):514–7.
18. Carlson CL. Effectiveness of the World Health Organization cancer pain relief guidelines: an integrative review. J Pain Res. 2016;9:515–34.
19. Bandieri E, Romero M, Ripamonti CI, Artioli F, Sichetti D, Fanizza C, Santini D, Cavanna L, Melotti B, Conte PF, Roila F, Cascinu S, Bruera E, Tognoni G, Luppi M. Randomized trial of low-dose morphine versus weak opioids in moderate cancer pain. J Clin Oncol. 2016;34(5):436–42.
20. Fredheim OM, Brelin S, Hjermstad MJ, Loge JH, Aass N, Johannesen TB, Skurtveit S. Prescriptions of analgesics during complete disease trajectories in patients who are diagnosed with and die from cancer within the five-year period 2005–2009. Eur J Pain. 2017;21(3):530–40.
21. Brooks P, Emery P, Evans JF, Fenner H, Hawkey CJ, Patrono C, Smolen J, Breedveld F, Day R, Dougados M, Ehrich EW, Gijon-Baños J, Kvien TK, Van Rijswijk MH, Warner T, Zeidler H. Interpreting the clinical significance of the differential inhibition of cyclooxygenase-1 and cyclooxygenase-2. Rheumatology (Oxford). 1999;38(8):779–88.
22. Oniga SD, Pacureanu L, Stoica CI, Palage MD, Crăciun A, Rusu LR, Crisan EL, Araniciu C. COX inhibition profile and molecular docking studies of some 2-(trimethoxyphenyl)-thiazoles. Molecules. 2017;22(9):E1507.
23. Venkat K, Brown MD, Barkin R. Nonsteroidal anti-inflammatory drugs and gastroduodenal injury. Am J Ther. 1998;5(4):263–72.
24. Delmas PD. Non-steroidal anti-inflammatory drugs and renal function. Br J Rheumatol. 1995;34(Suppl 1):25–8.

25. Zhang J, Ding EL, Song Y. Adverse effects of cyclooxygenase 2 inhibitors on renal and arrhythmia events: meta-analysis of randomized trials. JAMA. 2006;296(13):1619–32.

26. Griswold DE, Adams JL. Constitutive cyclooxygenase (COX-1) and inducible cyclooxygenase (COX-2): rationale for selective inhibition and progress to date. Med Res Rev. 1996;16(2):181–206.

27. Mukherjee D, Nissen SE, Topol EJ. Risk of cardiovascular events associated with selective COX-2 inhibitors. JAMA. 2001; 286(8):954–9.

28. Walker C, Biasucci LM. Cardiovascular safety of non-steroidal anti-inflammatory drugs revisited. Postgrad Med. 2018;130(1): 55–71.

29. Ross JS, Krumholz HM. Bringing Vioxx back to market. BMJ. 2018;360:k242.

30. Kearney PM, Baigent C, Godwin J, Halls H, Emberson JR, Patrono C. Do selective cyclo-oxygenase-2 inhibitors and traditional non-steroidal anti-inflammatory drugs increase the risk of atherothrombosis? Meta-analysis of randomised trials. BMJ. 2006;332(7553):1302–8.

31. Constance JE, Campbell SC, Somani AA, Yellepeddi V, Owens KH, Sherwin CMT. Pharmacokinetics, pharmacodynamics and pharmacogenetics associated with nonsteroidal anti-inflammatory drugs and opioids in pediatric cancer patients. Expert Opin Drug Metab Toxicol. 2017;13(7):715–24.

32. Armstrong P, Wilkinson P, McCorry NK. Use of parecoxib by continuous subcutaneous infusion for cancer pain in a hospice population. BMJ Support Palliat Care. 2018;8(1):25–9.

33. McNicol E, Strassels SA, Goudas L, Lau J, Carr DB. NSAIDS or paracetamol, alone or combined with opioids, for cancer pain. Cochrane Database Syst Rev. 2005;1:CD005180.

34. Strawson J. Nonsteroidal anti-inflammatory drugs and cancer pain. Curr Opin Support Palliat Care. 2018;12(2):102–7.

35. Cooper TE, Heathcote LC, Anderson B, Grégoire MC, Ljungman G, Eccleston C. Non-steroidal anti-inflammatory drugs (NSAIDs) for cancer-related pain in children and adolescents. Cochrane Database Syst Rev. 2017;7:CD012563.

36. Derry S, Wiffen PJ, Moore RA, McNicol ED, Bell RF, Carr DB, McIntyre M, Wee B. Oral nonsteroidal anti-inflammatory drugs (NSAIDs) for cancer pain in adults. Cochrane Database Syst Rev. 2017;7:CD012638.

37. Hooijmans CR, Geessink FJ, Ritskes-Hoitinga M, Scheffer GJ. A systematic review and meta-analysis of the ability of analgesic drugs to reduce metastasis in experimental cancer models. Pain. 2015;156(10):1835–44.

38. Grabosch SM, Shariff OM, Helm CW. Non-steroidal anti-inflammatory agents to induce regression and prevent the progression of cervical intraepithelial neoplasia. Cochrane Database Syst Rev. 2018;2:CD004121.

39. Lu Y, Liu XF, Liu TR, Fan RF, Xu YC, Zhang XZ, Liu LL. Celecoxib exerts antitumor effects in HL-60 acute leukemia cells and inhibits autophagy by affecting lysosome function. Biomed Pharmacother. 2016;84:1551–7.

40. Lu L, Shi L, Zeng J, Wen Z. Aspirin as a potential modality for the chemoprevention of breast cancer: a dose-response meta-analysis of cohort studies from 857,831 participants. Oncotarget. 2017;8(25):40389–401.

41. Jóźwiak-Bebenista M, Nowak JZ. Paracetamol: mechanism of action, applications and safety concern. Acta Pol Pharm. 2014;71(1):11–23.

42. Alloui A, Chassaing C, Schmidt J, Ardid D, Dubray C, Cloarec A, Eschalier A. Paracetamol exerts a spinal, tropisetron-reversible, antinociceptive effect in an inflammatory pain model in rats. Eur J Pharmacol. 2002;443(1–3):71–7.

43. Bujalska M. Effect of nitric oxide synthase inhibition on antinociceptive action of different doses of acetaminophen. Pol J Pharmacol. 2004;56(5):605–10.

44. Zygmunt PM, Ermund A, Movahed P, Andersson DA, Simonsen C, Jönsson BA, Blomgren A, Birnir B, Bevan S, Eschalier A, Mallet C, Gomis A, Högestätt ED. Monoacylglycerols activate TRPV1--a link between phospholipase C and TRPV1. PLoS One. 2013;8(12):e81618.

45. Hinz B, Brune K. Paracetamol and cyclooxygenase inhibition: is there a cause for concern? Ann Rheum Dis. 2012;71(1):20–5.

46. Hinz B, Cheremina O, Brune K. Acetaminophen (paracetamol) is a selective cyclooxygenase-2 inhibitor in man. FASEB J. 2008;22(2):383–90.

47. Hinz B, Dormann H, Brune K. More pronounced inhibition of cyclooxygenase 2, increase in blood pressure, and reduction of heart rate by treatment with diclofenac compared with celecoxib and rofecoxib. Arthritis Rheum. 2006;54(1):282–91.

48. Wiffen PJ, Derry S, Moore RA, McNicol ED, Bell RF, Carr DB, McIntyre M, Wee B. Oral paracetamol (acetaminophen) for cancer pain. Cochrane Database Syst Rev. 2017;7:CD012637.

49. Israel FJ, Parker G, Charles M, Reymond L. Lack of benefit from paracetamol (acetaminophen) for palliative cancer patients requiring high-dose strong opioids: a randomized, double-blind, placebo-controlled, crossover trial. J Pain Symptom Manag. 2010;39(3):548–54.

50. Naito M, Sato T, Nakamura T, Yamanashi T, Miura H, Tsutsui A, Watanabe M. Pain management using acetaminophen throughout postoperative course of laparoscopic colorectal surgery: a case-matched control study. Ann Med Surg (Lond). 2017;17:38–42.

51. Ohkura Y, Haruta S, Shindoh J, Tanaka T, Ueno M, Udagawa H. Effectiveness of postoperative intravenous acetaminophen (Acelio) after gastrectomy: a propensity score-matched analysis. Medicine (Baltimore). 2016;95(44):e5352.

52. Artime CA, Aijazi H, Zhang H, Syed T, Cai C, Gumbert SD, Ferrario L, Normand KC, Williams GW, Hagberg CA. Scheduled intravenous acetaminophen improves patient satisfaction with postcraniotomy pain management: a prospective, randomized, placebo-controlled, double-blind study. J Neurosurg Anesthesiol. 2018;30(3):231–6.

53. Ohkura Y, Shindoh J, Ueno M, Iizuka T, Haruta S, Udagawa H. A new postoperative pain management (intravenous acetaminophen: Acelio®) leads to enhanced recovery after esophagectomy: a propensity score-matched analysis. Surg Today. 2018;48(5):502–9.

54. Amiri HR, Mirzaei M, Beig Mohammadi MT, Tavakoli F. Multi-modal preemptive analgesia with pregabalin, acetaminophen, naproxen, and dextromethorphan in radical neck dissection surgery: a randomized clinical trial. Anesth Pain Med. 2016;6(4):e33526.

55. Amiri HR, Mirzaei M, Pournaghi M, Fathi F. Three-agent preemptive analgesia, pregabalin-acetaminophen-naproxen, in laparotomy for cancer: a randomized clinical trial. Anesth Pain Med. 2016;7(2):e33269.

56. Mour G, Feinfeld DA, Caraccio T, McGuigan M. Acute renal dysfunction in acetaminophen poisoning. Ren Fail. 2005;27(4):381–3.

57. Lee WM. Acetaminophen-related acute liver failure in the United States. Hepatol Res. 2008;38(Suppl 1):S3–8.

58. Bunchorntavakul C, Reddy KR. Acetaminophen (APAP or N-acetyl-p-aminophenol) and acute liver failure. Clin Liver Dis. 2018;22(2):325–46.

59. Faria J, Barbosa J, Moreira R, Queirós O, Carvalho F, Dinis-Oliveira RJ. Comparative pharmacology and toxicology of tramadol and tapentadol. Eur J Pain. 2018;22(5):827–44.

60. Raffa RB, Buschmann H, Christoph T, Eichenbaum G, Englberger W, Flores CM, Hertrampf T, Kögel B, Schiene K, Straßburger W, Terlinden R, Tzschentke TM. Mechanistic and functional differentiation of tapentadol and tramadol. Expert Opin Pharmacother. 2012;13(10):1437–49.

61. Wiffen PJ, Derry S, Moore RA. Tramadol with or without paracetamol (acetaminophen) for cancer pain. Cochrane Database Syst Rev. 2017;5:CD012508.

62. O'Donnell JB, Ekman EF, Spalding WM, Bhadra P, McCabe D, Berger MF. The effectiveness of a weak opioid medication versus a cyclo-oxygenase-2 (COX-2) selective non-steroidal anti-

inflammatory drug in treating flare-up of chronic low-back pain: results from two randomized, double-blind, 6-week studies. J Int Med Res. 2009;37(6):1789–802.

63. Moore RA, McQuay HJ. Single-patient data meta-analysis of 3453 postoperative patients: oral tramadol versus placebo, codeine and combination analgesics. Pain. 1997;69(3):287–94.

64. Murphy DL, Lebin JA, Severtson SG, Olsen HA, Dasgupta N, Dart RC. Comparative rates of mortality and serious adverse effects among commonly prescribed opioid analgesics. Drug Saf. 2018;41(8):787–95.

65. Srinivas NR. Differential consequences of tramadol in overdosing: dilemma of a polymorphic cytochrome P450 2D6-mediated substrate. J Pain Palliat Care Pharmacother. 2015;29(3):272–5.

66. No authors listed. "Weak" opioid analgesics. Codeine, dihydrocodeine and tramadol: no less risky than morphine. Prescrire Int. 2016;25(168):45–50.

67. Vicencio-Rosas E, Pérez-Guillé MG, Flores-Pérez C, Flores-Pérez J, Trujillo-Jiménez F, Chávez-Pacheco JL. Buprenorphine and pain treatment in pediatric patients: an update. J Pain Res. 2018;11:549–59.

68. Al-Hasani R, Bruchas MR. Molecular mechanisms of opioid receptor-dependent signaling and behavior. Anesthesiology. 2011;115(6):1363–81.

69. Ondrovics M, Hoelbl-Kovacic A, Fux DA. Opioids: modulators of angiogenesis in wound healing and cancer. Oncotarget. 2017;8(15):25783–96.

70. Plein LM, Rittner HL. Opioids and the immune system - friend or foe. Br J Pharmacol. 2018;175(14):2717–25.

71. Yang Y. Cancer immunotherapy: harnessing the immune system to battle cancer. J Clin Invest. 2015;125(9):3335–7.

72. Copenhaver DJ, Karvelas NB, Fishman SM. Risk management for opioid prescribing in the treatment of patients with pain from cancer or terminal illness: inadvertent oversight or taboo? Anesth Analg. 2017;125(5):1610–5.

73. White LD, Hodge A, Vlok R, Hurtado G, Eastern K, Melhuish TM. Efficacy and adverse effects of buprenorphine in acute pain management: systematic review and meta-analysis of randomised controlled trials. Br J Anaesth. 2018;120(4):668–78.

74. Davis MP. Twelve reasons for considering buprenorphine as a frontline analgesic in the management of pain. J Support Oncol. 2012;10(6):209–19.

75. Wiffen PJ, Wee B, Derry S, Bell RF, Moore RA. Opioids for cancer pain - an overview of Cochrane reviews. Cochrane Database Syst Rev. 2017;7:CD012592.

76. Kessler ER, Shah M, Gruschkus SK, Raju A. Cost and quality implications of opioid-based postsurgical pain control using administrative claims data from a large health system: opioid-related adverse events and their impact on clinical and economic outcomes. Pharmacotherapy. 2013;33(4):383–91.

77. Paice JA, Portenoy R, Lacchetti C, Campbell T, Cheville A, Citron M, Constine LS, Cooper A, Glare P, Keefe F, Koyyalagunta L, Levy M, Miaskowski C, Otis-Green S, Sloan P, Bruera E. Management of chronic pain in survivors of adult cancers: American Society of Clinical Oncology Clinical Practice Guideline. J Clin Oncol. 2016;34(27):3325–45.

78. Beecher HK. Relationship of significance of wound to pain experienced. JAMA. 1956;161(17):1609–13.

79. Hooten WM. Chronic pain and mental health disorders: shared neural mechanisms, epidemiology, and treatment. Mayo Clin Proc. 2016;91(7):955–70.

80. Linden W, Vodermaier A, Mackenzie R, Greig D. Anxiety and depression after cancer diagnosis: prevalence rates by cancer type, gender, and age. J Affect Disord. 2012;141(2–3):343–51.

81. Wasan AD, Michna E, Edwards RR, Katz JN, Nedeljkovic SS, Dolman AJ, Janfaza D, Isaac Z, Jamison RN. Psychiatric comorbidity is associated prospectively with diminished opioid analgesia and increased opioid misuse in patients with chronic low back pain. Anesthesiology. 2015;123(4):861–72.

82. Pinquart M, Duberstein PR. Depression and cancer mortality: a meta-analysis. Psychol Med. 2010;40(11):1797–810.

83. Onghena P, Van Houdenhove B. Antidepressant-induced analgesia in chronic non-malignant pain: a meta-analysis of 39 placebo-controlled studies. Pain. 1992;49(2):205–19.

84. Fishbain DA, Cutler RB, Rosomoff HL, Rosomoff RS. Do antidepressants have an analgesic effect in psychogenic pain and somatoform pain disorder? A meta-analysis. Psychosom Med. 1998;60(4):503–9.

85. Obata H. Analgesic mechanisms of antidepressants for neuropathic pain. Int J Mol Sci. 2017;18(11):E2483.

86. Finnerup NB, Attal N, Haroutounian S, McNicol E, Baron R, Dworkin RH, Gilron I, Haanpää M, Hansson P, Jensen TS, Kamerman PR, Lund K, Moore A, Raja SN, Rice AS, Rowbotham M, Sena E, Siddall P, Smith BH, Wallace M. Pharmacotherapy for neuropathic pain in adults: a systematic review and meta-analysis. Lancet Neurol. 2015;14(2):162–73.

87. Kimura M, Saito S, Obata H. Dexmedetomidine decreases hyperalgesia in neuropathic pain by increasing acetylcholine in the spinal cord. Neurosci Lett. 2012;529(1):70–4.

88. Hiroki T, Suto T, Saito S, Obata H. Repeated administration of amitriptyline in neuropathic pain: modulation of the noradrenergic descending inhibitory system. Anesth Analg. 2017;125(4):1281–8.

89. Dick IE, Brochu RM, Purohit Y, Kaczorowski GJ, Martin WJ, Priest BT. Sodium channel blockade may contribute to the analgesic efficacy of antidepressants. J Pain. 2007;8(4):315–24.

90. Barygin OI, Nagaeva EI, Tikhonov DB, Belinskaya DA, Vanchakova NP, Shestakova NN. Inhibition of the NMDA and AMPA receptor channels by antidepressants and antipsychotics. Brain Res. 1660;2017:58–66.

91. Yokogawa F, Kiuchi Y, Ishikawa Y, Otsuka N, Masuda Y, Oguchi K, Hosoyamada A. An investigation of monoamine receptors involved in antinociceptive effects of antidepressants. Anesth Analg. 2002;95(1):163–8.

92. Antkiewicz-Michaluk L, Romańska I, Michaluk J, Vetulani J. Role of calcium channels in effects of antidepressant drugs on responsiveness to pain. Psychopharmacology. 1991;105(2):269–74.

93. Galeotti N, Ghelardini C, Bartolini A. Involvement of potassium channels in amitriptyline and clomipramine analgesia. Neuropharmacology. 2001;40(1):75–84.

94. Phillis JW, Wu PH. Adenosine mediates sedative action of various centrally active drugs. Med Hypotheses. 1982;9(4):361–7.

95. McCarson KE, Duric V, Reisman SA, Winter M, Enna SJ. GABA(B) receptor function and subunit expression in the rat spinal cord as indicators of stress and the antinociceptive response to antidepressants. Brain Res. 2006;1068(1):109–17.

96. Isenberg KE, Cicero TJ. Possible involvement of opiate receptors in the pharmacological profiles of antidepressant compounds. Eur J Pharmacol. 1984;103(1–2):57–63.

97. Hirayama Y, Ishitani K, Sato Y, Iyama S, Takada K, Murase K, Kuroda H, Nagamachi Y, Konuma Y, Fujimi A, Sagawa T, Ono K, Horiguchi H, Terui T, Koike K, Kusakabe T, Sato T, Takimoto R, Kobune M, Kato J. Effect of duloxetine in Japanese patients with chemotherapy-induced peripheral neuropathy: a pilot randomized trial. Int J Clin Oncol. 2015;20(5):866–71.

98. Piccolo J, Kolesar JM. Prevention and treatment of chemotherapy-induced peripheral neuropathy. Am J Health Syst Pharm. 2014;71(1):19–25.

99. Hershman DL, Lacchetti C, Dworkin RH, Lavoie Smith EM, Bleeker J, Cavaletti G, Chauhan C, Gavin P, Lavino A, Lustberg MB, Paice J, Schneider B, Smith ML, Smith T, Terstriep S, Wagner-Johnston N, Bak K, Loprinzi CL, American Society of Clinical Oncology. Prevention and management of chemotherapy-induced peripheral neuropathy in survivors of adult cancers: American Society of Clinical Oncology clinical practice guideline. J Clin Oncol. 2014;32(18):1941–67.

100. Aziz MT, Good BL, Lowe DK. Serotonin-norepinephrine reuptake inhibitors for the management of chemotherapy-induced peripheral neuropathy. Ann Pharmacother. 2014;48(5):626–32.

101. Katsuyama S, Aso H, Otowa A, Yagi T, Kishikawa Y, Komatsu T, Sakurada T, Nakamura H. Antinociceptive effects of the serotonin and noradrenaline reuptake inhibitors milnacipran and duloxetine on vincristine-induced neuropathic pain model in mice. ISRN Pain. 2014;2014:915464.

102. Durand JP, Deplanque G, Montheil V, Gornet JM, Scotte F, Mir O, Cessot A, Coriat R, Raymond E, Mitry E, Herait P, Yataghene Y, Goldwasser F. Efficacy of venlafaxine for the prevention and relief of oxaliplatin-induced acute neurotoxicity: results of EFFOX, a randomized, double-blind, placebo-controlled phase III trial. Ann Oncol. 2012;23(1):200–5.

103. Nishishinya B, Urrútia G, Walitt B, Rodriguez A, Bonfill X, Alegre C, Darko G. Amitriptyline in the treatment of fibromyalgia: a systematic review of its efficacy. Rheumatology (Oxford). 2008;47(12):1741–6.

104. Kaur S, Pandhi P, Dutta P. Painful diabetic neuropathy: an update. Ann Neurosci. 2011;18(4):168–75.

105. Kautio AL, Haanpää M, Saarto T, Kalso E. Amitriptyline in the treatment of chemotherapy-induced neuropathic symptoms. J Pain Symptom Manag. 2008;35(1):31–9.

106. Hammack JE, Michalak JC, Loprinzi CL, Sloan JA, Novotny PJ, Soori GS, Tirona MT, Rowland KM Jr, Stella PJ, Johnson JA. Phase III evaluation of nortriptyline for alleviation of symptoms of cis-platinum-induced peripheral neuropathy. Pain. 2002;98(1–2):195–203.

107. Kautio AL, Haanpää M, Leminen A, Kalso E, Kautiainen H, Saarto T. Amitriptyline in the prevention of chemotherapy-induced neuropathic symptoms. Anticancer Res. 2009;29(7):2601–6.

108. Hughes S, Lacasse J, Fuller RR, Spaulding-Givens J. Adverse effects and treatment satisfaction among online users of four antidepressants. Psychiatry Res. 2017;255:78–86.

109. Rowbotham MC, Goli V, Kunz NR, Lei D. Venlafaxine extended release in the treatment of painful diabetic neuropathy: a double-blind, placebo-controlled study. Pain. 2004;110(3):697–706.

110. Zygmunt M, Sapa J. Muscle relaxants--the current position in the treatment of spasticity in orthopedics. Ortop Traumatol Rehabil. 2015;17(4):423–30.

111. Patiño-Camacho SI, Déciga Campos M, Beltrán-Villalobos K, Castro-Vidal DA, Montiel-Ruiz RM, Flores-Murrieta FJ. Low doses of tizanidine synergize the anti-nociceptive and anti-inflammatory effects of ketorolac or naproxen while reducing of side effects. Eur J Pharmacol. 2017;805:51–7.

112. Lee S, Zhao X, Hatch M, Chun S, Chang E. Central neuropathic pain in spinal cord injury. Crit Rev Phys Rehabil Med. 2013;25(3–4):159–72.

113. Talakoub R, Abbasi S, Maghami E, Zavareh SM. The effect of oral tizanidine on postoperative pain relief after elective laparoscopic cholecystectomy. Adv Biomed Res. 2016;5:19.

114. Mastenbroek TC, Kramp-Hendriks BJ, Kallewaard JW, Vonk JM. Multimodal intrathecal analgesia in refractory cancer pain. Scand J Pain. 2017;14:39–43.

115. Kumru H, Kofler M, Flores MC, Portell E, Robles V, Leon N, Vidal J. Effect of intrathecal baclofen on evoked pain perception: an evoked potentials and quantitative thermal testing study. Eur J Pain. 2013;17(7):1039–47.

116. Nemeth BA, Montero RJ, Halanski MA, Noonan KJ. Epidural baclofen for the management of postoperative pain in children with cerebral palsy. J Pediatr Orthop. 2015;35(6):571–5.

117. Yenigün D, Ekiz T, Yuzer GF, Tasoglu O, Aslan MD, Ozgirgin N. Severe pain, spasticity, and heterotopic ossification in a patient with spinal cord injury: a vicious circle and management with baclofen pump. Pain Physician. 2014;17(6):E794–5.

118. Khurana SR, Garg DS. Spasticity and the use of intrathecal baclofen in patients with spinal cord injury. Phys Med Rehabil Clin N Am. 2014;25(3):655–9.

119. Pai A, Heining M. Ketamine. Continuing Educ Anaesth Crit Care Pain. 2007;7(2):59–63.

120. Bredlau AL, Thakur R, Korones DN, Dworkin RH. Ketamine for pain in adults and children with cancer: a systematic review and synthesis of the literature. Pain Med. 2013;14(10):1505–17.

121. Bell RF, Eccleston C, Kalso EA. Ketamine as an adjuvant to opioids for cancer pain. Cochrane Database Syst Rev. 2017;6:CD003351.

122. Fallon MT, Wilcock A, Kelly CA, Paul J, Lewsley LA, Norrie J, Laird BJA. Oral ketamine vs placebo in patients with cancer-related neuropathic pain: a randomized clinical trial. JAMA Oncol. 2018;4(6):870–2.

123. Kopsky DJ, Keppel Hesselink JM, Bhaskar A, Hariton G, Romanenko V, Casale R. Analgesic effects of topical ketamine. Minerva Anestesiol. 2015;81(4):440–9.

124. Knezevic NN, Tverdohleb T, Nikibin F, Knezevic I, Candido KD. Management of chronic neuropathic pain with single and compounded topical analgesics. Pain Manag. 2017;7(6):537–58.

125. Singh V, Gillespie TW, Harvey RD. Intranasal ketamine and its potential role in cancer-related pain. Pharmacotherapy. 2018;38(3):390–401.

126. White PF, Schüttler J, Shafer A, Stanski DR, Horai Y, Trevor AJ. Comparative pharmacology of the ketamine isomers. Studies in volunteers. Br J Anaesth. 1985;57(2):197–203.

127. White PF, Way WL, Trevor AJ. Ketamine-its pharmacology and therapeutic uses. Anesthesiology. 1982;56(2):119–36.

128. Liebe T, Li S, Lord A, Colic L, Krause AL, Batra A, Kretzschmar MA, Sweeney-Reed CM, Behnisch G, Schott BH, Walter M. Factors influencing the cardiovascular response to subanesthetic ketamine: a randomized, placebo-controlled trial. Int J Neuropsychopharmacol. 2017;20(11):909–18.

129. Sener S, Eken C, Schultz CH, Serinken M, Ozsarac M. Ketamine with and without midazolam for emergency department sedation in adults: a randomized controlled trial. Ann Emerg Med. 2011;57(2):109–14.

130. Hutchinson MR, Zhang Y, Brown K, Coats BD, Shridhar M, Sholar PW, Patel SJ, Crysdale NY, Harrison JA, Maier SF, Rice KC, Watkins LR. Non-stereoselective reversal of neuropathic pain by naloxone and naltrexone: involvement of toll-like receptor 4 (TLR4). Eur J Neurosci. 2008;28(1):20–9.

131. Block L, Björklund U, Westerlund A, Jörneberg P, Biber B, Hansson E. A new concept affecting restoration of inflammation-reactive astrocytes. Neuroscience. 2013;250:536–45.

132. Gold MS, Dackis CA, Pottash AL, Sternbach HH, Annitto WJ, Martin D, Dackis MP. Naltrexone, opiate addiction, and endorphins. Med Res Rev. 1982;2(3):211–46.

133. Zagon IS, McLaughlin PJ. Gene-peptide relationships in the developing rat brain: the response of preproenkephalin mRNA and [Met5]-enkephalin to acute opioid antagonist (naltrexone) exposure. Brain Res Mol Brain Res. 1995;33(1):111–20.

134. Paquette J, Olmstead MC. Ultra-low dose naltrexone enhances cannabinoid-induced antinociception. Behav Pharmacol. 2005;16(8):597–603.

135. Liu SL, Li YH, Shi GY, Chen YH, Huang CW, Hong JS, Wu HL. A novel inhibitory effect of naloxone on macrophage activation and atherosclerosis formation in mice. J Am Coll Cardiol. 2006;48(9):1871–9.

136. Younger J, Parkitny L, McLain D. The use of low-dose naltrexone (LDN) as a novel anti-inflammatory treatment for chronic pain. Clin Rheumatol. 2014;33(4):451–9.

137. Ringerike T, Pike E, Nevjar J, Klemp M. The use of naltrexone in low doses beyond the approved indication. Research overview; 2015.

138. Raknes G, Småbrekke L. Low-dose naltrexone and opioid consumption: a drug utilization cohort study based on data from the Norwegian prescription database. Pharmacoepidemiol Drug Saf. 2017;26(6):685–93.

139. Patten DK, Schultz BG, Berlau DJ. The safety and efficacy of low-dose naltrexone in the management of chronic pain and inflammation in multiple sclerosis, fibromyalgia, Crohn's disease, and other chronic pain disorders. Pharmacotherapy. 2018;38(3):382–9.

140. Liu WM, Scott KA, Dennis JL, Kaminska E, Levett AJ, Dalgleish AG. Naltrexone at low doses upregulates a unique gene expression not seen with normal doses: implications for its use in cancer therapy. Int J Oncol. 2016;49(2):793–802.

141. Donahue RN, McLaughlin PJ, Zagon IS. Low-dose naltrexone suppresses ovarian cancer and exhibits enhanced inhibition in combination with cisplatin. Exp Biol Med (Maywood). 2011;236(7):883–95.

142. Turel AP, Oh KH, Zagon IS, McLaughlin PJ. Low dose naltrexone for treatment of multiple sclerosis: a retrospective chart review of safety and tolerability. J Clin Psychopharmacol. 2015;35(5):609–11.

143. Segal D, Macdonald JK, Chande N. Low dose naltrexone for induction of remission in Crohn's disease. Cochrane Database Syst Rev. 2014;2:CD010410.

144. Mitchell JE. Naltrexone and hepatotoxicity. Lancet. 1986;1(8491):1215.

145. Smith JP, Field D, Bingaman SI, Evans R, Mauger DT. Safety and tolerability of low-dose naltrexone therapy in children with moderate to severe Crohn's disease: a pilot study. J Clin Gastroenterol. 2013;47(4):339–45.

146. Yen MH, Ko HC, Tang FI, Lu RB, Hong JS. Study of hepatotoxicity of naltrexone in the treatment of alcoholism. Alcohol. 2006;38(2):117–20.

147. Adcock IM, Cosio B, Tsaprouni L, Barnes PJ, Ito K. Redox regulation of histone deacetylases and glucocorticoid-mediated inhibition of the inflammatory response. Antioxid Redox Signal. 2005;7(1–2):144–52.

148. Chow E, Loblaw A, Harris K, Doyle M, Goh P, Chiu H, Panzarella T, Tsao M, Barnes EA, Sinclair E, Farhadian M, Danjoux C. Dexamethasone for the prophylaxis of radiation-induced pain flare after palliative radiotherapy for bone metastases: a pilot study. Support Care Cancer. 2007;15(6):643–7.

149. Roth P, Happold C, Weller M. Corticosteroid use in neuro-oncology: an update. Neurooncol Pract. 2015;2(1):6–12.

150. Yang H, Seon J, Sung PS, Oh JS, Lee HL, Jang B, Chun HJ, Jang JW, Bae SH, Choi JY, Yoon SK. Dexamethasone prophylaxis to alleviate postembolization syndrome after transarterial chemoembolization for hepatocellular carcinoma: a randomized, double-blinded, placebo-controlled study. J Vasc Interv Radiol. 2017;28(11):1503–11.

151. Haywood A, Good P, Khan S, Leupp A, Jenkins-Marsh S, Rickett K, Hardy JR. Corticosteroids for the management of cancer-related pain in adults. Cochrane Database Syst Rev. 2015;4:CD010756.

152. Todd FD 2nd, Miller CA, Yates AJ, Mervis LJ. Steroid-induced remission in primary malignant lymphoma of the central nervous system. Surg Neurol. 1986;26(1):79–84.

153. Ryken TC, McDermott M, Robinson PD, Ammirati M, Andrews DW, Asher AL, Burri SH, Cobbs CS, Gaspar LE, Kondziolka D, Linskey ME, Loeffler JS, Mehta MP, Mikkelsen T, Olson JJ, Paleologos NA, Patchell RA, Kalkanis SN. The role of steroids in the management of brain metastases: a systematic review and evidence-based clinical practice guideline. J Neuro-Oncol. 2010;96(1):103–14.

154. Ly KI, Wen PY. Clinical relevance of steroid use in neuro-oncology. Curr Neurol Neurosci Rep. 2017;17(1):5.

155. Dietrich J, Rao K, Pastorino S, Kesari S. Corticosteroids in brain cancer patients: benefits and pitfalls. Expert Rev Clin Pharmacol. 2011;4(2):233–42.

156. Markman M, Sheidler V, Ettinger DS, Quaskey SA, Mellits ED. Antiemetic efficacy of dexamethasone. Randomized, double-blind, crossover study with prochlorperazine in patients receiving cancer chemotherapy. N Engl J Med. 1984;311(9):549–52.

157. Koehler PJ. Use of corticosteroids in neuro-oncology. Anti-Cancer Drugs. 1995;6(1):19–33.

158. Yang Q, Zhang Z, Xin W, Li A. Preoperative intravenous glucocorticoids can decrease acute pain and postoperative nausea and vomiting after total hip arthroplasty: a PRISMA-compliant meta-analysis. Medicine (Baltimore). 2017;96(47):e8804.

159. Clayburgh D, Stott W, Bolognone R, Palmer A, Achim V, Troob S, Li R, Brickman D, Graville D, Andersen P, Gross ND. A randomized controlled trial of corticosteroids for pain after transoral robotic surgery. Laryngoscope. 2017;127(11):2558–64.

160. Hui D, Kilgore K, Frisbee-Hume S, Park M, Tsao A, Delgado Guay M, Lu C, William W Jr, Pisters K, Eapen G, Fossella F, Amin S, Bruera E. Dexamethasone for dyspnea in cancer patients: a pilot double-blind, randomized, controlled trial. J Pain Symptom Manage. 2016;52(1):8–16.

161. Aljebab F, Choonara I, Conroy S. Systematic review of the toxicity of short-course oral corticosteroids in children. Arch Dis Child. 2016;101(4):365–70.

162. Ravindran V, Rachapalli S, Choy EH. Safety of medium- to long-term glucocorticoid therapy in rheumatoid arthritis: a meta-analysis. Rheumatology (Oxford). 2009;48(7):807–11.

163. Alles SRA, Smith PA. Etiology and pharmacology of neuropathic pain. Pharmacol Rev. 2018;70(2):315–47.

164. Chen J, Li L, Chen SR, Chen H, Xie JD, Sirrieh RE, MacLean DM, Zhang Y, Zhou MH, Jayaraman V, Pan HL. The $\alpha 2\delta$-1-NMDA receptor complex is critically involved in neuropathic pain development and gabapentin therapeutic actions. Cell Rep. 2018;22(9):2307–21.

165. Rao RD, Michalak JC, Sloan JA, Loprinzi CL, Soori GS, Nikcevich DA, Warner DO, Novotny P, Kutteh LA, Wong GY, North Central Cancer Treatment Group. Efficacy of gabapentin in the management of chemotherapy-induced peripheral neuropathy: a phase 3 randomized, double-blind, placebo-controlled, crossover trial (N00C3). Cancer. 2007;110(9):2110–8.

166. Saif MW, Syrigos K, Kaley K, Isufi I. Role of pregabalin in treatment of oxaliplatin-induced sensory neuropathy. Anticancer Res. 2010;30(7):2927–33.

167. Heir GM, Masterson M. Bilateral glossopharyngeal neuropathy following chemo and radiation therapy for a primitive neuroectodermal tumour. J Oral Rehabil. 2016;43(2):154–8.

168. Jordan RI, Mulvey MR, Bennett MI. A critical appraisal of gabapentinoids for pain in cancer patients. Curr Opin Support Palliat Care. 2018;12(2):108–17.

169. Doleman B, Heinink TP, Read DJ, Faleiro RJ, Lund JN, Williams JP. A systematic review and meta-regression analysis of prophylactic gabapentin for postoperative pain. Anaesthesia. 2015;70(10):1186–204.

170. Zencirci B. Analgesic efficacy of oral gabapentin added to standard epidural corticosteroids in patients with failed back surgery. Clin Pharmacol. 2010;2:207–11.

171. Drug Enforcement Administration, Department of Justice. Schedules of controlled substances: placement of pregabalin into schedule V. Final rule. Fed Regist. 2005;70(144):43633–5.

172. Patorno E, Bohn RL, Wahl PM, Avorn J, Patrick AR, Liu J, Schneeweiss S. Anticonvulsant medications and the risk of suicide, attempted suicide, or violent death. JAMA. 2010;303(14):1401–9.

173. Ghodke-Puranik Y, Thorn CF, Lamba JK, Leeder JS, Song W, Birnbaum AK, Altman RB, Klein TE. Valproic acid pathway: pharmacokinetics and pharmacodynamics. Pharmacogenet Genomics. 2013;23(4):236–41.

174. Matsushita Y, Araki K, Omotuyi OI, Mukae T, Ueda H. HDAC inhibitors restore C-fibre sensitivity in experimental neuropathic pain model. Br J Pharmacol. 2013;170(5):991–8.

175. Rodriguez-Menendez V, Gilardini A, Bossi M, Canta A, Oggioni N, Carozzi V, Tremolizzo L, Cavaletti G. Valproate protective effects on cisplatin-induced peripheral neuropathy: an in vitro and in vivo study. Anticancer Res. 2008;28(1A):335–42.

176. Wadia RJ, Stolar M, Grens C, Ehrlich BE, Chao HH. The prevention of chemotherapy induced peripheral neuropathy by concurrent treatment with drugs used for bipolar disease: a retrospective chart analysis in human cancer patients. Oncotarget. 2017;9(7):7322–31.

177. Rauck R, Busch M, Marriott T. Effectiveness of a heated lidocaine/tetracaine topical patch for pain associated with myofascial trigger points: results of an open-label pilot study. Pain Pract. 2013;13(7):533–8.

178. Cheng YJ. Lidocaine skin patch (Lidopat® 5%) is effective in the treatment of traumatic rib fractures: a prospective double-blinded and vehicle-controlled study. Med Princ Pract. 2016;25(1):36–9.

179. van den Heuvel SAS, van der Wal SEI, Smedes LA, Radema SA, van Alfen N, Vissers KCP, Steegers MAH. Intravenous lidocaine: old-school drug, new purpose-reduction of intractable pain in patients with chemotherapy induced peripheral neuropathy. Pain Res Manag. 2017;2017:8053474.

180. Ho MLJ, Kerr SJ, Stevens J. Intravenous lidocaine infusions for 48 hours in open colorectal surgery: a prospective, randomized, double-blinded, placebo-controlled trial. Korean J Anesthesiol. 2018;71(1):57–65.

181. Kamei J, Nozaki C, Saitoh A. Effect of mexiletine on vincristine-induced painful neuropathy in mice. Eur J Pharmacol. 2006;536(1–2):123–7.

182. Egashira N, Hirakawa S, Kawashiri T, Yano T, Ikesue H, Oishi R. Mexiletine reverses oxaliplatin-induced neuropathic pain in rats. J Pharmacol Sci. 2010;112(4):473–6.

183. Argyriou AA, Chroni E, Polychronopoulos P, Iconomou G, Koutras A, Makatsoris T, Gerolymos MK, Gourzis P, Assimakopoulos K, Kalofonos HP. Efficacy of oxcarbazepine for prophylaxis against cumulative oxaliplatin-induced neuropathy. Neurology. 2006;67(12):2253–5.

184. von Delius S, Eckel F, Wagenpfeil S, Mayr M, Stock K, Kullmann F, Obermeier F, Erdmann J, Schmelz R, Quasthoff S, Adelsberger H, Bredenkamp R, Schmid RM, Lersch C. Carbamazepine for prevention of oxaliplatin-related neurotoxicity in patients with advanced colorectal cancer: final results of a randomised, controlled, multicenter phase II study. Investig New Drugs. 2007;25(2):173–80.

185. Carroll IR, Kaplan KM, Mackey SC. Mexiletine therapy for chronic pain: survival analysis identifies factors predicting clinical success. J Pain Symptom Manag. 2008;35(3):321–6.

186. Pachman DR, Barton DL, Watson JC, Loprinzi CL. Chemotherapy-induced peripheral neuropathy: prevention and treatment. Clin Pharmacol Ther. 2011;90(3):377–87.

187. Deandrea S, Montanari M, Moja L, Apolone G. Prevalence of undertreatment in cancer pain. A review of published literature. Ann Oncol. 2008;19(12):1985–91.

188. Gulati A, Shah R, Puttanniah V, Hung J, Malhotra V. A retrospective review and treatment paradigm of interventional therapies for patients suffering from intractable thoracic chest wall pain in the oncologic population. Pain Med. 2015;16(4):802–10.

189. Hutson N, Hung J, Puttanniah V, Lis E, Laufer I, Gulati A. Interventional pain management for sacroiliac tumors in the oncologic population: a case series and paradigm approach. Pain Med. 2016;18(5):959–68.

190. Neal JM. Ultrasound-guided regional anesthesia and patient safety: update of an evidence-based analysis. Reg Anesth Pain Med. 2016;41(2):195–204.

191. McDermott G, Korba E, Mata U, Jaigirdar M, Narayanan N, Boylan J, Conlon N. Should we stop doing blind transversus abdominis plane blocks? Br J Anaesth. 2012;108(3):499–502.

192. Nader A, Kendall MC, De Oliveria GS, Chen JQ, Vanderby B, Rosenow JM, Bendok BR. Ultrasound-guided trigeminal nerve block via the pterygopalatine fossa: an effective treatment for trigeminal neuralgia and atypical facial pain. Pain Physician. 2013;16(5):E537–45.

193. Siegenthaler A, Moriggl B, Mlekusch S, Schliessbach J, Haug M, Curatolo M, Eichenberger U. Ultrasound-guided suprascapular nerve block, description of a novel supraclavicular approach. Reg Anesth Pain Med. 2012;37(3):325–8.

194. Wijayasinghe N, Duriaud HM, Kehlet H, Andersen KG. Ultrasound guided intercostobrachial nerve blockade in patients with persistent pain after breast cancer surgery: a pilot study. Pain Physician. 2016;19(2):E309–18.

195. Wisotzky E, Saini V, Kao C. Ultrasound-guided intercostobrachial nerve block for intercostobrachial neuralgia in breast cancer patients: a case series. PM R. 2016;8(3):273–7.

196. Thomassen I, van Suijlekom JA, van de Gaag A, Ponten JE, Nienhuijs SW. Ultrasound-guided ilioinguinal/iliohypogastric nerve blocks for chronic pain after inguinal hernia repair. Hernia. 2013;17(3):329–32.

197. Hong M, Kim Y, Park J, Hong H. Management of pudendal neuralgia using ultrasound-guided pulsed radiofrequency: a report of two cases and discussion of pudendal nerve block techniques. J Anesth. 2015;30(2):356–9.

198. Saranteas T, Anagnostis G, Paraskeuopoulos T, Koulalis D, Kokkalis Z, Nakou M, Anagnostopoulou S, Kostopanagiotou G. Anatomy and clinical implications of the ultrasound-guided subsartorial saphenous nerve block. Reg Anesth Pain Med. 2011;36(4):399–402.

199. Malik T. Ultrasound-guided paravertebral neurolytic block: a report of two cases. Pain Pract. 2013;14(4):346–9.

200. Blanco R, Parras T, McDonnell JG, Prats-Galino A. Serratus plane block: a novel ultrasound-guided thoracic wall nerve block. Anaesthesia. 2013;68(11):1107–13.

201. Zocca JA, Chen GH, Puttanniah VG, Hung JC, Gulati A. Ultrasound-guided serratus plane block for treatment of postmastectomy pain syndromes in breast cancer patients: a case series. Pain Pract. 2017;17(1):141–6.

202. Piracha MM, Thorp SL, Puttanniah V, Gulati A. "A tale of two planes": deep versus superficial serratus plane block for postmastectomy pain syndrome. Reg Anesth Pain Med. 2017;42(2):259–62.

203. Abdallah FW, MacLean D, Madjdpour C, Cil T, Bhatia A, Brull R. Pectoralis and serratus fascial plane blocks each provide early analgesic benefits following ambulatory breast cancer surgery: a retrospective propensity-matched cohort study. Anesth Analg. 2017;125(1):294–302.

204. Hebbard PD, Barrington MJ, Vasey C. Ultrasound-guided continuous oblique subcostal transversus abdominis plane blockade: description of anatomy and clinical technique. Reg Anesth Pain Med. 2010;35(5):436–41.

205. Blomstedt PC, Bergenheim AT. Technical difficulties and perioperative complications of retrogasserian glycerol rhizotomy for trigeminal neuralgia. Stereotact Funct Neurosurg. 2002;79(3–4):168–81.

206. Ischia S, Luzzani A, Polati E, Ischia A. Percutaneous controlled thermocoagulation in the treatment of trigeminal neuralgia. Clin J Pain. 1990;6(2):96–104.

207. Gunduz OH, Kenis-Coskun O. Ganglion blocks as a treatment of pain: current perspectives. J Pain Res. 2017;10:2815–26.

208. Pather N, Partab P, Singh B, Satyapal KS. Cervico-thoracic ganglion: its clinical implications. Clin Anat. 2006;19(4):323–6.

209. Ghai A, Kaushik T, Kumar R, Wadhera S. Chemical ablation of stellate ganglion for head and neck cancer pain. Acta Anaesthesiol Belg. 2016;67(1):6–8.

210. Guo JR, Guo W, Jin XJ, Yu J, Jin BW, Xu F, Liu Y. Effects of stellate ganglionic block on hemodynamic changes and intrapulmonary shunt in perioperative patients with esophageal cancer. Eur Rev Med Pharmacol Sci. 2014;18(24):3864–9.

211. Park JH, Min YS, Chun SM, Seo KS. Effects of stellate ganglion block on breast cancer-related lymphedema: comparison of various injectates. Pain Physician. 2015;18(1):93–9.

212. Kambadakone A, Thabet A, Gervais DA, Mueller PR, Arellano RS. CT-guided celiac plexus neurolysis: a review of anat-

omy, indications, technique, and tips for successful treatment. Radiographics. 2011;31(6):1599–621.

213. Cao J, He Y, Liu H, Wang S, Zhao B, Zheng X, Yang K, Xie D. Effectiveness of percutaneous celiac plexus ablation in the treatment of severe cancer pain in upper abdomen and evaluation of health economics. Am J Hosp Palliat Care. 2017;34(2):142–7.

214. Shwita AH, Amr YM, Okab MI. Comparative study of the effects of the retrocrural celiac plexus block versus splanchnic nerve block, C-arm guided, for upper gastrointestinal tract tumors on pain relief and the quality of life at a six-month follow up. Korean J Pain. 2015;28(1):22–31.

215. Nitschke AM, Ray CE Jr. Percutaneous neurolytic celiac plexus block. Semin Intervent Radiol. 2013;30(3):318–21.

216. Seicean A. Celiac plexus neurolysis in pancreatic cancer: the endoscopic ultrasound approach. World J Gastroenterol. 2014;20(1):110–7.

217. Koyyalagunta D, Engle MP, Yu J, Feng L, Novy DM. The effectiveness of alcohol versus phenol based splanchnic nerve neurolysis for the treatment of intra-abdominal cancer pain. Pain Physician. 2016;19(4):281–92.

218. Staats PS, Hekmat H, Sauter P, Lillemoe K. The effects of alcohol celiac plexus block, pain, and mood on longevity in patients with unresectable pancreatic cancer: a double-blind, randomized, placebo-controlled study. Pain Med. 2001;2(1):28–34.

219. Fujii-Lau LL, Bamlet WR, Eldrige JS, Chari ST, Gleeson FC, Abu Dayyeh BK, Clain JE, Pearson RK, Petersen BT, Rajan E, Topazian MD, Vege SS, Wang KK, Wiersema MJ, Levy MJ. Impact of celiac neurolysis on survival in patients with pancreatic cancer. Gastrointest Endosc. 2015;82(1):46–56.

220. Oh TK, Lee WJ, Woo SM, Kim NW, Yim J, Kim DH. Impact of celiac plexus neurolysis on survival in patients with unresectable pancreatic cancer: a retrospective, propensity score matching analysis. Pain Physician. 2017;20(3):E357–65.

221. Minaga K, Kitano M, Imai H, Miyata T, Kudo M. Acute spinal cord infarction after EUS-guided celiac plexus neurolysis. Gastrointest Endosc. 2016;83(5):1039–40.

222. Koker IH, Aralasmak A, Unver N, Asil T, Senturk H. Spinal cord ischemia after endoscopic ultrasound guided celiac plexus neurolysis: case report and review of the literature. Scand J Gastroenterol. 2017;52(10):1158–61.

223. Heindel W, Ernst S, Manshausen G, Gawenda M, Siemens P, Krahe T, Walter M, Lackner K. CT-guided lumbar sympathectomy: results and analysis of factors influencing the outcome. Cardiovasc Intervent Radiol. 1998;21(4):319–23.

224. Sze DY, Mackey SC. MR guidance of sympathetic nerve blockade: measurement of vasomotor response initial experience in seven patients. Radiology. 2002;223(2):574–80.

225. Hong JH, Oh MJ. Comparison of multilevel with single level injection during lumbar sympathetic ganglion block: efficacy of sympatholysis and incidence of psoas muscle injection. Korean J Pain. 2010;23(2):131–6.

226. Abramov R. Lumbar sympathetic treatment in the management of lower limb pain. Curr Pain Headache Rep. 2014;18(4):403.

227. Carroll I, Clark JD, Mackey S. Sympathetic block with botulinum toxin to treat complex regional pain syndrome. Ann Neurol. 2009;65(3):348–51.

228. Feigl GC, Dreu M, Ulz H, Breschan C, Maier C, Likar R. Susceptibility of the genitofemoral and lateral femoral cutaneous nerves to complications from lumbar sympathetic blocks: is there a morphological reason? Br J Anaesth. 2014;112(6):1098–104.

229. Sniderman M, Raghavendra M, Holtman JR Jr. Priapism following a lumbar sympathetic nerve block. Pain Med. 2011;12(7):1046–8.

230. Dirim A, Kumsar S. Iatrogenic ureteral injury due to lumbar sympathetic block. Scand J Urol Nephrol. 2008;42(4):395–6.

231. Kraima AC, van Schaik J, Susan S, van de Velde CJ, Hamming JF, Lakke EA, DeRuiter MC. New insights in the neuroanatomy of the human adult superior hypogastric plexus and hypogastric nerves. Auton Neurosci. 2015;189:60–7.

232. Plancarte R, Amescua C, Patt RB, Aldrete JA. Superior hypogastric plexus block for pelvic cancer pain. Anesthesiology. 1990;73(2):236–9.

233. Cariati M, De Martini G, Pretolesi F, Roy MT. CT-guided superior hypogastric plexus block. J Comput Assist Tomogr. 2002;26(3):428–31.

234. Turker G, Basagan-Mogol E, Gurbet A, Ozturk C, Uckunkaya N, Sahin S. A new technique for superior hypogastric plexus block: the posteromedian transdiscal approach. Tohoku J Exp Med. 2005;206(3):277–81.

235. Mishra S, Bhatnagar S, Gupta D, Thulkar S. Anterior ultrasound-guided superior hypogastric plexus neurolysis in pelvic cancer pain. Anaesth Intensive Care. 2008;36(5):732–5.

236. de Leon-Casasola OA, Kent E, Lema MJ. Neurolytic superior hypogastric plexus block for chronic pelvic pain associated with cancer. Pain. 1993;54(2):145–51.

237. Scott-Warren JT, Hill V, Rajasekaran A. Ganglion impar blockade: a review. Curr Pain Headache Rep. 2013;17(1):306.

238. Foye PM. Ganglion impar blocks via coccygeal versus sacrococcygeal joints. Reg Anesth Pain Med. 2008;33(3):279–80.

239. Huang JJ. Another modified approach to the ganglion of Walther block (ganglion of impar). J Clin Anesth. 2003;15(4):282–3.

240. Agarwal-Kozlowski K, Lorke DE, Habermann CR, Am Esch JS, Beck H. CT-guided blocks and neuroablation of the ganglion impar (Walther) in perineal pain: anatomy, technique, safety, and efficacy. Clin J Pain. 2009;25(7):570–6.

241. Lin CS, Cheng JK, Hsu YW, Chen CC, Lao HC, Huang CJ, Cheng PH, Narouze S. Ultrasound-guided ganglion impar block: a technical report. Pain Med. 2010;11(3):390–4.

242. Marker DR, U-Thainual P, Ungi T, Flammang AJ, Fichtinger G, Iordachita II, Carrino JA, Fritz J. MR-guided perineural injection of the ganglion impar: technical considerations and feasibility. Skelet Radiol. 2016;45(5):591–7.

243. Gunduz OH, Sencan S, Kenis-Coskun O. Pain relief due to transsacrococcygeal ganglion impar block in chronic coccygodynia: a pilot study. Pain Med. 2015;16(7):1278–81.

244. Adas C, Ozdemir U, Toman H, Luleci N, Luleci E, Adas H. Transsacrococcygeal approach to ganglion impar: radiofrequency application for the treatment of chronic intractable coccydynia. J Pain Res. 2016;9:1173–7.

245. McCormick Z, Kennedy DJ, Garvan C, Rivers E, Temme K, Margolis S, Zander E, Rohr A, Smith MC, Plastaras C. Comparison of pain score reduction using triamcinolone vs. betamethasone in transforaminal epidural steroid injections for lumbosacral radicular pain. Am J Phys Med Rehabil. 2015;94(12):1058–64.

246. Kennedy DJ, Plastaras C, Casey E, Visco CJ, Rittenberg JD, Conrad B, Sigler J, Dreyfuss P. Comparative effectiveness of lumbar transforaminal epidural steroid injections with particulate versus nonparticulate corticosteroids for lumbar radicular pain due to intervertebral disc herniation: a prospective, randomized, double-blind trial. Pain Med. 2014;15(4):548–55.

247. Ploumis A, Christodoulou P, Wood KB, Varvarousis D, Sarni JL, Beris A. Caudal vs transforaminal epidural steroid injections as short-term (6 months) pain relief in lumbar spinal stenosis patients with sciatica. Pain Med. 2014;15(3):379–85.

248. Wei G, Liang J, Chen B, Zhou C, Ru N, Chen J, Zhang F. Comparison of transforaminal verse interlaminar epidural steroid injection in low back pain with lumbosacral radicular pain: a meta-analysis of the literature. Int Orthop. 2016;40(12):2533–45.

249. Beyaz SG. Comparison of transforaminal and interlaminar epidural steroid injections for the treatment of chronic lumbar pain. Braz J Anesthesiol. 2017;67(1):21–7.

250. El-Yahchouchi CA, Plastaras CT, Maus TP, Carr CM, McCormick ZL, Geske JR, Smuck M, Pingree MJ, Kennedy DJ. Adverse event rates associated with transforaminal and interlaminar epidural steroid injections: a multi-institutional study. Pain Med. 2016;17(2):239–49.

251. Ertas IE, Sehirali S, Ozsezgin Ocek S, Sanci M, Arbak G, Yildirim Y. The effectiveness of subcutaneously implanted epidural ports for relief of severe pain in patients with advanced-stage gynecological cancer: a prospective study. Agri. 2014;26(1):8–14.

252. van Boekel RL, Vissers KC, van de Vossenberg G, de Baat-Ananta M, van der Sande R, Scheffer GJ, Steegers MA. Comparison of epidural or regional analgesia and patient-controlled analgesia: a critical analysis of patient data by the acute pain service in a university hospital. Clin J Pain. 2016;32(8):681–8.

253. Candido K, Stevens RA. Intrathecal neurolytic blocks for the relief of cancer pain. Best Pract Res Clin Anaesthesiol. 2003;17(3):407–28.

254. Hay C. Subarachnoid alcohol block in the control of intractable pain: report of results in 252 patients. Anesth Analg. 1962;41:12–6.

255. Wood KM. The use of phenol as a neurolytic agent: a review. Pain. 1978;5(3):205–29.

256. Heavner JE, Racz GB. Gross and microscopic lesions produced by phenol neurolytic procedures. In: Racz GB, editor. Techniques of neurolysis. Boston: Kluwer Academic; 1989. p. 27–33.

257. Xie W, Strong JA, Zhang JM. Active nerve regeneration with failed target reinnervation drives persistent neuropathic pain. eNeuro. 2017;4(1)

258. Deer TR, Smith HS, Cousins M, Doleys DM, Levy RM, Rathmell JP, Staats PS, Wallace M, Webster LR. Consensus guidelines for the selection and implantation of patients with noncancer pain for intrathecal drug delivery. Pain Physician. 2010;13(3):E175–213.

259. Burton AW, Conroy B, Garcia E, Solanki D, Williams CG. Illicit substance abuse via an implanted intrathecal pump. Anesthesiology. 1998;89(5):1264–7.

260. Gebhardt R, Ludwig M, Kirsner S, Kisling K, Kosturakis AK. Implanted intrathecal drug delivery systems and radiation treatment. Pain Med. 2013;14(3):398–402.

261. Smith TJ, Staats PS, Deer T, Stearns LJ, Rauck RL, Boortz-Marx RL, Buchser E, Català E, Bryce DA, Coyne PJ, Pool GE, Implantable Drug Delivery Systems Study Group. Randomized clinical trial of an implantable drug delivery system compared with comprehensive medical management for refractory cancer pain: impact on pain, drug-related toxicity, and survival. J Clin Oncol. 2002;20(19):4040–9.

262. Deer TR, Pope JE, Hayek SM, Bux A, Buchser E, Eldabe S, De Andrés JA, Erdek M, Patin D, Grider JS, Doleys DM, Jacobs MS, Yaksh TL, Poree L, Wallace MS, Prager J, Rauck R, DeLeon O, Diwan S, Falowski SM, Gazelka HM, Kim P, Leong M, Levy RM, McDowell G II, McRoberts P, Naidu R, Narouze S, Perruchoud C, Rosen SM, Rosenberg WS, Saulino M, Staats P, Stearns LJ, Willis D, Krames E, Huntoon M, Mekhail N. The Polyanalgesic Consensus Conference (PACC): recommendations on intrathecal drug infusion systems best practices and guidelines. Neuromodulation. 2017;20(2):96–132.

263. McGuire D, Bowersox S, Fellmann JD, Luther RR. Sympatholysis after neuron-specific, N-type, voltage-sensitive calcium channel blockade: first demonstration of N-channel function in humans. J Cardiovasc Pharmacol. 1997;30(3):400–3.

264. Staats PS, Yearwood T, Charapata SG, Presley RW, Wallace MS, Byas-Smith M, Fisher R, Bryce DA, Mangieri EA, Luther RR, Mayo M, McGuire D, Ellis D. Intrathecal ziconotide in the treatment of refractory pain in patients with cancer or AIDS: a randomized controlled trial. JAMA. 2004;291(1):63–70.

265. Wallace MS, Rauck RL, Deer T. Ziconotide combination intrathecal therapy: rationale and evidence. Clin J Pain. 2010;26(7):635–44.

266. Shields DE, Aclan J, Szatkowski A. Chemical stability of admixtures containing ziconotide 25 mcg/mL and morphine sulfate 10 mg/mL or 20 mg/mL during simulated Intrathecal administration. Int J Pharm Compd. 2008;12(6):553–7.

267. Shields DE, Aclan J, Szatkowski A. Chemical stability of admixtures combining ziconotide with fentanyl or sufentanil during simulated intrathecal administration. Int J Pharm Compd. 2008;12(5):463–6.

268. Robert J, Sorrieul J, Rossignol E, Beaussart H, Kieffer H, Folliard C, Dupoiron D, Devys C. Chemical stability of morphine, ropivacaine, and ziconotide in combination for intrathecal analgesia. Int J Pharm Compd. 2017;21(4):347–51.

269. Staats PS, Yearwood T, Charapata SG, et al. Intrathecal ziconotide in the treatment of refractory pain in patients with cancer or AIDS: a randomized controlled trial. JAMA. 2004;291:63–70.

270. Hettiarachchi HD, Hsu Y, Harris TJ Jr, Penn R, Linninger AA. The effect of pulsatile flow on intrathecal drug delivery in the spinal canal. Ann Biomed Eng. 2011;39(10):2592–602.

271. Hsu Y, Hettiarachchi HD, Zhu DC, Linninger AA. The frequency and magnitude of cerebrospinal fluid pulsations influence intrathecal drug distribution: key factors for interpatient variability. Anesth Analg. 2012;115(2):386–94.

272. Bernards CM. Cerebrospinal fluid and spinal cord distribution of baclofen and bupivacaine during slow intrathecal infusion in pigs. Anesthesiology. 2006;105(1):169–78.

273. Wallace M, Yaksh TL. Characteristics of distribution of morphine and metabolites in cerebrospinal fluid and plasma with chronic intrathecal morphine infusion in humans. Anesth Analg. 2012;115(4):797–804.

274. Tangen KM, Hsu Y, Zhu DC, Linninger AA. CNS wide simulation of flow resistance and drug transport due to spinal microanatomy. J Biomech. 2015;48(10):2144–54.

275. Sigg J, Sonntag JC, Li J. Solubility and stability of intrathecal baclofen solutions at high concentrations: implications for chronic use in the SynchroMed VR infusion system; 2009.

276. Deer TR, Prager J, Levy R, Rathmell J, Buchser E, Burton A, Caraway D, Cousins M, De Andrés J, Diwan S, Erdek M, Grigsby E, Huntoon M, Jacobs MS, Kim P, Kumar K, Leong M, Liem L, McDowell GC 2nd, Panchal S, Rauck R, Saulino M, Sitzman BT, Staats P, Stanton-Hicks M, Stearns L, Wallace M, Willis KD, Witt W, Yaksh T, Mekhail N. Polyanalgesic consensus conference – 2012: consensus on diagnosis, detection, and treatment of catheter-tip granulomas (inflammatory masses). Neuromodulation. 2012;15(5):483–95.

277. Cabbell KL, Taren JA, Sagher O. Spinal cord compression by catheter granulomas in high-dose intrathecal morphine therapy: case report. Neurosurgery. 1998;42(5):1176–80.

278. Jackson TP, Lonergan DF, Todd RD, Martin PR. Intentional intrathecal opioid detoxification in 3 patients: characterization of the intrathecal opioid withdrawal syndrome. Pain Pract. 2013;13(4):297–309.

279. Lee HM, Ruggoo V, Graudins A. Intrathecal clonidine pump failure causing acute withdrawal syndrome with 'stress-induced' cardiomyopathy. J Med Toxicol. 2016;12(1):134–8.

280. Mohammed I, Hussain A. Intrathecal baclofen withdrawal syndrome- a life-threatening complication of baclofen pump: a case report. BMC Clin Pharmacol. 2004;4:6.

281. Klimo P Jr, Kestle JR, Schmidt MH. Clinical trials and evidence-based medicine for metastatic spine disease. Neurosurg Clin N Am. 2004;15(4):549–64.

282. Kassamali RH, Ganeshan A, Hoey ET, Crowe PM, Douis H, Henderson J. Pain management in spinal metastases: the role of percutaneous vertebral augmentation. Ann Oncol. 2011;22(4):782–6.

283. Kam NM, Maingard J, Kok HK, Ranatunga D, Brooks D, Torreggiani WC, Munk PL, Lee MJ, Chandra RV, Asadi H. Combined vertebral augmentation and radiofrequency ablation in the management of spinal metastases: an update. Curr Treat Options in Oncol. 2017;18(12):74.

284. Munk PL, Rashid F, Heran MK, Papirny M, Liu DM, Malfair D, Badii M, Clarkson PW. Combined cementoplasty and radiofrequency ablation in the treatment of painful neoplastic lesions of bone. J Vasc Interv Radiol. 2009;20(7):903–11.

285. Reyes M, Georgy M, Brook L, Ortiz O, Brook A, Agarwal V, Muto M, Manfre L, Marcia S, Georgy BA. Multicenter clinical and imaging evaluation of targeted radiofrequency ablation (t-RFA) and cement augmentation of neoplastic vertebral lesions. J Neurointerv Surg. 2018;10(2):176–82.

286. Kobayashi T, Arai Y, Takeuchi Y, Nakajima Y, Shioyama Y, Sone M, Tanigawa N, Matsui O, Kadoya M, Inaba Y, Japan Interventional Radiology in Oncology Study Group (JIVROSG). Phase I/II clinical study of percutaneous vertebroplasty (PVP) as palliation for painful malignant vertebral compression fractures (PMVCF): JIVROSG-0202. Ann Oncol. 2009;20(12):1943–7.

287. Berenson J, Pflugmacher R, Jarzem P, Zonder J, Schechtman K, Tillman JB, Bastian L, Ashraf T, Vrionis F, Cancer Patient Fracture Evaluation (CAFE) Investigators. Balloon kyphoplasty versus non-surgical fracture management for treatment of painful vertebral body compression fractures in patients with cancer: a multicentre, randomised controlled trial. Lancet Oncol. 2011;12(3):225–35.

288. Ontario HQ. Vertebral augmentation involving vertebroplasty or kyphoplasty for cancer-related vertebral compression fractures: an economic analysis. Ont Health Technol Assess Ser. 2016;16(12):1–34.

289. Tsoumakidou G, Too CW, Koch G, Caudrelier J, Cazzato RL, Garnon J, Gangi A. CIRSE guidelines on percutaneous vertebral augmentation. Cardiovasc Intervent Radiol. 2017;40(3):331–42.

290. Chew C, Craig L, Edwards R, Moss J, O'Dwyer PJ. Safety and efficacy of percutaneous vertebroplasty in malignancy: a systematic review. Clin Radiol. 2011;66(1):63–72.

291. Halpin RJ, Bendok BR, Liu JC. Minimally invasive treatments for spinal metastases: vertebroplasty, kyphoplasty, and radiofrequency ablation. J Support Oncol. 2004;2(4):339–51.

292. Deibert CP, Gandhoke GS, Paschel EE, Gerszten PC. A longitudinal cohort investigation of the development of symptomatic adjacent level compression fractures following balloon-assisted kyphoplasty in a series of 726 patients. Pain Physician. 2016;19(8):E1167–72.

293. Li G, Xue M, Chen W, Yi S. Efficacy and safety of radiofrequency ablation for lung cancers: a systematic review and meta-analysis. Eur J Radiol. 2018;100:92–8.

294. Chung SR, Suh CH, Baek JH, Park HS, Choi YJ, Lee JH. Safety of radiofrequency ablation of benign thyroid nodules and recurrent thyroid cancers: a systematic review and meta-analysis. Int J Hyperth. 2017;33(8):920–30.

295. Kurup AN, Morris JM, Callstrom MR. Ablation of musculoskeletal metastases. AJR Am J Roentgenol. 2017;209(4):713–21.

296. Puijk RS, Ruarus AH, Scheffer HJ, Vroomen LGPH, van Tilborg AAJM, de Vries JJJ, Berger FH, van den Tol PMP, Meijerink MR. Percutaneous liver tumour ablation: image guidance, endpoint assessment, and quality control. Can Assoc Radiol J. 2018;69(1):51–62.

297. Maciolek KA, Abel EJ, Best SL, Emamekhoo H, Averill SL, Ziemlewicz TJ, Lubner MG, Hinshaw JL, Lee FT Jr, Wells SA. Percutaneous microwave ablation for local control of metastatic renal cell carcinoma. Abdom Radiol (NY). 2018;43(9):2446–54.

298. Yoong J, Chandra RV, William L, Franco M, Goldschlager T, Runacres F, Poon P. Percutaneous sacroplasty for painful bone metastases: a case report. Pain Pract. 2017;17(7):945–51.

299. Dmytriw AA, Talla K, Smith R. Percutaneous sacroplasty for the management of painful pathologic fracture in a multiple myeloma patient: case report and review of the literature. Neuroradiol J. 2017;30(1):80–3.

300. Cho S, Park HS, Kim DY, Kim CH, Chung RK, Kim YJ. Percutaneous sacroplasty under fluoroscopic guidance combined with epidurogram for sacral insufficiency fracture resulting from metastatic tumor and osteoporosis. Pain Physician. 2016;19(3):E473–80.

301. Agarwal V, Sreedher G, Weiss KR, Hughes MA. Sacroplasty for symptomatic sacral hemangioma: a novel treatment approach. A case report. Interv Neuroradiol. 2013;19(2):245–9.

302. Moussazadeh N, Laufer I, Werner T, Krol G, Boland P, Bilsky MH, Lis E. Sacroplasty for cancer-associated insufficiency fractures. Neurosurgery. 2015;76(4):446–50.

303. Pereira LP, Clarençon F, Cormier E, Rose M, Jean B, Le Jean L, Chiras J. Safety and effectiveness of percutaneous sacroplasty: a single-centre experience in 58 consecutive patients with tumours or osteoporotic insufficient fractures treated under fluoroscopic guidance. Eur Radiol. 2013;23(10):2764–72.

304. Chai T, Suleiman ZA, Roldan CJ. Unilateral lower extremity pain due to malignancy managed with cordotomy: a case report. PMR. 2017;S1934-1482(17):31293–5.

305. Feizerfan A, Antrobus JHL. Role of percutaneous cervical cordotomy in cancer pain management. Contin Educ Anaesth Crit Care Pain. 2014;14(1):23–6.

306. Kanpolat Y. The surgical treatment of chronic pain: destructive therapies in the spinal cord. Neurosurg Clin N Am. 2004;15(3):307–17.

307. Fitzgibbon DR. Percutaneous CT-guided C1-2 cordotomy for intractable cancer pain. Curr Pain Headache Rep. 2009;13(4):253–5.

308. Nashold BS Jr, el-Naggar A, Mawaffak Abdulhak M, Ovelmen-Levitt J, Cosman E. Trigeminal nucleus caudalis dorsal root entry zone: a new surgical approach. Stereotact Funct Neurosurg. 1992;59(1–4):45–51.

309. Kanpolat Y, Tuna H, Bozkurt M, Elhan AH. Spinal and nucleus caudalis dorsal root entry zone operations for chronic pain. Neurosurgery. 2008;62(3):235–42.. – Review of the anatomy and excellent description of the approach to stereotactic destruction

310. Sjoquist O. Studies on pain conduction in trigeminal nerve. A contribution to the treatment of facial pain. Acta Psychiatr Neurol Suppl. 1938;17(9):139.

311. Hitchcock E. Stereotactic trigeminal tractotomy. Ann Clin Res. 1970;2(2):131–5.

312. Crue BL, Carregal EJA, Felsoory A. Percutaneous stereotactic radiofrequency trigeminal tractotomy with neurophysiological recordings. Stereotact Funct Neurosurg. 1972;34(6):389–97.

313. Kanpolat Y, Kahilogullari G, Ugur HC, Elhan AH. Computed tomography-guided percutaneous trigeminal tractotomy-nucleotomy. Neurosurgery. 2008;63(1):147–53.

314. Sindou M, Goutelle A. Surgical posterior rhizotomies for the treatment of pain. In: Krayenbuhl H, editor. Advances and technical standards in neurosurgery, vol. 10. Vienna: Springer; 1983. p. 147–83.

315. Schvarcz JR. Functional exploration of the spinomedullary junction. Acta Neurochir Suppl. 1977;24:179–85.

316. Al-Chaer ED, Lawand NB, Westlund KN, Willis WD. Visceral nociceptive input into the ventral posterolateral nucleus of the thalamus: a new function for the dorsal column pathway. J Neurophysiol. 1996;76(4):2661–74.

317. Shealy CN, Tyner CF, Taslitz N. Physiological evidence of bilateral spinal projections of pain fibers in cats and monkeys. J Neurosurg. 1966;24:708.

318. Gildenberg PL, Hirshberg RM. Limited myelotomy for the treatment of intractable cancer pain. J Neurol Neurosurg Psychiatry. 1984;47(1):94–6.

319. Nauta HJ, Hewitt E, Westlund KN, Willis WD Jr. Surgical interruption of a midline dorsal column visceral pain pathway. Case report and review of the literature. J Neurosurg. 1997;86(3):538–42.

320. Tonezzer T, Caffaro LAM, Menon KRS, Brandini da Silva FC, Moran de Brito CM, Sarri AJ, Casarotto RA. Effects of transcutaneous electrical nerve stimulation on chemotherapy-induced peripheral neuropathy symptoms (CIPN): a preliminary case-control study. J Phys Ther Sci. 2017;29(4):685–92.

321. Lee JE, Anderson CM, Perkhounkova Y, Sleeuwenhoek BM, Louison RR. Transcutaneous electrical nerve stimulation reduces resting pain in head and neck cancer patients: a randomized and placebo-controlled double-blind pilot study. Cancer Nurs. 2019;42(3):218–28.

322. Loh J, Gulati A. The use of transcutaneous electrical nerve stimulation (TENS) in a major cancer center for the treatment of severe cancer-related pain and associated disability. Pain Med. 2015;16(6):1204–10.

323. Loh J, Gulati A. Transcutaneous electrical nerve stimulation for treatment of sarcoma cancer pain. Pain Manag. 2013;3(3):189–99.

324. Hou L, Zhou C, Wu Y, Yu Y, Hu Y. Transcutaneous electrical acupoint stimulation (TEAS) relieved cancer-related fatigue in non-small cell lung cancer (NSCLC) patients after chemotherapy. J Thorac Dis. 2017;9(7):1959–66.

325. Choi YD, Lee JH. Edema and pain reduction using transcutaneous electrical nerve stimulation treatment. J Phys Ther Sci. 2016;28(11):3084–7.

326. Hou L, Gu F, Gao G, Zhou C. Transcutaneous electrical acupoint stimulation (TEAS) ameliorates chemotherapy-induced bone marrow suppression in lung cancer patients. J Thorac Dis. 2017;9(3):809–17.

327. Wong R, Major P, Sagar S. Phase 2 study of acupuncture-like transcutaneous nerve stimulation for chemotherapy-induced peripheral neuropathy. Integr Cancer Ther. 2016;15(2):153–64.

328. Xie J, Chen LH, Ning ZY, Zhang CY, Chen H, Chen Z, Meng ZQ, Zhu XY. Effect of transcutaneous electrical acupoint stimulation combined with palonosetron on chemotherapy-induced nausea and vomiting: a single-blind, randomized, controlled trial. Chin J Cancer. 2017;36(1):6.

329. Smith TJ, Coyne PJ, Parker GL, Dodson P, Ramakrishnan V. Pilot trial of a patient-specific cutaneous electrostimulation device (MC5-A Calmare®) for chemotherapy-induced peripheral neuropathy. J Pain Symptom Manag. 2010;40(6):883–91.

330. Lee SC, Park KS, Moon JY, Kim EJ, Kim YC, Seo H, Sung JK, Lee DJ. An exploratory study on the effectiveness of "Calmare therapy" in patients with cancer-related neuropathic pain: a pilot study. Eur J Oncol Nurs. 2016;21:1–7.

331. Tomasello C, Pinto RM, Mennini C, Conicella E, Stoppa F, Raucci U. Scrambler therapy efficacy and safety for neuropathic pain correlated with chemotherapy-induced peripheral neuropathy in adolescents: a preliminary study. Pediatr Blood Cancer. 2018;65(7):e27064.

332. Greenlee H, Crew KD, Capodice J, Awad D, Buono D, Shi Z, Jeffres A, Wyse S, Whitman W, Trivedi MS, Kalinsky K, Hershman DL. Randomized sham-controlled pilot trial of weekly electro-acupuncture for the prevention of taxane-induced peripheral neuropathy in women with early stage breast cancer. Breast Cancer Res Treat. 2016;156(3):453–64.

333. Hsiao HT, Chien HJ, Lin YC, Liu YC. Transcutaneous electrical nerve stimulator of 5000 Hz frequency provides better analgesia than that of 100 Hz frequency in mice muscle pain model. Kaohsiung J Med Sci. 2017;33(4):165–70.

334. Shealy CN, Mortimer JT, Reswick JB. Electrical inhibition of pain by stimulation of the dorsal columns: preliminary clinical report. Anesth Analg. 1967;46(4):489–91.

335. Peng L, Min S, Zejun Z, Wei K, Bennett MI. Spinal cord stimulation for cancer-related pain in adults. Cochrane Database Syst Rev. 2015;6:CD009389.

336. Xing F, Yong RJ, Kaye AD, Urman RD. Intrathecal drug delivery and spinal cord stimulation for the treatment of cancer pain. Curr Pain Headache Rep. 2018;22(2):11.

337. Wall PD, Sweet WH. Temporary abolition of pain in man. Science. 1967;155(3758):108–9.

338. Haugland M, Sinkjaer T. Interfacing the body's own sensing receptors into neural prosthesis devices. Technol Health Care. 1999;7(6):393–9.

339. Monti E. Peripheral nerve stimulation: a percutaneous minimally invasive approach. Neuromodulation. 2004;7(3):193–6.

340. Slavin KV, Colpan ME, Munawar N, Wess C, Nersesyan H. Trigeminal and occipital peripheral nerve stimulation for craniofacial pain: a single-institution experience and review of the literature. Neurosurg Focus. 2006;21(6):E5.

341. Huntoon MA, Burgher AH. Ultrasound-guided permanent implantation of peripheral nerve stimulation (PNS) system for neuropathic pain of the extremities: original cases and outcomes. Pain Med. 2009;10(8):1369–77.

342. Deer T, Pope J, Benyamin R, Vallejo R, Friedman A, Caraway D, Staats P, Grigsby E, Porter McRoberts W, McJunkin T, Shubin R, Vahedifar P, Tavanaiepour D, Levy R, Kapural L, Mekhail N. Prospective, multicenter, randomized, double-blinded, partial crossover study to assess the safety and efficacy of the novel Neuromodulation system in the treatment of patients with chronic pain of peripheral nerve origin. Neuromodulation. 2016;19(1):91–100.

343. Verrills P, Vivian D, Mitchell B, Barnard A. Peripheral nerve field stimulation for chronic pain: 100 cases and review of the literature. Pain Med. 2011;12(9):1395–405.

344. Paicius RM, Bernstein CA, Lempert-Cohen C. Peripheral nerve field stimulation in chronic abdominal pain. Pain Physician. 2006;9(3):261–6.

345. Levi V, Messina G, Franzini A, Zanin L, Castelli N, Dones I. Peripheral nerve field stimulation (PNFS) as a treatment option for intractable radiation-induced facial neuropathic pain in a survivor of laryngeal cancer: a case report. World Neurosurg. 2016;91:671.

346. US Department of Health and Human Services. 2008 physical activity guidelines for Americans. http://www.health.gov/PAGuidelines.

347. Speck RM, Courneya KS, Mâsse LC, Duval S, Schmitz KH. An update of controlled physical activity trials in cancer survivors: a systematic review and meta-analysis. J Cancer Surviv. 2010;4(2):87–100.

348. Ohira T, Schmitz KH, Ahmed RL, Yee D. Effects of weight training on quality of life in recent breast cancer survivors: the Weight Training for Breast Cancer Survivors (WTBS) study. Cancer. 2006;106(9):2076–83.

349. Espíndula RC, Nadas GB, Rosa MID, Foster C, Araújo FC, Grande AJ. Pilates for breast cancer: a systematic review and meta-analysis. Rev Assoc Med Bras (1992). 2017;63(11):1006–12.

350. Mishra SI, Scherer RW, Snyder C, Geigle PM, Berlanstein DR, Topaloglu O. Exercise interventions on health-related quality of life for people with cancer during active treatment. Cochrane Database Syst Rev. 2012;8:CD008465.

351. Lahart IM, Metsios GS, Nevill AM, Carmichael AR. Physical activity for women with breast cancer after adjuvant therapy. Cochrane Database Syst Rev. 2018;1:CD011292.

352. Mishra SI, Scherer RW, Geigle PM, Berlanstein DR, Topaloglu O, Gotay CC, Snyder C. Exercise interventions on health-related quality of life for cancer survivors. Cochrane Database Syst Rev. 2012;8:CD007566.

353. Cormie P, Newton RU, Spry N, Joseph D, Taaffe DR, Galvão DA. Safety and efficacy of resistance exercise in prostate cancer patients with bone metastases. Prostate Cancer Prostatic Dis. 2013;16(4):328–35.

354. Galvão DA, Nosaka K, Taaffe DR, Spry N, Kristjanson LJ, McGuigan MR, Suzuki K, Yamaya K, Newton RU. Resistance training and reduction of treatment side effects in prostate cancer patients. Med Sci Sports Exerc. 2006;38(12):2045–52.

355. Al-Majid S, Waters H. The biological mechanisms of cancer-related skeletal muscle wasting: the role of progressive resistance exercise. Biol Res Nurs. 2008;10(1):7–20.

356. Kang DW, Lee EY, An KY, Min J, Jeon JY, Courneya KS. Associations between physical activity and comorbidities in Korean cancer survivors. J Cancer Surviv. 2018;12(4):441–9.

357. Schmitz KH, Speck RM. Risks and benefits of physical activity among breast cancer survivors who have completed treatment. Womens Health (Lond). 2010;6(2):221–38.

358. Nelson NL. Breast cancer-related lymphedema and resistance exercise: a systematic review. J Strength Cond Res. 2016;30(9):2656–65.

359. Ruiz JR, Sui X, Lobelo F, Lee DC, Morrow JR Jr, Jackson AW, Hébert JR, Matthews CE, Sjöström M, Blair SN. Muscular strength and adiposity as predictors of adulthood cancer mortality in men. Cancer Epidemiol Biomark Prev. 2009;18(5):1468–76.

360. Markes M, Brockow T, Resch KL. Exercise for women receiving adjuvant therapy for breast cancer. Cochrane Database Syst Rev. 2006;4:CD005001.

361. Furmaniak AC, Menig M, Markes MH. Exercise for women receiving adjuvant therapy for breast cancer. Cochrane Database Syst Rev. 2016;9:CD005001.

362. Ottenbacher A, Yu M, Moser RP, Phillips SM, Alfano C, Perna FM. Population estimates of meeting strength training and aerobic guidelines, by gender and cancer survivorship status: findings from the Health Information National Trends Survey (HINTS). J Phys Act Health. 2015;12(5):675–9.

363. Bourke L, Homer KE, Thaha MA, Steed L, Rosario DJ, Robb KA, Saxton JM, Taylor SJ. Interventions for promoting habitual exercise in people living with and beyond cancer. Cochrane Database Syst Rev. 2013;9:CD010192.

364. Andersen C, Rorth M, Ejlertsen B, Adamsen L. Exercise despite pain--breast cancer patient experiences of muscle and joint pain during adjuvant chemotherapy and concurrent participation in an exercise intervention. Eur J Cancer Care (Engl). 2014;23(5):653–67.

365. Sheill G, Guinan E, Neill LO, Hevey D, Hussey J. The views of patients with metastatic prostate cancer towards physical activity: a qualitative exploration. Support Care Cancer. 2018;26(6):1747–54.

366. Jensen BT, Jensen JB, Laustsen S, Petersen AK, Søndergaard I, Borre M. Multidisciplinary rehabilitation can impact on health-related quality of life outcome in radical cystectomy: secondary reported outcome of a randomized controlled trial. J Multidiscip Healthc. 2014;7:301–11.

367. Mirandola D, Miccinesi G, Muraca MG, Belardi S, Giuggioli R, Sgambati E, Manetti M, Monaci M, Marini M. Longitudinal assessment of the impact of adapted physical activity on upper limb disability and quality of life in breast cancer survivors from an Italian cohort. Support Care Cancer. 2018;26(2):329–32.

368. Jensen BT, Petersen AK, Jensen JB, Laustsen S, Borre M. Efficacy of a multiprofessional rehabilitation programme in radical cystectomy pathways: a prospective randomized controlled trial. Scand J Urol. 2015;49(2):133–41.

369. Cho Y, Do J, Jung S, Kwon O, Jeon JY. Effects of a physical therapy program combined with manual lymphatic drainage on shoulder function, quality of life, lymphedema incidence, and pain in breast cancer patients with axillary web syndrome following axillary dissection. Support Care Cancer. 2016;24(5):2047–57.

370. Cheville AL, Rhudy L, Basford JR, Griffin JM, Flores AM. How receptive are patients with late stage cancer to rehabilitation services and what are the sources of their resistance? Arch Phys Med Rehabil. 2017;98(2):203–10.

371. Nishigori H, Ishii M, Kokado Y, Fujimoto K, Higashiyama H. Effectiveness of pelvic floor rehabilitation for bowel dysfunction after intersphincteric resection for lower rectal cancer. World J Surg. 2018;42(10):3415–21.

372. Chen SC, Huang BS, Chung CY, Lin CY, Fan KH, Chang JT, Wu SC. Effects of a swallowing exercise education program on dysphagia-specific health-related quality of life in oral cavity cancer patients post-treatment: a randomized controlled trial. Support Care Cancer. 2018;26(8):2919–28.

373. Maher C, Mendonca RJ. Impact of an activity-based program on health, quality of life, and occupational performance of women diagnosed with cancer. Am J Occup Ther. 2018;72(2):1–8.

374. Ferrer RA, Huedo-Medina TB, Johnson BT, Ryan S, Pescatello LS. Exercise interventions for cancer survivors: a meta-analysis of quality of life outcomes. Ann Behav Med. 2011;41(1):32–47.

375. Rick O, Dauelsberg T, Kalusche-Bontemps EM. Oncological rehabilitation. Oncol Res Treat. 2017;40(12):772–7.

376. De Groef A, Van Kampen M, Vervloesem N, Dieltjens E, Christiaens MR, Neven P, Vos L, De Vrieze T, Geraerts I, Devoogdt N. Effect of myofascial techniques for treatment of persistent arm pain after breast cancer treatment: randomized controlled trial. Clin Rehabil. 2018;32(4):451–61.

377. De Groef A, Van Kampen M, Vervloesem N, De Geyter S, Christiaens MR, Neven P, Vos L, De Vrieze T, Geraerts I, Devoogdt N. Myofascial techniques have no additional beneficial effects to a standard physical therapy programme for upper limb pain after breast cancer surgery: a randomized controlled trial. Clin Rehabil. 2017;31(12):1625–35.

378. Baxter GD, Liu L, Petrich S, Gisselman AS, Chapple C, Anders JJ, Tumilty S. Low level laser therapy (Photobiomodulation therapy) for breast cancer-related lymphedema: a systematic review. BMC Cancer. 2017;17(1):833.

379. Castro-Martín E, Ortiz-Comino L, Gallart-Aragón T, Esteban-Moreno B, Arroyo-Morales M, Galiano-Castillo N. Myofascial induction effects on neck-shoulder pain in breast cancer survivors: randomized, single-blind, placebo-controlled crossover design. Arch Phys Med Rehabil. 2017;98(5):832–40.

380. Imperatori A, Grande A, Castiglioni M, Gasperini L, Faini A, Spampatti S, Nardecchia E, Terzaghi L, Dominioni L, Rotolo N. Chest pain control with kinesiology taping after lobectomy for lung cancer: initial results of a randomized placebo-controlled study. Interact Cardiovasc Thorac Surg. 2016;23(2):223–30.

381. Burgess C, Cornelius V, Love S, Graham J, Richards M, Ramirez A. Depression and anxiety in women with early breast cancer: five year observational cohort study. BMJ. 2005;330(7493):702.

382. Tighe M, Molassiotis A, Morris J, Richardson J. Coping, meaning and symptom experience: a narrative approach to the overwhelming impacts of breast cancer in the first year following diagnosis. Eur J Oncol Nurs. 2011;15(3):226–32.

383. Jazzar U, Yong S, Klaassen Z, Huo J, Hughes BD, Esparza E, Mehta HB, Kim SP, Tyler DS, Freedland SJ, Kamat AM, Wolf DV, Williams SB. Impact of psychiatric illness on decreased survival in elderly patients with bladder cancer in the United States. Cancer. 2018;124(15):3127–35.

384. Satin JR, Linden W, Phillips MJ. Depression as a predictor of disease progression and mortality in cancer patients: a meta-analysis. Cancer. 2009;115(22):5349–61.

385. Barber B, Dergousoff J, Slater L, Harris J, O'Connell D, El-Hakim H, Biron VL, Mitchell N, Seikaly H. Depression and survival in patients with head and neck cancer: a systematic review. JAMA Otolaryngol Head Neck Surg. 2016;142(3):284–8.

386. Lattie EG, Antoni MH, Millon T, Kamp J, Walker MR. MBMD coping styles and psychiatric indicators and response to a multidisciplinary pain treatment program. J Clin Psychol Med Settings. 2013;20(4):515–25.

387. Holmes A, Christelis N, Arnold C. Depression and chronic pain. Med J Aust. 2013;199(6 Suppl):S17–20.

388. Turk DC, Fillingim RB, Ohrbach R, Patel KV. Assessment of psychosocial and functional impact of chronic pain. J Pain. 2016;17(9 Suppl):T21–49.

389. Fawzy FI, Fawzy NW, Hyun CS, Elashoff R, Guthrie D, Fahey JL, Morton DL. Malignant melanoma. Effects of an early structured psychiatric intervention, coping, and affective state on recurrence and survival 6 years later. Arch Gen Psychiatry. 1993;50(9):681–9.

390. Spiegel D, Bloom JR, Kraemer HC, Gottheil E. Effect of psychosocial treatment on survival of patients with metastatic breast cancer. Lancet. 1989;2(8668):888–91.

391. Xia Y, Tong G, Feng R, Chai J, Cheng J, Wang D. Psychosocial and behavioral interventions and cancer patient survival again: hints of an adjusted meta-analysis. Integr Cancer Ther. 2014;13(4):301–9.

392. Giese-Davis J, Collie K, Rancourt KMS, Neri E, Kraemer HC, Spiegel D. Decrease in depression symptoms is associated with

longer survival in patients with metastatic breast cancer: a secondary analysis. J Clin Oncol. 2011;29(4):413–20.

393. Mulick A, Walker J, Puntis S, Burke K, Symeonides S, Gourley C, Wanat M, Frost C, Sharpe M. Does depression treatment improve the survival of depressed patients with cancer? A long-term follow-up of participants in the SMaRT Oncology-2 and 3 trials. Lancet Psychiatry. 2018;5(4):321–6.

394. Dobson K, Dozios DJA. Historical and philosophical bases of the cognitive behavioral therapy. In: Dobson KS, editor. Handbook of cognitive behavioral therapies. 3rd ed. New York, NY: Guilford Press; 2010. p. 3–38.

395. Folkman S, Moskowitz JT. Stress, positive emotion, and coping. Cur Dir Psych Sci. 2000;9(4):115–8.

396. McGinn L, Sanderson W. What allows cognitive behavioral therapy to be brief: overview, efficacy and crucial factors facilitating brief treatment. Psychol Sci Pract. 2001;8(1):23–37.

397. Dalton JA, Keefe FJ, Carlson J, Youngblood R. Tailoring cognitive-behavioral treatment for cancer pain. Pain Manag Nurs. 2004;5(1):3–18.

398. Anderson KO, Cohen MZ, Mendoza TR, Guo H, Harle MT, Cleeland CS. Brief cognitive-behavioral audiotape interventions for cancer-related pain: immediate but not long-term effectiveness. Cancer. 2006;107(1):207–14.

399. Kwekkeboom KL, Abbott-Anderson K, Cherwin C, Roiland R, Serlin RC, Ward SE. Pilot randomized controlled trial of a patient-controlled cognitive-behavioral intervention for the pain, fatigue, and sleep disturbance symptom cluster in cancer. J Pain Symptom Manag. 2012;44(6):810–22.

400. Phianmongkhol Y, Thongubon K, Woottiluk P. Effectiveness of cognitive behavioral therapy techniques for control of pain in lung cancer patients: an integrated review. Asian Pac J Cancer Prev. 2015;16(14):6033–8603.

401. Chiesa A, Serretti A. Mindfulness-based interventions for chronic pain: a systematic review of the evidence. J Altern Complement Med. 2011;17(1):83–93.

402. Reiner K, Tibi L, Lipsitz JD. Do mindfulness-based interventions reduce pain intensity? A critical review of the literature. Pain Med. 2013;14(2):230–42.

403. Johannsen M, O'Connor M, O'Toole MS, Jensen AB, Hojris I, Zachariae R. Efficacy of mindfulness-based cognitive therapy on late post-treatment pain in women treated for primary breast cancer: a randomized controlled trial. J Clin Oncol. 2016;34(28):3390–9.

404. Kabat-Zinn J. An outpatient program in behavioral medicine for chronic pain patients based on the practice of mindfulness meditation: theoretical considerations and preliminary results. Gen Hosp Psychiatry. 1982;4(1):33–47.

405. Baer RA, Carmody J, Hunsinger M. Weekly change in mindfulness and perceived stress in a mindfulness-based stress reduction program. J Clin Psychol. 2012;68(7):755–65.

406. Elvery N, Jensen MP, Ehde DM, Day MA. Pain catastrophizing, mindfulness, and pain acceptance: what's the difference? Clin J Pain. 2017;33(6):485–95.

407. Turner JA, Anderson ML, Balderson BH, Cook AJ, Sherman KJ, Cherkin DC. Mindfulness-based stress reduction and cognitive behavioral therapy for chronic low back pain: similar effects on mindfulness, catastrophizing, self-efficacy, and acceptance in a randomized controlled trial. Pain. 2016;157(11):2434–44.

408. Johannsen M, O'Connor M, O'Toole MS, Jensen AB, Zachariae R. Mindfulness-based cognitive therapy and persistent pain in women treated for primary breast cancer: exploring possible statistical mediators: results from a randomized controlled trial. Clin J Pain. 2018;34(1):59–67.

409. Reich RR, Lengacher CA, Alinat CB, Kip KE, Paterson C, Ramesar S, Han HS, Ismail-Khan R, Johnson-Mallard V, Moscoso M, Budhrani-Shani P, Shivers S, Cox CE, Goodman M, Park J. Mindfulness-based stress reduction in post-treatment breast cancer patients: immediate and sustained effects across multiple symptom clusters. J Pain Symptom Manag. 2017;53(1):85–95.

410. National Center for Complementary and Integrative Health. Complementary, Alternative, or Integrative Health: What's In a Name? nccam.nih.gov/health/whatiscam.

411. Greenlee H, DuPont-Reyes MJ, Balneaves LG, Carlson LE, Cohen MR, Deng G, Johnson JA, Mumber M, Seely D, Zick SM, Boyce LM, Tripathy D. Clinical practice guidelines on the evidence-based use of integrative therapies during and after breast cancer treatment. CA Cancer J Clin. 2017;67(3):194–232.

412. Armstrong K, Lanni T Jr, Anderson MM, Patricolo GE. Integrative medicine and the oncology patient: options and benefits. Support Care Cancer. 2018;26(7):2267–73.

413. Greenlee H, Balneaves LG, Carlson LE, Cohen M, Deng G, Hershman D, Mumber M, Perlmutter J, Seely D, Sen A, Zick SM, Tripathy D, Society for Integrative Oncology. Clinical practice guidelines on the use of integrative therapies as supportive care in patients treated for breast cancer. J Natl Cancer Inst Monogr. 2014;2014(50):346–58.

414. US Preventive Services Task Force. Grade definitions; 2008. http://www.uspreventiveservicestaskforce.org/uspstf/grades.htm.

415. Shen Y, Liu L, Chiang JS, Meng Z, Garcia MK, Chen Z, Peng H, Bei W, Zhao Q, Spelman AR, Cohen L. Randomized, placebo-controlled trial of K1 acupoint acustimulation to prevent cisplatin-induced or oxaliplatin-induced nausea. Cancer. 2015;121(1):84–92.

416. Gan TJ, Jiao KR, Zenn M, Georgiade G. A randomized controlled comparison of electro-acupoint stimulation or ondansetron versus placebo for the prevention of postoperative nausea and vomiting. Anesth Analg. 2004;99(4):1070–5.

417. Bao T, Cai L, Giles JT, Gould J, Tarpinian K, Betts K, Medeiros M, Jeter S, Tait N, Chumsri S, Armstrong DK, Tan M, Folkerd E, Dowsett M, Singh H, Tkaczuk K, Stearns V. A dual-center randomized controlled double blind trial assessing the effect of acupuncture in reducing musculoskeletal symptoms in breast cancer patients taking aromatase inhibitors. Breast Cancer Res Treat. 2013;138(1):167–74.

418. Crew KD, Capodice JL, Greenlee H, Apollo A, Jacobson JS, Raptis G, Blozie K, Sierra A, Hershman DL. Pilot study of acupuncture for the treatment of joint symptoms related to adjuvant aromatase inhibitor therapy in postmenopausal breast cancer patients. J Cancer Surviv. 2007;1(4):283–91.

419. Crew KD, Capodice JL, Greenlee H, Brafman L, Fuentes D, Awad D, Yann Tsai W, Hershman DL. Randomized, blinded, sham-controlled trial of acupuncture for the management of aromatase inhibitor-associated joint symptoms in women with early-stage breast cancer. J Clin Oncol. 2010;28(7):1154–60.

420. Oh B, Kimble B, Costa DS, Davis E, McLean A, Orme K, Beith J. Acupuncture for treatment of arthralgia secondary to aromatase inhibitor therapy in women with early breast cancer: pilot study. Acupunct Med. 2013;31(3):264–71.

421. Mao JJ, Farrar JT, Bruner D, Zee J, Bowman M, Seluzicki C, DeMichele A, Xie SX. Electroacupuncture for fatigue, sleep, and psychological distress in breast cancer patients with aromatase inhibitor-related arthralgia: a randomized trial. Cancer. 2014;120(23):3744–51.

422. Paley CA, Johnson MI, Tashani OA, Bagnall AM. Acupuncture for cancer pain in adults. Cochrane Database Syst Rev. 2015;(10):CD007753.

423. Hu C, Zhang H, Wu W, Yu W, Li Y, Bai J, Luo B, Li S. Acupuncture for pain management in cancer: a systematic review and meta-analysis. Evid Based Complement Alternat Med. 2016;2016:1720239.

424. Melchart D, Weidenhammer W, Streng A, Reitmayr S, Hoppe A, Ernst E, Linde K. Prospective investigation of adverse effects of acupuncture in 97,733 patients. Arch Intern Med. 2004;164(1):104–5.
425. Witt CM, Pach D, Brinkhaus B, Wruck K, Tag B, Mank S, Willich SN. Safety of acupuncture: results of a prospective observational study with 229,230 patients and introduction of a medical information and consent form. Forsch Komplementmed. 2009;16(2):91–7.
426. Healing Touch Program. What Is Healing Touch? https://www.healingtouchprogram.com/about/what-is-healing-touch.
427. Post-White J, Kinney ME, Savik K, Gau JB, Wilcox C, Lerner I. Therapeutic massage and healing touch improve symptoms in cancer. Integr Cancer Ther. 2003;2(4):332–44.
428. McGilvery C, Reed J. Step-by-step massage: a guide to massage techniques for health, relaxation and vitality. Detroit, MI: Treasure Press; 1994.
429. Hughes D, Ladas E, Rooney D, Kelly K. Massage therapy as a supportive care intervention for children with cancer. Oncol Nurs Forum. 2008;35(3):431–42.
430. Billhult A, Lindholm C, Gunnarsson R, Stener-Victorin E. The effect of massage on immune function and stress in women with breast cancer--a randomized controlled trial. Auton Neurosci. 2009;150(1–2):111–5.
431. Lee PL, Tam KW, Yeh ML, Wu WW. Acupoint stimulation, massage therapy and expressive writing for breast cancer: a systematic review and meta-analysis of randomized controlled trials. Complement Ther Med. 2016;27:87–101.
432. Foley NC, Bhogal SK, Teasell RW, Bureau Y, Speechley MR. Estimates of quality and reliability with the physiotherapy evidence-based database scale to assess the methodology of randomized controlled trials of pharmacological and nonpharmacological interventions. Phys Ther. 2006;86(6):817–24.
433. Shin ES, Seo KH, Lee SH, Jang JE, Jung YM, Kim MJ, Yeon JY. Massage with or without aromatherapy for symptom relief in people with cancer. Cochrane Database Syst Rev. 2016;(6):CD009873.
434. Izgu N, Ozdemir L, Bugdayci Basal F. Effect of aromatherapy massage on chemotherapy-induced peripheral neuropathic pain and fatigue in patients receiving oxaliplatin: an open label quasi-randomized controlled pilot study. Cancer Nurs. 2019;42(2):139–47.
435. Lopez G, Liu W, Milbury K, Spelman A, Wei Q, Bruera E, Cohen L. The effects of oncology massage on symptom self-report for cancer patients and their caregivers. Support Care Cancer. 2017;25(12):3645–50.
436. Jane SW, Chen SL, Wilkie DJ, Lin YC, Foreman SW, Beaton RD, Fan JY, Lu MY, Wang YY, Lin YH, Liao MN. Effects of massage on pain, mood status, relaxation, and sleep in Taiwanese patients with metastatic bone pain: a randomized clinical trial. Pain. 2011;152(10):2432–42.
437. Wilcock A, Manderson C, Weller R, Walker G, Carr D, Carey AM, Broadhurst D, Mew J, Ernst E. Does aromatherapy massage benefit patients with cancer attending a specialist palliative care day centre? Palliat Med. 2004;18(4):287–90.
438. National Center for Complementary and Integrative Health. Yoga. nccih.nih.gov/health/yoga.
439. Smith KB, Pukall CF. An evidence-based review of yoga as a complementary intervention for patients with cancer. Psychooncology. 2009;18(5):465–75.
440. Buffart LM, van Uffelen JG, Riphagen II, Brug J, van Mechelen W, Brown WJ, Chinapaw MJ. Physical and psychosocial benefits of yoga in cancer patients and survivors, a systematic review and meta-analysis of randomized controlled trials. BMC Cancer. 2012;12:559.
441. Wayne PM, Lee MS, Novakowski J, Osypiuk K, Ligibel J, Carlson LE, Song R. Tai Chi and Qigong for cancer-related symptoms and quality of life: a systematic review and meta-analysis. J Cancer Surviv. 2018;12(2):256–67.
442. Danhauer SC, Addington EL, Sohl SJ, Chaoul A, Cohen L. Review of yoga therapy during cancer treatment. Support Care Cancer. 2017;25(4):1357–72.
443. Carlson LE, Zelinski E, Toivonen K, Flynn M, Qureshi M, Piedalue KA, Grant R. Mind-body therapies in cancer: what is the latest evidence? Curr Oncol Rep. 2017;19(10):67.
444. Derry HM, Jaremka LM, Bennett JM, Peng J, Andridge R, Shapiro C, Malarkey WB, Emery CF, Layman R, Mrozek E, Glaser R, Kiecolt-Glaser JK. Yoga and self-reported cognitive problems in breast cancer survivors: a randomized controlled trial. Psychooncology. 2015;24(8):958–66.
445. Littman AJ, Bertram LC, Ceballos R, Ulrich CM, Ramaprasad J, McGregor B, McTiernan A. Randomized controlled pilot trial of yoga in overweight and obese breast cancer survivors: effects on quality of life and anthropometric measures. Support Care Cancer. 2012;20(2):267–77.
446. Cohen L, Warneke C, Fouladi RT, Rodriguez MA, Chaoul-Reich A. Psychological adjustment and sleep quality in a randomized trial of the effects of a Tibetan yoga intervention in patients with lymphoma. Cancer. 2004;100(10):2253–60.
447. Peppone LJ, Janelsins MC, Kamen C, Mohile SG, Sprod LK, Gewandter JS, Kirshner JJ, Gaur R, Ruzich J, Esparaz BT, Mustian KM. The effect of YOCAS©® yoga for musculoskeletal symptoms among breast cancer survivors on hormonal therapy. Breast Cancer Res Treat. 2015;150(3):597–604.
448. Adair M, Murphy B, Yarlagadda S, Deng J, Dietrich MS, Ridner SH. Feasibility and preliminary efficacy of tailored yoga in survivors of head and neck cancer: a pilot study. Integr Cancer Ther. 2018;17(3):774–84.
449. Cramer H, Ward L, Saper R, Fishbein D, Dobos G, Lauche R. The safety of yoga: a systematic review and meta-analysis of randomized controlled trials. Am J Epidemiol. 2015;182(4):281–93.
450. Cramer H, Lauche R, Klose P, Lange S, Langhorst J, Dobos GJ. Yoga for improving health-related quality of life, mental health and cancer-related symptoms in women diagnosed with breast cancer. Cochrane Database Syst Rev. 2017;1:CD010802.
451. Kiecolt-Glaser JK, Bennett JM, Andridge R, Peng J, Shapiro CL, Malarkey WB, Emery CF, Layman R, Mrozek EE, Glaser R. Yoga's impact on inflammation, mood, and fatigue in breast cancer survivors: a randomized controlled trial. J Clin Oncol. 2014;32(10):1040–9.
452. Mustian KM, Sprod LK, Janelsins M, Peppone LJ, Palesh OG, Chandwani K, Reddy PS, Melnik MK, Heckler C, Morrow GR. Multicenter, randomized controlled trial of yoga for sleep quality among cancer survivors. J Clin Oncol. 2013;31(26):3233–41.
453. Bower JE, Garet D, Sternlieb B, Ganz PA, Irwin MR, Olmstead R, Greendale G. Yoga for persistent fatigue in breast cancer survivors: a randomized controlled trial. Cancer. 2012;118(15):3766–75.
454. Potié A, Roelants F, Pospiech A, Momeni M, Watremez C. Hypnosis in the perioperative management of breast cancer surgery: clinical benefits and potential implications. Anesthesiol Res Pract. 2016;2016:2942416.
455. National Cancer Institute. Topics in Integrative, Alternative, and Complementary Therapies (PDQ)-Patient Version. cancer.gov/about-cancer/treatment/cam/patient/cam-topics-pdq.
456. Taylor S, Harley C, Ziegler L, Brown J, Velikova G. Interventions for sexual problems following treatment for breast cancer: a systematic review. Breast Cancer Res Treat. 2011;130(3):711–24.
457. Del Casale A, Ferracuti S, Rapinesi C, Serata D, Caltagirone SS, Savoja V, Piacentino D, Callovini G, Manfredi G, Sani G, Kotzalidis GD, Girardi P. Pain perception and hypnosis: findings from recent functional neuroimaging studies. Int J Clin Exp Hypn. 2015;63(2):144–70.

458. Adachi T, Fujino H, Nakae A, Mashimo T, Sasaki J. A meta-analysis of hypnosis for chronic pain problems: a comparison between hypnosis, standard care, and other psychological interventions. Int J Clin Exp Hypn. 2014;62(1):1–28.

459. Montgomery GH, David D, Kangas M, Green S, Sucala M, Bovbjerg DH, Hallquist MN, Schnur JB. Randomized controlled trial of a cognitive-behavioral therapy plus hypnosis intervention to control fatigue in patients undergoing radiotherapy for breast cancer. J Clin Oncol. 2014;32(6):557–63.

460. Jensen MP. Hypnosis for chronic pain management: a new hope. Pain. 2009;146(3):235–7.

461. Montgomery GH, Bovbjerg DH, Schnur JB, David D, Goldfarb A, Weltz CR, Schechter C, Graff-Zivin J, Tatrow K, Price DD, Silverstein JH. A randomized clinical trial of a brief hypnosis intervention to control side effects in breast surgery patients. J Natl Cancer Inst. 2007;99(17):1304–12.

462. Montgomery GH, Kangas M, David D, Hallquist MN, Green S, Bovbjerg DH, Schnur JB. Fatigue during breast cancer radiotherapy: an initial randomized study of cognitive-behavioral therapy plus hypnosis. Health Psychol. 2009;28(3):317–22.

463. Wortzel J, Spiegel D. Hypnosis in cancer care. Am J Clin Hypn. 2017;60(1):4–17.

464. Montgomery GH, Weltz CR, Seltz M, Bovbjerg DH. Brief presurgery hypnosis reduces distress and pain in excisional breast biopsy patients. Int J Clin Exp Hypn. 2002;50(1):17–32.

465. Lahoud MJ, Kourie HR, Antoun J, El Osta L, Ghosn M. Road map for pain management in pancreatic cancer: a review. World J Gastrointest Oncol. 2016;8(8):599–606.

466. Mendoza ME, Capafons A, Gralow JR, Syrjala KL, Suárez-Rodríguez JM, Fann JR, Jensen MP. Randomized controlled trial of the Valencia model of waking hypnosis plus CBT for pain, fatigue, and sleep management in patients with cancer and cancer survivors. Psychooncology. 2017;26(11):1832–8.

467. Brugnoli MP, Pesce G, Pasin E, Basile MF, Tamburin S, Polati E. The role of clinical hypnosis and self-hypnosis to relief pain and anxiety in severe chronic diseases in palliative care: a 2-year long-term follow-up of treatment in a nonrandomized clinical trial. Ann Palliat Med. 2018;7(1):17–31.

468. Berlière M, Roelants F, Watremez C, Docquier MA, Piette N, Lamerant S, Megevand V, Van Maanen A, Piette P, Gerday A, Duhoux FP. The advantages of hypnosis intervention on breast cancer surgery and adjuvant therapy. Breast. 2018;37:114–8.

469. Jochimsen PR, Lawton RL, VerSteeg K, Noyes R Jr. Effect of benzopyranoperidine, a delta-9-THC congener, on pain. Clin Pharmacol Ther. 1978;24(2):223–7.

470. Compton WM, Han B, Hughes A, Jones CM, Blanco C. Use of marijuana for medical purposes among adults in the United States. JAMA. 2017;317(2):209–11.

471. Pergam SA, Woodfield MC, Lee CM, Cheng GS, Baker KK, Marquis SR, Fann JR. Cannabis use among patients at a comprehensive cancer center in a state with legalized medicinal and recreational use. Cancer. 2017;123(22):4488–97.

472. Whiting PF, Wolff RF, Deshpande S, Di Nisio M, Duffy S, Hernandez AV, Keurentjes JC, Lang S, Misso K, Ryder S, Schmidlkofer S, Westwood M, Kleijnen J. Cannabinoids for medical use: a systematic review and meta-analysis. JAMA. 2015;313(24):2456–73.

473. Kramer JL. Medical marijuana for cancer. CA Cancer J Clin. 2015;65(2):109–22.

474. Blake A, Wan BA, Malek L, DeAngelis C, Diaz P, Lao N, Chow E, O'Hearn S. A selective review of medical cannabis in cancer pain management. Ann Palliat Med. 2017;6(Suppl 2):S215–22.

475. Boehnke KF, Litinas E, Clauw DJ. Medical cannabis use is associated with decreased opiate medication use in a retrospective cross-sectional survey of patients with chronic pain. J Pain. 2016;17(6):739–44.

476. Andreae MH, Carter GM, Shaparin N, Suslov K, Ellis RJ, Ware MA, Abrams DI, Prasad H, Wilsey B, Indyk D, Johnson M, Sacks HS. Inhaled cannabis for chronic neuropathic pain: a meta-analysis of individual patient data. J Pain. 2015;16(12):1221–32.

477. Johnson JR, Burnell-Nugent M, Lossignol D, Ganae-Motan ED, Potts R, Fallon MT. Multicenter, double-blind, randomized, placebo-controlled, parallel-group study of the efficacy, safety, and tolerability of THC:CBD extract and THC extract in patients with intractable cancer-related pain. J Pain Symptom Manag. 2010;39(2):167–79.

478. Portenoy RK, Ganae-Motan ED, Allende S, Yanagihara R, Shaiova L, Weinstein S, McQuade R, Wright S, Fallon MT. Nabiximols for opioid-treated cancer patients with poorly-controlled chronic pain: a randomized, placebo-controlled, graded-dose trial. J Pain. 2012;13(5):438–49.

479. Lichtman AH, Lux EA, McQuade R, Rossetti S, Sanchez R, Sun W, Wright S, Kornyeyeva E, Fallon MT. Results of a double-blind, randomized, placebo-controlled study of nabiximols oromucosal spray as an adjunctive therapy in advanced cancer patients with chronic uncontrolled pain. J Pain Symptom Manag. 2018;55(2):179–88.

480. Zhang MW, Ho RC. The cannabis dilemma: a review of its associated risks and clinical efficacy. J Addict. 2015;2015:707596.

481. Noyes R Jr, Brunk SF, Baram DA, Canter A. Analgesic effect of delta-9-tetrahydrocannabinol. J Clin Pharmacol. 1975;15(2–3):139–43.

482. Lynch ME, Cesar-Rittenberg P, Hohmann AG. A double-blind, placebo-controlled, crossover pilot trial with extension using an oral mucosal cannabinoid extract for treatment of chemotherapy-induced neuropathic pain. J Pain Symptom Manag. 2014;47(1):166–73.

Cervical Radicular Pain

Carl Noe and Gabor Racz

Introduction

Cervical radicular pain, or cervical radiculitis, is pain in the distribution of one or more cervical nerve root(s). It may be caused by the mechanical effects of disc herniation, degenerative or neoplastic changes leading to stenosis of the neural foramen/lateral recess, the chemical effects related to extravasation of nucleus pulposus, acute herpes zoster or postherpetic neuralgia (PHN), epidural scarring, as well as sensitization of various pathways in the peripheral and central nervous systems. Cervical radiculopathy is related to radiculitis, but encompasses other symptoms and signs of nerve root pathology including sensory loss, weakness, reflex changes, dysesthesias, or paresthesias. Cervical myelopathy is associated with compression of the spinal cord or spinal cord disease.

Anatomy

Knowledge of cervical spine anatomy is important for establishing an accurate diagnosis and for performing interventional procedures safely. External anatomic landmarks of the posterior neck include the greater external occipital protuberance, the superior nuchal line, and the C7 dorsal spinous process. The bony cervical spine consists of seven vertebrae. The atlas (first cervical vertebra) has unique anatomy and does not have a vertebral body but rather has a bony ring structure with lateral masses. The atlanto-occipital joint is active in flexion, and extension and upper neck pain with flexion may be due to arthritis of these joints. The axis (second cervical vertebra) also has a unique anatomy including the dens (odontoid process) that extends superiorly and artic-

ulates with the anterior arch of the atlas as the medial atlanto-axial joint, allowing rotation of the cervical spine. The lateral atlanto-axial joints involved with rotation are much more anterior compared to lower cervical facet joints. Upper neck pain with rotation may be due to arthritis in the lateral C1–C2 joints. Patients with rheumatoid arthritis may have C1–C2 subluxation, superior migration of the odontoid, or subaxial subluxation. The axis also has the foramen transversarium on each side that carries the vertebral artery. The ligaments of the upper cervical spine that are external to the spine include the atlanto-occipital, anterior atlanto-occipital, and anterior atlanto-occipital ligaments. Internally, the transverse ligament binds the odontoid to the anterior arch of the atlas. The bilateral alar ligaments attach the odontoid to the anterior bone of the foramen magnum. The accessory atlantoaxial ligament connects the occipital bone to the atlas and axis as a unit.

The C3–C6 cervical vertebra are more similar to each other anatomically. The anterior column of the mid- and lower cervical spine is comprised of the anterior longitudinal ligaments, the anterior two-thirds of the annulus fibrosus, and intervertebral discs. Discs are present from C2 to C7. The middle vertebral column is comprised of the posterior longitudinal ligament and the posterior one-third of the annulus fibrosis and disc. The posterior column consists of the pedicles, transverse processes, facet joints, lamina, and dorsal spinous processes. The anterior tubercle of the C6 vertebra transverse process is named Chassaignac's tubercle and lies between the carotid and vertebral arteries. The C7 cervical vertebra, also known as the vertebra prominens (due to its prominent spinous process), has several variations of the foramen transversarium anatomy, and the vertebral artery usually does not pass through the foramen at this level. The C7 spinous process is the most prominent cervical spinous process.

The brain stem extends inferiorly to the level of the axis. Compression of the lower brain stem may result from craniocervical junction abnormalities. These may be congenital or acquired and may involve the occipital bone, foramen

C. Noe
Department of Anesthesiology and Pain Management, University of Texas Southwestern Medical center, Dallas, TX, USA

G. Racz (✉)
Texas Tech University Health Sciences Center, Lubbock, TX, USA
e-mail: gaborr@epimedint.com

© Springer Nature Switzerland AG 2019
Y. Khelemsky et al. (eds.), *Academic Pain Medicine*, https://doi.org/10.1007/978-3-030-18005-8_29

magnum, atlas, and axis. Neck pain and headache (not limited to the occiput) may be the primary symptoms of craniocervical junction abnormalities (as well as abnormalities in other areas of the upper cervical spine), and surgical treatment may be required.

The first seven cervical nerve roots exit above the corresponding vertebral body, and the C8 nerve root exits below the C7 vertebral body. The C1 root is classified as a motor nerve root and does not have an assigned dermatome. The nerve may have multiple rootlets and variations with respect to ventral and dorsal roots. Multiple connections with the spinal accessory nerve have been reported [1]. The C2 nerve exits the spinal canal and lies posterior to the lateral C1–C2 joint as opposed to the C3–C8 nerves that lie anterior to their respective facet joints in a bony foramen [2].

The C2 root supplies muscles involved with neck flexion and extension. The medial branch of its dorsal primary ramus becomes the greater occipital nerve. The C3 nerve supplies muscles controlling lateral flexion. The C3 dorsal root ganglion (DRG) and root lie more posterior than the DRG at lower levels. The C3 level is more prone to injury from procedures related to the use of oblique fluoroscopic views without lateral views to confirm placement. Also, parallax can occur when the neural foramina do not line up to be superimposed. As a consequence, the needle is positioned based not on the intended side but on the opposite side which may be too anterior. Also, excessively large radiofrequency thermocoagulation lesions have been associated with motor deficits and paralysis. Cold radiofrequency lesions have been associated with winged scapula as a complication.

The C4 nerve supplies muscles for shoulder elevation. The dermatome is in the lower neck and upper shoulder area. The sclerotome includes the upper scapula and clavicle area. The C5–C8 roots contribute to the brachial plexus that has five roots (C5–C8 plus T1). The roots form superior, middle, and inferior trunks that continue as divisions as they pass laterally. The trunks form posterior, lateral, and medial cords before forming branches including the median, radial, ulnar, musculocutaneous, and axillary nerves. The C5 root myotome abducts the arm at the shoulder. The dermatome is over the shoulder and the sclerotome includes the shoulder. The C6 root supplies muscles for elbow flexion and wrist extension. The dermatome includes the lateral forearm and thumb.C5 and C6 innervate muscles around the shoulder girdle and axilla including the supraspinatus, deltoid, and pectoralis minor. Trigger points in muscles are often missed on physical examination, but myofascial pain can be diagnosed by palpation and can mimic radicular pain. The C7 root supplies muscles for elbow extension and wrist flexion. The dermatome is in the mid-hand and the sclerotome is in the mid-forearm. The C8 root supplies muscles for thumb extension. The dermatome is in the medial hand and the sclerotome is deep to the dermatome.

The vertebral artery courses through a series foramina transversarium superiorly from C6 to C3. The artery flows supero-laterally to C3 and passes superiorly through the foramen transversarium of C2 and C1 and then medially into the spinal canal. The vertebral artery has branches that supply the cord and nerve roots. These branches are vulnerable to injury during transforaminal injections. Epidural veins vary in number in the cervical epidural space at different levels and within the anterior or posterior epidural space [3]. The venous plexus is denser posteriorly below C7, and this contributes to the practice of entering the C7–T1 epidural space for procedures.

Causes and Differentiation from Neck Pain and Somatic Nerve Pain

As mentioned earlier, cervical radicular pain results from physical or chemical insult of the nerve roots that may be caused by fracture, disc herniation, spondylosis, spondylolisthesis, foraminal stenosis, central spinal stenosis, tumor, vascular malformation, spinal cord pathology, multiple sclerosis, brachial plexus avulsion, herpes zoster, and other conditions. Table 29.1 details a differential diagnosis of cervical radiculopathy.

Myelopathy, which results from compression of the spinal cord, should be excluded early in the work-up. The diagnosis of myelopathy is largely clinical and based on upper motor neuron symptoms and exam findings such as shock-like sensations with cervical flexion (e.g., Lhermitte's sign), gait disturbance, clumsiness, weakness, spasticity, and extremity pain. Physical examination findings of dysfunctional tandem gait (heel to toe walking), altered muscle tone, spastic motor weakness, hyperreflexia, and pathological reflexes such as Hoffman's and Babinski may also be present. Bladder and bowel dysfunction may also occur. The treatment is often surgical.

Palpation of the scalene muscles is a useful examination for identifying patients with mid and lower cervical radicular

Table 29.1 Differential diagnosis of lumbar radiculopathy

Cardiac pain
Carpal tunnel syndrome
Cubital tunnel syndrome
Herpes zoster
Tumor
Parsonage-Turner syndrome
Complex regional pain syndrome
Thoracic outlet syndrome
Cervical myelopathy
Rotator cuff/shoulder pain
Myofascial pain
Facet-mediated pain

pain due to thoracic outlet syndrome. This may respond to an interscalene block or injection of these muscles [6].

Scapular pain, parascapular pain, and rhomboid pain are common with cervical radicular pain with disc pathology at C5 and C6. Trigger points may represent cervical radicular pain in these areas. Also, referred pain from cervical facet joints and other structures may masquerade as radicular pain and produce pain and muscle spasm of the shoulder and upper chest.

History Taking and Neurologic Examination

The history should include the pain location, onset, duration, severity, and change in severity over time. Additional information for the history of present illness includes quality, timing, context, aggravating and alleviating factors, associated signs and symptoms, and the effect of the pain on physical and psychological function. The past medical history should include previous treatments and underlying or coexisting diseases and conditions, especially malignancies and infections. Medication history, especially blood thinners, surgeries, hospitalizations, and allergies are important. Occupational requirements and disability status should be documented. A review of symptoms should include specific questions about numbness, weakness, allodynia, lancinating pain, urinary or bowel dysfunction, as well as gait and clumsiness. The physical exam should include cranial nerves, inspection of the neck and upper extremity, cervical and upper extremity range of motion, and palpation of the painful area. The neurologic examination should include inspection for atrophy, muscle tone, sensory, and motor exams of the upper and lower extremities. Reflexes of the biceps, triceps, and brachioradialis should be performed. Hoffman's and Babinski tests for pathological reflexes are important signs of upper motor neuron disease in myelopathy.

The C2 root is associated with pain in the occipital area and sometimes behind the eyes due to the communication of the nucleus caudalis of C2 with the sphenopalatine ganglion.

The C3 and C4 roots are associated with pain in the neck and trapezius. The medial branches of C2 and C3 may refer to pain to the eyes and face via the trigeminocervical complex (TCC) and potentially trigger underlying primary headache disorders. The trapezius and sternocleidomastoid are innervated by the accessory nerve, which has a contribution from C1 to C5. Pain from these muscles may also be referred to the head/face via the TCC and similarly trigger or potentiate primary headaches. The C5 root is associated with pain in the shoulder and lateral upper extremity and weakness in the deltoid. The C6 root is associated with pain in the lateral forearm and base of the thumb, weakness in the biceps, and blunting of the biceps reflex. The C7 root is associated with pain in the posterior forearm and middle finger and weakness in the triceps and blunting of the triceps reflex. C8 and T1 contribute to the ulnar nerve and innervate the medial hand and hand intrinsic muscles.

History that points toward cervical radiculopathy includes arm pain with numbness and/or weakness, previous documented episode of radicular pain, and radiating pain with coughing, sneezing, or Valsalva maneuver. History that points away from cervical radicular pain includes neck pain only, history of neuropathy in lower extremities, peripheral nerve entrapment, and complex regional pain syndrome symptoms. Physical exam findings that point toward cervical radicular pain include positive Spurling's test, upper limb tension test, shoulder abduction test, painful neural flossing maneuvers (Fig. 29.1), asymmetrically blunted reflexes in the affected arm, and numbness and weakness in the same nerve root distribution. Physical exam findings that point away from cervical radicular pain include signs of complex regional pain syndrome, normal sensorimotor and reflex exams, and myofascial tenderness that reproduces the patient's pain.

A systematic review found that no single provocative test had both a high sensitivity and high specificity [7]. The Spurling's test, neck traction test (lifting the head and relieving pain), and Valsalva maneuver were found to be highly specific. The upper limb tension test is highly sensitive. This test is performed in the supine position. The examiner follows

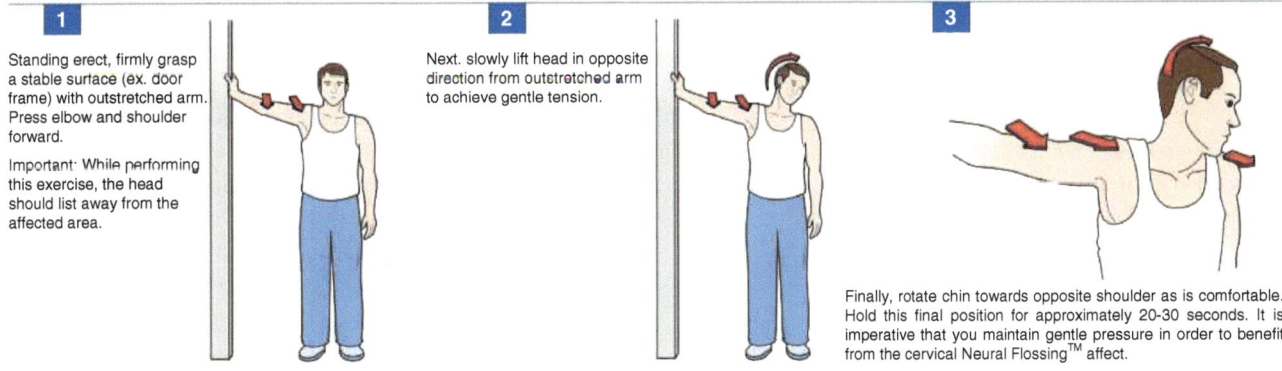

1 Standing erect, firmly grasp a stable surface (ex. door frame) with outstretched arm. Press elbow and shoulder forward.

Important: While performing this exercise, the head should list away from the affected area.

2 Next, slowly lift head in opposite direction from outstretched arm to achieve gentle tension.

3 Finally, rotate chin towards opposite shoulder as is comfortable. Hold this final position for approximately 20-30 seconds. It is imperative that you maintain gentle pressure in order to benefit from the cervical Neural Flossing™ affect.

Fig. 29.1 Cervical neural flossing exercises

a sequence of steps: scapular depression, shoulder abduction, forearm supination and digit extension, shoulder lateral elevation, elbow extension, and cervical side bending. This test is positive if pain is reproduced, elbow extension associated pain is different from one arm to the other by 10 degrees or more, or contralateral side bending increases symptoms or ipsilateral bending decreases symptoms. The shoulder abduction test has moderate to high specificity and the maneuver complements tests that provoke pain. The patient is seated and asked to place both hands on top of their head. Pain from cervical radiculitis should improve with this maneuver.

Imaging

The American College of Radiology recommends a cervical spine series of x-rays as an initial study including lateral, anteroposterior, and oblique views. Disc-space narrowing, subchondral sclerosis, and osteophyte formation can be evaluated on lateral views. Attention to comparing disc height at one level to adjacent levels is important [8]. Foraminal stenosis can be evaluated on oblique views. Attention to comparing the symptomatic side to the asymptomatic side is important. A swimmer's view with the arms in front of the patient can give a better lateral image of the C7 level. CT imaging may be required to visualize C7 adequately. Flexion and extension and lateral bending films can be used to diagnose instability. Computerized tomography (CT) is a good imaging technique for bone and fractures. It is frequently adequate for disc herniation in patients who are unable to have an MRI. CT with myelography is excellent for visualizing disc herniation and evaluation of the subarachnoid space. MRI is indicated in patients with neurologic findings with normal x-rays. In a study of asymptomatic subjects, 10% of patients under age 40 had disc herniations, and in patients over 40, 20% have foraminal stenosis and 8% had disc herniations [9]. Because of this, it is unadvisable to rely solely on imaging for diagnosing cervical radicular pain. Many surgeons insist on having recent MRI images performed before any surgical procedure. For interventional pain procedures, imaging within the past year may be adequate as long as the pain syndrome is essentially the same as it was at the time of the imaging. MR neurography is a test for neural pathology using MRI scanning and techniques to reduce the signal of non-neural structures [10]. Bone scans are used to localize tumor, infection, and inflammation. Bone density tests are important for patients who are being evaluated for hardware placement.

Electrodiagnostic Studies

Electrodiagnostic studies do not measure pain, but they are useful tests particularly when information from the patient history, physical examination, or imaging is inconclusive.

The specificity of EMG for diagnosing radiculopathy has been reported to be 77%, while average sensitivity was 73% [11]. For mild to moderate radiculopathy, the sensitivity was lower, 40%. For moderate to severe radiculopathy, the sensitivity was higher, 80%. The diagnosis changed in only 2/60 cases with the addition of clinical information. Intra-rater reproducibility was 80%, 87% for radiculopathy and 73% for normal studies. Inter-rater agreement was 63%, 70% for radiculopathy and 53% for normal studies. Inter-rater agreement for denervation was 90% and re-innervation was only 60%. Positive sharp waves and fibrillation potentials occur 2–3 weeks after the onset of radiculopathy, so studies performed before this may yield falsely negative results. EMG studies are of unknown value in patients with an unclear diagnosis of cervical radiculopathy after clinical examination and imaging [12].

Natural History and Relevance to Management

The vast majority of patients with cervical radicular pain improve, but data regarding natural history is limited [12]. The prognosis for acute radicular pain is much better than it is for chronic radicular pain. This is relevant to management, since the risk and costs of treatment need to be minimized for self-limiting conditions. Also, the evidence-based data guiding treatment for cervical radicular pain is limited. However, patients with pain are motivated to seek relief, and physicians should appropriately match the risks, costs, and efficacy of treatment option recommendations to the severity and duration of complaints and disability.

Medical Management

Indomethacin has been shown to be superior to placebo for radicular pain [13]. In a trial comparing morphine, nortriptyline, and the combination of the two drugs, nortriptyline alone was more effective than placebo, morphine alone, or the combination [14]. The combination of gabapentin and NSAID is more effective than NSAID alone [15]. Oral corticosteroid was superior to gabapentinoids in patients with MRI evidence of nerve root compression [16]. Several studies of non-pharmacological treatment have also been reported. In a trial comparing nonsteroidal anti-inflammatory drugs (NSAID) to acupuncture, no difference was found, and both treatments were associated with improvement [17]. In a trial of a semihard collar, rest for 3–6 weeks and physiotherapy for 6 weeks with home exercise were more effective than a "wait-and-see treatment" for cervical radiculopathy [18]. A Cochrane review endorses cervical stretching, strengthening, and stabilization exercises for acute radiculopathy but the quality of evidence is low and the benefit is small [19].

Interventional Management

Indications for injections for cervical radicular pain include pain that has not responded to non-pharmacological treatment and medications. Pre-procedural imaging should show spinal fluid around the cord at the narrowest point in the canal to insure adequate volume for injected fluid. Contraindications include local infection, allergy to medications required to perform the procedure, unstable medical or psychiatric status, and concurrent use of anticoagulant medications. Local tumor is a relative contraindication, especially if it is vascular. Informed consent should include failure to reduce pain or worsening of pain, nerve damage including paralysis, epidural hematoma, infection, seizure, persistent leak of spinal fluid which may require surgery, breathing, and/or heart problems including cardiac arrest. Monitoring should include pulse oximetry, EKG, noninvasive blood pressure, and respiratory rate. Routine use of sedation for these procedures is not recommended and deep sedation should be avoided [20].

Cervical transforaminal epidural steroid injections (CTESI) have been used as an alternative to selective nerve root blocks and interlaminar epidural steroid injections. One of the initial studies of transforaminal epidural steroid injections showed impressive results in patients with lumbar radicular pain. The control group received trigger point injections. At an average of 15-month follow-up, the success rate was 84% versus 48% [21]. However, in a subgroup analysis of another study, transforaminal injections were not significantly beneficial in patients with spinal stenosis [22]. A randomized trial reported no difference between transforaminal cervical transforaminal steroid injections and controls [23]. In another study of cervical transforaminal epidural steroid injections versus facet injections, no difference was shown [24]. Transforaminal injections can be considered in patients with potential surgical pathology [25]. Favorable outcome after CTFESI cannot be predicted based on radiologic or clinical findings [26]. Use of selective nerve root blocks or transforaminal epidural steroid injections to predict surgical levels and outcomes in the cervical spine is controversial. It is imperative to note that due to the potential for catastrophic complications and questionable outcomes, use of both cervical selective nerve root blocks and cervical transforaminal epidural injections has come under considerable scrutiny [27, 28]. If performed, use of non-particulate steroids is mandatory for these procedures [29].

Interlaminar epidural steroid injections have also been used to treat cervical radicular pain. Superior results with cervical epidural steroid injections compared to steroid injection around cervical muscles as a control group have been reported [30]. Medications and epidural steroid injections have been studied in a trial comparing medication alone (gabapentin and or nortriptyline), cervical epidural steroid injections, and the combination of medications and epidural steroid injections [31]. The primary end point in the study was relief of arm pain. That was not improved to a significantly different level in any group. However, the combination group was improved in other important outcomes such as neck pain. In a study of interlaminar epidural steroid injections versus perineural injection of conditioned autologous serum, the results were similar [32]. Overall, there is good evidence for radiculitis secondary to disc herniation for cervical interlaminar epidural steroid injections (CIESI) using a combination of steroid and local anesthetic [33]. There does not appear to be significant difference in outcomes between midline and paramedian approaches for CIESI [34]. Figure 29.2 shows an example of appropriate needle position for an interlaminar epidural steroid injection.

Epidural catheter techniques have also been developed to treat cervical radicular pain [35]. Crock pioneered surgical foraminotomies and observed the correlation between successful decompression and perineural venous dilatation [36].

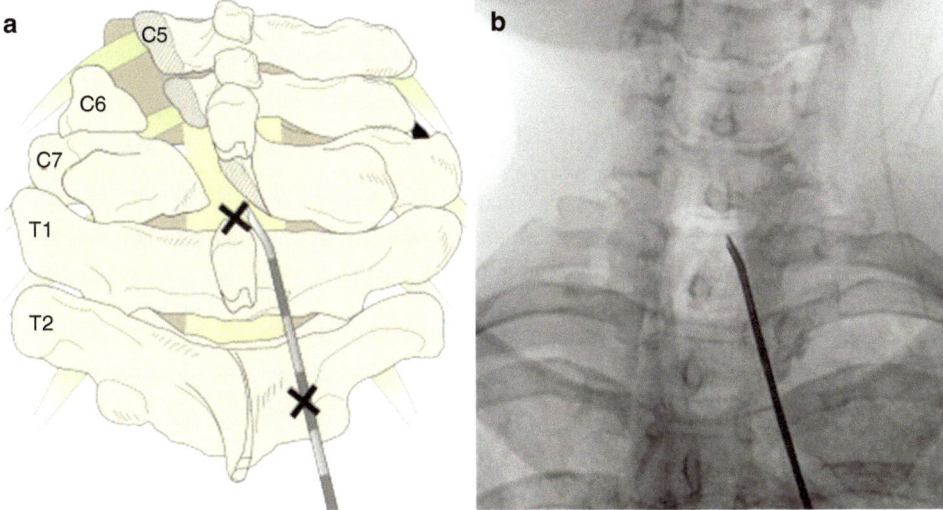

Fig. 29.2 (**a**) Needle in good final position with the bevel facing the symptomatic side (left). (**b**) Fluoroscopic image of needle placement for cervical epidural

This led to the fluid foraminotomy concept of the lysis of adhesions technique [37–39]. Lysis of adhesions addresses inflammation with corticosteroid and restriction with epidurography and fluid foraminotomy by opening foramina with fluid injection. Contrast runoff has been shown to correlate with outcomes [40]. Also, epidurographic improvement after the procedure has been correlated with improvement in outcomes [41].

Surgical Treatment

Surgery is inevitably necessary with spinal instability or significant neurologic compromise. For single-level cervical radiculopathy, anterior cervical discectomy and anterior cervical discectomy with fusion are similarly effective operations [12]. An interbody graft may improve sagittal alignment. Anterior cervical discectomies with fusion with and without a plate are similarly effective operations for single-level cervical radiculopathy related to degenerative disease. For foraminal disc herniation and radiculopathy, anterior cervical discectomy and fusion and posterolateral fusion are comparable operations. For single-level cervical radiculopathy from central and paracentral nerve root compression and spondylosis, anterior cervical discectomy and fusion are recommended over posterolateral fusion surgery. Total disc arthroplasty is equivalent to anterior cervical disc and fusion for single-level radiculopathy from degenerative disease. Surgery is an option for single-level disease radiculopathy and has good short- and long-term outcomes [12]. However, the Cochrane library reviews state that data from trials of surgery for cervical spondylotic radiculopathy and myelopathy are inadequate to make conclusions about long-term outcomes [42]. Surgery may provide better short-term relief than physiotherapy and cervical collar immobilization. Cervical myelopathy patients improve after surgery, but long-term results are not certain [42]. In summary, surgical treatment has variable and uncertain outcomes; therefore, appropriate patient selection and surgical skill are critical.

Complications of Cervical Epidural Injections

Complications from cervical interventional pain management procedures include total spinal block (if local anesthetic is used), spinal cord injury, vertebral artery injury or embolization, nerve root injury, paralysis, and death. Informed consent and a solid indication for performing procedures are important. Epidural hematoma may occur acutely and require emergent surgical drainage. Abscess formation may occur later and usually requires surgical drainage and antibiotic treatment for *Staphylococcus*. Infection from contamination of steroid preparations is possible if the steroid is

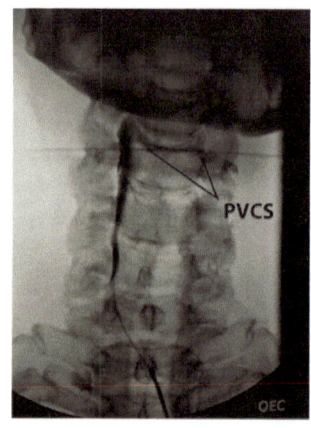

Fig. 29.3 Perivenous counter spread (PVCS) showing contrast spreading next to epidural veins to the opposite side without flowing out of neural foramen

sourced from compounding pharmacies. Non-particulate, preservative-free corticosteroids have been the main source of fungal and other atypical infections [43]. The use of a sharp needle is one potential risk factor for complications related to transforaminal injections and other injections. A survey regarding the safety of transforaminal cervical epidural steroid injections, which had a relatively low response rate of 21%, still captured 78 complications, including 16 vertebrobasilar infarcts, 12 spinal cord infarcts, and 2 patients with both [44].

Nerve puncture and dissection with injection can also occur with sharp needles. Perforation of the vertebral artery and intra-arterial injection of toxic doses of contrast, local anesthetic, or steroid can occur [45, 46]. When performing cervical epidural procedures, perivenous counter spread (PVCS) can occur by injectate tracking across the epidural space in the spaces adjacent to veins and collecting and loculating on the opposite side from the catheter (Figs. 29.3) [47]. Rotation can also be used along with flexion to open the foramina and relieve pressure from loculation. Physicians should be prepared to manage pain and numbness during and after procedures that may be related to PVCS [48]. Spinal cord ischemia may result from spinal cord compression, loculation of injected fluid, expanding loculation from hyperosmolar solution (hypertonic saline), embolization of particulate steroid, intraneural injection, and intracordal injection. Catheter shearing is a complication of catheter techniques when the catheter is withdrawn for repositioning. Needle modifications have reduced this problem significantly.

Expert Discussion: Medicolegal Pitfalls

These cases are presented as examples of complications of epidural procedures resulting in medicolegal action.

The first patient had a history of five previous failed surgeries, three lumbar and two cervical fusions at C4/C5 and C6/C7. The patient had severe C6 radiculopathy and had a series of single shot epidural steroid injections by a nonboard-certified physician. The physician used the wrong template for the operative note, and while the fluoroscopic images showed proper needle placement, the medical record documented a hanging drop technique in the sitting position. The patient experienced 2 weeks of pain relief and returned for a second injection 3 weeks later. The wrong template was again used, and a transforaminal epidural steroid injection was documented in the medical record. However, the fluoroscopy images again showed a properly placed interlaminar epidural steroid injection. In the recovery area, the patient complained of pain and then numbness. After the patient left, the staff tried to contact the patient but received no answer. The patient developed arm weakness and returned 3 weeks later for a third injection. The physician ordered an MRI that revealed a syrinx. On the epidurogram of the second interlaminar injection, contrast was present in the scar area, but not flowing through the neural foramina. The record keeping was indefensible and the jury awarded a substantial verdict to the plaintiff.

The second case began with a patient who had occipital neuralgia and failed C2 nerve surgery and nerve blocks. She underwent an upper cervical lysis of adhesions procedure after which she experienced severe pain. She was medicated with fentanyl and midazolam for several hours and discharged. The next day, she developed arm paralysis and was admitted. The day after that, she developed upper and lower extremity hemiplegia, from which she recovered after 5 months. The importance of contrast runoff through neural foramen and PVCS was not known at the time of the complication. Ten years later, the case went to court and a defense verdict was reached.

The third case involved a patient who underwent an upper thoracic epidural injection and developed a spinal headache. The patient was treated with an epidural blood patch at the level of the previous puncture. The patient developed back and leg pain with loss of bladder function. An MRI showed an epidural hematoma, but the neurosurgeon attributed it to the epidural blood patch. The hematoma expanded and the patient became paralyzed. Surgery was delayed due to the thought that the blood patch was the source of all of the blood in the epidural space.

In the final example, a patient underwent a thoracic lysis of adhesions procedure. The patient developed numbness in both legs, and the following epidurogram was sent to the author (GBR). Flexion rotation exercises were performed. An MRI was obtained that showed no new lesions. The patient made a full recovery after 1 month. Being able to communicate with colleagues in a collegial, timely manner is an important way to reduce harms to patients [49].

References

1. Campos D, Goerck ML, Ellwanger JH, Corbellini RO, Hoelscher RH, Souza MS, Rieger AJ. Anatomy of the first spinal nerve – a review. J Morphol Sci. 2012;29(2):65–8.
2. Bilge O. An anatomic and morphometric study of C2 nerve root ganglion and its corresponding foramen. Spine. 2004;29(5):495–9.
3. Clemens H. Die Venensysteme der Menschlichen Wirbelsaule. Morphologie and Functionelle Bedeutung. Berlin: Walter de Gruyter & Co., plate 1; 1961.
4. McCarron RF, Wimpee MW, Hudkins PG, Laros GS. The inflammatory effect of nucleus pulposus. A possible element in the pathogenesis of low back pain. Spine. 1987;12:760–4.
5. Lohman C, Gilbert K, Sobczak S, Brismée J, James C, Day M, Smith M, Taylor L, Dugailly P, Pendergrass T, Sizer P. Young Investigator Award Winner: Cervical Nerve Root Displacement and Strain During Upper Limb Neural Tension Testing: Part 1: A Minimally Invasive Assessment in Unembalmed Cadavers. Spine. 2015;40(11):793–800. https://doi.org/10.1097/BRS.0000000000000686.
6. Racz GB, Noe CE, editors. Techniques of neurolysis. Springer; 2016. p. 140. https://doi.org/10.1007/978-3-319-27607-6 E-Book ISBN 978-3-319-27607-6; Hardcover ISBN 978-3-319-27605-2.
7. Rubenstein S, Pool J, Tulder M, Riphagen I, deVet H. A systematic review of the diagnostic accuracy of provocative tests of the neck for diagnosing cervical radiculopathy. Eur Spine J. 2007;16(3):307–19.
8. American College of Radiology. ACR Appropriateness Criteria. Chronic neck pain. http://www.acr.org/SecondaryMainMenuCategories/quality_safety/app_criteria/pdf/ExpertPanelonMusculoskeletalImaging/ChronicNeckPainDoc9.aspx. Accessed July 6, 2010.
9. Boden SD, McCowin PR, Davis DO, Dina TS, Mark AS, Wiesel SL. Abnormal magnetic-resonance scans of the cervical spine in asymptomatic subjects. A prospective investigation. J Bone Joint Surg (Am Vol). 1990;72(8):1178–84.
10. Chhabra A, Zhao L, Carrino JA, et al. MR neurography: advances. Radiol Res Pract. 2013;2013:809568. https://doi.org/10.1155/2013/809568.
11. Narayanaswami P, Geisbush T, Jones L, Weiss M, Mozaffar T, Rutkove S. Confirmation bias and specificity of electromyography for radiculopathy. Neurology. 2015;84(14 Supplement):P3.164.
12. Bono CM et al. The North American Spine Society. Evidence-based clinical guidelines for multidisciplinary spine care diagnosis and treatment of cervical radiculopathy from degenerative disorders. Spine J. 2011;11(1):64–72. ISBN:1-929988-25-7.
13. Jacobs J, Grayson M. Trial of an anti-inflammatory agent (indomethacin) in low Back pain with and without radicular involvement. Br Med J. 1968;3:158. https://doi.org/10.1136/bmj.3.5611.158.
14. Khorami S, Cui L, Nackers L, Max M. Morphine, nortriptyline and their combination vs. placebo in patients with chronic lumbar root pain. PAIN. 2007;130(1):66–75. https://doi.org/10.1016/j.pain.2006.10.029.
15. Shahverdi F, Roointan R, Afkari H, Barmi F, Shahryar M. Evaluation of the efficacy and safety of gabapentin in treatment of lumbar radiculopathy; a randomized clinical trial. IOSR J Pharm. 2016;6(6):01–3.
16. Sangbong K, Sungguk K, Jaejung K, Tacbum O. The effectiveness of oral corticosteroids for management of lumbar radiating pain: randomized, controlled trial study. Clin Orthop Surg. 2016;8:262–7. https://doi.org/10.4055/cios.2016.8.3.262.
17. Zencirci B, Yuksel K, Gumusalan Y. Effectiveness of acupuncture with NSAID medication in the management of acute discogenic radicular pain: a randomised, controlled trial. J Anesth Clinic Res. 2012;3:203.

18. Kuijper A, Tans B, Beelen J, Nollet A, deVisser F. Cervical collar or physiotherapy versus wait and see policy for recent onset cervical radiculopathy: randomised trial. BMJ. 2009;339:b3883.

19. Gross A, Kay T, Paquin J, Blanchette S, Lalonde P, Christie T, Dupont G, Graham N, Burnie S, Gelly G, Goldsmith C, Forget M, Hoving J, Brontfort G, Santaguida P, Cervical Overview Group. Exercises for mechanical neck disorders. Cochrane Database Syst Rev. 2015;(1):CD004250. https://doi.org/10.1002/14651858. CD004250.pub5.

20. Bogduk N. Practice guidelines for spinal diagnostic and treatment procedures. 2nd ed. Spine Intervention Society, San Francisco; 2013. p. 3–4.

21. Vad B, Bhat A, Lutz G, Cammisa F. Transforaminal epidural steroid injections in lumbosacral radiculopathy a prospective randomized study. Spine. 2002;27(1):11–6.

22. Freidly J, Comstock B, Turner J, Heagerty P, Deyo R, Sullivan S, Bauer Z, Bresnahan B, Avins A, Nedeljkovic S, Nerenz D, Standaert C, Kessler L, Akuthota V, Annaswamy T, Chen A, Diehn F, Firtch W, Gerges F, Gilligan C, Goldberg H, Kennedy D, Mandel S, Tyburski M, Saders W, Sibell D, Smuck M, Wasan A, Won L, Jarvik J. A randomized trial of epidural glucocorticoid injections for spinal stenosis. N Engl J Med. 2014;371:11–21. https://doi.org/10.1056/NEJMoa1313265.

23. Anderberg L, Annertz M, Persson L, Brandt L, Säveland H. Transforaminal steroid injections for the treatment of cervical radiculopathy: a prospective and randomised study. Eur Spine J. 2007;16(3):321–8. https://doi.org/10.1007/s00586-006-0142-8.

24. Bureau NJ, Dagher JH, Shedid D, Li M, Brassard P, Leduc BE. Transforaminal versus intraarticular facet corticosteroid injections for the treatment of cervical radiculopathy: a randomized, double-blind, controlled study. Am J Neuroradiol. 2014;35(8):1467–74.

25. Costndi S, Gerges A, Yashar E, Zeyed Y, Atalla J, Looka M, Mekhail N. Cervical transforaminal epidural steroid injections: diagnostic and therapeutic value regional anesthesia and pain medicine. Reg Anesth Pain Med. 2015;40(6):674–80.

26. Klessinger S, et al. Response to transforaminal injection of steroids and correlation to mri findings in patients with cervical radicular pain or radiculopathy due to disc herniation or spondylosis. Pain Med. 2014;15(6):929–37.

27. Manchikanti L, et al. Cervical radicular pain: the role of interlaminar and transforaminal epidural injections. Curr Pain Headache Rep. 2014;18(1):389.

28. Schneider BJ, et al. Safety and complications of cervical epidural steroid injections. Phys Med Rehabil Clin N Am. 2018;29(1):155–69.

29. Feeley IH, et al. Particulate and non-particulate steroids in spinal epidurals: a systematic review and meta-analysis. Eur Spine J. 2017;26(2):336–44.

30. Stav A, Ovadia L, Sternbert A, Kaadan M, Weksler N. Cervical epidural steroid injection for cervicobrachialgia. Acta Anaesthesiol Scand. 1993;37:562–6. https://doi.org/10.1111/j.1399-6576.1993. tb03765.x.

31. Cohen SP, Hayek S, Semenov Y, Pasquina PF, White RL, Veizi E, Huang JH, Kurihara C, Zhao Z, Guthmiller KB, Griffith SR, Verdun AV, Giampetro DM, Vorobeychik Y. Epidural steroid injections, conservative treatment, or combination treatment for cervical radicular pain: a multicenter, randomized, comparative-effectiveness study. Anesthesiology. 2014;121(5):1045–55.

32. Goni V, Singh J, Gopinathan N, Behera P, Batra Y, Arjun R, Guled U, Vardhan H. Efficacy of epidural perineural injection of autologous conditioned serum in unilateral cervical radiculopathy: a pilot study. Spine. 2015;40(16):E915–21.

33. Diwan S, Manchikanti L, Benyamin RM, et al. Effectiveness of cervical epidural injections in the management of chronic neck and upper extremity pain. Pain Physician. 2012;15:E405–34.

34. Yoon JY, Kwon JW, Yoon YC, Lee J. Cervical interlaminar epidural steroid injection for unilateral cervical radiculopathy: comparison of midline and paramedian approaches for efficacy. Korean J Radiol. 2015;16:604–12.

35. Racz GB, Heavner JE, Singleton W, Carline M. Hypertonic saline and corticosteroid injected epidurally for pain control. In: Racz GB, editor. Techniques of neurolysis. 1st ed. Boston: Kluwer Academic publishers; 1989. p. 84.

36. Crock HV. Nerve root canal decompression. Lumbar perineural venous dilatation as an indicator of its efficacy. Acta Orthopaedica Scandinavica. 1994;65(2):225–7.

37. Ji GY, Oh CH, Won KS, Han IB, Ha Y, Shin DA, Kim KN. Randomized controlled study of percutaneous epidural neuroplasty using Racz catheter and epidural steroid injection in cervical disc disease. Pain Physician. 2016;19(2):39–48.

38. Park C, Lee S, Lee S. Preliminary results of the clinical effectiveness of percutaneous adhesiolysis using a Racz catheter in the management of chronic pain due to cervical central stenosis. Pain Physician. 2013;16(4):353–8.

39. Moon DE, Park HJ, Kim YH. Assessment of clinical outcomes of cervical epidural neuroplasty using a Racz-catheter and predictive factors of efficacy in patients with cervical spinal pain. Pain Physician. 2015;18(2):E163–70.

40. Han Y, Lee M, Min Ji Cho M, Park H, Moon D, Kim Y. Contrast runoff correlates with the clinical outcome of cervical epidural neuroplasty using a Racz catheter. Pain Physician. 2016;19(7):E1035–40.. ISSN 2150-1149

41. Kim JH, Jung HJ, Nahm FS, Lee PB. Does improvement in epidurography following percutaneous epidural neuroplasty correspond to patient outcome? Pain Pract. 2015;15:407–13. https://doi.org/10.1111/papr.12197.

42. Nikolaidis I, Fouyas IP, Sandercock PAG, Statham PF. Surgery for cervical radiculopathy or myelopathy. Cochrane Database Syst Rev. 2010;(1):CD001466. https://doi.org/10.1002/14651858. CD001466.pub3.

43. Epstein NE. The risks of epidural and transforaminal steroid injections in the spine: commentary and a comprehensive review of the literature. Surg Neurol Int. 2013;4(Suppl 2):S74–93. https://doi.org/10.4103/2152-7806.109446.

44. Scanlon GC, Moeller-Bertram T, Romanowsky SM, Wallace MS. Cervical transforaminal epidural steroid injections more dangerous than we think? Spine. 2007;32(11):1249–56.

45. Seelander D, Sjostrand J. Longitudinal spread of intraneurally injected local anesthetics. An experimental study of the initial neural distribution following intraneural injections. Acta Anaesthesiol Scand. 1978;22:622–34.

46. Seelander D, Dhuner KG, Lundborg G. Peripheral nerve injury due to injection needles used for regional anesthesia. An experimental study of the acute effects of needle point trauma. Acta Anaesthesiol Scand. 1977;21:182–8.

47. Racz GB, Heavner JE. Cervical spinal canal loculation and secondary ischemic cord injury--PVCS--perivenous counter spread-danger sign! Pain Practice. 2008;8(5):399–403.

48. Smith HK, Racz GB, Heavner JE. Peri-venous counter spread-be prepared. Pain Physician. 2010;13:1–6.

49. Racz GB, Apicella E, Vohra P. Collegial communication and problem-solving: intraspinal canal manipulation. Pain Pract. 2013;13:667–70. https://doi.org/10.1111/papr.12057.

Lowell Shih, Alopi Patel, and Sudhir Diwan

Anatomy

The cervical spinal column is composed of seven vertebrae, and beginning below the second cervical level, vertebral bodies are separated by intervertebral discs. Cervical discs are unique because their main function is to allow for rotation of the head and neck and they are relatively void of weight-bearing responsibilities. An increased range of rotation is primarily accomplished because cervical intervertebral discs have a crescent-shaped annulus fibrosis that is thick anteriorly and tapers in width as it approaches the uncovertebral region [1]. This is in contrast to lumbar intervertebral discs that carry a significant weight-bearing burden and therefore contain both a large water-based matrix (known as the nucleus pulposus) and a fully circumferential annulus fibrosis to withstand extensive compressive force. Irrespective of anatomic location, intervertebral disc degeneration can be a significant source of pain. The nociceptive fibers that supply the dural sac and dural root nerve sleeve innervate the outer 1/3 of the annulus fibrosis, and are responsible for pain transmission from the disc [2].

The first cervical vertebra (C1) is known as the atlas. It is characterized by a lack of a true body, and its large lateral masses form the inferior portion of the atlanto-occipital (AO) joint, which serves to help support the base of the skull. The second cervical vertebra (C2), otherwise known as the axis, is most recognizable by an upward central lengthening known as the odontoid process or dens. The relationship between the odontoid process and the anterior arch of C1 is responsible for the majority of head and neck rotation. The AO and the AA

L. Shih (✉)
Department of Pain Management, Ochsner Health Center, Covington, LA, USA
e-mail: Lowell.Shih@Ochsner.org

A. Patel
Icahn School of Medicine at Mount Sinai, New York, NY, USA

S. Diwan
Manhattan Spine and Pain Medicine, Lenox Hill Hospital, New York, NY, USA

joints are both anatomically considered anterior joints and are innervated by branches of the ventral rami of C1 and C2, lacking innervation by medial branches of the dorsal cervical rami. Instead, the medial branch of the dorsal ramus of C2, which distally becomes the greater occipital nerve, is responsible for sensory and motor innervation to the occiput, and plays a key role in the pathology of cervicogenic headaches [2, 3].

Cervical facet (zygapophysial) joints are true synovial joints that are posteriorly oriented with the longitudinal axis at an approximately 45° angle. They are innervated by the medial branches of the primary dorsal rami of the cervical spinal nerves (Fig. 30.1). Lateral branches of the primary dorsal rami are responsible for innervation of the multifidus muscles, sensation to the skin, and other paraspinal musculature of the neck [2].

Innervation to the C2/C3 facet joint is unique because the dorsal ramus of the C3 spinal nerve gives off two separate medial branches and both branches innervate the C2/C3 facet. The larger and cephalad branch, which is also known as the third occipital nerve (TON), is the main nociceptive source of the C2/C3 facet, but it also contributes to cutaneous innervation of the occiput. The second branch of the dorsal rami of C3 is smaller and also innervates the C3/C4 facet joint [2, 3]. In conjunction with the greater occipital nerve, the third occipital nerve also contributes to cervicogenic headaches. Beginning with the C3/C4 and continuing to C7/T1, each medial branch is responsible for innervating a facet joint one level above and one level below its origin. In other words, the C5 medial branch nerve, which comes of the C5 spinal nerve, innervates the C4/C5 facet joint and the C5/C6 fact joint. From the perspective of the facet joint, each joint is innervated by one medial branch from the top aspect of the joint and one medial branch nerve from lower aspect. For example, the C5/C6 facet joint receives innervation from the medial branches of C5 and C6. The dual innervation of the facet joint means that blocking either the C5 or C6 medial branch alone will not provide appropriate analgesia [2, 3]. Thus, in order to abolish nociceptive input from the C5/C6 facet joint, the medial branches of both C5 and C6 must be anesthetized.

© Springer Nature Switzerland AG 2019
Y. Khelemsky et al. (eds.), *Academic Pain Medicine*, https://doi.org/10.1007/978-3-030-18005-8_30

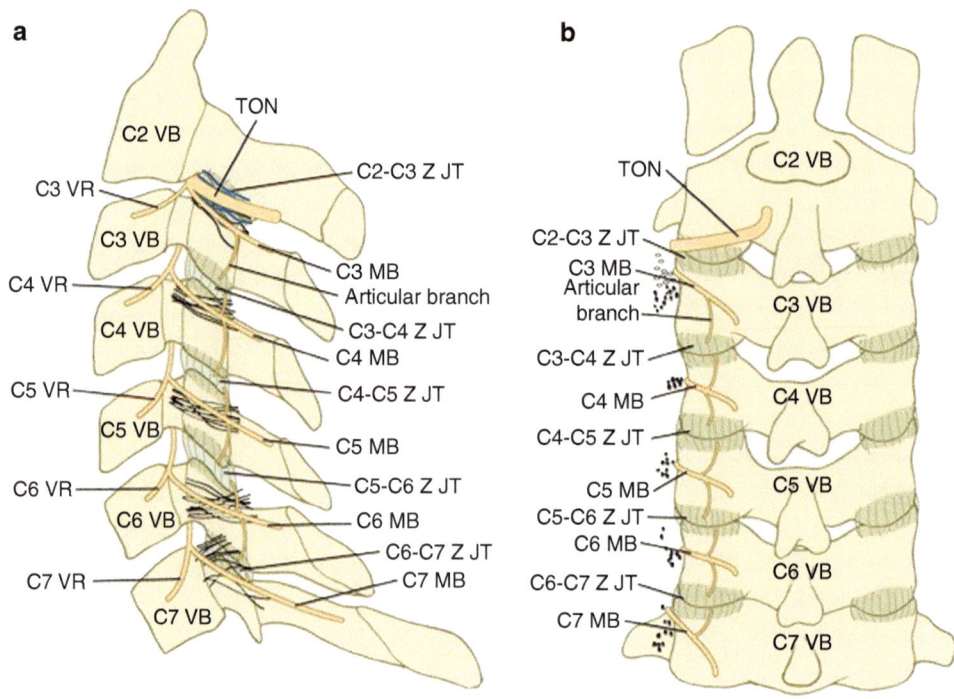

Fig. 30.1 (**a**) Lateral depiction of the cervical spine with location of the cervical medial branches. (**b**) AP depiction of the cervical spine with anatomy of the cervical medial branches

Risk Factors: Etiologic and Prognostic

In the general population, the 12-month prevalence of neck pain ranges from 30% to 50%, and neck pain may restrict activities of daily living in up to 11% of patients [4]. A systemic search and critical review by The Bone and Joint Decade 2000–2010 Task Force on Neck Pain and Its Associated Disorders concluded that the prevalence of neck pain increases with older age; however evidence on whether age itself is a risk factor is equivocal [5].

The task force was able to identify a variety of other risk factors associated with neck pain in the general population. Their review showed consistent evidence that neck pain often coincides with other musculoskeletal complaints such as low back pain, as well as with headache and poor self-rated health. Other risk factors of neck pain that were identified include gender (Female>Male), prior history of neck pain, genetics, and poor psychological health. They also were unable to identify any conclusive evidence that cervical degenerative disc disease is a risk factor for neck pain [5].

Multiple factors have been identified that may influence recovery, pain intensity, and neck function. It appears that neck in patients older than 40 or concomitant low back pain is associated with an unfavorable prognosis. From the perspective of long-term prognosis (52 weeks), an inciting traumatic event and duration of neck pain for greater than 13 weeks after initial presentation seemed to indicate that patients with stable but chronic neck pain and/or recurrent neck pain may also have a poor long-term prognosis [6].

History Taking: Use and Limitations

The initial approach to taking a history in a patient with neck pain should be to place an emphasis on ruling out any serious underlying etiology such as instability or malignancy. Some potential symptoms that may signal primary or metastatic malignancy as a cause of neck pain include history of malignancy, pain starting after the age of 50, continuous pain that is independent of posture or movement, and night-time pain. The presentation of one or more of these symptoms in combination with a review of symptoms positive for unintentional weight loss, fever, nausea/vomiting, dysphagia, or frequent coughing warrants an expeditious work-up [4].

Facetogenic neck pain can present as axial neck pain that may or may not radiate to the head (including the face), shoulders, and upper back. Unfortunately, the utility of history taking is hampered by the fact that the clinical presentation of cervical facetogenic neck pain is similar to axial neck pain caused by other etiologies such as spinal stenosis, muscle strain, or discogenic pain. Furthermore, there is no current evidence to significantly support the relationship of any particular signs or symptoms with cervical facet disease [7].

Differentiation of Neck Pain and Somatic Referring Pain from Radicular Pain and Radiculopathy

Cervical spinal pain is defined as pain that is perceived to arise from the cervical vertebral column or its surrounding structures. The borders of cervical spinal pain extended superiorly to the superior nuchal line, inferiorly to the first thoracic spinous process, and laterally in sagittal planes tangential to the lateral borders of the neck [8].

Common sources of cervical spinal pain include the facet (e.g., zygapophysial) joints, intervertebral discs, and surrounding ligaments and muscles. Cervical pain may present as either axial neck pain or as referred pain to the head, shoulder, scapula, and upper arm, and it is typically described as sharp, cramping, throbbing or aching in nature. The distinguishing characteristic of referred spinal pain, in comparison to radicular pain, is that referred spinal is initiated by stimulation of nerve endings of afferent fibers that innervate the vertebrae and surrounding structures. Radicular pain arises from pathologies affecting the spinal nerves [8].

Herniation of the nucleus pulposus or osteophytes from severely degenerated facet joints can cause compression of the dorsal nerve root leading to radicular pain. Cervical radicular pain is defined as pain arising in a limb that is caused by activation of nociceptive afferent fibers in a spinal nerve or its root. The underlying pathology can be attributed to either direct mechanical compression, ischemia, or inflammatory insult resulting in a lesion that compromises the dorsal root ganglion [8]. Patients with radicular neck pain often describe shooting, stabbing, or burning pain that radiates into one or both upper extremities in a dermatomal distribution. Radicular pain must further be delineated from radiculopathy. In patients with radiculopathy, there may be subjective sensations of numbness or weakness in the affected extremity; however there must also be an objective determination of loss of sensory and/or motor function determined by physical exam [8, 9].

For all patients with neck pain, a detailed history should focus on detection of neurologic abnormalities such as numbness, weakness, changes in reflexes, gait instability, and bladder and/or bowel dysfunction. Physical exam should include evaluation of upper and lower extremity reflexes, muscle strength, cutaneous sensation, and reproduction of pain with palpation or other provocative maneuvers (i.e., Spurling's, neck extension, etc.). It is important to compare lower extremity neurological reflex arcs to the upper extremity, as lower cervical spinal cord lesions may not always produce signs of upper motor neuron involvement in the upper extremity.

Treatment of neck pain should start with conservative management. Physical therapy exercises including stretching and strengthening of the cervical muscles should be started as soon as the patient can tolerate; however overall benefit of therapy may be influenced by the acuity of neck pain and whether there is a radicular component to the patient's pain. A Cochrane review of 27 randomized controlled trials on exercises for mechanical neck disorders concluded that cervico-scapulothoracic strengthening and stabilization may

be beneficial for reducing pain and improving function in patients with cervicogenic headache and radiculopathy; however overall, there was no high-quality evidence supporting exercise for chronic neck pain [10].

Nonsteroidal anti-inflammatory drugs (NSAIDs), acetaminophen, and muscle relaxants are all first-line pharmacologic therapies. Chronic opioid therapy should be avoided. Interventional options include trigger point injections for myofascial pain, occipital nerve blocks for pain referred to the head, and cervical medial branch blocks followed by radiofrequency ablation for facetogenic neck pain (including headache/pain in the head/face arising from the cervical spine). Epidural steroid injections may be indicated in the presence of radicular pain.

Mechanisms of Referred Pain Perceived as Headache

Referred pain is pain that is perceived in a region that is different from the anatomic source. Pain presenting as a headache that is referred from the cervical spine is known as a cervicogenic headache. These types of headaches typically present unilaterally, begin in the occipital region, are often described as constant, dull, and aching, and radiating up the back of the head and refer to the temporal and frontal part of the hemicranium [11]. The primary mechanism of cervicogenic headaches involves converging inputs between cervical and trigeminal afferent signals in the trigeminocervical nucleus (Fig. 30.2). Specifically, nociceptive afferent signals from the C1–C3 spinal nerves converge with afferent signals from adjacent cervical nerves and the ophthalmic division of the trigeminal nerve [12]. This significant junction of afferent signals is the source for referral of cervical pain to the head. Furthermore, in addition to the direct referral of pain from the neck to the head, primary headache disorders, such as migraines, may be triggered and potentiated by nociceptive input from the neck. Such input may be due to cervical etiologies or to secondary sensitization of neck structures by chronic headache. These hyperexcitable peripheral structures may, in turn, augment the headache – creating a vicious positive feedback loop [13–16].

Cervical facet joints are the most common source of pain that originates in the neck that can be perceived as a headache. Inflammation and resultant nociceptive signaling and stimulation of cervical spinal nerves that innervate the AO joint, lateral AA joints, C2/3 facet joint, and C2/3 intervertebral disc can all produce referred pain that presents as a cervicogenic headache [12]. Bogduk and Govind conducted a review of studies in an attempt to map the distribution of referred pain from joints in the neck and found that pain from the AA joint is usually localized around occipital and suboccipital regions with a referral pattern to the vertex of the head, orbit, and ipsilateral ear. The C2/C3 facet joint can also present with focal pain in the occipital region with a referral pattern that extends across the parietal region of the skull that can extend to the frontal region and orbit. Finally, they found that referred pain originating from the C3/C4 facet joint can be felt in the occiput and the upper and lateral cervical regions of the neck (Fig. 30.3) [12].

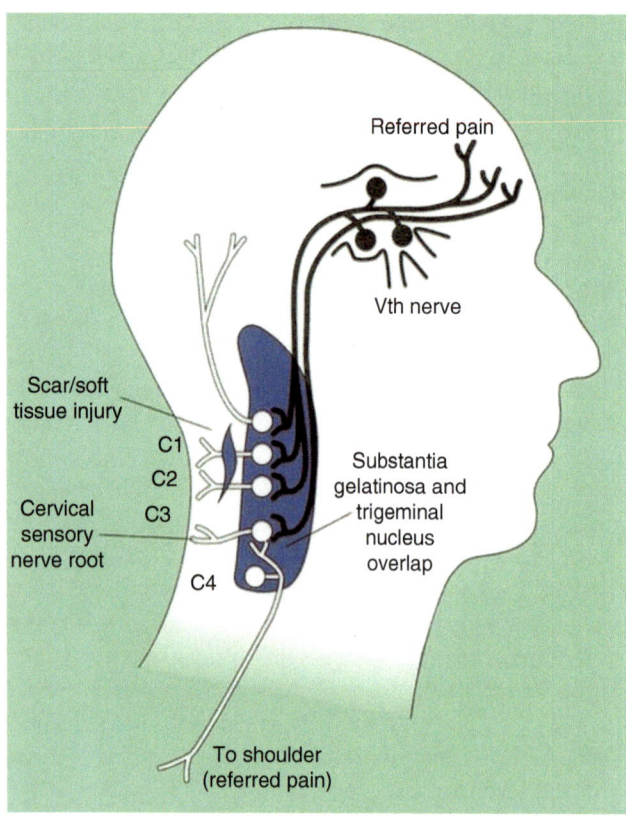

Fig. 30.2 Mechanism of cervical pain referral to the head and face, as well as mechanism of triggering of primary headaches and facial pain syndromes by cervical input

Whiplash

Whiplash injury is a common term used to describe cervical spinal pain that is caused by an injury involving sudden acceleration or deceleration of the head and neck with regard to the trunk. Following whiplash injury, the facet joints are the most common source of chronic neck pain, but pain from surrounding musculature and ligaments can also be contributory [17]. The diagnosis of whiplash injury is a clinical diagnosis that presents with appropriate traumatic history as previously described and neck pain that worsened by repetitive or prolonged use of neck and shoulder girdle muscles [11].

Most people who are involved in sudden acceleration/ deceleration accidents do not develop neck pain; however in patients who present with pain following whiplash injury, the most common presenting symptom is neck pain and followed closely by neck stiffness, headache, lower back pain, and shoulder pain [18]. Between 60% and 85% of people who develop acute neck pain following whiplash injury completely recover, up to 40% can develop mild, chronic neck pain, and 5–10% will have permanent, partial, or total disability. Full recovery can be seen in about half of all patients with whiplash injury within 3 months of the initial event and nearly 75% of patients who make a full recovery will do so within 1 year [17].

Imaging

As previously discussed, a thorough history and physical exam is the first step in ruling out 'red flags' and detecting any neurologic abnormalities. Medical imaging is useful if a patient with neck pain has an unclear diagnosis or as a tool to rule out severe pathology. Initial screening should start with

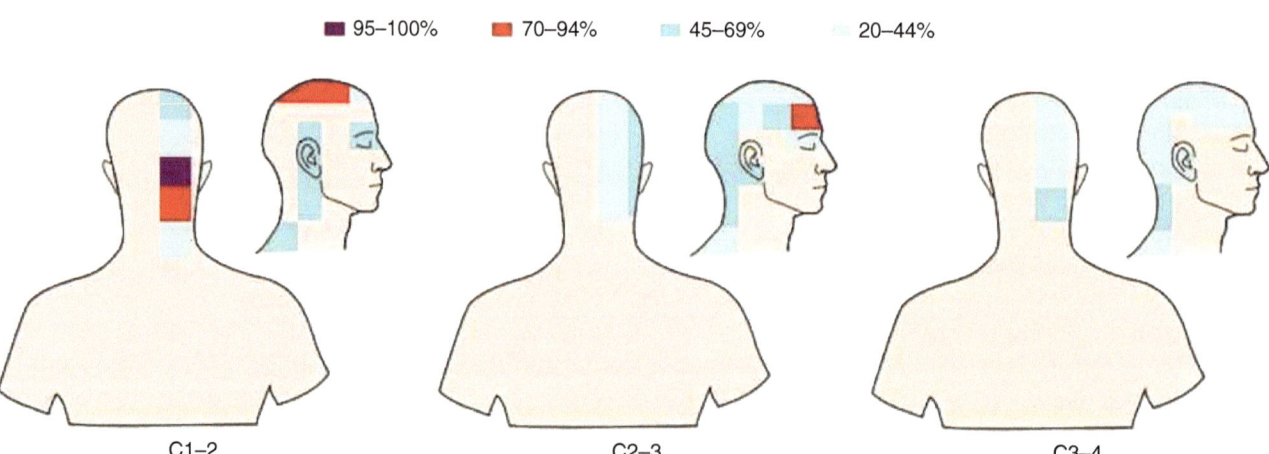

Fig. 30.3 Areas of referred pain from the cervical facets. Colored areas represent various frequencies of pain relief after controlled blocks at C1–C2, C2–C3 and C3–C4. For example, blocks at C2–C3 resulted in pain relief of the supraorbital region in 70–94% of patients

plain radiography to evaluate spinal alignment, postoperative hardware, to exclude bony tumor or fracture, and to detect abnormal bony lesions or osteoarthritis. Radiographic images should include flexion and extension views to detect any abnormal vertebral motion or instability [7]. The most important limitations of plain radiography is its inability to identify herniated intervertebral discs, neuroforaminal stenosis, and tumors in the spinal cord or epidural space [19].

Magnetic resonance imaging (MRI) is the most commonly used method of advanced spinal imaging. It provides further insight into pathology involving intervertebral discs, spinal cord and nerve roots, and ligamentous, osseous, muscle, and soft tissue surrounding the cervical spine [20]. MRI is particularly useful to evaluate the presence and severity of degenerative disc disease and neuroforaminal stenosis in a patient who presents with radicular pain or radiculopathy. Abnormalities within the intrathecal or epidural space such as central canal stenosis, hematoma or abscess formation, or presence of tumor can also be assessed.

One of the major limitations of MRI in the assessment of pain, is that findings often do not coincide with clinical presentation. Nakashima et al. conducted a large prospective study evaluating asymptomatic patients with cervical MRI. They demonstrated that significant disc herniations were present in 88% of asymptomatic subjects, and the frequency, number of bulging discs, and average size of disc displacement increased with age [21]. This data underscores the importance of correlating imaging with the history and physical exam and that clinical decision-making should not be solely based on radiologic findings.

Computed topography (CT) is an alternative imaging modality to MRI that may be useful in patients in whom an MRI is contraindicated, in patients with bone tumors, or in suspected traumatic cervical spine fracture. It allows superb visualization of the foramina. CT myelography is considered by many radiologists to be the gold standard of advanced spinal imaging and is especially useful for evaluation of congenital abnormalities or in patients with prior cervical surgery; however it is typically a secondary modality, due to its invasiveness and associated complications such as post-dural puncture headache, infection, and nerve injury [19].

Invasive Tests

Chronic axial neck pain may be due to numerous etiologies. One way to determine whether neck pain is of facetogenic origin is to perform diagnostic medial branch blocks. Sehgal et al. performed a systematic review of prospective and retrospective studies that evaluated diagnostic medial branch blocks in patients with chronic neck pain (>3 months). They observed that in one study single or uncontrolled cervical medial branch blocks had as high as a 45% false-positive rate

[22]. Ideally, multiple diagnostic injections should be performed to mitigate the placebo effect and possible false-positive response, and the gold standard diagnostic technique is one that controls with a placebo. However, in clinical practice, ethical and cost implications render placebo-controlled injections impractical; thus controlled comparative blocks with both short- and long-acting local anesthetics are typically employed [22].

This was exemplified by Manchikanti et al. who conducted a randomized controlled double-blind study where patients with chronic axial neck pain underwent comparative diagnostic medial branch blocks with 0.5 ml of 1% lidocaine followed 3–4 weeks later with 0.5 ml 0.25% bupivacaine. Patients who had at least 80% pain relief following both sets of diagnostic blocks were then treated with therapeutic medial branch blocks consisting of either bupivacaine or bupivacaine and betamethasone, with 85% of patients treated with bupivacaine and 93% treated with bupivacaine and betamethasone exhibiting over 50% pain relief over a 2 year period [23].

Discography is another method to aid in the diagnosis of axial neck pain and serves two main purposes. First, it allows clinicians to investigate for intervertebral disc disruption in patients with persistent neck pain with a normal MRI and second, it can help determine which intervertebral disc is symptomatic in a patient with multiple levels of disc disease confirmed on MRI [19]. Schellhas et al. compared MRI and discography in both asymptomatic patients and patients with chronic neck pain and found that in asymptomatic patients, 17 out of 20 discs appearing normal on MRI had discographically confirmed annular tears. They also found that in the patients with chronic neck pain, 10 out of 11 discs that appeared normal on MRI proved to have annular tears on discogram [24].

Medial Branch Neurotomy

Cervical medial branch neurotomy represents a treatment option for patients with chronic axial neck pain caused by facet joint arthropathy. Radiofrequency produces a small area of tissue coagulation around the active tip of an electrode and allows for a controlled method of destructive thermal neurolysis. In further detail, the mechanism of action of radiofrequency ablation is that it prevents neuronal nociceptive transmission by denaturing components of Aδ and C nerve fibers while leaving the medial branch nerve itself anatomically intact [25]. After verifying appropriate placement of the probes with fluoroscopy (Fig. 30.4), but prior to thermal ablation, low voltage stimulation should be applied to the RF electrode to assess for sensory or motor conduction to avoid damage to the nerve roots.

Medial branch neurotomy with radiofrequency ablation should be considered for a longer duration of pain relief

224																																																																																																																																																																																																																																																																																																																																																																																																																																																																																																																																																																																																																																																																																																																																																																																																																																																																																																																																																																																																																																																																																																																																																																																																																																																																																																																																																																																																																																																																																																																																																																																																																																																																																																																																																																																																																																																																																																																																																																																																																																																																																																																																																																																																																																																																																																																																																																																																				L. Shih et al.

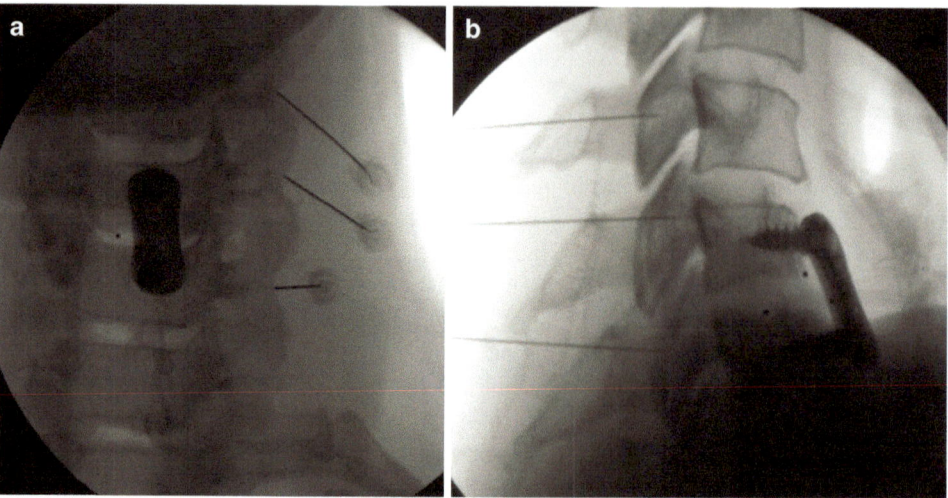

Fig. 30.4 (**a**) AP view of needle placement for RF ablation of cervical medial branches (C4–C6). (**b**) Lateral view of needle placement for RF ablation of cervical medial branches. Note: the needles at C4 (top level) and C6 (lowest level) should likely be advanced more anteriorly (lateral projection) for optimal positioning

following two positive diagnostic blocks with short- and long-acting local anesthetics (i.e., lidocaine and bupivacaine) that identify the medial branch as the source of neck pain. Lord et al. conducted a randomized, double-blinded trial comparing RF neurotomy of cervical medial branches at 80 °C with RF probe placement without thermal lesioning. In the study, treatment was only considered successful if the patients received complete pain relief. They concluded that not only was RF neurotomy clinically and statistically more efficacious than the control but, in patients with chronic facetogenic neck pain confirmed with a double-blind, placebo-controlled local anesthetic, RF neurotomy with multiple lesions of target nerves can provide long-lasting pain relief [26].

The efficacy of radiofrequency ablation of cervical medial branch nerves can further be illustrated by Engel et al.'s systemic literature review of neurotomy for chronic facetogenic neck pain. In that review the authors found evidence that cervical RF ablation results in 63% of patients being pain-free at 6 months and 38% pain-free at 12 months [25]. Similar to Lord et al., these results can only be interpreted with the consideration that all patients must have had successful comparative double diagnostic medial branch injections with 100% relief prior to radiofrequency. Equally as important to realize is that cervical medial branch neurotomy is a therapeutic but by no means a curative treatment for neck pain caused by cervical facet arthropathy. Currently, there is no known technique or intervention to prevent or reverse the process of degenerative zygapophysial joint disease [25].

Surgical Treatment

Surgical consultation for neck pain may be indicated in patients who have failed conservative and minimally invasive interventional treatment. Generally speaking, patients with refractory axial neck pain associated with instability, radiculopathy, or myelopathy should be considered candidates for surgical intervention. However a gray area exists for patients with chronic axial neck pain with nonradicular symptoms. One study looked at the clinical outcomes in anterior cervical discectomy and fusion in patients with chronic mechanical axial neck pain that lacked surgical indication for symptoms of radiculopathy or myelopathy. The study showed that greater than 80% of subjects who underwent surgery reported an improvement in pain and greater than 85% of subjects reported a 50% improvement in functionality [27]. Although these results are promising, further investigation is warranted to determine the long-term benefit of surgical intervention in patients with axial neck pain without signs or symptoms of spinal cord or nerve root compression.

References

1. Mercer S, Bogduk N. The ligaments and annulus fibrosus of human adult cervical intervertebral discs. Spine (Phila Pa 1976). 1999;24(7):619–28.
2. Manchikanti L, Singh V. Interventional techniques in chronic spinal pain. Pain Physician. 2007; Jan;10(1):7–111.
3. Bogduk N. The clinical anatomy of the cervical dorsal rami. Spine (Phila Pa 1976). 1982;7(4):319–30.
4. Van EM, Patijn J, Lataster A, Mekhail N, Van Zundert J. 5. Cervical facet pain. Pain Pract. 2010;10(2):113–23.
5. Hogg-Johnson S, van der Velde G, Carroll LJ, Holm LW, David Cassidy J, Guzman J, et al. The burden and determinants of neck pain in the general population results of the bone and joint decade 2000 –2010 task force on neck pain and its associated disorders. Spine (Phila Pa 1976). 2000;33(4S):39–51.
6. Hoving JL, De Vet HCW, Twisk JWR, Devillé WLJM, Van Der Windt D, Koes BW, et al. Prognostic factors for neck pain in general practice. Pain. 2004;110(3):639–45.
7. Kirpalani D, Mitra R. Cervical facet joint dysfunction: a review. Arch Phys Med Rehabil. 2008;89:770–4.
8. Merskey H, Bogduk N, editors. Classification of chronic pain. Descriptions of chronic pain syndromes and definitions of pain terms: IASP Press; Seattle, Washington, 1994. p. i–xvi.

9. Van Zundert J, Huntoon M, Patijn J, Lataster A, Mekhail N, Van Kleef M. 4. Cervical radicular pain. Pain Pract. 2010;10:1–17.

10. Gross A, Tm K, Jp P, Blanchette S, Lalonde P, Christie T, et al. Exercises for mechanical neck disorders (Review). Cochrane Database Syst Rev. 2015;(1)

11. Livingstone C, Murali R, Jannetta. Secondary neuralgia (trigeminal) from central nervous system lesions (11–2). In: Rovit RL, et al., editors. Trigeminal neuralgia. Baltimore: Williams Wilkins; 1994. p. 699–710.

12. Bogduk N, Govind J. Cervicogenic headache: an assessment of the evidence on clinical diagnosis, invasive tests, and treatment. Lancet Neurol. 2009;8:959–68.

13. Koppen H, van Veldhoven PLJ. Migraineurs with exercise-triggered attacks have a distinct migraine. J Headache Pain. 2013;14:99.

14. Pradhan S, Choudhury S. Clinical characterization of neck pain in migraine. Neurol India. 2018;66(2):377.

15. Gandolfi M, Geroin C, Valè N, Marchioretto F, Turrina A, Dimitrova E, et al. Does myofascial and trigger point treatment reduce pain and analgesic intake in patients undergoing onabotulinumtoxinA injection due to chronic intractable migraine? Eur J Phys Rehabil Med. 2018;54(1):1–12.

16. Varlibas A, Erdemoglu AK. Altered trigeminal system excitability in menstrual migraine patients. J Headache Pain. 2009;10(4):277–82.

17. Schofferman J, Bogduk N, Slosar P. Chronic whiplash and whiplash-associated disorders: an evidence-based approach. J Am Acad Orthop Surg. 2007;15:596–606.

18. McClune T, Burton AK, Waddell G. Whiplash associated disorders: a review of the literature to guide patient information and advice. Emerg Med J. 2002;19(6):499–506.

19. Mink JH, Gordon RE, Deutsch AL. The cervical spine: Radiologist's perspective. Phys Med Rehabil Clin N Am. 2003;14(3):493–548.

20. Modic MT, Masaryk TJ, Mulopulos GP, Bundschuh C, Han JS, Bohlman H. Cervical radiculopathy: prospective evaluation with surface coil MR imaging, CT with metrizamide, and metrizamide myelography. Radiology. 1986;161(3):753–9.

21. Nakashima H, Yukawa Y, Suda K, Yamagata M, Ueta T, Kato F. Abnormal findings on magnetic resonance images of the cervical spines in 1211 asymptomatic subjects. Spine (Phila Pa 1976). 2015;40(6):392–8.

22. Sehgal N, Dunbar EE, Shah RV, Colson J. Systematic review of diagnostic utility of facet (zygapophysial) joint injections in chronic spinal pain: an update. Pain Physician. 2007;10(1):213–28.

23. Manchikanti L, Singh V, Falco FJ, Cash KA, Fellows B. Comparative outcomes of a 2-year follow-up of cervical medial branch blocks in management of chronic neck pain: a randomized, double-blind controlled trial. Pain Physician. 2010;13(5):437–50.

24. Schellhas KP, Smith MD, Gundry CR, Pollei SR. Cervical discogenic pain. Prospective correlation of magnetic resonance imaging and discography in asymptomatic subjects and pain sufferers. Spine (Phila Pa 1976). 1996;21(3):300–11; discussion 311–2

25. Engel A, Rappard G, King W, Kennedy DJ. The effectiveness and risks of fluoroscopically-guided cervical medial branch thermal radiofrequency neurotomy: a systematic review with comprehensive analysis of the published data. Pain Med. 2016;17(4):658–69.

26. Lord SM, Barnsley L, Wallis BJ, McDonald GJ, Bogduk N. Percutaneous radio-frequency neurotomy for chronic cervical zygapophyseal-joint pain. N Engl J Med. 1996;335(23):1721–6.

27. Garvey TA, Transfeldt EE, Malcolm JR, Kos P. Outcome of anterior cervical discectomy and fusion as perceived by patients treated for dominant axial-mechanical cervical spine pain. Spine (Phila Pa 1976). 2002;27(17):1887–94.

Lumbar Radiculopathy

31

Ramsin M. Benyamin, William J. Smith, James Lieber, and Ricardo Vallejo

Introduction

Radicular pain refers to pain perceived in the limb or trunk by ectopic activation of nociceptors in a spinal nerve or the associated nerve root [1]. This condition has been documented for millennia with early Germanic and Britannic civilizations referred to it as witch's shot and elf's arrow, attributing the pain to mystical origins. Descriptions of radicular pain are found in the book of Genesis and the Talmud, as well. Ancient Greek and Egyptian societies demystified the pathology somewhat, with Hippocrates noting the phenomenon of claudication with the pain [2]. The physiological underpinnings were still a mystery until Domenico Cotugno's famous De Ischiade Nervosa Commentarius in 1764. From this point forward, the advancements in understanding and treatment of lumbar radicular pain begin to develop more rapidly. The mid-nineteenth century saw Virchow's discovery of disc involvement in sciatica, the straight-leg raise by Lasègue, and finally the first laminectomy by either MacEwen or Horsley in 1887.

A Brief Preface on Terminology

Often lumbar radicular pain is accompanied by radiculopathy, but they are two distinct pathologies [3]. Additionally, radiculitis is another pathology which presents identically yet may have a distinctly different etiology. As such, these conditions should be defined separately and their differences highlighted prior to exploration of the diagnosis and treatment modalities undertaken in this chapter.

- Radicular pain is defined by the International Association for the Study of Pain (IASP) as "Pain perceived as arising in a limb or the trunk wall caused by ectopic activation of nociceptive afferent fibers in a spinal nerve or its roots or other neuropathic mechanisms" [1].
- Radiculopathy is defined by the IASP as "Objective loss of sensory and/or motor function as a result of conduction block in axons of a spinal nerve or its roots" [1].
- Radiculitis is pain perceived as arising in the limb or the trunk wall caused by ectopic activation of nociceptive afferent fibers in a spinal nerve or its roots due to non-compressive inflammatory conditions.

For the duration of this chapter, the three pathologies discussed above, radiculopathy, radicular pain, and radiculitis, will be collectively referred to as lumbar radiculopathic syndromes.

Anatomy

As stated above, radicular pain, radiculopathy, and radiculitis originate in the spinal nerves and spinal nerve roots [1]. Specifically, lumbar radicular pain affects the nerves and their roots from the L1 to L5 vertebrae.

- Spinal nerves extend from the spinal cord to the periphery through intervertebral foramina in the posterolateral direction.
- Dorsal roots contain primary afferent axons from pseudounipolar neurons with cell bodies outside the spinal cord in the dorsal root ganglion (DRG) [4].
  - Contain Aδ and C fibers
  - Synapses in dorsal horn to second-order neuron, which decussates anteriorly to the spinothalamic tract

R. M. Benyamin (✉)
Millennium Pain Center, Bloomington, IL, USA

College of Medicine, University of Illinois, Urbana, IL, USA
e-mail: RBenyamin@millenniumpaincenter.com

W. J. Smith
Millennium Pain Center, Bloomington, IL, USA

J. Lieber
College of Medicine, University of Illinois, Urbana, IL, USA

R. Vallejo
Millennium Pain Center, Bloomington, IL, USA

Illinois Wesleyan University, Bloomington, IL, USA

© Springer Nature Switzerland AG 2019
Y. Khelemsky et al. (eds.), *Academic Pain Medicine*, https://doi.org/10.1007/978-3-030-18005-8_31

Table 31.1 Lumbar dermatomal patterns

Disc/nerve root affected	Pain	Sensory loss	Affected muscles
L1	Inguinal	Inguinal	None
L2	Groin, thigh (ant.)	Anterior and medial thigh	Flexion of thigh on trunk (iliopsoas muscle)
L3	Thigh (ant.)	Medial thigh and knee	Flexion of thigh on trunk (iliopsoas muscle) Extension of lower leg on knee (quadriceps) Adduction of leg (hip adductors)
L4	Lower leg (medial)	Medial lower leg	Extension of lower leg on knee (quadriceps) Adduction of leg (hip adductors) Extension and inversion of foot at ankle (tibialis anterior)
L5	Thigh (lat.), lower leg, foot (dorsal)	Lateral lower leg, dorsal foot, hallux	Flexion extension of toes Dorsiflexion of ankle (ankle dorsiflexor) Eversion and inversion of ankle Abduction of leg (hip abductors)
S1	Thigh (pos.), lower leg (pos.), heel	Dorsal foot and lateral foot, lateral ankle, lateral two toes	Flexion of toes Plantar flexion of foot and flexion of lower leg at the knee (gastrocnemius) Flexion of the knee and extension of the hip (biceps femoris) Extension and lateral rotation of the hip (gluteus maximus)

Adapted from Tarulli and Raynor [7]

- Nerve roots have distinct organizational difference from peripheral nerves.
  - Arranged in parallel without dense connective tissue [5]
  - Lack epineural covering [5]
  - Results in increased risk for mechanical stretch and compression injuries [5]
- Anterior to the spinal cord and associated nerve roots are intervertebral discs.
  - Fill spaces between adjacent vertebral bodies
  - Serve to cushion and bear axial load in the lumbar spine [4]
- Intervertebral discs comprised of a nucleus surrounded by a matrix containing proteins, water, and trace amounts of collagen [4].
  - Nucleus pulposus lies in the center of the disc and is surrounded by the annulus fibrosus [4].
  - Annulus fibrosus is collagen rich and highly ordered [4] and serves to withstand compression forces that displace the disc outward.
- The pain and sensorimotor loss associated with lumbar radiculopathic syndromes often follow a dermatomal pattern based on the disc level of cause of the pain (Table 31.1).

Causes and Differentiation from Low-Back Pain and Somatic Referred Pain

Given their identical presentation of symptoms, it is the etiology of radiculopathic syndromes where the difference between radicular pain, radiculopathy, and radiculitis is seen. As such, the causes of the radiating pain often accompanied by sensorimotor loss will be divided into two groups: radicular pain/radiculopathy and radiculitis. While the latter is

Table 31.2 Causes of radiculopathic pain

Radicular pain and radiculopathy causes		Radiculitis
Musculoskeletal	Neoplastic	Infectious
Spinal stenosis/foraminal stenosis – *these are descriptive terms and do not refer to any particular etiology (typically secondary to discs, facets, ligamentum flavum)* Intervertebral disc herniation Bulging intervertebral disc Spondylosis Spondylolisthesis Piriformis syndrome [7] Paget's disease [9] Failed back surgery syndrome (FBSS)	Primary tumors Ependymoma Schwannoma Neurofibroma Lymphoma Lipoma Dermoid Epidermoid Hemangioblastoma Paraganglioma Ganglioma Osteoma Plasmacytoma Metastatic tumors Leptomeningeal metastasis	Herpes zoster Spinal abscess HIV/AIDS Lyme disease Mycobacterium *Inflammatory* Diabetes mellitus Sarcoidosis Guillain-Barré syndrome *Vascular* Arachnoiditis Arteriovenous malformation Radiation-induced vascular occlusion Nerve root infarction due to vasculitis

important, the former are much more common. Radicular pain and radiculopathy causes can be further divided into two groups: musculoskeletal and neoplastic. The causes are listed in Table 31.2.

Musculoskeletal and neoplastic causes of radicular pain and radiculopathy involve mechanical compression of the spinal nerve or associated nerve root. In the case of neoplastic etiologies, a mechanical compression is due to a tumor [6]. In musculoskeletal etiologies, however, the structure causing the compression is a displaced or diseased biological tissue, usually bone or cartilage [7, 8]. The varying causes of radiculitis, on the other hand, stem not from mechanical compression, but rather from an immune inflammatory response, as is the case with all infectious causes presented below.

Of the etiologies listed in Table 31.2, intervertebral disc herniation and bulging discs are the most common causes of radicular pain and radiculopathy [7]. The annulus fibrosus of the disc weakens and succumbs to compressive forces, extends posterolaterally, and causes compression on the spinal cord or nerve root [7]. The difference between the two being that in a bulging disc the nucleus pulposus is still intact, while disc herniations are characterized by the nucleus breeching the annulus fibrosus.

Other common mechanical compression pathologies include spondylosis/spondylolisthesis, piriformis syndrome [7], Paget's disease, among others [8, 9].

- Spondylosis and spondylolisthesis are degenerative diseases of the vertebra, with the latter being characterized by the vertebra being displaced; facet joint hypertrophy may compromise the space available for nerve roots.
- Piriformis syndrome is characterized by inflammation of the piriformis muscle compressing the sciatic nerve.
- Paget's disease causes diseased bone to expand compressing the nerve root and DRG at the foramina [9].
- Ependymomas, schwannomas, neurofibroma, ganglioneuromas, and other primary tumors of neural structures can cause compression throughout the spinal cord, nerve root, dorsal root ganglion (DRG), and peripheral nerve pathways.
- Granulomas accumulating from sarcoidosis can also result in irritation of the nerve root.

The presence of somatic referred pain creates difficulty in diagnosis and treatment of these conditions. Normally recognizable by its intensity and localization, somatic pain becomes more of a confounding variable when it is referred to other regions of the body [10].

Somatic referred pain often occurs in the facets and discs where nociceptive nerve endings are activated to signal pain, but produce a referred pain distribution to other body regions. One clinical sign that points to a somatic component of pain is a lack of neurological involvement. Given that somatic referred pain originates from nociceptive neurons and does not implicate the nerve root, common neurological signs, such as claudication and paresthesia, are not seen.

History and Neurologic Examination: Reliability, Validity, and Limitations

For patients under the age of 50, the most common cause of radicular pain is lumbar disc herniation. After the age of 50, the pain is more likely attributed to age-related degenerative disorders such as spinal stenosis [8]. To identify these pathologies, the most common diagnostic tests are neurodynamic in nature. These are designed to manipulate the lumbar spine in a way that increases the compression on the affected nerve. These tests include:

- Straight leg raise/Lasègue's sign [12, 13]
  - The patient is placed supine. The physician extends the knee of the patient's normal leg. Using one hand to keep the knee extended, the ankle is supported and used to lift the leg by flexing at the hip [11].
  - This is continued until pain and sensory loss is felt, indicating a positive test, or tightness and pain is felt in the thigh, indicating a negative result.
  - Placing the patient supine when performing the test is preferred to having the patient seated during the test [14].
  - The test shows high levels of test-retest reliability and intraobserver and interobserver reliability [11] and receives a grade of A from the North American Spine Society indicating good evidence for use of the test [14].
- Bell test
  - Patient is in the standing position, and the physician manually applies pressure between spinous processes in an effort to exacerbate compression on the nerve root(s), thus increasing symptoms.
  - A positive test is marked by increased pain and sensory loss in the leg following the painful dermatome.
  - The test is considered negative if the patient only exhibits pain in the lower back.
  - While it has shown some clinical value [13], the North American Spine Society (NASS) has deemed the procedure requiring more evidence [12, 14].
- Hyperextension test
  - The patient is standing for the test. The patient is mobilized into a state of increased extension of the torso at the hips [13].
  - The test is positive if the pain is recreated/exacerbated in the legs and negative if the pain is localized to the low back.
  - Similar to the Bell test, the hyperextension test has been deemed inconclusive by the North American Spine Society's clinical guidelines [12, 14].
- Femoral nerve stretch test
  - Patient is prone and the knee passively flexed causing the relevant nerve and associated nerve roots to be pulled downward.
  - The test is positive if anterior thigh pain is present.
  - Studies have shown that this test actually causes minimal movement in the nerve root [15] and as such has been given the label of inconclusive by NASS [12, 14].
- Reflex response
  - Common reflexes such as the patellar, Achilles, and hallux are evaluated to diagnose and localize the presence of radiculopathy and its associated disc herniation.

– Radiculopathy and associated lumbar disc herniation are suspected if the reflex is diminished or not present; however these tests require more research to support their diagnostic abilities [12, 14, 16].

If the patient shows a positive result for these tests or shows a negative result in the above tests but still presents with the sensorimotor-deficit characteristic of radiculopathy, electrodiagnostic testing and imaging must be employed.

Medical Imaging and Electrodiagnostic Testing: Indication and Validity

Diagnostic imaging allows for confirmation of a positive result of neurodynamic tests and identification of other structural abnormalities when neurodynamic tests are inconclusive. In the case of a positive neurodynamic test indicating a pathology such as lumbar disc herniation, radicular pain symptoms may be treated with conservative therapy and are likely to resolve within 6–12 weeks [8]. Imaging should be considered at any point when deemed clinically appropriate. Magnetic resonance imaging (MRI) is considered the most appropriate noninvasive test to confirm the diagnosis. However, in cases where MRI is inconclusive or contraindicated, other imaging modalities such as computed tomography (CT) or myelography may be employed to elucidate the underlying pathology [12, 14].

In both compressive and non-compressive causes of radiculopathy, electrodiagnostic tools may be utilized. These include electromyography (EMG) and electrical impedance myography (EIM). The North American Spine Society recommends EMG as a diagnostic tool to confirm radiculopathy when other conditions are present [12, 14]. Additionally, these two electrodiagnostic tools have shown efficacy in diagnosing general radiculopathy regardless of etiology [17, 18].

Finally, in the case of certain infectious etiologies, patients presenting with radicular symptoms should undergo standard hematological and immunological testing to determine the cause of their radiculopathy.

Commonly Used Interventions: Evidence-Based

Paramount in the treatment of lumbar radicular pain is a transparent and informed dialogue with the patient regarding the treatment options and the known outcomes. The first step presented to the patient should always be conservative therapeutic methods.

Initial Approaches

The first step in this treatment process is anti-inflammatory medications to reduce any swelling in the area that is causing the radicular pain and physical therapy [19]. Common anti-inflammatory medications used are cox-2 inhibitors such as meloxicam, which has shown high effectiveness in pain reduction when compared to placebo or other nonsteroidal anti-inflammatory agents (NSAIDs) [20]. In combination with physical therapy techniques, a randomized clinical trial showed 79% of patients reported pain relief compared to 59% of patients who received pharmacological intervention alone [17]. Other commonly used medications include acetaminophen, steroids, gabapentinoids (e.g., gabapentin and pregabalin), tricyclic antidepressants (typically amitriptyline/nortriptyline at doses of 10–25 mg at night), anticonvulsants, muscle relaxants, and duloxetine [21–24]. It is important to note that the evidence base for these medications for this specific indication is hardly robust. If the patient fails to obtain relief from these conservative treatment methodologies or if the pain is severe, interventional approaches should be considered.

Procedures

Epidural corticosteroid injections (ESI) have generated a debate regarding their efficacy. However, when evidence from high-quality studies is employed, it is clear that these procedures are effective and safe modalities for the management of *radicular pain* [25–29]. One reason for possible poor outcomes described in some reviews is the use of ESIs for indications for which they are known to be less effective, such as spinal stenosis or "low back pain" [26]. Furthermore, the imaging modality used for guiding needle placement is not consistent across studies, with many performing ESIs without image guidance, which significantly decreases the probability of a successful injection [26]. The three main approaches, caudal, parasagittal interlaminar, and transforaminal, have been studied in an attempt to find benefit to one over the other. However, multiple studies have found there to be no increase in efficacy between the three approach options [12, 28, 30, 31].

Another technique that is employed in the treatment of radiculopathic syndromes is selective nerve root blocks (SNRB) [32–34]. Traditionally a diagnostic tool, studies into the therapeutic benefit of this treatment have shown its efficacy as a short-term option for patients suffering from lumbar radiculopathy and radicular pain. Relief generally appears immediately [32, 33] with the duration of pain relief reported as lasting 2 months [34] to greater than 1 year [32].

One advantage of the SNRB is the reduced dosage of therapeutic agent needed in comparison to ESIs [34]. Given their efficacy in patients who are indicated for surgery [33, 34], the SNRB can serve as a powerful tool in pain reduction.

Spinal cord stimulation (SCS) and dorsal root ganglion (DRG) stimulation may be both employed in the treatment of certain types of radicular pain [35–40]. A comprehensive discussion of these modalities may be found in the chapter dedicated to this topic.

Surgical Treatment: Indications and Efficacy

Surgical intervention for lumbar radiculopathic syndromes is dependent on the etiology involved. Given that lumbar disc herniation and other mechanical causes such as stenosis of the spinal canal or foramina are the most common etiologies, surgeries to address these issues are more commonly performed. Before undergoing any surgical intervention, the patient should be explained the full range of outcomes possible from the surgery.

In cases of lumbar disc herniation, the required surgical intervention is a discectomy or microdiscectomy [12]. The timeline regarding surgical intervention is debated. As stated above it should only be considered after conservative therapy has failed. Several studies have shown that patient outcomes improve when surgery is undertaken between 6 months and 1 year after symptoms arise [12, 41, 42].

One portion of the pivotal Spine Patient Outcomes Research Trial (SPORT) included any patients with greater than 6 weeks of lumbar radiculopathy symptoms presenting for discectomy [43]. At the 8-year follow-up, the study reported primary outcomes including SF36 Bodily Pain, SF36 Physical Function, and Oswestry Disability Index. These three surveys aim to assess not only the patient's level of pain but also their ability to complete various physical tasks, giving a more holistic view of their response to a treatment. The mean baseline SF36 BP and PF scores were 28.3 and 39.5, respectively. When interpreting both these surveys, it is important to remember that scores are reported between 0 and 100 where higher scores correspond to less severe symptoms. The baseline value for the Oswestry Disability Index was 46.9 on a scale of 0–100 as well, with lower scores on the ODI mean less severe symptoms.

Across all three of these metrics, no significant difference was seen between surgical intervention (open discectomy) and conventional medical management (active physical therapy, education/counseling with home exercise instruction, and nonsteroidal anti-inflammatory) at 8 years. The SF36 BP score increased from 40.9 on average for the surgical group to 69.2 and from 40.2 for the conventional medical management group to 68.5. The 8-year SF36 PF scores were 75.8 (+36.3) and 74.2 (+34.7) for the surgical and conventional

groups, respectively. ODI scores decreased for both groups to a final value of 16.3 (−30.6) and 20.5 (−26.4) for the surgical and conventional groups, respectively [43].

While the primary intent to treat outcomes indicated no significant difference between surgical intervention and conventional medical management, the secondary outcomes measuring satisfaction with symptoms and self-rated improvement were significantly higher in the surgical treatment group compared to conventional medical management. Despite their statistical significance, the surgical treatment group only scored 6.9% higher on satisfaction with symptoms and 4.1% higher on self-rated improvement [43]. This matches with previous studies findings, including the first large back surgery study in 1982 (Weber, H), which found no significant difference in patients reporting "no pain" between surgical and nonsurgical groups at the 4- and 10-year follow-up evaluation [44]. The Maine Lumbar Study, however, found statistical significance between sciatica patients treated with discectomy versus conventional medical management. At 5 years, surgical patients had better outcomes across measures of low back pain improvement, leg pain improvement, and patient satisfaction [45].

The SPORT study also reported that dural tears were the most common complication occurring with surgery and that roughly 5% of patients in the randomized cohorts and 3% in the observational cohort. At 8 years after surgery, 15% of patients required reoperation, and 85% of these reoperations were for recurrent herniations at the same level [43]. The study reports 7% and 11% rates of recurrent herniation in the randomized and observational cohorts, respectively [43]. While it is difficult to pin down a true rate of re-herniation, it is estimated to be between 5% and 15% [46]. Other complications can include iatrogenic neurological deficits due to compression of the cord or new-onset radiculitis [47] and failed back surgery syndrome. Other less common complications include wrong-level surgery, nerve root injuries, wound infection, and damage to vasculature, ureter, or intestines [43, 46]. Ultimately, these complications and the outcome in the aforementioned studies should all be discussed with the patients prior to their decision to undergo a discectomy.

The other major surgical intervention performed on patients with lumbar radiculopathic syndromes is decompressive laminectomy with or without fusion. This surgery can be used to alleviate radicular symptoms due to herniated discs [48], degenerative spondylolisthesis [49], or lumbar spinal stenosis [50]. In addition to evaluating discectomy, the SPORT trial evaluated laminectomy with and without lumbar fusion for spondylolisthesis and stenosis [49, 50]. Both trials found results that favor the use of laminectomy over conventional medical management for the treatment of lumbar spinal stenosis and lumbar degenerative spondylolisthesis at 4-year follow-up [49, 50]. While the SPORT trial is the most sophisticated and comprehensive trial performed to date, the study design and statistical analysis of both the randomized and observation cohorts together cast doubt on the conclusions.

As with discectomies, the leading complication is dural tear [48, 49, 50]; however with laminectomies, reoperation rates are reported between 13% and 15% across several large patient population studies [49, 50, 51]. In the cases of reoperation, >50% are for a second decompression surgery [51]. In addition to these common complications, the same set of standard complications mentioned with discectomy and with any invasive surgery are relevant and should be considered.

While these surgeries are the most common for alleviating radiculopathic syndromes, other surgeries may be required depending on the etiology. In the case of neoplastic causes, removal of tumor must be performed surgically and vascular etiologies may require surgery to repair the malformation. Ultimately, the decision to undergo surgery should rest entirely on the patient's fully informed consent. The emphasis cannot be stressed enough that all nonoperative conservative measures should be undertaken prior to surgical intervention in the case of lumbar radiculopathy, radicular pain, and radiculitis.

References

1. Merskey H, Bogduk N, editors. Classification of chronic pain. Descriptions of chronic pain syndromes and definition of pain terms. Seattle: IASP Press; 1994.
2. Truumees E. A history of lumbar disc herniation from Hippocrates to the 1990s. Clin Orth Rel Res. 2015;473:1885–95.
3. Bogduk N. On the definitions and physiology of back pain, referred pain, and radicular pain. Pain. 2009;147:17–9.
4. Manchikanti L, Singh V. Spinal anatomy for the Interventionalist. In: Interventional techniques in chronic spinal pain. Paducah, KY: ASIPP Publishing; 2007. p. 33–56.
5. Goldstein B. Anatomic issues related to cervical and lumbosacral radiculopathy. Phys Med Rehabil Clin N Am. 2002;13:423–37.
6. Kleiner JB, Donaldson WF 3rd, Curd JG, Thorne RP. Extraspinal causes of lumbosacral radiculopathy. J Bone Joint Surg Am. 1991;73(6):817–21.
7. Tarulli AW, Raynor EM. Lumbosacral radiculopathy. Neurol Clin. 2007;25(2):387–405.
8. Boxem KV, Cheng J, Patijn J, et al. Evidence based medicine: evidence-based interventional pain medicine according to clinical diagnostics. Chapter 11: lumbosacral radicular pain. Pain Pract. 2010;10(4):339–58.
9. Poncelet A. The neurologic complications of Paget's disease. J Bone Miner Res. 1999;14.(suppl:88–91.
10. Abrams B, et al., editors. Practical management of pain. 3rd ed. St. Louis, MO: Mosby/Harcourt Health Sciences; 2000.
11. Jensen OH. The level-diagnosis of a lower lumbar disc herniation: the value of sensibility and motor testing. Clin Rheumatol. 1987;6:564–9.
12. Kreiner DS, Hwang S, Easa JW, et al. Evidence-based clinical guidelines for multidisciplinary spine care: clinical guidelines for diagnosis and treatment of lumbar disc herniation with radiculopathy: North American Spine Society; Burr Ridge, Illinois 2012.
13. Poiraudeau S, Foltz V, Drapé JL, et al. Value of the bell test and the hyperextension test for diagnosis in sciatica associated with dis herniation: comparison with Lasègue's sign and the crossed Lasègue's sign. Rheymatology. 2001;40(4):460–6.
14. Kreiner DS, Hwang SW, Easa JE, et al. An evidence-based clinical guideline for the diagnosis and treatment of lumbar disc herniation with radiculopathy. Spine J. 2014;14:180–91.
15. Christodoulides AN. Ipsilateral sciatica on femoral nerve stretch test is pathognomonic of an L4/5 disc protrusion. J Bone Joint Surg. 1989;71-B:88–9.
16. Kortelainen P, Puranen J, Koivisto E, et al. Symptoms and signs of sciatica and their relation to the localization of the lumbar disc herniation. Spine. 1985;10:88–92.
17. Spieker AJ, Narayanaswami P, Fleming L, et al. Electrical impedance myography in the diagnosis of radiculopathy. Muscle Nerve. 2013;48:800–5.
18. Barr K. Electrodiagnosis of lumbar radiculopathy. Phys Med Rehabil Clin N Am. 2013;24:79–91.
19. Luijsterburg PA, Lamers LM, Verhagen AP, et al. Cost effectiveness of physical therapy and general practitioner care for sciatica. Spine. 2007;32(18):1942–8.
20. Dreiser RL, Le Parc JM, Vélicitat P, Lleu PL. Oral meloxicam is effective in acute sciatica: two randomized, double-blind trials versus placebo or diclofenac. Inflamm Res. 2001;Suppl 1:S17–23.
21. Ko S, Kim S, Kim J, Oh T. The effectiveness of oral corticosteroids for management of lumbar radiating pain: randomized, controlled trial study. Clin Orthop Surg. 2016;8(3):262–7.
22. Vanelderen P, Van Zundert J, Kozicz T, et al. Effect of minocycline on lumbar radicular neuropathic pain: a randomized, placebo-controlled, double-blind clinical trial with amitriptyline as a comparator. Anesthesiology. 2015;122(2):399–406.
23. Schukro RP, Oehmke MJ, Geroldinger A, Heinze G, Kress HG, Pramhas S. Efficacy of duloxetine in chronic low back pain with neuropathic component: a randomized, double-blind, placebo-controlled crossover trial. Anesthesiology. 2016;124(1):150–8.
24. Dosenovic S, Jelicic Kadic A, Miljanovic M, et al. Interventions for neuropathic pain: an overview of systematic reviews. Anesth Analg. 2017;125(2):643–52.
25. Benoist M, Boulu P, Hayem G. Epidural Steroid Injections in the management of low-back pain with radiculopathy: an update of their efficacy and safety. Eur Spine J. 2012;21(2):204–13.
26. Manchikanti L, Knezevic NN, Boswell MV, Kaye AD, Hirsch JA. Epidural Steroid Injections for lumbar radiculopathy and spinal stenosis: a comparative systematic review and meta-analysis. Pain Physician. 2016;19(3):E365–410.
27. Staal JB, de Bie R, de Vet HC, Hildebrandt J, Nelemans P. Injection therapy for subacute and chronic low-back pain. Cochrane Database Syst Rev. 2008;16(3)
28. Kaye AD, Manchikanti L, Abdi S, et al. Efficacy of epidural injections in managing chronic spinal pain: a best evidence synthesis. Pain Physician. 2015;18(6):E939–1004.
29. Rivera CE. Lumbar epidural steroid injections. Phys Med Rehabil Clin N Am. 2018;29(1):73–92.
30. Liu J, Zhou H, Lu L, et al. The effectiveness of transforaminal versus caudal routes for epidural steroid injections in managing lumbosacral radicular pain: a systematic review and meta-analysis. Medicine (Baltimore). 2016;95(18):e3373.
31. Hashemi SM, Aryani MR, Momenzadeh S, et al. Comparison of transforaminal and parasagittal epidural steroid injections in patients with radicular low Back pain. Anesth Pain Med. 2015;5(5):e26652.
32. Narozny M, Zanetti M, Boos N. Therapeutic efficacy of selective nerve root blocks in the treatment of lumbar radicular leg pain. Swiss Med Weekly. 2001;131:75–80.
33. Blankenbaker D, De Smet A, Stanczak J, Fine J. Lumbar radiculopathy: treatment with selective lumbar nerve blocks—comparison of effectiveness of triamcinolone and betamethasone injectable suspensions. Radiology. 2005;237:738–41.
34. Pfirrman C, Oberholzer P, Zanetti M, Boos N, Trudell D, Resnick D, Hodler J. Selective nerve root blocks for the treatment of sciatica: evaluation of injection site and effectiveness—a study with patients and cadavers. Radiology. 2001;221:704–11.

35. Zucco F, Ciampichini R, Lavano A. Et. al. cost-effectiveness and cost-utility analysis of spinal cord stimulation in patients with failed back surgery syndrome: results from the PRECISE study. Neuromodulation. 2015;18(4):266–76.
36. Taylor RS, Desai MJ, Rigoard P, Taylor RJ. Predictors of pain relief following spinal cord stimulation in chronic back and leg pain and failed back surgery syndrome: a systematic review and meta-regression analysis. Pain Prac. 2014;14(6):489–505.
37. Batier C, Privat JM, Seignarbieux F. Posterior spinal cord neurostimulation in lumbar radiculitis pain. Apropos of 14 cases. Agressologie. 1989;30(3):137.
38. Reverberi C, Dario A, Barolat G. Spinal cord stimulation (SCS) in conjunction with peripheral nerve field stimulation (PNfS) for the treatment of complex pain in failed back surgery syndrome (FBSS). Neuromodulation. 2012;16:78–83.
39. Atallah J, Armah F, Wong D, Weis P, Fahy B. Use of spinal cord stimulator for treatment of lumbar radiculopathy in a patient with severe kyphoscoliosis. Pain Physician. 2008;11:555–9.
40. Deer TR, Levy RM, Kramer J, et al. Dorsal root ganglion stimulation yielded higher treatment success rate for complex regional pain syndrome and causalgia at 3 and 12 months: a randomized comparative trial. Pain. 2017;158(4):669–81.
41. Ng LCL, Sell P. Predictive value of the duration of sciatica for lumbar discectomy. J Bone Joint Surg Am. 2004;86(4):546–9.
42. Nygaard O, Kloster R, Solberg T. Duration of leg pain as a predictor of outcome after surgery for lumbar disc herniation: a prospective cohort study with 1-year follow up. J Neurosurg. 2000;92(2):131–4.
43. Lurie J, Tosteson T, Tosteson A. Surgical versus non-operative treatment for lumbar disc herniation: eight-year results for the spine patient outcomes research trial (SPORT). Spine. 2014;39(1):3–16.
44. Weber H. Lumbar disc herniation: a controlled, prospective study with ten years of observation. Spine. 1983;8(2):131–40.
45. Atlas SJ, Keller RB, Chang Y, et al. Surgical and nonsurgical management of sciatica secondary to a lumbar disc herniation. Five-year outcomes from the Maine lumbar spine study. Spine. 2001;26(10):1179–87.
46. Bruggeman A, Decker R. Surgical treatment and outcomes of lumbar radiculopathy. Phys Med Rehab Clinics N Am. 2011;22(1): 161–78.
47. Ghobrial GM, Williams KA Jr, Arnold P, Fehlings M, Harrop JS. Iatrogenic neurologic deficit after lumbar spine surgery: a review. Clin Neurol Neurosurg. 2015;139:76–80.
48. Albert TJ, Mesa JJ, Eng K, McIntosh TC, Balderston RA. Health outcome assessment before and after lumbar laminectomy for radiculopathy. Spine. 1996;21(8):960–2.
49. Weinstein J, Lurie J, Tosteson T, et al. Surgical compared with nonoperative treatment for lumbar degenerative spondylolisthesis. Four-year results in the spine patient outcomes research trial (SPORT) randomized and observational cohorts. J Bone Joint Surg Am. 2009;91(6):1295–304.
50. Weinstein J, Tosteson T, Lurie J, et al. Surgical versus nonoperative treatment for lumbar spinal stenosis four-year results of the spine patient outcomes research trial (SPORT). Spine. 2010;35(14):1329–38.
51. Bydon M, Macki M, Abt NB, et al. Clinical and surgical outcomes after lumbar laminectomy: an analysis of 500 patients. Surg Neuol Int. 2015;6(Suppl 4):S190–3.

Low Back Pain

Sapan Shah, Julia H. Ding, and Anis Dizdarević

Introduction

Low back pain is among the most common complaints for which patients seek medical care [1]. It is a major contributor to disability, personal suffering, and socioeconomic costs. Low back pain is frequently categorized based on duration as acute, subacute, and chronic [2]. Acute pain is pain felt immediately after the onset of symptoms following trauma and tissue injury. If the acute symptoms worsen or do not improve, or the improvement plateaus short of complete elimination of symptoms, then the pain transitions into a subacute phase. If this pain process continues further, beyond the expected healing timeline, the pain can then be categorized as chronic. Pain in subacute or chronic phases may involve a persistent state of inflammation affecting joints, nerves, and muscles.

Anatomy

Low back pain, generally, is a nonspecific term that refers to pain in the lumbosacral region. The vertebral column is comprised of a series of vertebrae (7 cervical, 12 thoracic, 5 lumbar, and 5 fused sacral and 3–5 fused coccygeal elements). The functional spinal unit in the cervical, thoracic, and lumbar regions is comprised of two adjacent vertebral bodies separated by an intervertebral disc (IVD) and articulated by paired posterior facet (zygapophysial) joints. Bony elements of each vertebrae form a neural arch that encircles the spinal canal, which houses the spinal cord. The neural arch is defined posteriorly by the spinous process, spinal laminae, and ligamentum flavum and laterally by the pedicles and

intervertebral foramina. The sacroiliac joints transmit the forces applied to the spinal column to the lower extremities. These joints are the largest joints in the body and connect the torso and the lower extremities.

The IVDs absorb energy and distribute weight between spinal segments. The IVDs are composed of nucleus pulposus (NP) centrally and annulus fibrosus (AF) circumferentially. Both the NP and AF are composed of sparse cells in an intercellular matrix, though the cell morphologies and matrix compositions differ. The NP consists of chondrocyte-like cells in a jellylike matrix, whereas the AF is made of fibrocyte-like cells in a collagen-rich matrix. IVDs are largely avascular. Innervation of the IVD is complex and derived from multiple spinal segments including the sinuvertebral nerve, segmental spinal nerve, gray ramus communicans, and sympathetic trunk.

Facet joints are formed by the articulation of the inferior and superior articular processes of adjacent vertebrae. Facet joints are diarthrodial synovial joints. The cartilage covers the sliding surfaces, and a ligamentous capsule guides and limits the translation and rotation of the adjacent vertebra. As true of all synovial joints, injury to the cartilage structure will elicit an inflammatory response that can lead to chronic pain. Innervation of the facet joint is derived from the medial branch of the posterior primary ramus of the gray ramus communicans (Figs. 32.1 and 32.2).

Differentiation of Low Back Pain and Referred Somatic Pain from Radicular Pain

The IVD has been shown to be the cause of pain in 26–42% of patients with chronic low back pain without radicular symptoms, although this is not without controversy [3]. Disc herniation occurs when the NP extends beyond the disc margin, causing an inflammatory reaction when the herniated NP extends to an adjacent spinal nerve.

S. Shah · J. H. Ding
Department of Anesthesiology, Columbia University Medical Center, New York-Presbyterian Hospital, New York, NY, USA

A. Dizdarević (✉)
Department of Anesthesiology and Pain Medicine, Columbia University Medical Center, New York, NY, USA

© Springer Nature Switzerland AG 2019
Y. Khelemsky et al. (eds.), *Academic Pain Medicine*, https://doi.org/10.1007/978-3-030-18005-8_32

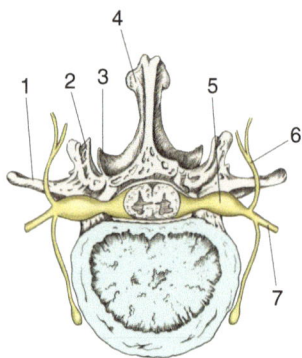

Fig. 32.1 Lumbar spinal cross section with bony and neural anatomy. (1) Transverse process, (2) superior articular process, (3) inferior articular process, (4) spinous process, (5) dorsal root ganglion, (6) dorsal ramus, (7) ventral ramus

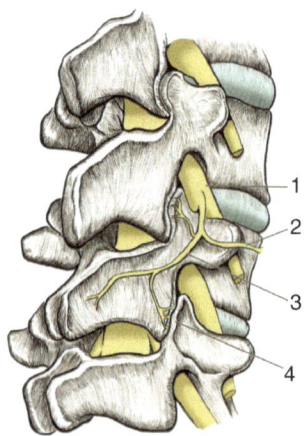

Fig. 32.2 Facet joint anatomy and innervation. (1) Lumbar nerve root, (2) lateral branch, (3) medial branch, (4) facet joint

Facet joint pain has been shown to be a cause of pain in up to 36% or more of patients with chronic low back pain [4]. Furthermore, hypertrophy of the facet joint can reduce the size of intervertebral foramina (e.g., foraminal stenosis), causing nerve root compression and radicular pain or radiculopathy. Typical characteristics of facet pain include exacerbated pain with palpation over facet joints, referred pain, and positive provocative maneuvers, such as Kemp's test. Findings on radiographic imaging are variable and often non-diagnostic; in older patients, frequently some degree of facet arthropathy is present (Fig. 32.3).

Radicular pain in the distribution of a spinal nerve may result from physical compression or other irritation of the nerve roots or dorsal root ganglion (DRG). This is distinct from radiculopathy, which also encompasses numbness, weakness, or loss of reflexes.

Referred somatic pain is pain perceived in a region innervated by nerves other than those innervating the painful area. Referred pain from lumbar disc and facet joints can mimic radicular pain radiating into the buttocks and thighs, but typically not below the knees.

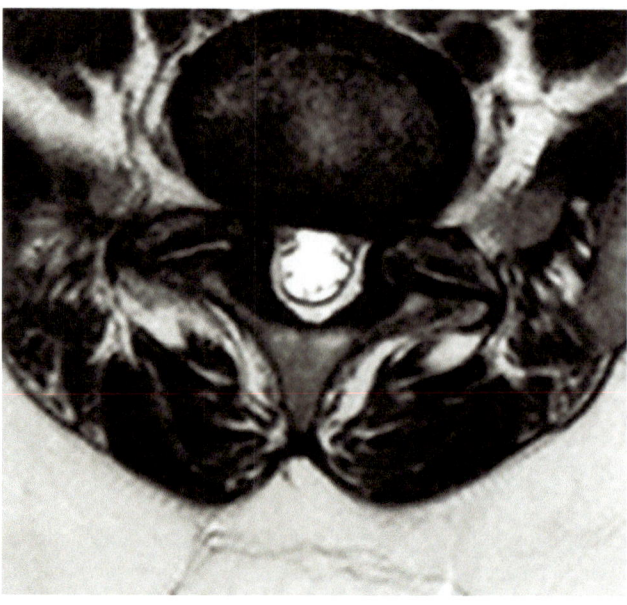

Fig. 32.3 MRI findings, lumbar facet joint arthropathy, T2 images

History

Patients presenting with low back pain should undergo a thorough history and physical exam to aid in diagnosis and to rule out "red flag" features.

A detailed history should include the following elements:

- Location of pain.
- Radiation (especially in a dermatomal distribution).
- Onset (history of trauma).
- Quality (characteristics such as aching, burning, or lancinating).
- Severity.
- Aggravating and alleviating factors.
- Previous treatments trialed.
- Effect on daily function and ability to sleep at night.
- Associated physical or psychological factors.
- Constitutional symptoms: fever, malaise, or weight loss.
- Neurologic symptoms: numbness, weakness, bowel or bladder dysfunction.

"Red flag" features requiring immediate attention and further workup include the following:

- Extremes of age
- History of trauma
- Infection
- Malignancy
- Constitutional symptoms
- Systemic illness
- Unrelenting pain
- Worsening neurologic deficits

Physical Examination and Conventional Medical Imaging

A complete physical exam should be performed, with attention given to the neurologic exam including assessment of gait, posture, spinal range of motion, local and paraspinal tenderness, and sensory and motor strength exams. Specific tests should be performed for nerve root irritation, facet syndrome, and sacroiliac joint dysfunction. No abnormalities in the neurologic exam are found in the majority of patients who present with acute low back pain without radicular symptoms.

Imaging studies used in the diagnosis of low back pain include plain radiography, computed tomography (CT), and magnetic resonance imaging (MRI). It is important to understand the limitations of imaging in the absence red flags. Anatomic changes will be present in a substantial portion of the population, increasing with age. It has been shown that 90% of asymptomatic patients over 50 years old will have some evidence of disc degeneration on MRI studies [5]. In patients with axial lower back pain, imaging studies have a low sensitivity and specificity as a diagnostic test unless a red flag is noted (e.g., infection, fracture, tumor, or metastases). In patients suffering from radicular pain or a radiculopathy, imaging may occasionally correlate with the symptoms. Routine imaging may not be needed in patients with acute back pain less than 4 weeks of duration without "red flag" features. Routine imaging may also not be needed in patients suffering an exacerbation or recurrence of pain which they readily identify as their usual pain.

- Plain radiography
- Can be used to assess bony spinal anatomy and reliably diagnose fractures, deformities, and spondylolisthesis.
- Common abnormal findings in asymptomatic patients include lumbar lordosis, disc space narrowing, arthritic changes, and vertebral end plate ossification.
- Advantages: relatively inexpensive, wide availability, and ease of performance.
- Disadvantages: inability to visualize soft tissue structures such as herniated disc, nerve compression, and soft tissue neoplasms.
- Computed tomography
- Used to evaluate osseous details especially the facet joints and lateral recesses and to diagnose fractures, tumors involving the spine, dislocations, and spondylolisthesis
- Not reliable in diagnosing soft tissue lesions such as herniated disc, epidural scar tissue, or soft tissue neoplasms
- Advantages: higher-resolution images, ability to manipulate and reconstruct views in any plane, excellent visualization of foramina
- Disadvantages: motion artifact and radiation exposure
- Magnetic resonance imaging
- Gold standard in spinal imaging
- Superior soft tissue resolution which is used to evaluate the spinal canal, neural elements, and disc spaces
- Advantages: relatively safe without known biologic effects
- Disadvantages: prolonged exam time, claustrophobia, and contraindication with ferromagnetic implants

Invasive Tests

Invasive diagnostic testing may be used when history and physical and radiologic studies fail to yield a definitive diagnosis.

Intra-articular facet joint injection (historically) or medial branch nerve blocks (most common contemporary practice) may be used to identify if the facet(s) is/are the cause of pain and to provide short-term pain relief. In some patients, these blocks may also provide long-term benefit. However, like all medical interventions, these techniques may be associated with placebo effect in a certain percentage of patients. Patients who respond favorably to diagnostic facet joint injections or medial branch nerve blocks may be candidates for treatment with longer-lasting radiofrequency denervation [6].

Diagnostic discography is a procedure used in an attempt to precisely diagnose symptomatic discs in patients who have not responded to algorithmic treatment of their lower back pain. It is utilized secondary to the high rate of disc abnormalities seen in asymptomatic patients thus rendering MRI a weak diagnostic tool in therapeutic decision making when considering higher-risk treatments. Provocative discography involves injecting a small volume of radiographic contrast through a series of needles in the central portion of the IVD to reproduce the patient's typical pain. This test helps to determine the symptomatic disc and may be used to select patients for more invasive therapies including intradiscal electrothermal therapy (IDET), biacuplasty, spinal cord stimulation, or fusion surgery. The use of diagnostic discography to predict surgical outcomes is controversial, with limited evidence from randomized studies [7]. False-positive results may occur as disc stimulation may elicit pain in normal discs.

Natural History

The majority of episodes of low back pain resolve without treatment. However, it is now known that persistent lower back pain is present in 25% of patients 1 year after the initial episode. Up to 70% of acute back pain resolves by 6 weeks, and up to 90% resolves by 12 weeks. Beyond 12 weeks, recovery is less certain. Of patients suffering from low back pain for longer than 6 months, fewer than half will return to work. For patients disabled for 2 years, the rate of returning to work is almost zero.

Etiologic and Prognostic Risk Factors

Etiologic risk factors are those that contribute to the development of low back pain and depend largely on the patient's own characteristics and lifestyle. These can preemptively be used to stratify patients at highest risk and provide primary intervention [8]. Several common risk factors that have been identified include:

1. Certain patient lifestyle aspects, such as extended sitting, poor posture, smoking, and excessive alcohol consumption, are risk factors for low back pain [9].
2. Physical characteristics such as obesity and increased height have also been identified as risk factors for certain low back pain syndromes.
3. Hard physical labor including heavy lifting and postural stress may lead to sciatica from disc degeneration.
4. Additionally, both occupational and psychosocial factors play a major role in the development of back pain and are explored further below.
5. Genetic predisposition places individuals at an increased risk of low back pain.

Similarly, prognostic risk factors are those characteristics of the patient and the disease state that can determine future outcomes. Current studies show a complex interaction of prognostic factors that predict a disease course, and these can be used to track response to treatment and provide insight into future long-term outcomes. Factors related to the resolution or perpetuation of low back pain include:

1. Elevated baseline pain scores inherently confer an increased risk of continued pain, and as disease intensity increases, outcomes tend to worsen [10].
2. Almost all mental health disorders, including depression and anxiety, negatively affect low back pain severity.
3. A patient's belief that they will recover has incidentally been found to be one of the strongest predictors of improved outcomes [11].
4. Other poor prognostic factors include unemployment and extended disability leave.

Psychosocial and Occupational Factors Related to Low Back Pain and Chronicity

Current data supports the concept that chronic back pain is closely related to psychosocial factors including concurrent anxiety, depression, and psychological distress. A patient's social environment also has a large impact. It is important to identify these factors and other signs of fear, frustration, and isolation, as these all contribute to the overall disease state

and may require the engagement of a psychiatrist [12]. A patient's occupation has significant impact on their low back pain, as a physically demanding line of work may exacerbate the condition due to excess strain. An occupation with minimal physical expectations and extended leave and disability benefits is also a predictor of poor outcomes in a patient with low back pain [13].

The Diagnosis and Treatment of Specific Causes of Lumbar Spinal Pain

Interventional pain management procedures are typically indicated once the patient has failed in more conservative approaches consisting of medication and/or physical therapy. Interventional treatments of lower back pain have a favorable risk/benefit ratio. Based on the duration of therapeutic benefit, they could be repeated based on published guidelines to maintain control of painful symptoms and improve quality of life and functionality. Additionally, their importance in the management of pain is reinforced by the risks of common alternatives including surgery and prolonged treatment with opioids and other medications.

- Facet (zygapophyseal) joint pain – Treatment of facet joint pain includes intra-articular injections, medial branch nerve blocks, and percutaneous lumbar medial branch radiofrequency neurotomy. In addition to their therapeutic utility, medical branch blockade can also be diagnostic, as adequate pain relief can delineate the original source of pain. Current high-quality, randomized control trials support the use of this block in the lumbar region, as it has been shown to be both effective and cost-efficient in chronic low back pain that has been resistant to conservative therapies [14, 15].
- Sacroiliac joint pain – Treatment of pain from these joints is comparable to treatment of facet joint pain and similarly may also be of diagnostic value. Some authors have shown improvement of pain with sacral lateral branch neurotomy versus placebo, though the duration of this effect is limited [16]. Though there are studies showing improved pain relief and function status with sacroiliac joint interventions, the evidence is limited and varying, with room for further studies [17].
- Discogenic pain – Although a wide variety of interventions have been used to treat lumbar discogenic pain, only intradiscal electrothermal annuloplasty has been subject to controlled trials, which revealed a reduction in pain, increased return to work, and decreased opioid usage [18]. It must be noted that IDET carries a high failure rate, with up to 50% of patients receiving no benefit [19]. Biacuplasty has also been shown to have long-term benefit in appropriate selected patients [20].

Surgical Treatment

Although surgical techniques for treating low back pain vary between providers and institutions, the basic approach involves fusion to eliminate motion between spinal levels. This can be achieved with auto- or allogenic bone graft, or prosthetic material, being used to eliminate motion between transverse processes. Additionally, portions of a disc that may be causing pain are often removed to decompress nerve roots, and the space that is left may be filled with graft material. Alternatively, this technique may be supplemented with instrumentation, which involves the use of screws, rods, and/or plates to provide stability. Unfortunately, rigorous studies of all types of surgical treatment are extremely difficult to perform due to the inability to have a blinded placebo arm. Lastly, surgical procedures carry significant risk of not only failure to relieve pain but worsening of pain in addition to the perioperative risks. The use of surgery in benign pain conditions has been questioned for this reason.

Spondylolisthesis is a condition in which one vertebral body subluxates forward onto another and, in the case of low back pain, usually involves the L5 level. The fundamental feature of spondylolisthesis that justifies surgery is radicular pain, commonly caused by compression of a nerve root. Surgical intervention involves decompression of this nerve root, and anterior or posterior fusion of the spinal levels to maintain stability. This has been found to be more effective than conservative care, but only in a small portion of patients suffering from low back pain [21].

Although idiopathic lumbar back pain has been extensively treated with spinal fusion, there is an absence of evidence regarding the efficacy or long-term effects of this procedure. In fact, fusion has been found in some studies to be minimally or no more effective than other treatments including cognitive behavioral therapy and physiotherapy [22].

Discogenic low back pain, confirmed by positive provocation discography, is often treated with surgical intervention. Fusion with or without disc resection has widespread usage, with several studies demonstrating superior outcomes compared to conservative management [23].

Disc arthroplasty has gained popularity as a surgical intervention for low back pain. Rather than restricting movement at the joint level, this technique uses prostheses to restore joint mechanics and preserve motion in order to reduce pain and improve function. The development of this technology has been closely followed by several controlled trials and descriptive studies, demonstrating only minimal to modest improvement of pain and other outcomes compared to traditional fusion [24].

A final technique under development, coined dynamic stabilization, aims to employ prosthetic devices between lumbar spinous processes to limit extension without affecting flexion and other movements. These devices were originally used effectively to treat spinal stenosis; there is currently no evidence of effectiveness for their use in idiopathic back pain [25].

Medial Branch Neurotomy and Intradiscal Therapy

Medial branch neurotomy is the intervention of choice in a select group of low back pain patients, who have previously achieved complete resolution of pain after controlled, diagnostic blockade of these nerves. The Spine Intervention Society updated recommendations that describe diagnostic medial branch blockade as a diagnostic tool to determine the need for further radiofrequency neurotomy treatment [26]. Neurotomy entails placement of electrodes to target the medial branches of dorsal rami and coagulate these neural fibers. Under a caudally declined fluoroscopic view with slight lateral obliquity, the electrode is inserted parallel to the x-ray beam and lodged against the superior articular process. Once adequate location and depth are confirmed with fluoroscopic views, a matrix of lesions is produced across the anatomically determined location of neural fibers (Fig. 32.4). Patient selection is crucial to the success of medial branch neurotomy. When properly executed, the procedure can be highly effective at treating low back pain in certain patients. The evidence for medial branch neurotomy is variable, with many studies demonstrating both short- and long-term improvement in outcomes, while others still showed a lack of effectiveness [14]. If pain recurs, further neurotomy procedures may be performed, as studies have shown a high success rate and effective long-term pain relief with repeated neurotomies [27]. Procedural side effects include postprocedure neuritis, but this is typically a time-limited side

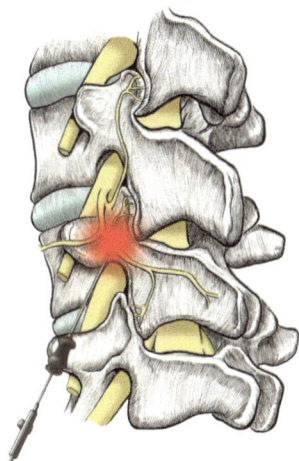

Fig. 32.4 Depiction of radiofrequency ablation of the medial branch neural fibers

effect. Other complications such as damage to other structures (such as spinal roots) are uncommon.

The most common form of intradiscal therapy is intradiscal electrothermal annuloplasty, which entails passage of an electrode into the annulus of a painful disc. The lesions produced by this method may help relieve back pain through several proposed mechanisms: denaturing collagen to strengthen the annulus, coagulation of nerve endings, or sealing of fissures. Although intradiscal therapy of this kind has a low success rate, it can greatly lower pain in those patients that are properly selected. Another commonly used intradiscal therapy involves thermal radiofrequency annuloplasty, which is a similar technique to IDET but with lower effectiveness [28]. Complications usually involve injury to the cauda equina, almost always due to operator error, as well as infection, disc herniation, and nerve root damage.

Multidisciplinary Therapy

Multidisciplinary management of chronic and recurrent low back pain in a compassionate and cost-effective manner will often require input from many providers in addition to the interventional pain management specialist. Medication management for chronic pain and exacerbations is extremely important and must be handled by well-qualified individuals to avoid the long-term risks, primarily of opioids, but also NSAIDs and other central nervous system depressants. Physiotherapists, psychologists, psychiatrists, occupational therapists, social workers, neurologists, and rehabilitation medicine specialists may all serve a role. Examples of common components and the evidence behind their use are provided:

- Physiotherapy: Physical rehabilitation is very commonly prescribed to patients with low back pain and has found good success for this disease. Exercise is recommended as a first-line therapy, and specifically core-strengthening exercises have good efficacy. Other commonly employed treatments including massage, manipulation, the McKenzie method, acupuncture, and transcutaneous electrical nerve stimulation (TENS) have all been found to be more effective than no treatment or even conventional pharmacologic treatments [29–33].
- Pharmacologic therapies: Acetaminophen has widespread use due to its relatively robust safety profile, but this has not been proven in any studies. NSAIDs are more effective than placebo and are largely used for acute low back pain [34]. There is short-term data to support the use of muscle relaxants for low back pain. Of the antidepressants studied, only tricyclic antidepressants have proven effective thus far. Tramadol has also been shown to be effective in the short-term treatment of low back pain [35]. Opioids have traditionally been used extensively;

however, there is no evidence to support their utility for the long-term management of low back pain (or any chronic non-cancer pain condition) and mounting evidence of associated mortality and morbidity [36].

- Interventional therapies: Although they have widespread use, other treatments such as trigger point injections have mixed outcomes [37]. Epidural steroid injections, via caudal or interlaminar routes, are also commonly used and are effective for radicular pain [38]. Additionally, epidural injections have moderate evidence in the treatment of discogenic pain and pain from spinal stenosis [39]. Another option for low back pain interventional management is spinal cord stimulator placement, which is more commonly used for spinal stenosis and neuropathic pain, but is also indicated for failed back surgery syndrome, chronic regional pain syndrome, and even angina [40]. The technique involves placement of electrodes, powered by a pulse generator, to deliver an electrical impulse through the epidural space and stimulate the dorsal vertebral columns. This in turn inhibits small nociceptive projections in the dorsal horn, blocking pain and creating a paresthesia effect. More recently, other mechanisms of action have been elucidated, including activation of GABA-B and adenosine a-1 receptors of pain modulation. The stimulation usually occurs in the 40–50 Hz range, though newer 10,000 Hz high-frequency stimulation has also proven to provide significant improvement in back pain, disability, and quality of life [41]. The technology behind spinal cord stimulation is rapidly evolving, and new developments are providing success with this opioid-sparing therapy. The addition of peripheral field stimulation to spinal cord stimulation provides another effective method of back pain control [42]. Finally, a new form of electrical neuromodulation involves eliciting lumbar multifidus muscle contraction and has also been shown to be an effective option for chronic mechanical low back pain [43].
- A final component of multimodal management includes behavioral training. Patient education is effective, as is fear-avoidance training administered by a psychiatrist. Cognitive behavioral therapy is a safe way to improve outcomes in patients with chronic low back pain [44].
- Above all, the critical component is an intense, multidisciplinary rehabilitation, which has been found to improve functional status and pain more than any other listed intervention [45].

References

1. Miller RD, Pardo MC, editors. Basics of anesthesia. 6th ed. Philadelphia: Elsevier Saunders; 2011.
2. Benzon HT, Raja SN, Liu SS, Fishman SM, Cohen SP, editors. Essentials of pain medicine. 3rd ed. Philadelphia: Elsevier Saunders; 2011.

3. Peng B-G. Pathophysiology, diagnosis, and treatment of discogenic low back pain. World J Orthop. 2013;4(2):42.
4. Manchikanti L, Boswell MV, Singh V, Pampati V, Damron KS, Beyer CD. Prevalence of facet joint pain in chronic spinal pain of cervical, thoracic, and lumbar regions. BMC Musculoskelet Disord. 2004;5:1–7.
5. Teraguchi M, Yoshimura N, Hashizume H, Muraki S, Yamada H, Minamide A, et al. Prevalence and distribution of intervertebral disc degeneration over the entire spine in a population-based cohort: the Wakayama Spine Study. Osteoarthr Cartil. 2014;22(1):104–10.
6. Cohen SP, Moon JY, Brummett CM, White RL, Larkin TM. Medial branch blocks or intra-articular injections as a prognostic tool before lumbar facet radiofrequency denervation: a multicenter, case-control study. Reg Anesth Pain Med. 2015;40(4):376–83.
7. Cohen SP, Hurley RW. The ability of diagnostic spinal injections to predict surgical outcomes. Anesth Analg. 2007;105(6):1756–75.
8. Heliövaara M. Risk factors for low back pain and sciatica. Ann Med. 1989;21(4):257–64.
9. Krishna VK, Sharma D, Samuel G. Epidemiological study for evaluation of etiology and risk factors in patients with low back Pain. Global Spine J. 2014;4(1_suppl). s-0034-1376533-s-0034-1376533.
10. Lionel KA. Risk factors forchronic low back pain. J Community Med Health Educ. 2014;4:271.
11. Cambell P. Prognostic indicators of low back pain in primary care: five-year prospective study. Jour Pain. 2013;14(8):873–83.
12. Fishman SM, et al. Bonica's management of pain. Philadelphia: Wolters Kluwer; 2009.
13. Fordyce WE. Behavioral methods for chronic pain and illness. St. Louis: Mosby; 1976.
14. Manchikanti L, et al. A systematic review and best evidence synthesis of the effectiveness of therapeutic facet joint interventions in managing chronic spinal pain. Pain Physician. 2015;18(4):E535–82.
15. Manchikanti L, et al. Therapeutic lumbar facet joint nerve blocks in the treatment of chronic low back pain: cost utility analysis based on a randomized controlled trial. Korean J Pain. 2018;31(1):27–38.
16. Cohen SP, et al. Randomized placebo controlled study evaluating lateral branch radiofrequency denervation for sacroiliac joint pain. Anesthesiology. 2008;109(2):279–88.
17. Simopoulos TT, et al. Systematic review of the diagnostic accuracy and therapeutic effectiveness of sacroiliac joint interventions. Pain Physician. 2015;18(5):E713–56.
18. Karasek M, Bogduk N. Twelve-month follow-up of a controlled trial of intradiscal thermal annuloplasty for back pain due to internal disc disruption. Spine. 2000;25(20):2601–7.
19. Freeman BJ, et al. A randomized, double-blind, controlled trial: intradiscal electrothermal therapy versus placebo for the treatment of chronic discogenic low back pain. Spine. 2005;30(21):2369–77.
20. Desai MJ, et al. Twelve-month follow-up of a randomized clinical trial comparing intradiscal biacuplasty to conventional medical management for discogenic lumbar back pain. Pain Med. 2017;18(4):751–63.
21. Mardjetko SM, Connolly PJ, Shott S. Degenerative lumbar spondylolisthesis: a meta-analysis of literature 1970–1993. Spine. 1994;19(20 Suppl):2256S–65S.
22. Brox JI, Sorensen R, Friis A, et al. Randomized clinical trial of lumbar instrumented fusion and cognitive intervention and exercises in patients with chronic low back pain, and disc degeneration. Spine. 2003;28(17):1913–21.
23. Greenough CG, Peterson MD, Hadlow S, et al. Instrumented posterolateral lumbar fusion. Results and comparison with anterior interbody fusion. Spine. 1998;23(4):479–86.
24. Mirza SK. Point of view: commentary on the research reports that led to Food and Drug Administration approval of an artificial disc. Spine. 2005;30(14):1561–4.
25. Zucherman JF, et al. A multicenter, prospective, randomized trial evaluating the X STOP interspinous process decompression system for the treatment of neurogenic intermittent claudication: two-year follow-up results. Spine. 2005;30(12):1351–8.
26. MacVicar J. Lumbar medial branch radiofrequency neurotomy in New Zealand. Pain Med. 2013;14(5):639–45.
27. Bogduk N. Practice guidelines for spinal diagnostic and treatment procedures. 2nd ed. San Francisco: International Spine Intervention Society; 2013.
28. Kapural L, Hayek S, Malak O, et al. Intradiscal thermal annuloplasty versus intradiscal radiofrequency ablation for the treatment of discogenic pain: a prospective matched control trial. Pain Med. 2005;6(6):425–31.
29. Imamura M, et al. Evidence-informed management of chronic low back pain with massage. Spine J. 2008;8(1):121–33.
30. Bronfort G, et al. Evidence-informed management of chronic low back pain with spinal manipulation and mobilization. Spine J. 2008;8(1):213–25.
31. May S, et al. Evidence-informed management of chronic low back pain with the McKenzie method. Spine J. 2008;8(1):134–41.
32. Ammendolia C, et al. Evidence-informed management of chronic low back pain with needle acupuncture. Spine J. 2008;8(1):160–72.
33. Poitras S, et al. Evidence-informed management of chronic low back pain with transcutaneous electrical nerve stimulation, interferential current, electrical muscle stimulation, ultrasound, and thermotherapy. Spine J. 2008;8(1):226–33.
34. Keller A, Hayden J, Bombardier C, et al. Effect sizes of nonsurgical treatments of nonspecific low-back pain. Eur Spine J. 2007;16(11):1776–88.
35. Schnitzer TJ, Gray WL, Paster RZ, et al. Efficacy of tramadol in treatment of chronic low back pain. J Rheumatol. 2000;27(3):772–8.
36. Koes BW. Pharmacotherapy for chronic non-specific low back pain: current and future options. Expert Opin Pharmacother. 2018;19(6):537–45.
37. Malanga G, et al. Evidence-informed management of chronic low back pain with trigger point injections. Spine J. 2008;8(1):243–52.
38. Benoist M, et al. Epidural steroid injections in the management of low-back pain with radiculopathy: an update of their efficacy and safety. Eur Spine J. 2012;21(2):204–13.
39. Pandey R. Efficacy of epidural steroid injection in management of lumbar prolapsed intervertebral disc. J Clin Diagn Res. 2016;10(7):RC05–11.
40. Barolat G. Spinal cord stimulation for chronic pain management. Arch Med Res. 2000;31:258–62.
41. Al-Kaisy A. 10 kHz High-Frequency Spinal Cord Stimulation for Chronic Axial Low Back Pain in Patients With No History of Spinal Surgery: A Preliminary, Prospective, Open Label and Proof-of-Concept Study. Neuromodulation. 2017;20(1):63–70.
42. Van Gorp EJ, Teernstra O, Aukes HJ, Hamm-Faber T, Bürger K, Kallewaard JW, Spincemaille G, Schapendonk JW, Vonhögen L, Bronkhorst E, Vissers KC. Long–term effect of peripheral nerve field stimulation as add-on therapy to spinal cord stimulation to treat low back pain in failed back surgery syndrome patients: a 12-month follow-up of a randomized controlled study. Neuromodulation. 2019; https://doi.org/10.1111/ner.12776.
43. Deckers K, et al. New Therapy for Refractory Chronic Mechanical Low Back Pain-Restorative Neurostimulation to Activate the Lumbar Multifidus: One Year Results of a Prospective Multicenter Clinical Trial. Neuromodulation. 2018;21(1):48–55.
44. Cherkin DC, et al. Effect of mindfulness-based stress reduction vs cognitive behavioral therapy or usual care on back pain and functional limitations in adults with chronic low back pain: a randomized clinical trial. JAMA. 2016;315(12):1240–9.
45. Guzman J, Esmail R, Karjalainen K, et al. Multidisciplinary rehabilitation for chronic back pain: systematic review. Brit Med J. 2001;322(7301):1511–6.

Musculoskeletal Pain Joint Pain: Upper Extremities

Melinda Aquino and Yuriy O. Ivanov

Epidemiology

According to the US Department of Labor, musculoskeletal disorders (MSD) affect the muscles, nerves, blood vessels, ligaments, and tendons and are among the most frequently reported causes of lost or restricted work time [1, 2]. The Bureau of Labor Statistics (BLS) reported in 2013 that MSD accounted for 33% of all worker injury and illness cases. The Centers for Disease Control and Prevention estimates that 54.4 million US adults suffer from arthritic pain. By 2040, an estimated 78 million (26%) of US adults ages 18 years or older are projected to have a diagnosis of arthritis [3].

In 2014, upper extremities affected by an injury or illness accounted for 346,170 cases or 32 cases per 10,000 full-time workers. Hands accounted for 40% of those cases, the most among upper extremities. Shoulder injuries caused workers to miss a median of 26 days of work, more than any other body part [4]. Among musculoskeletal complaints, shoulder pain is the third most common presenting complaint to primary care physicians and affects between 7% and 26% of adults [5].

Anatomy and Physiology

Shoulder

The shoulder girdle is a complex structure that is comprised of multiple articulations of the arm to the torso (Fig. 33.1). The main articulation is the glenohumeral (also referred to as *scapulohumeral*) joint. It connects the humerus and the socket of the glenoid and is the most mobile but least stable joint in the body [6]. The glenoid fossa is the lateral surface of the scapula that is made deeper by the glenoid labrum, an outpouching circular cartilaginous ligament (Fig. 33.2). This normally provides static stability to the glenohumeral joint. The labrum also gives rise to the glenohumeral capsule, which wraps around the head of the humerus, becoming thicker in the anterior shoulder to form glenohumeral ligaments [7]. The three glenohumeral ligaments are the superior, middle, and inferior and collectively prevent the head of the humerus from slipping off the glenoid fossa. The glenohumeral joint is further stabilized by the rotator cuff tendons of supraspinatus, infraspinatus, subscapularis, and teres minor muscles (Figs. 33.3 and 33.4). In addition, the long head of the biceps brachii muscle passes through the tendon sheath inside the capsule and attaches on the supraglenoid tubercle, providing further anterior stabilization of the shoulder.

The shoulder is attached to the thorax via the clavicle and the scapula. The other joints of the shoulder girdle are sternocostal, connecting the sternum with the ribs; sternoclavicular, connecting the manubrium of the sternum with the medial end of the clavicle; acromioclavicular, connecting the acromial process of the scapula with the lateral end of the clavicle; and scapulothoracic, connecting the scapula with the ribcage [6].

The acromioclavicular (AC) joint is a gliding (plane style) joint between the clavicle and scapula. It is covered by a synovial joint capsule and strengthened by the capsular ligaments [8]. It is also stabilized by the coracoacromial and coracoclavicular (CC) ligament, which is further made up of the conoid and trapezoid ligaments. These serve to prevent vertical translation of the clavicle [7].

The shoulder joint has multiple fluid-filled sacs or bursae that can become inflamed and cause irritation and pain. The most common of these is the subacromial bursa (Fig. 33.5). As the name suggests, it lies underneath the acromion, which is a common anatomical landmark for injections.

M. Aquino (✉)
Montefiore Medical Center, Albert Einstein College of Medicine, Bronx, NY, USA

Y. O. Ivanov
Department of Physical Medicine and Rehabilitation, Montefiore Medical Center, Bronx, NY, USA

© Springer Nature Switzerland AG 2019
Y. Khelemsky et al. (eds.), *Academic Pain Medicine*, https://doi.org/10.1007/978-3-030-18005-8_33

Fig. 33.1 Anatomy of
shoulder joint

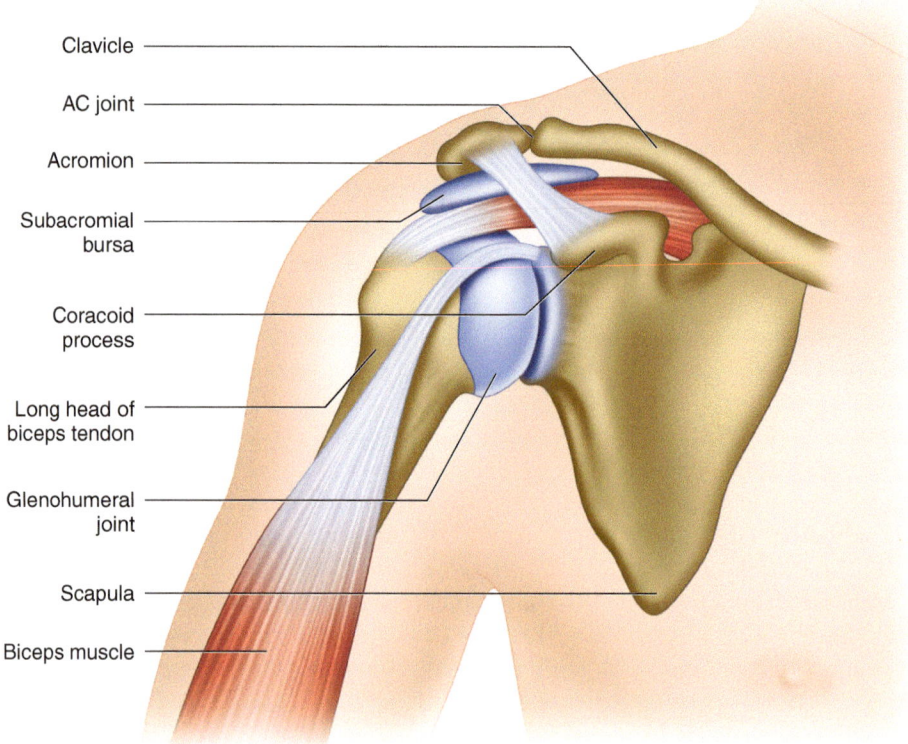

Clavicle

AC joint

Acromion

Subacromial
bursa

Coracoid
process

Long head of
biceps tendon

Glenohumeral
joint

Scapula

Biceps muscle

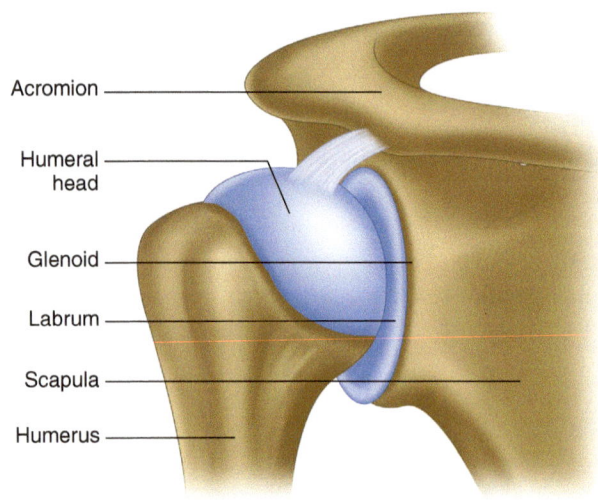

Acromion

Humeral
head

Glenoid

Labrum

Scapula

Humerus

Fig. 33.2 Anatomy of glenoid fossa

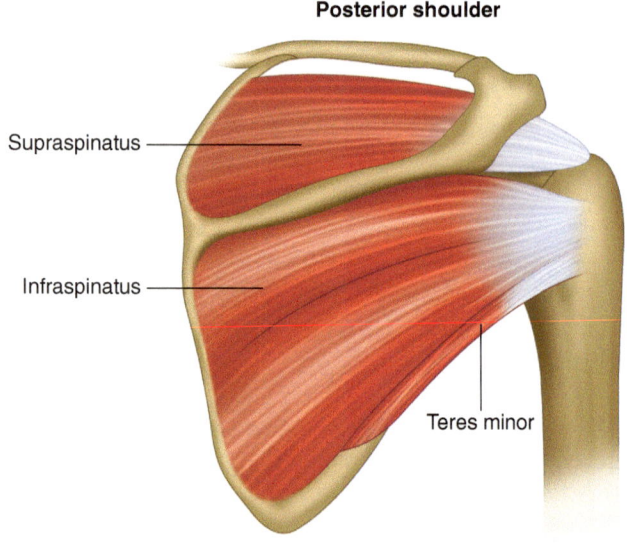

Posterior shoulder

Supraspinatus

Infraspinatus

Teres minor

Fig. 33.3 Anatomy of posterior shoulder

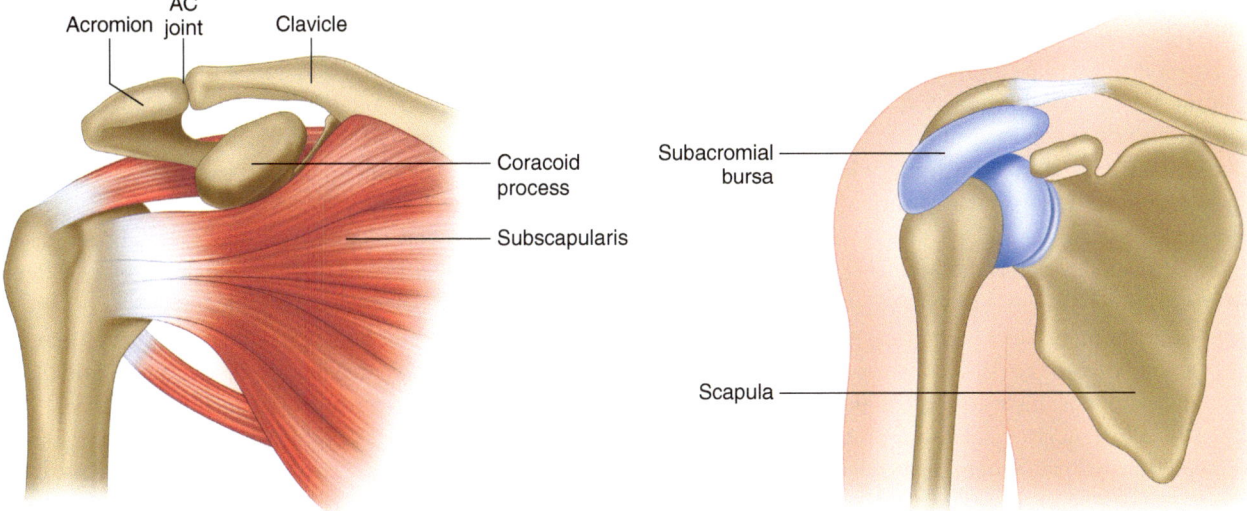

Fig. 33.4 Anatomy of anterior shoulder

Fig. 33.5 Subacromial bursa

Elbow

The elbow is a synovial joint that functions like a hinge, connecting the arm to the forearm. It is formed by the articulation of the humerus, the radius, and the ulna (Fig. 33.6). Being a synovial joint it is stabilized by a fibrous capsule, which is further strengthened by the medial (ulnar) and lateral (radial) collateral and annular ligaments. The elbow has several bursae, the most clinically relevant being the superficial olecranon bursa which lies between the olecranon and the subcutaneous tissue [9]. Slightly distal to the elbow joint, but still part of the capsule is the proximal radioulnar pivot joint. The annual ligament is responsible for maintaining the radial head in place on the radial notch of the ulna. The anatomical landmarks that are palpable and are important both for diagnosis and treatment of painful conditions affecting the elbow are the olecranon and the medial and lateral epicondyles. Normally, there is a slight deviation (5–15° as measured between the axis of the radius and humerus) of the supinated forearm away from the body. This is known as the carrying angle and it helps the arms to swing without hitting the hips while walking [10].

The cubital tunnel is found on the ulnar side of the elbow. It is formed by the flexor carpi ulnaris fascia and Osbourne's ligament, which connects the medial condyle to the olecranon. The ulnar nerve passes through the tunnel, compression or stretching of which results in cubital tunnel syndrome.

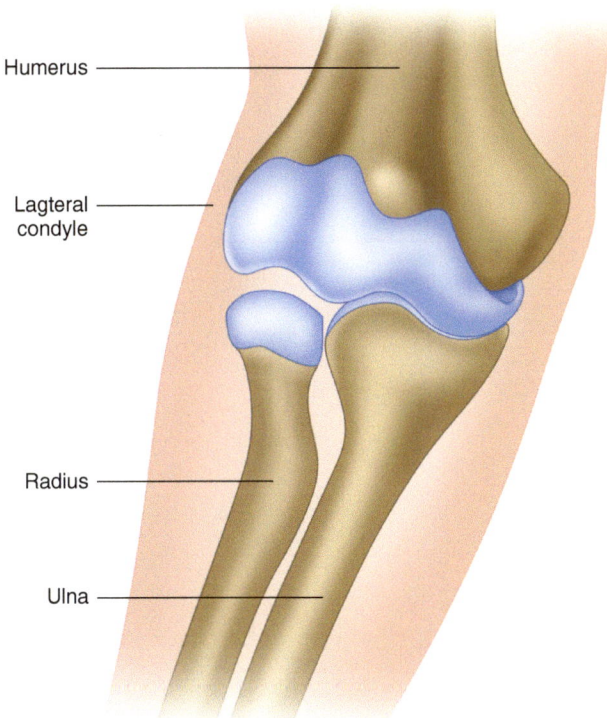

Fig. 33.6 Anatomy of elbow

Hand

The major articulations in the hand are the distal radioulnar joint, the carpals in the wrist, the metacarpals in the palm, and the phalanges in the fingers. Proximal to the wrist is the distal radioulnar joint, which is an articulation between the ulnar notch of the radius and the ulnar head [11].

The wrist (or the radiocarpal) joint is an ellipsoid (allows movement along two axes) synovial joint that is formed distally by the proximal row of carpal bones (except the pisiform) and proximally by the distal end of the radius and a fibrocartilaginous ligament called the articulating disk [12]. The actual wrist is made up of eight carpal bones, scaphoid, lunate, triquetrum, pisiform, hamate, capitate,

trapezoid, and trapezium, and five metacarpal bones (Figs. 33.7 and 33.8). There are also four ligaments which stabilize the wrist: palmar and dorsal radiocarpal ligaments and radial and ulnar collateral ligaments. Collectively, the ligaments act to unify the movement of the wrist and the corresponding bones and to prevent excess displacement in either direction.

The flexor retinaculum covers the carpal bones in the wrist and creates a tunnel through which a series of flexor tendons and the median nerve pass through.

Although a normal human hand has 5 fingers, there are only 14 phalanges, 5 proximal, 5 distal, and 4 middle, as the thumb does not have one. The interphalangeal (IP) joints are considered to be hinge joints and function via pulley systems. There are two tendon flexor systems, made

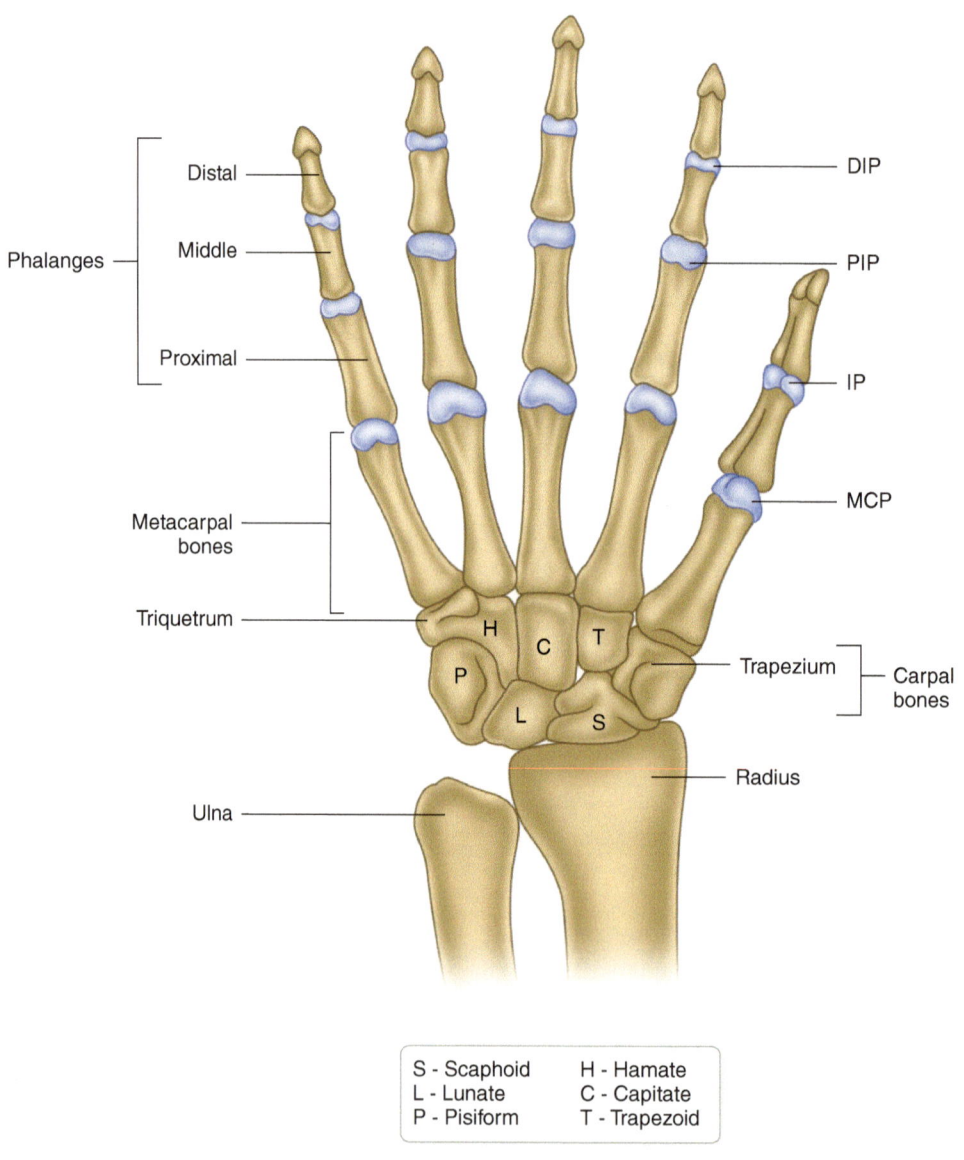

S - Scaphoid	H - Hamate
L - Lunate	C - Capitate
P - Pisiform	T - Trapezoid

Fig. 33.7 Anatomy of hand

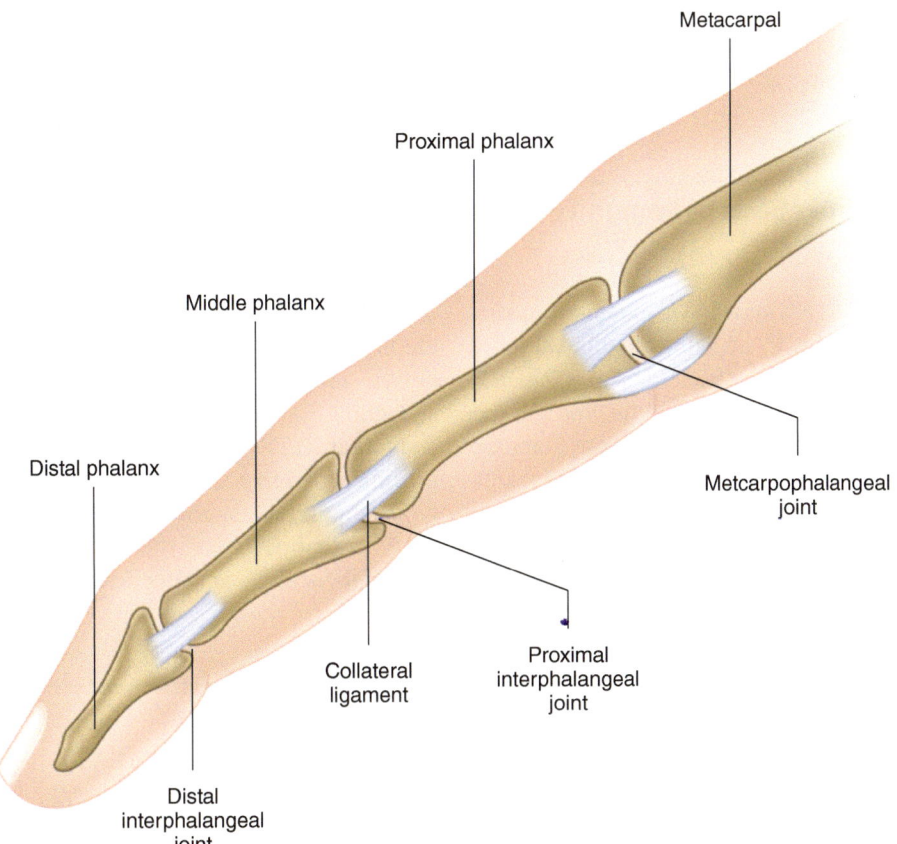

Metacarpal

Proximal phalanx

Middle phalanx

Distal phalanx

Metcarpophalangeal
joint

Collateral
ligament

Proximal
interphalangeal
joint

Distal
interphalangeal
joint

Fig. 33.8 Anatomy of finger

up of the flexor digitorum profundus (FDP) and flexor digitorum superficialis (FDS). Only one tendon is found in the extensor system – extensor digitorum communis (EDC) [7]. In the phalanges, there are distal and proximal inter-phalangeal joints (DIPs and PIPs); in the thumb, there is only an IP.

The carpal tunnel is found in the wrist. On the palmar surface, it is made up by the flexor retinaculum, which is attached to the pisiform and the hook of the hamate on the ulnar side of the wrist and the scaphoid and the trapezium on the radial side. On the dorsal surface, it is made up of the carpal bones. Four tendons of flexor digitorum profundus and superficialis pass through the tunnel, along with flexor pollicis longus tendon. The median nerve also passes through the tunnel, compression of which results in carpal tunnel syndrome.

The anatomical snuffbox is a triangular area on the dorso-lateral side of the wrist. It is formed by tendons of extensor pollicis longus medially and extensor pollicis brevis and abductor pollicis longus laterally. Inside the triangular snuff-box are the radial artery and dorsal cutaneous branch of the median nerve.

Mediators of Inflammation, Tissue Destruction, and Repair

Osteoarthritis and rheumatoid arthritis are the most common chronic, progressive diseases that cause pain and destruction of joints resulting in severe disability and deformity. An increasing amount of evidence points to inflammation, both local and systemic, as the cause of damage to joint and bones. Although the complete pathogenesis of arthritic joint disease has not been completely elucidated, there is general consen-sus that disruption of balance between cartilage and sub-chondral bone is caused by the presence of dysregulated mast cells [13]. Normally, there is equilibrium between bone catabolism and anabolism. This is driven and mediated by cytokines and growth factors that come from the mast cells and mediate cross talk between subchondral bone, cartilage, and synovia [13]. It has been observed that an increased number of localized activated mast cells are associated with arthritic changes in corresponding tissue. Unchecked activity of mast cell mediators can lead to reduced viscoelasticity of synovial fluid and degradation of hyaluronic acid. In addi-tion, mast cells release angiogenic mediators that lead to proliferation of new vasculature, typically seen in joint diseases. In short, excessive release of mast cell mediators, along with their proangiogenic, oxidative, and inflammatory effects, sets the stage for the classic manifestation of joint inflammation and pain [13].

Molecular and Cellular Basis of Immunity and Autoimmunity

Rheumatoid arthritis (RA) is a systemic autoimmune inflammatory disease [7]. It begins by affecting the joints through erosion of the synovial microvasculature and eventually leads to articular destruction via pannus formation. As this granulation tissue grows over cartilage, fibroblasts contained inside it invade and destroy the periarticular bone. In addition to fibroblast involvement, CD4+ T-lymphocytes are present and are involved in the inflammatory response on the synovial environment [7]. The exact cause of RA is still being investigated; however, it is known to have a genetic component. There is association of RA and major histocompatibility complex (MHC) subtypes.

Anatomy and Biomechanics of Joints and Muscles

Shoulder

The glenohumeral joint is responsible for the flexion, extension, internal and external rotation and abduction, and adduction of the arm. Normal range of motion of the shoulder joint is as follows: flexion 180°, extension 60°, abduction 180°, adduction 60°, internal rotation 90°, and external rotation 90°. There are numerous muscles that overlap in action to power and stabilize the shoulder joint.

Elbow

The elbow is functionally a hinge joint and is responsible for flexion and extension of the forearm. Pronator teres, biceps brachii, brachialis, and brachioradialis are responsible for flexion, whereas triceps and anconeus (considered by some to an extension of the triceps) perform extension. Supination and pronation occur nearby as part of the proximal radioulnar joint [14]. Supination is achieved by supinator and biceps brachii muscles. Pronator quadratus, pronator teres, and flexor carpi radialis function in pronation. Normal range of motion of the elbow joint is as follows: flexion 140°, extension 5°, supination 90°, and pronation 90°.

Hand

The wrist is able to move in flexion/extension and ulnar/radial deviation. Normal range of motion of the wrist joint is as follows: flexion 80°, extension 70°, ulnar deviation 30°, and radial deviation 20°. The thumb is able to flex, extend, adduct, abduct, oppose, and appose. Flexion is achieved by flexor pollicis brevis and longus, along with opponens pollicis and adductor pollicis. Extension is performed by extensor pollicis brevis and longus and abductor pollicis longus. The thumb has two sesamoid bones on the metacarpal bone, which serve to increase the force of muscle. Fingers move in flexion, extension, abduction, and adduction. Extension is performed by extensor digitorum communis (EDC), indicis proprius, and digiti minimi. Flexion is performed by flexor digitorum profundus (FDP), flexor digitorum superficialis (FDS), flexor digiti minimi (FDM), lumbricals and the dorsal and palmar interossei. Finger abduction and adduction is achieved by the interossei muscles.

Neurophysiology

Brachial Plexus

The brachial plexus (Fig. 33.9) originates from the roots of the spinal cord in the cervical spine at the level of C5-T1. The roots pass in between the scalene muscles in the neck and become trunks. The trunks are named based on their position and are called superior (from C5 and C6), middle (from C7), and inferior (from C8 and T1) trunks. They pass underneath the clavicle, after which point they each split into the anterior and posterior divisions. The divisions enter the axilla and become the lateral, posterior, and medial cords, which are named based on their location to the axillary artery. Distal to the axilla, the cords become the major nerve branches, radial, median, and ulnar nerves, along with the musculocutaneous and axillary nerves. Deep tendon reflexes are mediated by C5-C6 for biceps and by C6-C7 for triceps.

Psychosocial Aspects

As mentioned earlier, according to the Bureau of Labor Statistics upper extremity is the most commonly injured body part [4]. In turn, pain in the upper extremity can be a severe cause of disability. This can lead to the development of mood disorders such as anxiety and depression.

The shoulder is the most common body part where restriction of functional motion can lead to adhesive capsulitis. This

Fig. 33.9 Anatomy of brachial plexus

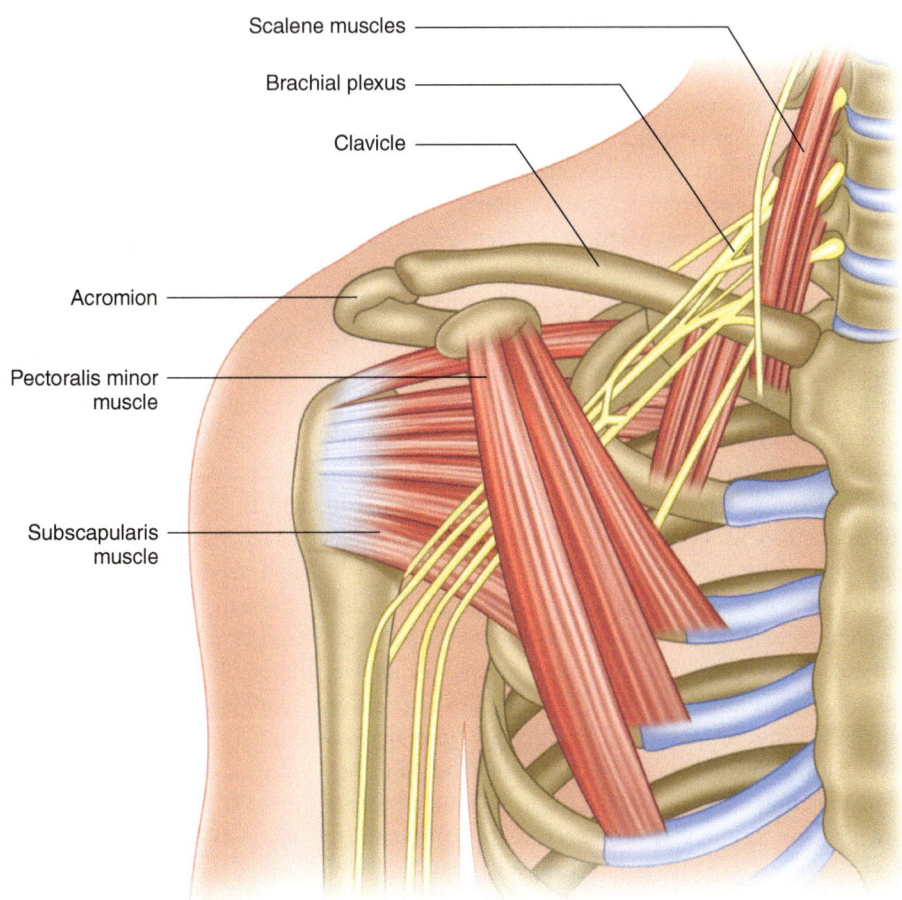

Scalene muscles

Brachial plexus

Clavicle

Acromion

Pectoralis minor muscle

Subscapularis muscle

influences activities of daily living (ADLs) and can limit job-related activities. Arthritis of the hands, whether it is inflammatory or degenerative, leads to progressive decline in function.

Each individual's experience of pain is influenced by many cognitive factors, such as beliefs surrounding pain, expectations of pain and treatment, and tendency to catastrophize the clinical situation [15]. However, whatever the person's baseline personality, upper extremity pain leads to disruption of mood and quality of life.

Classification and Clinical Characteristics of Musculoskeletal Diseases

Shoulder

Shoulder osteoarthritis presents as generalized pain inside the shoulder that is most severe with movement. It typically affects the entire joint, with loss of cartilage, bony remodeling, capsular stretching, and periarticular muscle weakness. Injury, misalignment due to muscle weakness or variation of anatomy along with advanced age and repetitive stress on the joint all lead to pain and destruction of the protective cartilage [17]. X-rays typically show irregular joint surfaces with joint space narrowing and osteophytes.

Subacromial bursitis is the inflammation of the bursa that lies deep to the deltoid muscle and the acromion. Patients report pain on the side and front of their shoulder that is worse with sleeping on the affected side with raising the arm to the side. This condition is often associated with the shoulder impingement syndrome.

Subacromial (shoulder) impingement syndrome typically affects the supraspinatus or long head of the biceps brachii tendon. Athletes who perform many overhead activities such as swimming, throwing or climbing are commonly affected by this condition. Provocative tests are Neer and Hawkins-Kennedy. During Neer's test, the examiner internally rotates the patient's fully extended arm and moves it passively through the full range of shoulder flexion. Hawkins-Kennedy test is performed with the patient's arm in front of them flexed at the elbow to 90°. The examiner rapidly internally rotates the arm by pushing it down to bring the wrist toward the floor. Any elicited pain in the anterior shoulder signifies a positive test.

Rotator cuff pathology often presents as a result of shoulder impingement syndrome. Pain is similarly reported in the anterior and lateral parts of the shoulder but is also associated with stiffness, weakness, and catching. Although macrotrauma can cause rotator cuff injuries, repetitive microtrauma and outlet impingement between the acromion and greater tuberosity of the humerus are more common [18]. With time patients develop chronic tendinopathy that can progress to tendon cuff tears [7]. Neer classified subacromial impingement syndrome into three stages. Stage 1 with edema and hemorrhage is considered to be reversible and occurs due to overuse in patients younger than 25 years old. Stage 2 is marked with fibrosis and tendonitis and affects patients between 25 and 40 years old. Stage 3 is found in patients older than 50 and is associated with acromioclavicular spurs and rotator cuff tears.

Rotator cuff tears can present as a sudden pain in the anterolateral shoulder or a dull achy sensation with loss or limited abduction of the arm. Over time, atrophy of the lateral shoulder muscles may develop. In addition to positive impingement tests, the empty can and drop arm tests may be positive. During the empty can test, the arm is held in front of the patient with the thumb pointed down. Pain and weakness in the arm signifies a positive test. If the examiner applies a down force and the patient drops their arm or is not able to maintain it in abduction and internal rotation, it is a positive drop arm test and indicates a complete tear of the cuff [7]. Radiographic imaging often shows cystic changes in the greater tuberosity of the humerus in impingement and flattening of the greater tuberosity in chronic tears. MRI is the gold standard and will show full or partial thickness tares [7].

Glenohumeral joint (GHJ) instability can be a cause of pain in the shoulder and can be classified as dislocation, subluxation or micro-instability [18]. Instability leads to increased motion of the humeral head in relation to the glenoid capsule and can result in dislocation or subluxation. During subluxation, there is incomplete separation of the humeral head from the glenoid fossa followed by immediate reduction. A dislocation, however, results in the shoulder being displaced from the socket. It requires manual or surgical correction. GHJ instability can be anterior (most common is anterior inferior) with the arm moving in direction of abduction and external rotation. This is typically found in young athletes and has a high risk of recurrence. The axillary nerve can be injured if the shoulder is dislocated completely [7]. Posterior GHJ instability is less common. Patients present with their arm in the adducted internally rotated position [7].

Glenoid labral tear is a painful condition caused by repetitive overhead sports activity or trauma. A common type is

the SLAP lesion: superior labral tear from anterior to posterior direction and is associated with pain, clicking and instability of the shoulder with overhead arm movement. O'Brien's test is used to screen for SLAP lesions and consists of two parts. Patient starts out with both arms outstretched in front with 90° shoulder flexion and pronation. Both arms are pushed downward. The second position is with the patient's arm in supination. If the same force is applied down and the pain is improved, the test is considered to be positive. However, the sensitivity and specificity of this test are highly variable, so imaging is typically necessary to make an accurate diagnosis.

Tendonitis is a common cause of pain in the shoulder due to tendon overuse. The two tendons that are typically affected are the supraspinatus and the long head of the biceps brachii. In the case of the supraspinatus tendonitis, patients report sharp pain with ROM, particularly with shoulder abduction and overhead activities [7]. This condition may be caused by calcium deposits with resultant irritation of the tendon and subsequent fusion of the synovial capsule with the shoulder bursa. In the case of the long head of biceps brachii tendon tendonitis, there is point tenderness in the bicipital groove and signs of impingement [7]. Provocative testing includes Yergason's test, shoulder pain with resisted supination of the wrist with the elbow fixed at 90°, and Speed's test – shoulder pain with resisted flexion of the shoulder against a supinated arm. Chronicity of this condition and age >40 are associated with biceps tendon rupture. A characteristic feature on the physical exam is the "Popeye sign," which is a "balling" of the biceps with contraction.

Adhesive capsulitis (AC), also known as "frozen shoulder," is both a standalone diagnosis (primary) and a sign of shoulder pathology (secondary). Most commonly it is secondary to an underlying shoulder problem, and other etiologies must be uncovered for successful treatment. It presents as painful active or passive motion of the shoulder. Because the shoulder joint is the most mobile large joint in the body, it depends heavily on the motion in all planes to deliver lubrication and nourishment to all parts of the joint capsule. Any limitation of this motion, either due to pain or injury will lead to a decreasing range of motion of the joint due the capsule thickening and tightening. There are three stages of AC: Stage 1 during initial inflammation and decreased ROM, lasting 3–9 months; Stage 2 with plateau of capsular pain and fibrosis of the capsule, lasting 4–12 months; and Stage 3 thawing stage with gradual return of ROM and decreased pain, lasting 12–42 months [5].

Acromioclavicular pain, although not as common as other conditions of the shoulder, must still be ruled out for a complete shoulder assessment. Patients generally complain of tenderness over the AC joint with palpation and ROM [7]. Pain can be due to arthritis, overuse or fall and sprain injuries. There are six types of AC joint sprains according to the

Rockwood classification [18]. They are graded based on the type of ligament involvement and clavicle displacement. Acromioclavicular joint separation occurs with type 4 and above grading. Provocative testing for AC joint pain is the Cross-chest test – AC joint pain with passive adduction of the arm across the midline of the chest is a positive test.

Sternoclavicular (SC) pathology is uncommon, with SC joint dislocation accounting for less than 1% of all joint dislocations [18]. However, it must be considered in a patient who presents with pain in the SC joint. Dislocations can either be anterior or posterior.

Parsonage-Turner syndrome is an uncommon neurological disorder characterized by rapid onset of severe pain in the shoulder and arm [19]. The cause is not musculoskeletal, but likely immune-mediated (exact causes are not yet known); however, it mimics many other types of shoulder pathologies. There is an acute phase with sudden onset of symptoms. After onset, however, symptoms are variable in the affected individuals: some have complete resolution of symptoms and others have recurrent episodes, yet others reach a chronic pain state of the shoulder. Weakness of the shoulder and arm muscles can also be present and if it persists can lead to atrophy.

Elbow

Medial epicondylitis is pain in the medial side of the elbow and is commonly known as golfer or pitcher's elbow. The cause is degenerative changes of the common flexor tendons, most frequently pronator teres and flexor carpi radialis (FCR) at the elbow due to valgus stress from repetitive activity [18]. On exam, there is tenderness around the medial epicondyle, over the tendon attachment sites. X-rays can reveal punctate calcifications in the regions of the flexor tendon origins [18].

Lateral epicondylitis is pain in the lateral side of the elbow and is commonly known as tennis elbow. It is exacerbated by activities that require repetitive wrist extension and forearm supination and is commonly due to overuse and poor sport technique [7]. In lateral epicondylitis, the origins of extensor carpi radialis brevis and extensor digitorum communis are affected. There is tenderness distal to the lateral epicondyle extensor origin and pain and weakness in grip strength [7]. Cozen's test is a positive indicator of the condition: pain in the lateral epicondyle with pronation and extension of the wrist against the examiner's resistance.

Olecranon bursitis is pain and swelling of the elbow due to olecranon bursa inflammation (Fig. 33.10). There are multiple etiologies, from overuse to trauma to inflammatory disorders. Infection must be ruled out if the joint appears inflamed.

Distal biceps tendonitis is not very common, but results from the overload of the tendon due to repetitive activity.

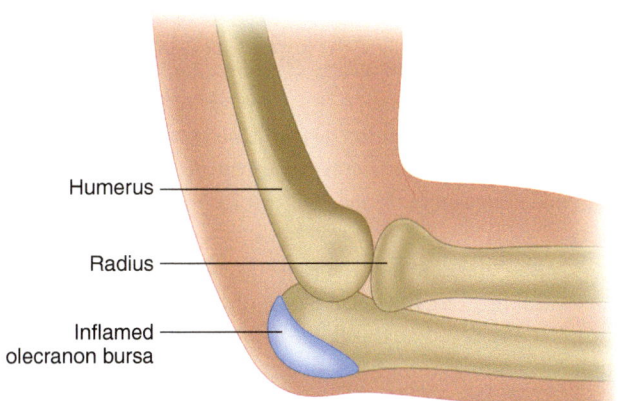

Fig. 33.10 Olecranon bursitis

Patients report antecubital fossa pain during repetitive bending activities and the follow-through phase of throwing [18]. Chronicity of the condition leads to microtearing of the distal biceps tendon and can eventually cause rupture.

Distal triceps tendonitis presents as pain at the back of the elbow with extension activities. Throwing, weight lifting and using a hammer can lead to inflammation of the tendon due to overuse [18]. Falling onto an outstretched hand or receiving a direct blow to the distal triceps brachii tendon can lead to a rupture or avulsion from the olecranon attachment site.

Collateral ligament strain can be due to medial (ulnar) (MCL) or lateral (radial) collateral ligament (LCL) sprain. LCL sprain occurs typically after elbow dislocation or a traumatic event. Patient presents with pain on the radial side and laxity during varus stress testing. MCL sprain results from repetitive microtrauma and/or a sudden throwing injury. Patients report pain over the antecubital fossa and the ulnar side of the elbow. MCL sprain typically present similarly to valgus extension overload of the elbow (VEO – see below) [7, 18].

Valgus extension overload of the elbow (VEO) is one of the most common disorders in overhead-throwing athletes. Patients complain of posterior elbow pain with locking during elbow extension and pain at the end range of ball throwing. The cause is olecranon osteophytes and loose bodies due to repetitive impingement of the posteromedial olecranon against the medial wall of the olecranon fossa [7, 18]. During the VEO test, the physician flexes the elbow to 30° and repetitively extends the elbow fully while applying a valgus stress test [7]. Pain at the end range of extension is significant for a positive VEO test.

Osteochondrosis of the capitellum, also known as Panner's disease, is a spontaneous necrosis and then regeneration and calcification of the entire capitellum (radial side of the humerus). It is typically observed in children between 7 and 10 years old and is frequently preceded by trauma or vascular impairment. Patients complain of dull achy pain and effusion in the radial side of the elbow that is relieved with rest [7, 18].

Osteochondritis dissecans of the capitellum differs from osteochondrosis in that it is observed in children 9 to 15 years old. This condition also affects the capitellum in a patchy distribution. Patients complain of pain, elbow locking, and contracture. It does not resolve like osteochondrosis does.

Cubital tunnel syndrome presents as pain with numbness and tingling along the ulnar aspect of the forearm with radiation into the fourth and fifth digits. It is caused by any irritation or compression of the ulnar nerve at the elbow [7, 18]. On exam, one might observe weakness of grip strength, muscle atrophy, and positive Tinel's sign at the elbow.

Hand

Flexor carpi tendonitis presents as pain in the wrist. Either the ulnar (FCU) or radial (FCR) flexor carpi tendons can be affected, leading to pain with wrist flexion and ulnar or radial deviation, respectively. This condition, just like any other tendonitis, is associated with overuse and microtrauma.

De Quervain's tenosynovitis (radial styloid tenosynovitis) is the most common tendonitis of the wrist and is typically seen in patients who perform frequent forceful gripping with ulnar deviation of the wrist or repetitive use of the thumb [18]. There is inflammation of abductor pollicis longus and extensor pollicis brevis tendons. Patients complain of pain on the radial side of the wrist. Finkelstein's test is pathognomonic for De Quervain's tenosynovitis [7, 18].

Ganglion cysts (e.g., "Bible cyst") can cause pain due to pressure exerted from collection of synovial fluid in the joint space. These typically occur on the dorsal surface of the wrist.

Kienbock's disease (osteonecrosis of the lunate) presents with pain and stiffness on the dorsal-ulnar side [7, 18]. On exam, there is tenderness over the lunate and decreased wrist ROM. This condition develops due to vascular compromise of the lunate, typically from repeated trauma. It leads to avascular necrosis with eventual collapse of the lunate [7, 18].

Triangular fibrocartilage complex (TFCC) injuries are characterized by pain over the ulnar side of the wrist that gets worse with movement of the wrist from side to side. It can result from falling on an outstretched hand or from overuse and degeneration.

Carpal tunnel syndrome is characterized by pain, numbness, and tingling in the first three digits and half of the fourth digit. Nighttime symptoms are frequently reported by patients due to the compression of the carpal tunnel from sleeping with the wrist bent. With time, weakness and atrophy may develop.

Trigger finger (stenosing tenosynovitis) is characterized by a catch of a digit in a flexed position and subsequent painful snap in extension. This is usually due to a painful nodule in the tendon. It is associated with repetitive trauma, diabetes, rheumatoid arthritis and gout [7].

Assessment of Activity and Severity of Rheumatic Disease

In 2010, the American College of Rheumatology and European League Against Rheumatism (ACR/EULAR) generated criteria for early diagnosis and classification of rheumatoid arthritis (RA), updating the 1987 criteria. The classification criteria for RA makes the diagnosis dependent on the score of certain factors, with the score greater than or equal to 6/10 being positive for RA. The factors that are assessed are joint involvement, serology, acute-phase reactants, and duration of symptoms [16]. Figure 33.11 depicts

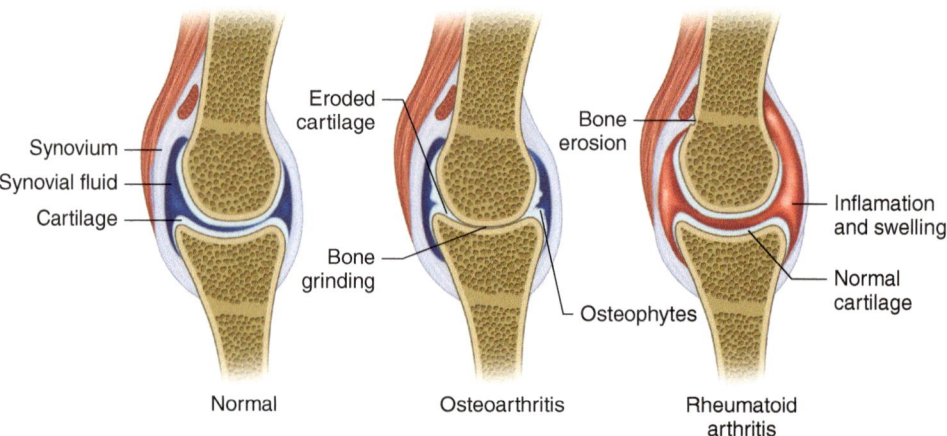

Fig. 33.11 Pathophysiologic changes in osteoarthritis and rheumatoid arthritis

Synovium
Synovial fluid
Cartilage

Eroded cartilage
Bone grinding

Bone erosion
Osteophytes

Inflamation and swelling
Normal cartilage

Normal   Osteoarthritis   Rheumatoid arthritis

pathophysiologic changes found in osteoarthritis and rheumatoid arthritis.

Treatment and Rehabilitation of Musculoskeletal Pain/Disability

Just like for any disease process, evaluation and proper diagnosis of the upper extremity is important in order to devise proper treatment and rehabilitation strategies. Although musculoskeletal causes of pain are the typical cause, other etiologies must be considered and ruled out before proceeding with treatment strategies. Cervical radiculopathy, brachial plexopathy, cancer, and infection should always be on the differential for causes of pain.

Lifestyle choices, the ability to comply with ongoing exercises, and social support systems all have a major impact on the outcome of treatment for musculoskeletal pain problems [17]. Therefore, treatment will depend on etiology, age, occupation, lifestyle and specific goals of the person. Patients who are suffering from pain will develop a muscle imbalance as they try to compensate and avoid irritating the painful area. This leads to a restricted range of motion (ROM) of the limb that must be addressed in order to prevent functional limitations in the future [18].

The goal of any pain treatment is to alleviate pain in order to improve quality of life. If possible, it is also important to resolve the underlying issue causing the pain, thereby preventing recurrence of the pain in the future. For acute injuries the general mantra has always been RICE – rest, ice, compression, and elevation. However, often by the time the patient is seen by a pain physician, the pain is a long-standing, chronic condition. Physical and occupational therapy are beneficial for all patients as long as the proper precautions are observed. Typical therapy techniques are muscle strengthening and stretching, passive and active ROM, modalities, ultrasound and transcutaneous electrical nerve stimulation (TENS). If the patient does not respond adequately to therapy, injections with a steroid and a local anesthetic can be performed into the joint or the area of the tender muscle or irritated nerve. These injections can be therapeutic for pain control and for facilitation of therapy. Various types of medications can be used to control pain. In chronic, advanced cases of osteoarthritis, as well as soft tissue pathologies, injections with hyaluronic acid products, platelet-rich plasma (PRP), and stem cells have been used with mixed long-term results. Splinting can be performed in some cases of pain such as carpal tunnel syndrome. Bracing and casting has been used for fractures and tendon injuries. Diagnostic peripheral nerve blocks, followed by radio-frequency nerve ablation, have been gaining momentum and popularity for longer and more precise pain control. Peripheral nerve stimulation with implantable devices has received FDA approval for post-stroke shoulder pain and is being trialed and performed on various other chronic pain syndromes. Finally, surgery can be performed and is sometimes curative for chronic, long-standing musculoskeletal pain. Whatever the method of chosen treatment, benefits and risks must be weighted and discussed with the patient in order to achieve proper goals of care and pain control.

References

1. Weinstein SI, Yelin EH, Watkins-Castillo SI. The big picture. 2014. Retrieved 10 Aug 2017, from http://www.boneandjointburden.org/2014-report/i0/big-picture.
2. United States Department of Labor. n.d. Retrieved 10 Aug 2017, from https://www.osha.gov/SLTC/ergonomics.
3. Prevalence Statistics. n.d. Retrieved 10 Aug 2017, from https://www.rheumatology.org/Learning-Center/Statistics/Prevalence-Statistics.
4. Type of injury or illness and body parts affected by nonfatal injuries and illnesses in 2014: The Economics Daily. (2015, December 2). Retrieved 10 Aug 2017, from https://www.bls.gov/opub/ted/2015/type-of-injury-or-illness-and-body-parts-affected-by-nonfatal-injuries-and-illnesses-in-2014.htm.
5. Holmes RE, Barfield WR, Woolf SK. Clinical evaluation of non-arthritic shoulder pain: diagnosis and treatment. Phys Sportsmed. 2015;43(3):262–8.
6. Kendall FP. Muscles: testing and function with posture and pain. Baltimore: Lippincott Williams & Wilkins; 2010. Print.
7. Cuccurullo S, Lee J. Physical medicine and rehabilitation board review. New York: Demos Medical; 2015. Print.
8. Shultz T, De Dobbeleer M. Acromioclavicular Joint. n.d. Retrieved 10 Aug 2017, from http://www.physio-pedia.com/Acromioclavicular_Joint.
9. Gaillard F, Bickle I. Elbow | Radiology reference article. n.d. Retrieved 10 Aug 2017, from https://radiopaedia.org/articles/elbow.
10. Goel A, Weerakkody Y. Carrying angle | radiology reference article. n.d. Retrieved 10 Aug 2017, from https://radiopaedia.org/articles/carrying-angle.
11. Jones O. 2017, March 27. The Radioulnar Joints. Retrieved 10 Aug 2017, from http://teachmeanatomy.info/upper-limb/joints/radioulnar-joints.
12. Jones O. 2017, April 15. The Wrist Joint. Retrieved 10 Aug 2017, from http://teachmeanatomy.info/upper-limb/joints/wrist-joint.
13. Fusco M, Skaper SD, Coaccioli S, Varrassi G, Paladini A. Degenerative joint diseases and neuroinflammation. Pain Pract. 2017;17(4):522–32.
14. Jones O. 2017, April 15. The Elbow Joint. Retrieved 10 Aug 2017, from http://teachmeanatomy.info/upper-limb/joints/elbow-joint.
15. Gatchel RJ, Schultz IZ, editors. Handbook of musculoskeletal pain and disability disorders in the workplace. New York: Springer-Verlag; 2014.
16. Aletaha D, Neogi T, Silman AJ, et al. 2010 rheumatoid arthritis classification criteria: an American College of Rheumatology/European League Against Rheumatism collaborative initiative. Arthritis Rheum. 2010;62(9):2569–81.
17. Barr KP. Review of upper and lower extremity musculoskeletal pain problems. Phys Med Rehabil Clin N Am. 2007;18(4):747–60, vi-vii.
18. Braddom RL, Chan L, Harrast MA. Physical medicine and rehabilitation. Philadelphia: Saunders/Elsevier; 2011. Print.
19. Parsonage Turner Syndrome. n.d. Retrieved 10 Aug 2017, from https://rarediseases.org/rare-diseases/parsonage-turner-syndrome.

Musculoskeletal Joint Pain: Lower Extremities

34

Paul K. Cheng and Magdalena Anitescu

Epidemiology

Musculoskeletal pain including lower extremity joint pain is extremely common and far-reaching. Musculoskeletal diseases affect more than 50% of people in the United States older than 18 years and 75% for those 65 and older [1]. In 2005, osteoarthritis, the most common joint pain disease, was estimated to affect 26.9 million in the United States [1]. It continues to be the leading cause of disability, lost work days, and impaired quality of life in the United States [2]. The cost of treating musculoskeletal diseases, including cost associated with pain treatment and disability, is greater than treatment for any other common health condition [1]. Per the Medical Expenditure Panel Survey for the 2 years, from 2009 to 2011, the Medical Expenditure Panel Survey showed that treatment of musculoskeletal disease costs a total of $796.3 billion [1].

Lower extremity joint pain makes up a large portion of musculoskeletal pain conditions. Foot and ankle pain alone affect between 15% and 24% of Americans older than 45 years of age, and osteoarthritis of the ankle affects 10% of people over 65 years old [3–6]. Lower extremity injuries account for 7% of all nonfatal injuries causing time away from work [7]. Lower extremity joint pain, more prevalent in older people, can affect the young, particularly athletes [8].

Anatomy and Physiology

Hip

The hip, a large ball and socket joint at the union of the femur and the pelvis (Fig. 34.1), is made up of a series of

P. K. Cheng
Departments of Pain Management and Neurosciences, Cleveland Clinic, Cleveland, OH, USA

M. Anitescu (✉)
Department of Anesthesia and Critical Care, University of Chicago Medicine, Chicago, IL, USA
e-mail: manitescu@dacc.uchicago.edu

ligaments (e.g., pubofemoral, iliofemoral, and ischiofemoral) that connect the ball-like femoral head to the socket-like acetabulum [7]. Their names correspond to the portion of the pelvis to which they attach. The ligaments form the joint capsule of the hip (Fig. 34.2). Linking the pelvis and the sacrum are three ligaments, starting with the most rostral sacroiliac ligament and then the sacrospinous ligament and finally the sacrotuberous ligament. Key portions of the skeleton act as external landmarks for various pain procedures including the elephant ear-like iliac crest, the anterior and posterior superior iliac spines, and the greater trochanter of the femur. The head and tip of the femur have different blood supplies: the tip is supplied by the obturator artery and the neck and body are supplied by the medial circumflex femoral artery (Fig. 34.2)

Knee

The knee (Fig. 34.3), considered a hinge joint, is found at the union of the femur to the tibia and fibula. Providing a cartilaginous structure inside the joint space are the semilunar medial and lateral menisci. There are four main ligaments of the knee, and the strength of each can be tested with special physical maneuvers.

- The anterior cruciate ligament (ACL) connects the lateral femoral condyle to the anterior horn of the medial meniscus. One test for an ACL tear is Lachman's test. With the knee flexed at 20 degrees, the lower leg is pulled forward while the thigh is stabilized and anterior translation is observed. In anterior drawer test, the knee is flexed at 90 degrees, the lower leg is pulled forward while stabilizing the foot, to see how far the tibial plateau translates anteriorly [9].
- The posterior cruciate ligament (PCL) connects the medial femoral condyle to the posterior aspect of the tibia. The main special test for the PCL is the posterior drawer test. With the knee flexed at 90 degrees, the lower leg is pushed posteriorly while the thigh is stabilized,

Fig. 34.1 Hip joint with ligaments – bony and ligamentous structure of the right hip, lateral view

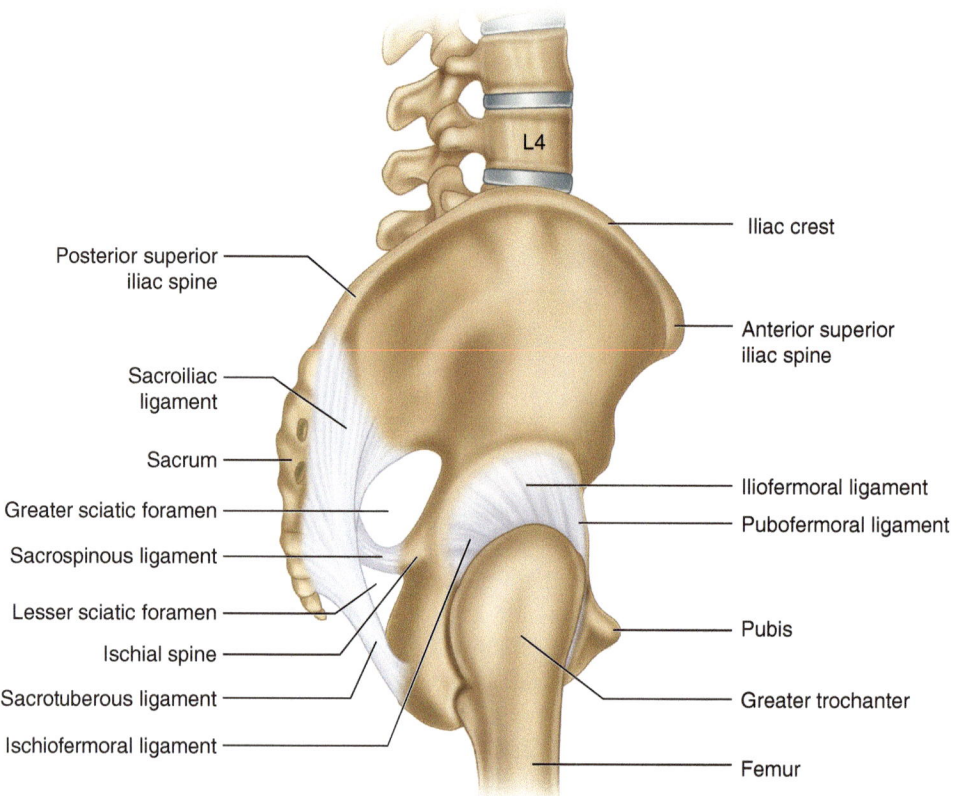

Iliac crest

Posterior superior iliac spine

Anterior superior iliac spine

Sacroiliac ligament

Sacrum

Iliofemoral ligament

Greater sciatic foramen

Pubofemoral ligament

Sacrospinous ligament

Lesser sciatic foramen

Ischial spine

Pubis

Sacrotuberous ligament

Greater trochanter

Ischiofemoral ligament

Femur

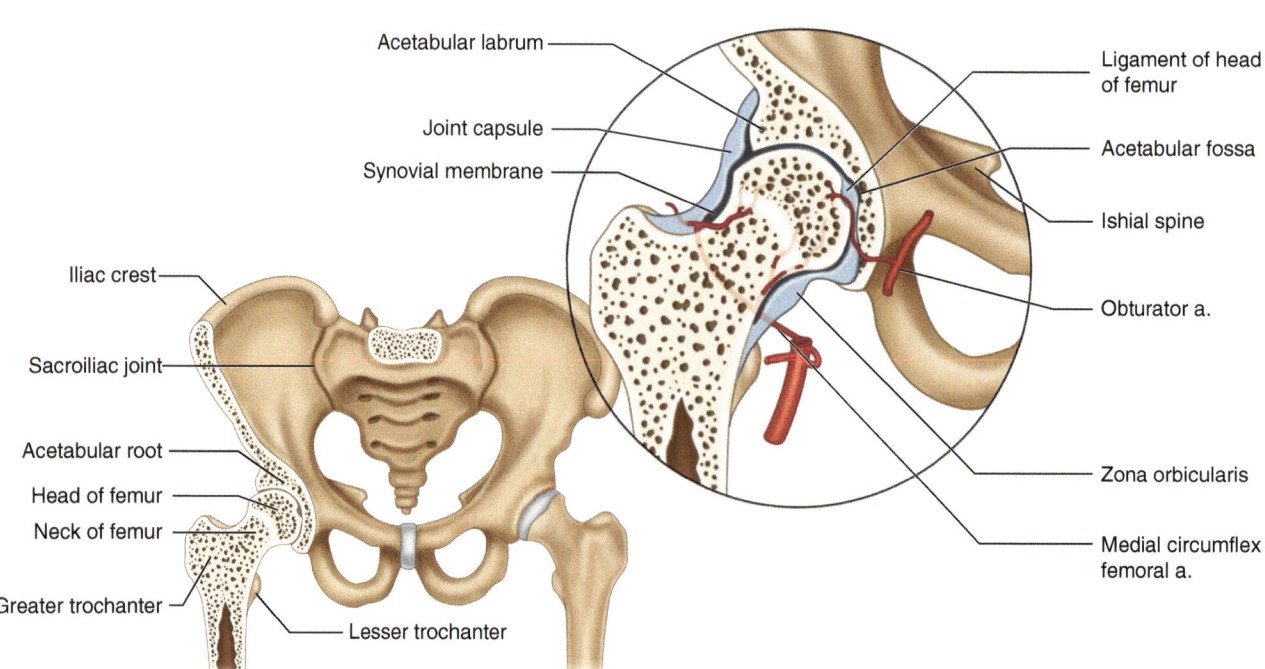

Acetabular labrum

Ligament of head of femur

Joint capsule

Acetabular fossa

Synovial membrane

Ishial spine

Iliac crest

Obturator a.

Sacroiliac joint

Acetabular root

Head of femur

Neck of femur

Zona orbicularis

Greater trochanter

Medial circumflex femoral a.

Lesser trochanter

Fig. 34.2 Hip cross-section and vascular supply – coronal cross-section of the right hip showing the joint as well as the key vascular supply of the neck and head of the femur

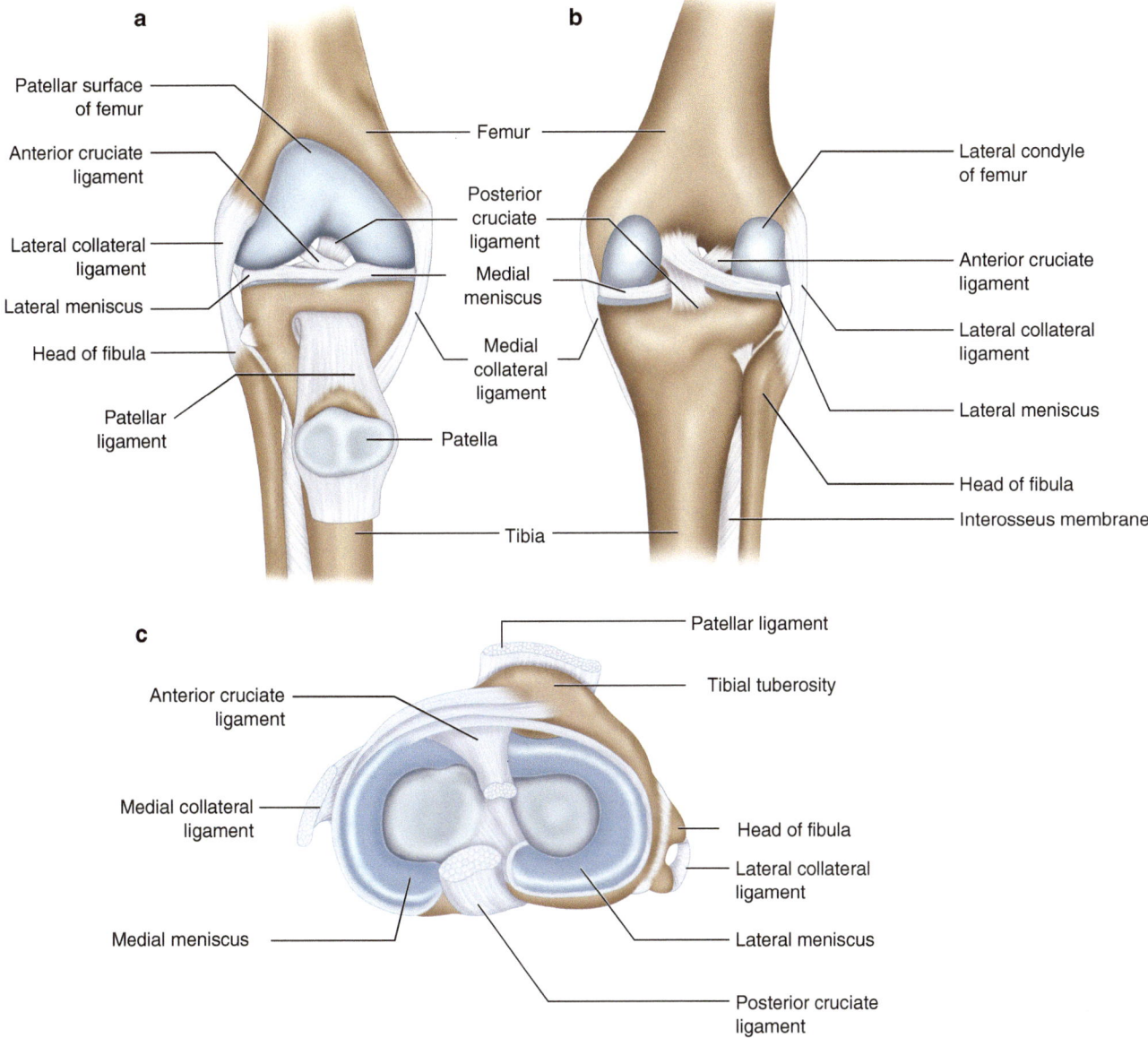

Fig. 34.3 Knee joint with ligaments. (**a**) Bony and ligamentous structure of the anterior knee, patella is reflected inferiorly. (**b**) Bony and ligamentous structure of the posterior knee. (**c**) Superior view of the knee showing inter-articular surface of the tibial head and the menisci

and the degree of posterior translation of the tibial plateau is evaluated.

- The medial collateral ligament (MCL) connects the medial femoral condyle to the medial aspect of the tibia. In testing, a valgus stress is applied to the knee in full extension and 30 degrees of flexion to evaluate for resultant movement or pain.
- The lateral collateral ligament (LCL) connects the lateral femoral condyle to the head of the fibula. In testing, a varus stress is applied to the knee in full extension and 30 degrees of flexion to evaluate for resultant movement or pain.

Along the anterior aspect of the knee lies the patella bone strapped rostrally by the quadriceps tendon and caudally by the patellar tendon where the patellar reflex can be elicited.

Ankle

The ankle (Fig. 34.4) is bound medially by a large deltoid ligament with four individual parts that connect the bones of the foot to the tibia and laterally by three key ligaments, the anterior talofibular ligament (ATFL), the pos-

Fig. 34.4 Ankle joint with ligaments – bony and ligamentous structure of the medial (**a**) and lateral (**b**) ankle

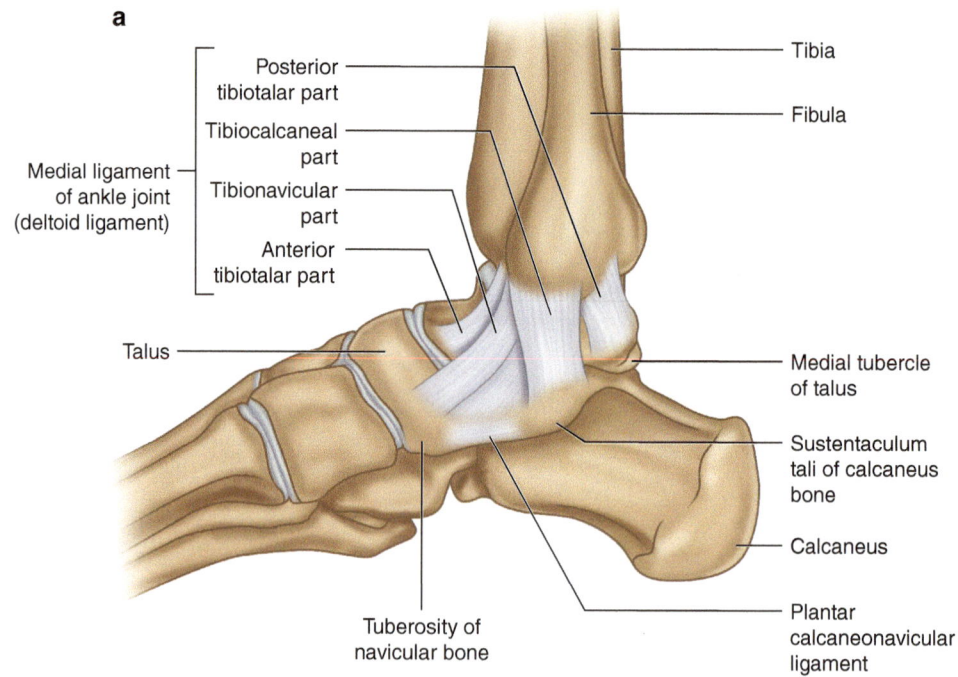

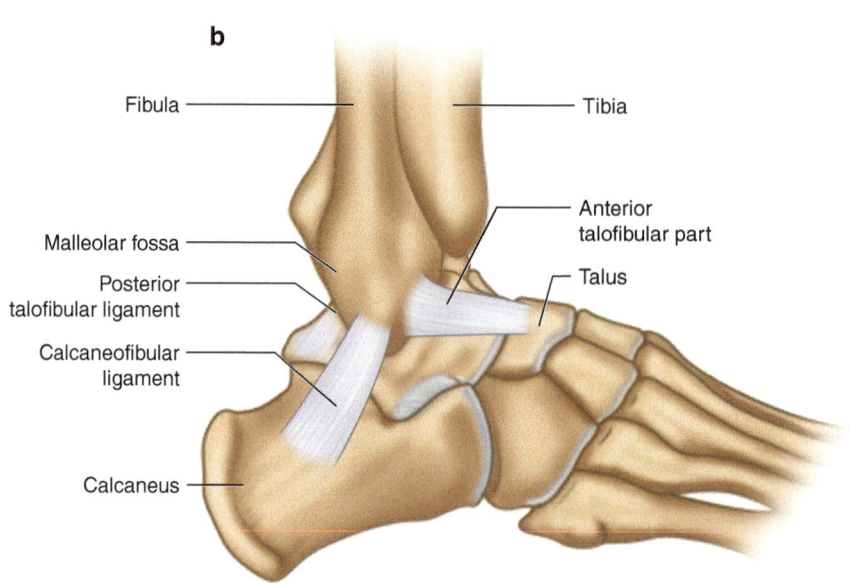

terior talofibular ligament (PTFL), and the calcaneofibular ligament. With eversion maneuvers the strength of the deltoid ligament is tested; with inversion maneuvers the calcaneofibular ligament is tested. Anterior drawer testing (by moving the foot anteriorly while stabilizing the leg) tests the ATFL, while posterior drawer testing (moving the foot posteriorly while stabilizing the leg) tests the PTFL.

Femoral Triangle

The femoral triangle (Fig. 34.5), located immediately below the inguinal line, is a key site for various procedures including a femoral nerve block and arterial/venous cannulation. The borders of the triangle are formed by the inguinal ligament, sartorius muscle, and the adductor longus muscle. The femoral vein is most medial, the femoral nerve is most lat-

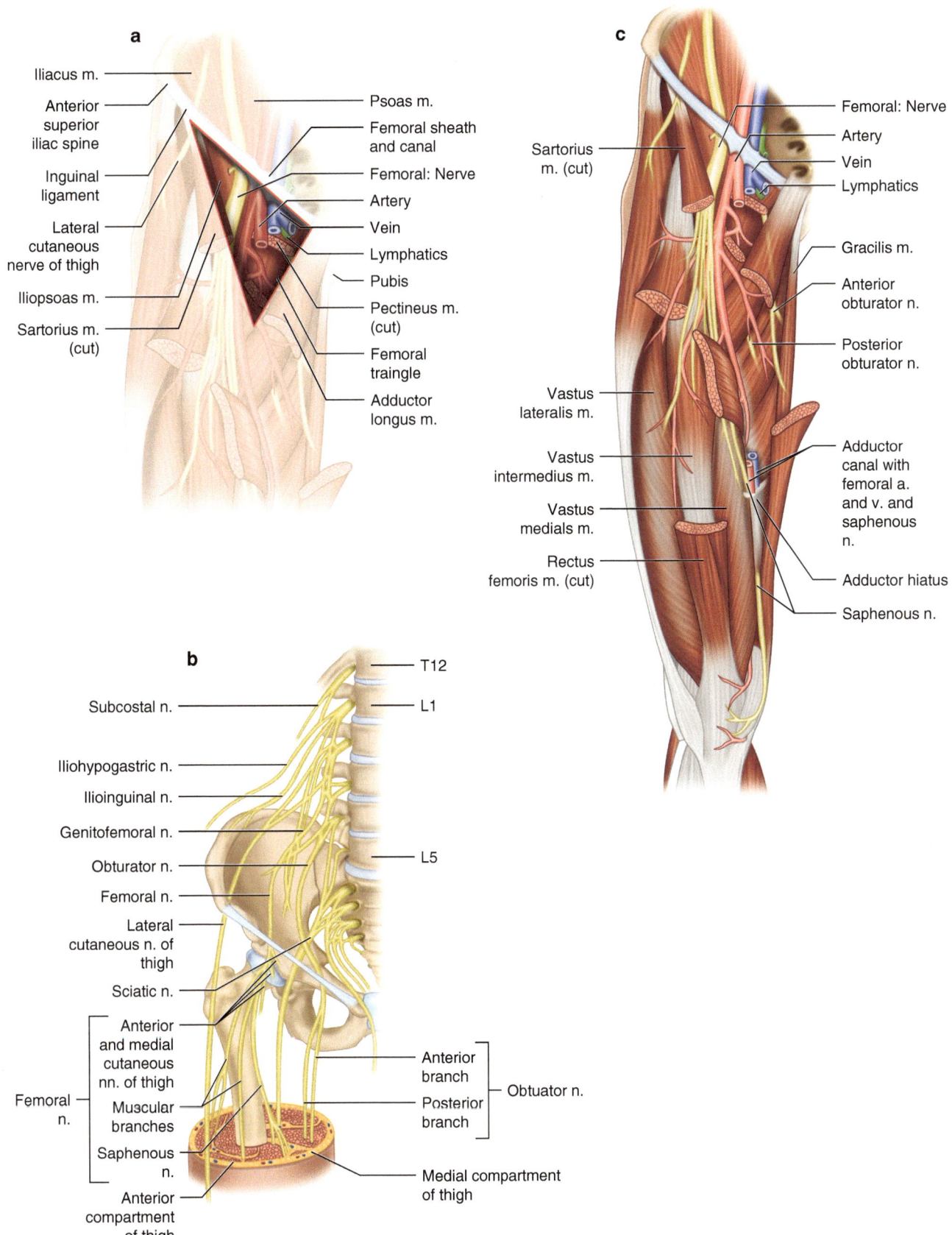

Fig. 34.5 Femoral triangle. (**a**) Femoral triangle of the right hip, (**b**) innervation of the thigh coming from the spinal roots, (**c**) neurovascular supply located in the femoral triangle

eral, and the femoral artery runs between the vein and nerve. A common mnemonic to remember the anatomic relationship is NAVeL, which describes the lateral to medial sequence of nerve-artery-vein-lymphatics.

Vascular Supply

The arterial supply of the lower extremity (Fig. 34.6) originates from the common iliac artery, which bifurcates into the internal and external iliac in the pelvis. The external iliac becomes the femoral artery at the inguinal line, the popliteal artery near the knee, and finally bifurcating into the anterior and posterior tibial arteries at the proximal tibia. The venous supply consists of two large veins into which multiple smaller veins drain. The great saphenous vein runs along most of the lower leg and thigh and becomes the femoral vein in the superior portion of the thigh.

Bursae

Throughout the lower extremity are bursae, fluid-filled sacs that pad areas of friction. Many bursae are located near the lower extremity joints, and inflammation of the bursae can cause pain.

Anatomy and Biomechanics of Joints and Muscles

Hip

As a ball-and-socket joint, the hip joint has the most planes of movement of all the lower extremity joints. It can flex, extend, rotate internally or externally, adduct, and abduct (Fig. 34.7). Flexion of the hip is enabled by the iliopsoas group (psoas major and iliacus), the sartorius, and rectus

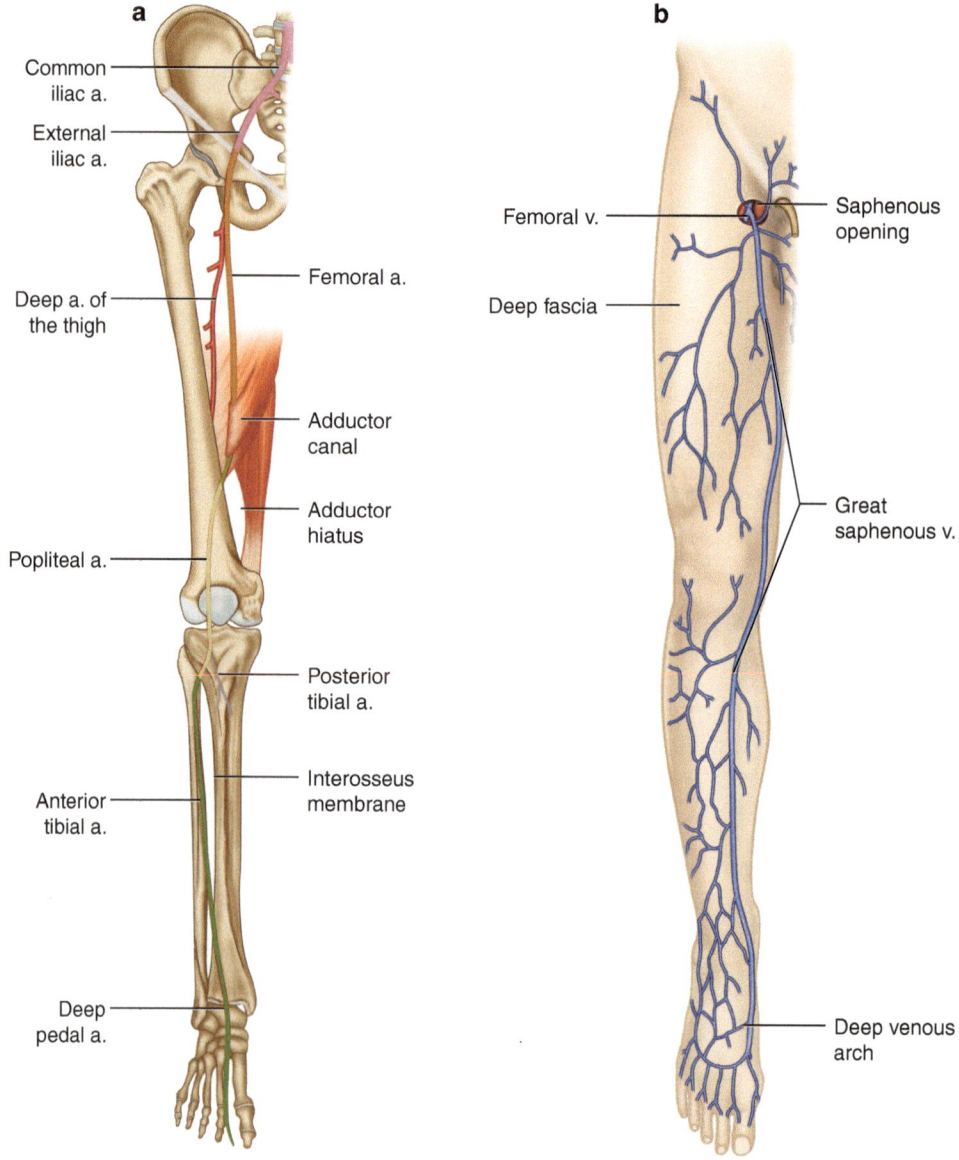

Fig. 34.6 Vascular supply to lower extremity. (**a**) Key arterial structures of the lower extremity. (**b**) Key superficial veins of the lower extremity

a

- Common iliac a.
- External iliac a.
- Deep a. of the thigh
- Femoral a.
- Adductor canal
- Adductor hiatus
- Popliteal a.
- Posterior tibial a.
- Interosseus membrane
- Anterior tibial a.
- Deep pedal a.

b

- Femoral v.
- Deep fascia
- Saphenous opening
- Great saphenous v.
- Deep venous arch

femoris (Fig. 34.5). Extension is performed by the large gluteus maximus with assistance from the hamstring group (e.g., semitendinosus, semimembranosus, biceps femoris).

Adduction is performed by the hip adductors (e.g., adductor brevis/longus/magnus, pectineus, and gracilis). Abduction of the hip is mediated by the gluteus minimus and medius, piriformis, obturator internus, and tensor fascia latae. Internal and external rotation is accomplished by many of the muscles scattered throughout the hip joint. The iliotibial band runs along the lateral aspect of the thigh and is a fibrous reinforcement of the fascia lata to which many of the hip muscles attach.

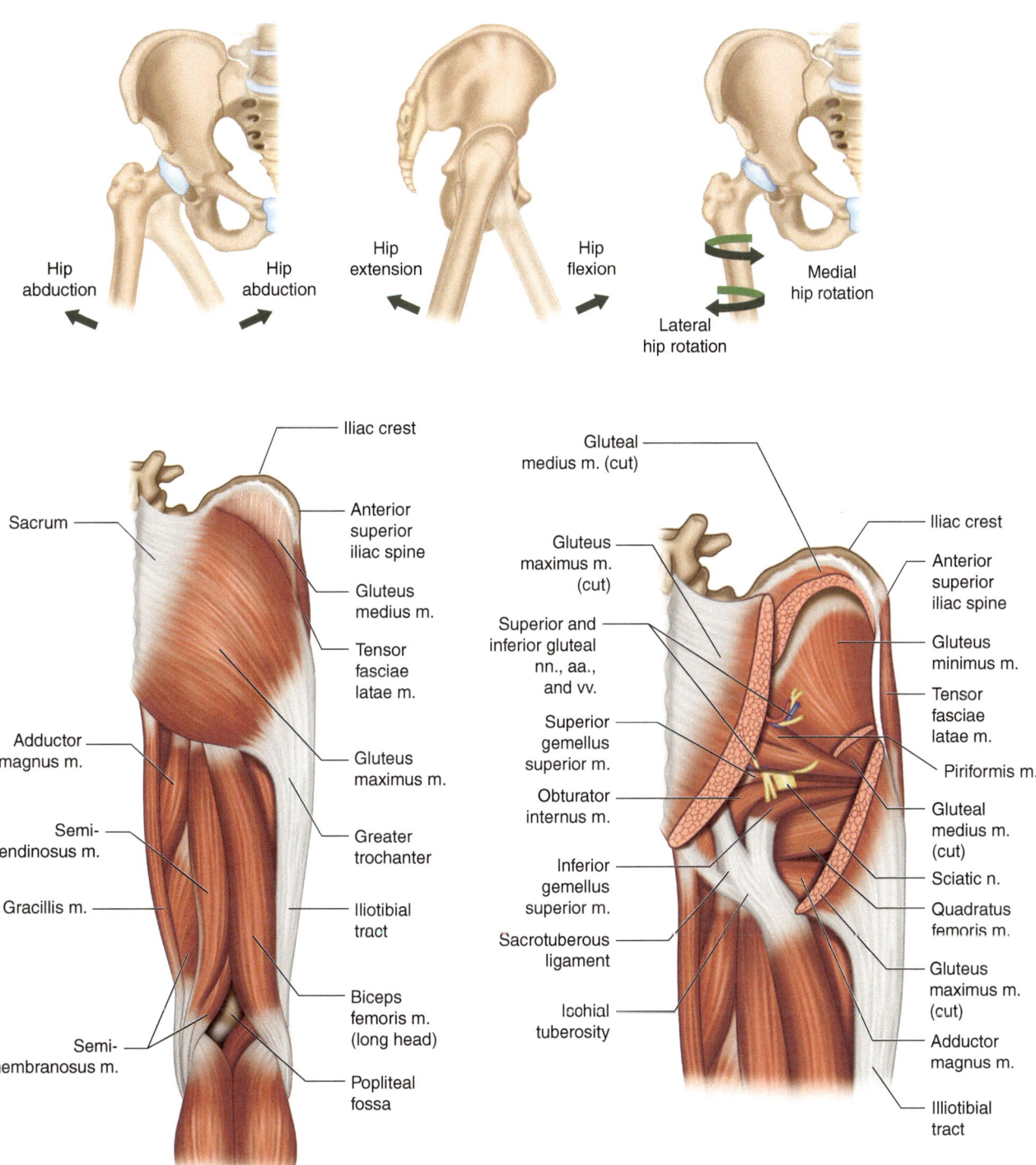

Fig. 34.7 Musculature surrounding hip. (**a**) Ranges of motion of the hip joint. (**b**) Posterior view of the hip and thigh musculature including the superficial gluteal muscle groups. (**c**) Deep gluteal muscle groups

Knee and Ankle

The knee is considered a modified hinge joint that can perform flexion and extension while maintaining stability under a large load of weight [7]. Muscles used in knee flexion are the three hamstring muscles (e.g., semitendinosus, semimembranosus, and biceps femoris), as well as the gracilis and sartorius (Figs. 34.7 and 34.8). The quadriceps group extends the knee and consists of four muscles: vastus medialis, intermedius, lateralis, and the rectus femoris (Fig. 34.5).

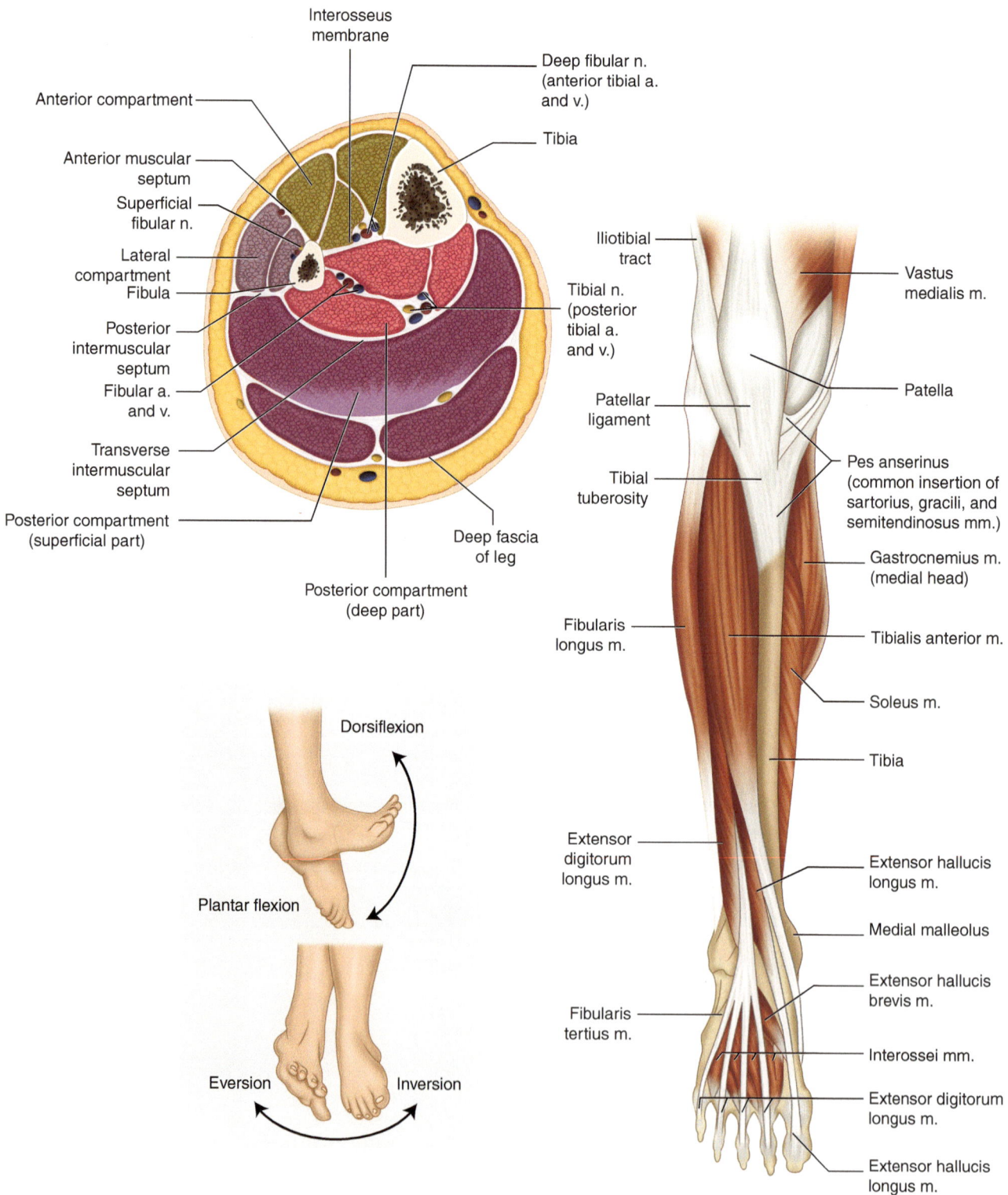

Fig. 34.8 Musculature of posterior leg (superficial) – posterior view of the musculature of the lower leg and ankle

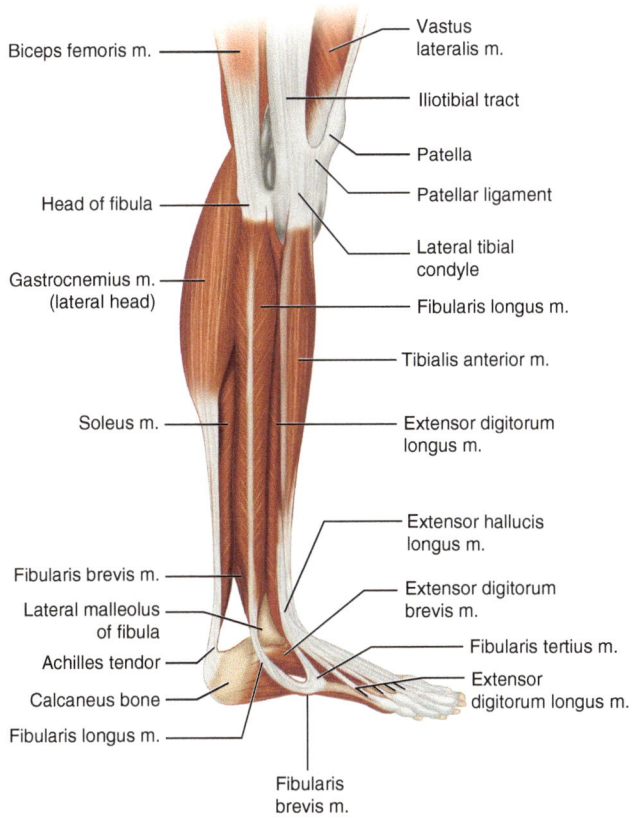

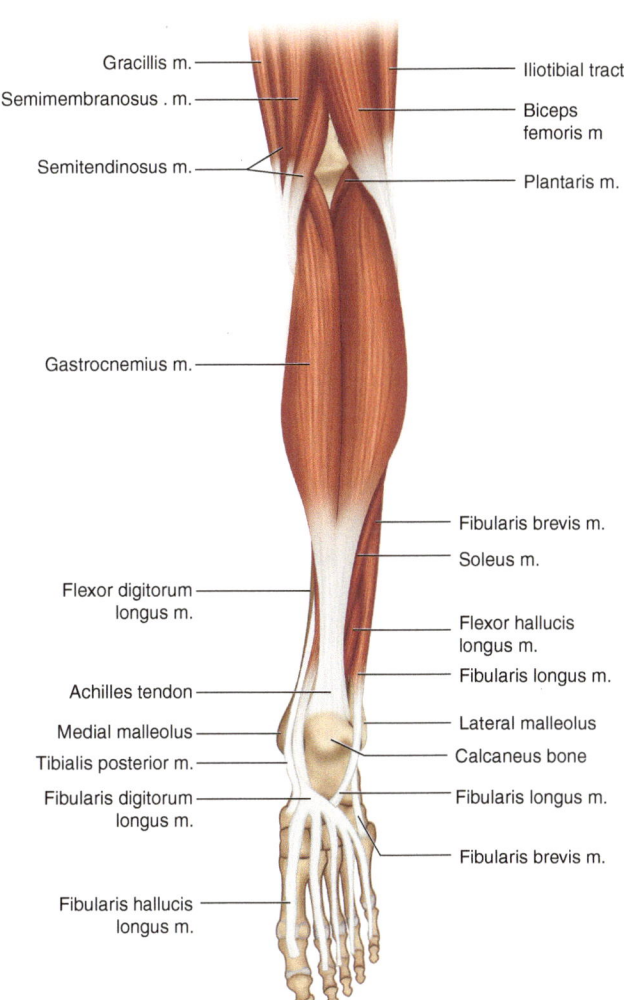

Fig. 34.9 Musculature surrounding anterior knee and ankle. (**a**) Cross section of the lower leg showing various compartments at the associated muscle groups. (**b**) Ranges of motion of the ankle. (**c**) Anterior view of the musculature in the lower leg

Fig. 34.10 Musculature surrounding lateral knee and ankle – lateral view of the musculature of the lower leg, ankle, and foot

The ankle has four motions: dorsiflexion, plantar flexion, inversion, and eversion (Figs. 34.9 and 34.10). Dorsiflexion is performed by tibialis anterior and the two extensors of the foot, extensor hallucis longus and extensor digitorum longus. Plantar flexion is accomplished by many muscles of the posterior compartment of the lower leg including the gastrocnemius, soleus, plantaris, and the flexors of the foot (e.g., flexor hallucis longus and flexor digitorum longus) (Figs. 34.10 and 34.11). The Achilles tendon, which connects the gastrocnemius, soleus, and plantaris to the calcaneus, is the site at which the plantar flexion reflex is elicited [7]. Inversion of the foot is caused by the two tibialis muscles, tibialis anterior and posterior. Eversion (Figs. 34.9 and 34.11) is activated by the fibularis muscles, longus, and brevis, also called the peroneus muscles (Fig. 34.10).

Joint Interdependence

A key to understanding lower extremity joint pain is that injury to one joint is often linked to injury of adjacent joints because all three joints are weight-bearing structures in a closed kinematic chain. Abnormalities of the ankle or foot,

for example, are often linked to injuries of the knee and hip because of this interdependence. Many individuals with abnormalities in foot structure subsequently develop osteoarthritis at the knee and hip [4].

Table 34.1 describes the common physical examination elements for evaluation of the lower extremity.

Neurophysiology

Nerve Distribution Around Joints

The sensory dermatomes of the lower extremity, as well as the innervation of each specific nerve, can be seen in Fig. 34.12. The lumbar plexus, formed from the anterior rami of L1–L4 (Fig. 34.13), lies between the psoas major and quadratus lumborum and gives rise to the major nerves of the hip and anterior thigh. The anterior divisions of L2–L4 form the obturator nerve which innervates the medial thigh. The

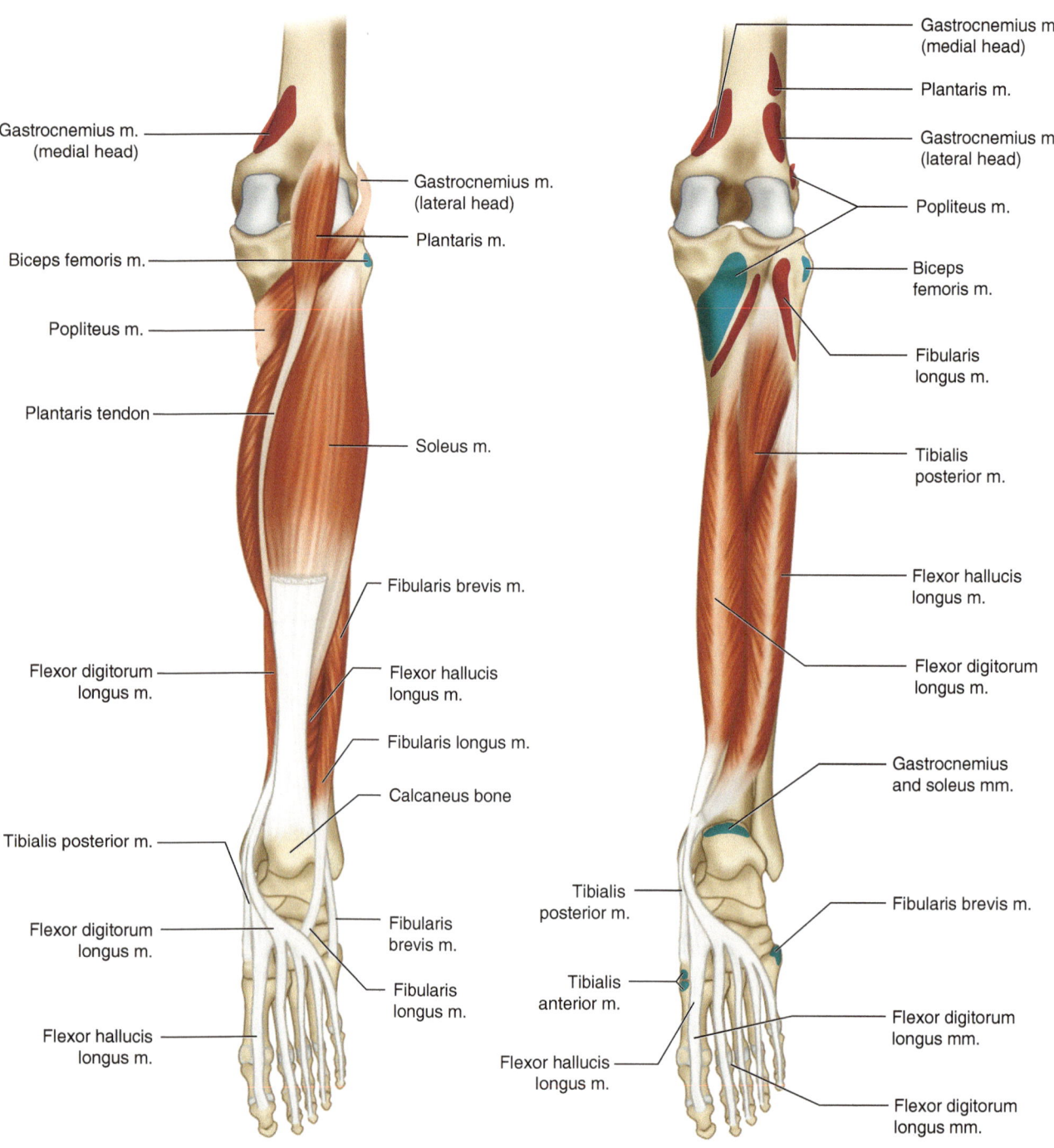

Fig. 34.11 Musculature of posterior leg (deep) – posterior view of the musculature of the lower leg with intermediate dissection (**a**) and deep dissection (**b**)

posterior division of the same lumbar nerves forms the femoral nerve positioned in the femoral triangle. The femoral nerve innervates the anterior thigh. The lateral femoral cutaneous nerve is formed from the posterior divisions of L2–L3 and innervates the lateral thigh.

The sacral plexus gives rise to the main nerves of the leg and the nerve corresponding to the posterior thigh.

The two key nerves that come from the sacral plexus are the posterior femoral cutaneous nerve sensory branches arising from S1–S3 and the sciatic nerve formed from branches of S1–S3 with input from L4–L5. The posterior femoral cutaneous nerve innervates the posterior of the thigh and knee. The sciatic nerve innervates all of the leg and foot below the knee except one small medial strip

Table 34.1 Physical Exam Special Tests for the lower extremity (personal table based on descriptions in Skinner and MvMahon [9])

Lower extremity joint	Physical exam maneuver	Tested structure	Technique
Hip	Patrick (FABER) test	Hip joint	With the patient supine, flex the hip and knee, and place the foot on the contralateral knee (which abducts and externally rotates the hip). This test is positive if groin pain is reproduced with this maneuver and indicates hip joint pathology such as OA as well as sacroiliac joint pathology. Of note this test is commonly called the FABER test, an acronym which stands for flexion, abduction, and externally rotate
Knee	Anterior drawer test	Anterior cruciate ligament	With patient supine and the knee bent at 90 degrees, anteriorly translate the lower leg while stabilizing the foot by sitting on it. This test is positive for ACL injury if a significant degree of laxity is appreciated with anterior translation
	Lachman's test	Anterior cruciate ligament	With patient supine and the knee bent at 20 degrees, anteriorly translate the lower leg while stabilizing the thigh. This test is positive for ACL injury if a significant degree of laxity is appreciated with anterior translation
	Posterior drawer test	Posterior cruciate ligament	With patient supine and the knee bent at 90 degrees, posteriorly translate the lower leg while stabilizing the foot by sitting on it. This test is positive for PCL injury if a significant degree of laxity is appreciated with posterior translation
	McMurray test	Meniscus	With the patient supine, perform passive flexion and extension of the knee while placing a varus or valgus stress. This test is positive for meniscus injury if a clunk is elicited along the joint line with flexion or extension
	Valgus stress	Medial collateral ligament	With the patient supine and the knee at 30 degrees of flexion, place pressure on the lateral aspect of the knee in order to open the medial knee to test laxity of the ligament. This test is positive for MCL injury if a significant degree of laxity is appreciated. This test can then be repeated at full extension of the knee. A positive test at full knee extension suggests injury to the posteromedial capsule in addition to MCL injury.
	Varus stress	Lateral collateral ligament	With the patient supine and the knee at 30 degrees of flexion, place pressure on the medial aspect of the knee in order to open the lateral knee to test laxity of the ligament. This test is positive for LCL injury if a significant degree of laxity is appreciated. This test can then be repeated at full extension of the knee. A positive test at full knee extension suggests injury to the posterolateral capsule in addition to LCL injury.
Ankle	Anterior drawer test	Anterior talofibular ligament	With patient in sitting position and the foot relaxed, translate the foot anteriorly while stabilizing the lower leg. This test is positive for ATFL injury if a significant degree of laxity is appreciated with anterior translation.
	Talar tilt test	Anterior talofibular ligament (ankle in plantar flexion), calcaneofibular ligament (ankle in neural or dorsiflexion position)	With patient in sitting position and the foot relaxed, invert the foot while stabilizing the lower leg. This test is positive for ATFL injury if a significant degree of laxity is appreciated with inversion while the ankle is plantarflexed. This test is positive for CFL injury if a significant degree of laxity is appreciated with inversion while the ankle is in neutral or dorsiflexion position.
	Posterior drawer test	Calcaneofibular ligament	With patient in sitting position and the foot relaxed, translate the foot posteriorly while stabilizing the lower leg. This test is positive for CFL injury if a significant degree of laxity is appreciated with posterior translation.

which is supplied by the saphenous nerve (branch of femoral). The sciatic is formed from two major trunks, the tibial and the common fibular. The tibial trunk receives input from L4–S3, and the common fibular trunk receives input from L4–S2. The two trunks separate in the popliteal fossa into the tibial nerve and the common fibular (peroneal) nerve (Fig. 34.14). The tibial nerve gives off the medial sural nerve and then continues down the leg as the tibial nerve, finally terminating as the medial and lateral plantar nerves in the foot (Figs. 34.12, 34.13, 34.14, and 34.15). The common fibular nerve gives off the lateral sural nerve and then divides into the superficial and deep fibular nerve after it passes the head of the fibula (Fig. 34.14). The medial sural nerve (from tibial nerve)

and the lateral sural nerve (from common fibular nerve) come together to form the sural nerve which innervates the lateral aspect of the leg (Fig. 34.12).

The main nerve in the lower leg which does not originate from the sacral plexus is the saphenous nerve. It is the terminal branch of the femoral nerve and provides sensory innervation of the medial lower leg (Fig. 34.12).

Psychosocial Aspects

Like most pain conditions, lower extremity joint pain is highly influenced by co-existing psychiatric comorbidities and behavioral factors. Many patients with lower extremity mus-

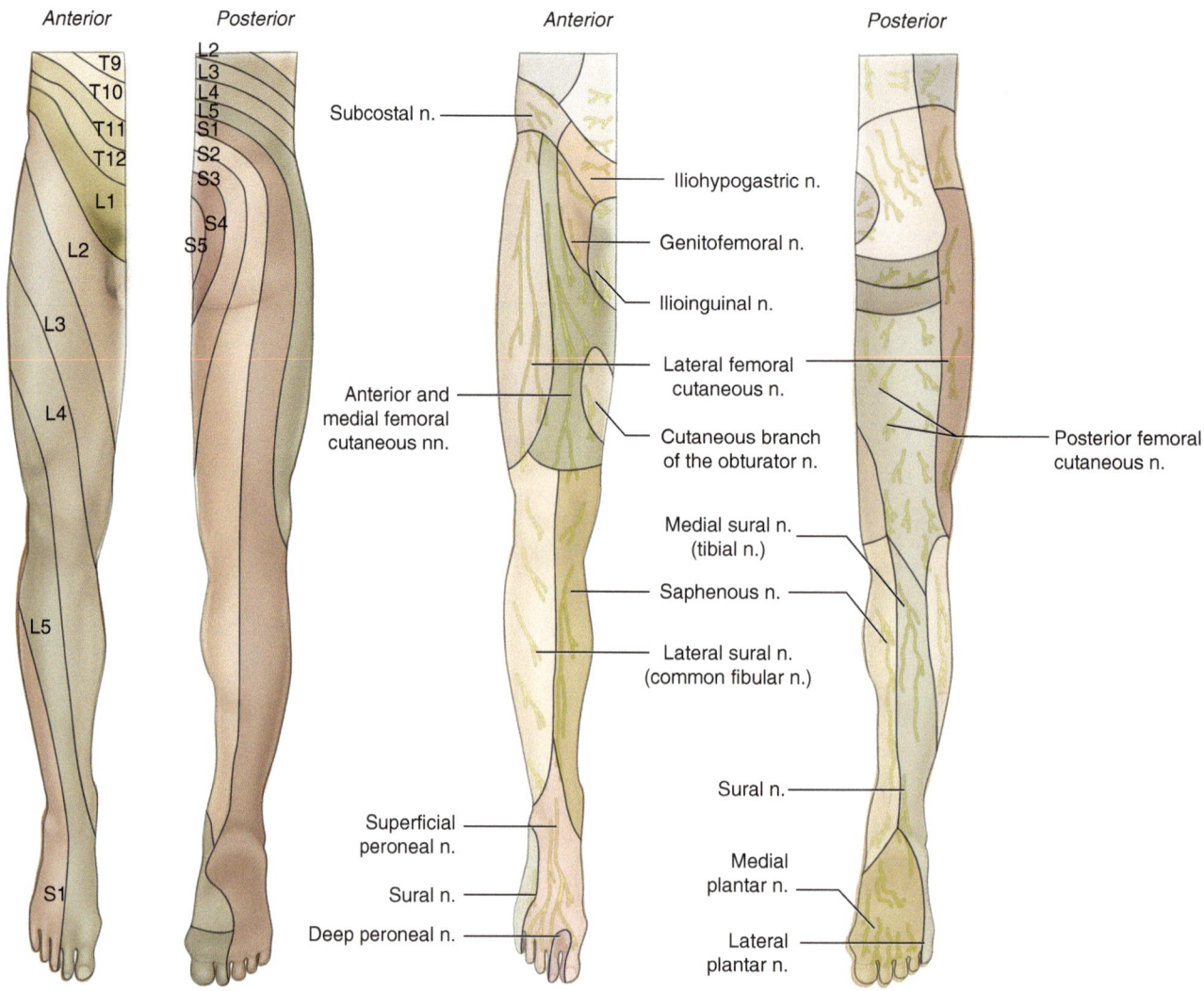

Fig. 34.12 Sensory dermatomes of lower extremity. (**a**) Dermatome of the entire lower extremity. (**b**) Terminal sensory nerve supply of the entire lower extremity

culoskeletal pain can develop mood disorders including anxiety and depression [7].

Pain is a taxing experience that drains resources and requires both adaptation and flexibility. Pain can cause avoidant and protective behaviors [7]. Each individual's experience of pain is influenced by many cognitive factors: beliefs surrounding pain, expectations of pain and treatment, and tendency to catastrophize the clinical situation [7].

Lower extremity joint pain can cause significant disability and affect activities of daily living [4]. Pain of the lower extremity joints can impede mobility causing frequent missed work days [10]. Many patients who develop lower extremity joint pain, particularly younger patients, are physically active and participate in sports. Their activity can quickly become limited by pain. Limiting participation in sports can significantly influence the psychological state of young adults suffering from musculoskeletal pain in the lower extremity.

Classification and Clinical Characteristics of Musculoskeletal Diseases

Hip

Hip osteoarthritis manifests as insidious onset hip pain during weight-bearing that waxes and wanes and improves with rest. There is typically a decrease in the range of motion. On radiography, loss of cartilage is visible and is sometimes accompanied by osseous hypertrophic changes. Osteoarthritis can exist concomitantly with bursitis or tendonitis [2, 11]. Risk factors for developing osteoarthritis are age over 50, congenital dislocation of the hip, slipped capital femoral epiphysis, Legg-Calve-Perthes disease, and positive family history [2, 11, 12].

In hip dislocation, the femoral head is displaced from the acetabulum, usually as a result of high-energy trauma.

Fig. 34.13 Innervation around hip joint, lumbar plexus. (**a**) Lumbosacral plexus showing specific nerve roots and corresponding nerves. (**b**) Nerves of the posterior hip

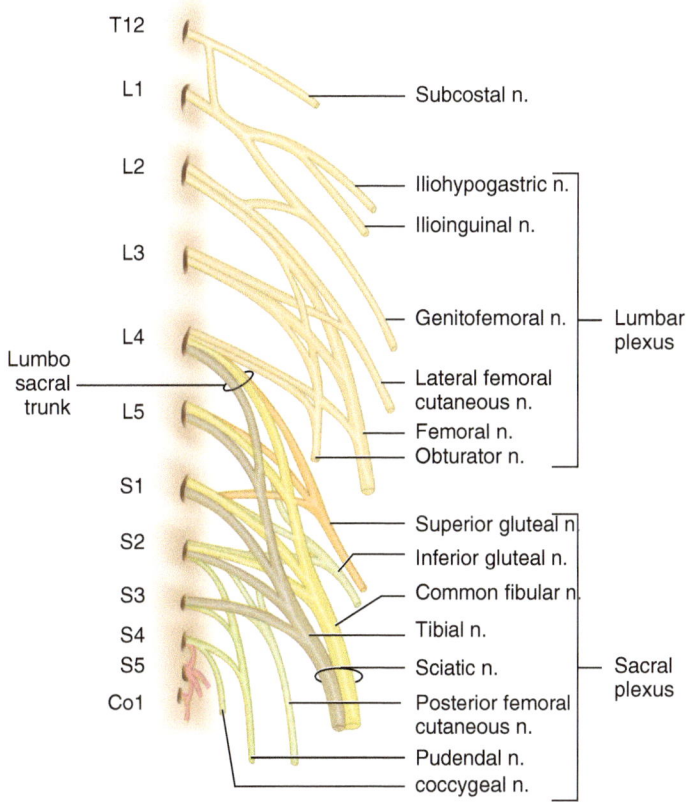

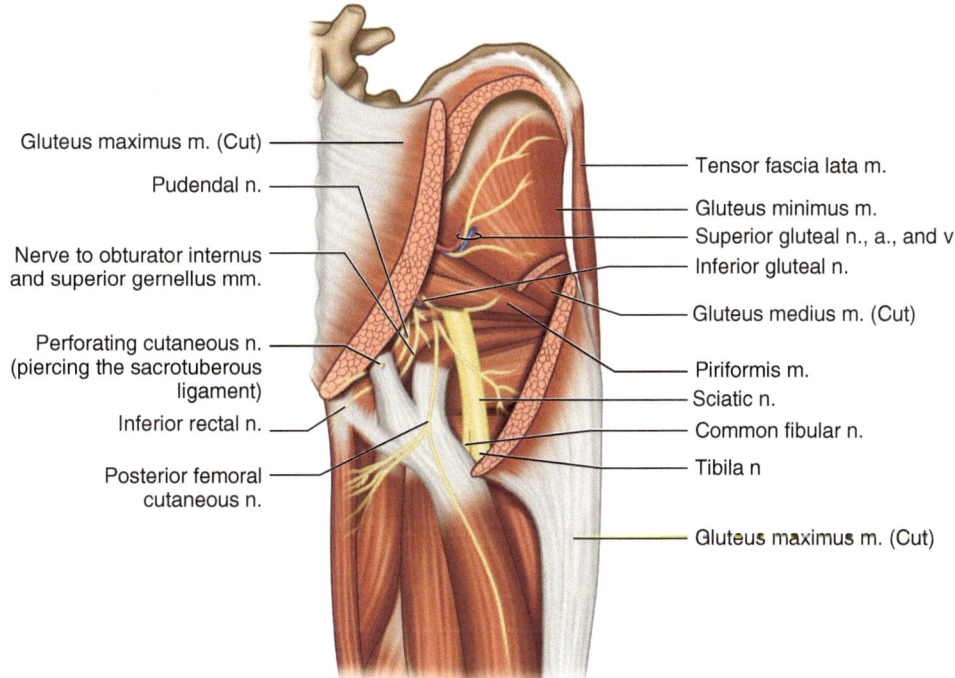

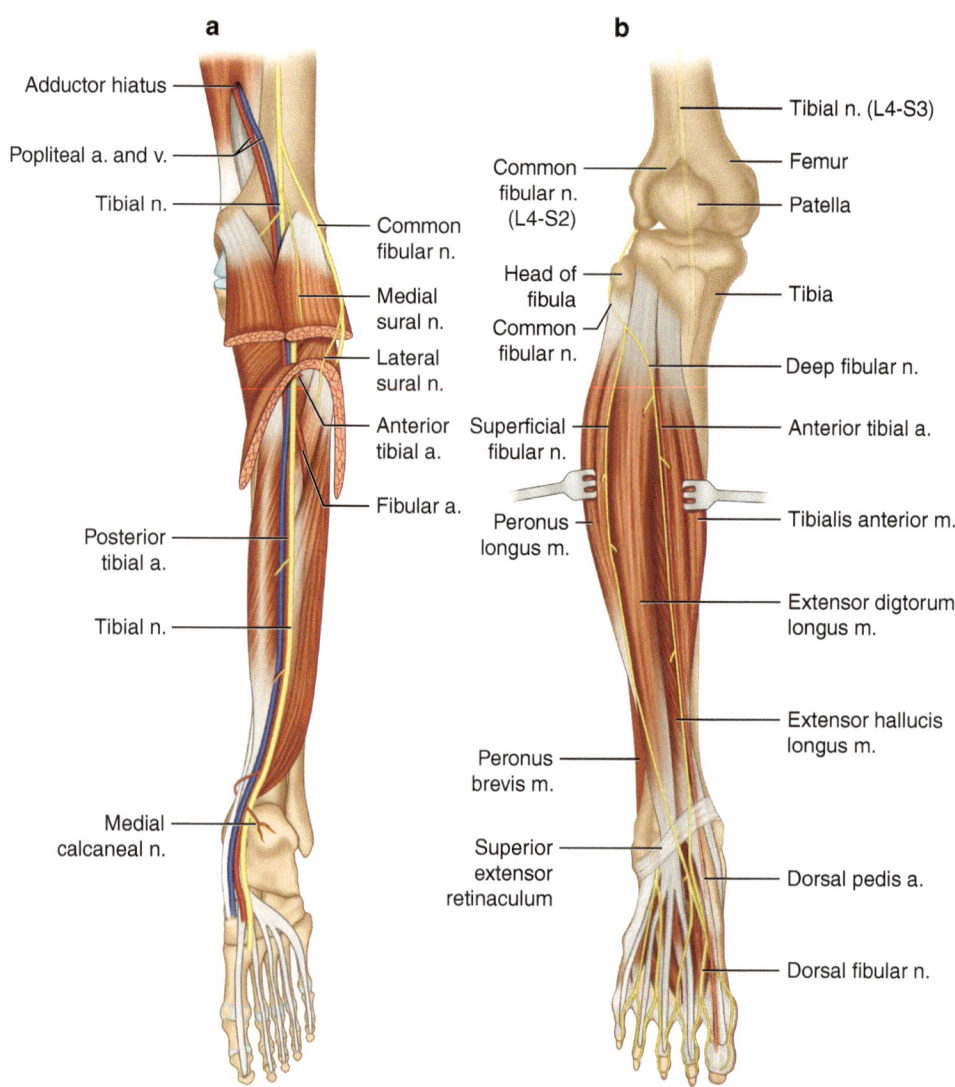

Fig. 34.14 Innervation around knee and ankle. Nerves surrounding the knee posterior view (**a**) and anterior view (**b**)

Dislocation is common in sports injuries or industrial or car accidents, which tend to cause more posterior dislocations of the hip [7]. Due to its proximity to nervous structures, hip dislocations can result in sciatic nerve injury [7].

Trochanteric bursitis results from repetitive movements such as running, gait disturbances, or direct trauma that inflames the bursa overlying the greater trochanter. Often trochanteric bursitis can be mistaken for pain in the hip joint itself [7]. It usually presents as lateral hip pain extending down the thigh, often over its lateral aspects, but not distal to the knee. Pain is worse with lying down on the affected side and is usually described as aching, but occasionally sharp. Pain is well-localized over the greater trochanter.

Femoroacetabular impingement is the result of abnormal anatomy that causes contact between the acetabulum and the femoral head-neck junction. It manifests as pain in the groin developing insidiously over months to years, usually in young to middle-aged physically active patients. Pain is worse with sitting and movements that require flexion and

internal rotation. Pain can frequently radiate to the buttocks or medial aspects of the knee [2, 12, 13].

Knee

Knee osteoarthritis is caused by noninflammatory progressive degeneration of the knee joint [11]. Osteoarthritis is one of the most common disorders of the knee. Risk factors include obesity, age greater than 50, and history of repetitive trauma or mechanical stress. On radiography, the joint space is narrowed and surrounded by osteophytes [7, 11]. The pain is difficult to localize, worsens with weight-bearing, and decreases range of movement over time. The cartilage degenerates and ligaments become lax. Patients tend to develop a greater loss of medial joint space, so a varus deviation of the knee can be seen chronically [11].

In knee bursitis, the various bursa at points of friction become inflamed with repetitive activity or trauma. Pain is

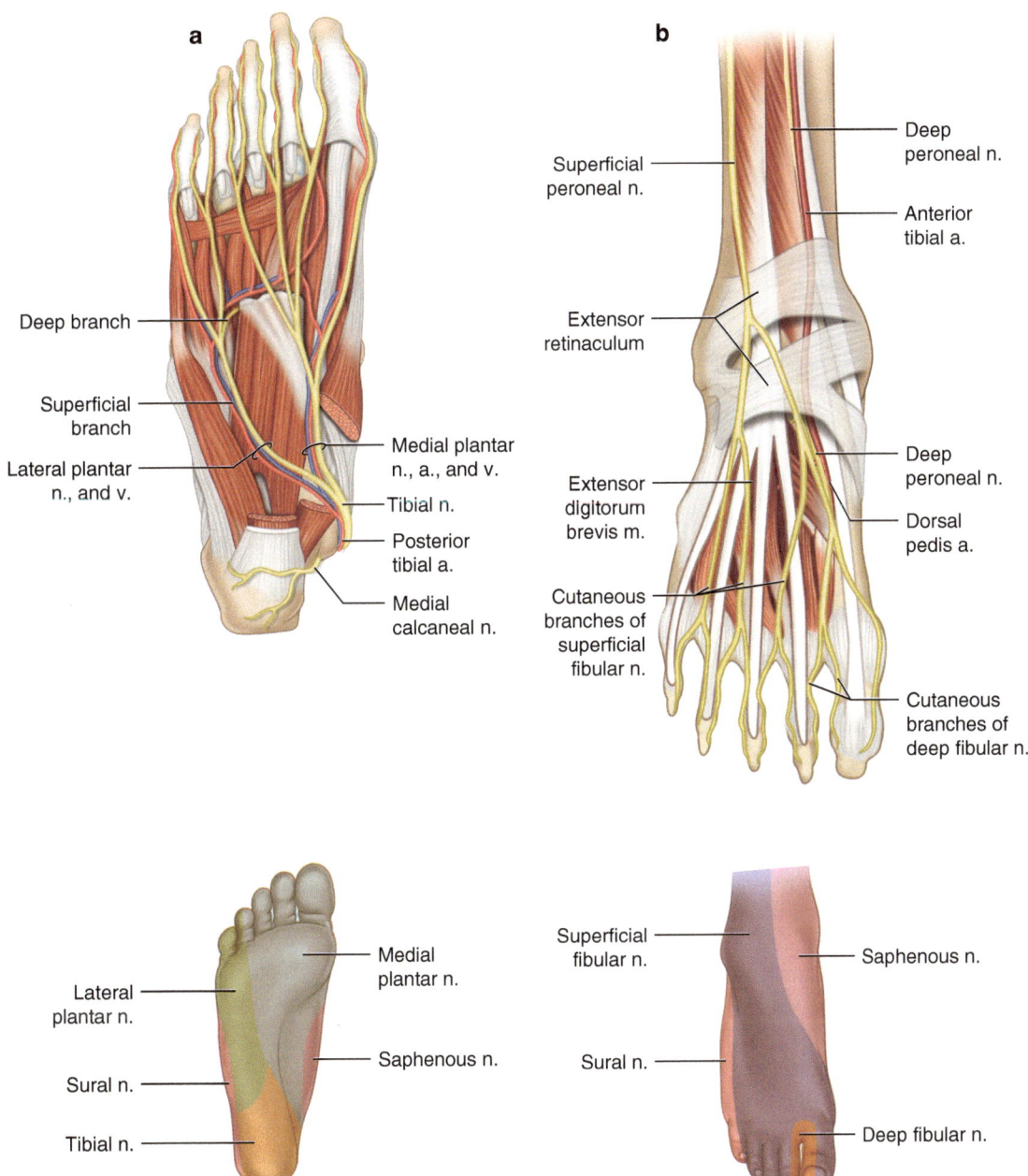

Fig. 34.15 Neurovascular supply of foot. Neurovascular structures of the plantar aspect of the foot (**a**) as well as the dorsal aspect (**b**) as well as sensory nerve distributions

well-localized over inflamed bursa and is usually present with knee movements and at rest [11]. Table 34.2 describes the clinically pertinent bursae of the knee.

Meniscus injury can result after axial loading of the knee combined with rotation or twisting, either from acute trauma or chronic wear and degeneration. Patients with meniscus tears feel a clicking or catching of the knee and pain in the joint capsule with movement [7]. A common sports injury, commonly known as the "unhappy triad," is concomitant tearing of the medial meniscus, anterior cruciate ligament

(ACL), and medial collateral ligament (MCL) (7). Meniscus injuries are classified by etiology (acute vs. degenerative), location (anterior, middle, posterior), and location in comparison to vascular supply (peripheral red zone near the meniscocapsular junction, intermediate red/white zone, and the most central white zone). The tears also can be classified based on the orientation within the meniscus itself: vertical, horizontal, radial or transverse, oblique, or complex [10]. On physical examination the joint line is tender, often with an effusion, and with a positive McMurray test during which

Table 34.2 Bursa of the knee (personal table based on discussions in Peng and Shankar [19])

Bursa	Location between	
Anserine	Pes anserinus	Tibia and medial collateral ligament
Subcutaneous prepatellar	Skin	Anterior surface of the patella
Suprapatellar	Quadriceps tendon	Femur
Subcutaneous infrapatellar	Skin	Tibial tuberosity
Deep infrapatellar	Patella tendon (ligament)	Anterior surface of tibia
Semimembranosus	Semimembranosus tendon	Medial head of the gastrocnemius
Popliteus	Popliteus tendon	Lateral condyle of tibia

forced flexion and rotation will elicit a clunk in the joint line if meniscus injury is present [9].

Knee Ligament Injury and Classification

Injury to the ligaments of the knee is graded based on the severity of injury: Grade 1, stretching of ligament with no detectable instability; Grade 2, fibers in continuity but further stretching can cause instability; and Grade 3, complete disruption of the ligament [7, 9]. The collateral and cruciate ligaments of the knee are the primary stabilizers of the joint itself, and any primary ligamentous injury can strain and potentially injure the secondary stabilizers of the knee including the menisci, iliotibial band, and biceps femoris [9].

MCL injury manifests with medial knee pain and valgus laxity at 30 degrees of flexion. Valgus or varus laxity at full extension would overlap with ACL and PCL injuries; therefore, testing laxity at 30 degrees can isolate the collateral ligaments [9, 11]. In chronic injuries, knee calcification in the MCL can be seen on MRI.

LCL injury is diagnosed from lateral knee pain and varus laxity at 30 degrees flexion. Incidence of concomitant perineal nerve injury is high. Isolated LCL injuries are quite rare and often occur with injury to other ligaments [9, 11].

ACL injury is caused by deceleration or rotational injury to the knee or application of a valgus force to an extended knee. Sudden changes of direction or hyperextension, such as during running and jumping, commonly cause ACL injury. Patients often will hear a "pop" and feel knee instability. Effusion is present within the first 12 hours; an anterior drawer test and a Lachman test will be positive. ACL injuries often have concomitant meniscus or ligament injury [9, 11].

PCL injury is caused by an anterior blow to the tibia with the knee flexed or a fall to the ground with foot plantarflexed. Edema of the joint and stiffness are common. Unlike ACL injuries, PCL injuries are not often associated with a "pop-ping" sensation. Individuals with a PCL tear can be asymptomatic if the injury is chronic or subacute [9].

Patellar dislocation is characterized by pain, edema, and tenderness over the medial border of the patella. Hemarthrosis may also be present [9]. Dislocation commonly affects women in the second decade of life. On physical examination, patients feel apprehension with the knee flexed and patella pushed laterally.

Quadriceps tendon injury is common in patients older than 40. Patients are unable to extend the knee likely because the patella rides in a lower position because of the injury. If the injury is untreated, the quadriceps will retract proximally. Quadriceps tendon injury is associated with gout, diabetes, and steroid use [9].

Patellar tendon injury is common in patients younger than 40. In these situations, patients are unable to extend the knee and the patella appears high-riding [9].

Patellar tendonitis is an overuse syndrome causing microtears to the patellar tendon and pain. Jumping sports have been implicated. This injury can also occur, less commonly, at the quadriceps insertion at the patella [11].

Osteochondral lesions/osteochondritis dissecans is a group of idiopathic diseases ranging from osteochondral fracture to pure cartilaginous injury. These injuries are associated with delimitation or fragmentation of the osteochondral area and are potentially reversible. They are differentiated into juvenile and adult forms. Patients will usually complain of a poorly localized ache in the posterolateral aspect of the medial femoral condyle. Less commonly, the lateral condyle may also be affected. Pain tends to be worse with stair climbing. Upon examination, patients who run regularly may have edema and crepitus of the knee [9].

Osgood-Schlatter disease, which can affect up to 20% of adolescents active in sports, is characterized by pronounced activity-induced pain at the tibial tuberosity. Repetitive use causes micro-tears or avulsion at epiphysis of the tibial tubercle [11].

Patellofemoral disorder is described as chronic anterior knee pain commonly experienced by young females in their second decade of life that is worse, but not severe, with weight-bearing and relieved with rest. This disorder is due to an imbalance of muscle strength when the lateral quadriceps overpower the medial quadriceps, causing patellar maltracking with flexion and extension of knee. Specifically, quadriceps contraction drives the patella into femoral condyles constraining the patellofemoral joint. Activities that place pressure on the patella or force it onto the femur can worsen pain including walking, running, and climbing stairs or hills. Patellofemoral disorder is a diagnosis of exclusion and is thought by some to increase risk for osteoarthritis [9, 11, 14].

Iliotibial band syndrome or bursitis is characterized by lateral knee pain with tenderness after palpation of the lateral epicondyle particularly at 30 degrees knee flexion. It is due to inflammation at the point where the iliotibial band contacts the lateral epicondyle. Iliotibial band syndrome commonly affects runners and cyclists [9].

Ankle and Foot

Ankle sprains result when ligaments tear after sudden stretching or recurrent trauma. Ankle sprains can cause functional instability, chronic pain, and inability to return to prior normal level of performance [11]. Most commonly, sprains are caused by inversion or eversion during sports or stepping off an uneven surface [7]. Ankle sprains have three grades: Grade 1, stretching and micro-tears of the ligament with mild tenderness and edema; Grade 2, partial tear of the ligament with moderate pain and edema and mild instability; Grade 3, complete tear, significant swelling and instability, and inability to support weight [7].

Lateral ankle ligamentous injury comprises 85% of ankle sprains [11]. Anterior talofibular ligament (ATFL) injuries are caused by inversion while in plantar flexion and calcaneofibular ligament (CFL) injuries by inversion while the foot is dorsiflexed. The anterior drawer test will be positive with ATFL sprains. The talar tilt test, which puts inversion stress on the heel, tests the ATFL with the ankle in plantar flexion and the CFL in neutral or dorsiflexion position [9].

Medial ankle ligamentous injury is rare and comprises just 5% of all ankle sprains [9, 11]. Eversion stress can damage the deltoid ligament [9].

The syndesmotic ligament, which connects the tibia to the fibula, can be injured with external rotational force. Patients generally have extensive swelling approximately 2 cm proximal to the ankle joint and pain with squeezing of the tibia and fibula together [7].

Osteochondral lesions of the talus/osteochondritis dissecans lesions are characterized by several months of pain in the posteromedial or anterolateral ankle following a routine sprain. They are caused by defects in the cartilage and subchondral bone in the talar dome and thought to be associated with mild ischemia. Patient also can have a sensation of locking if a loose flap of cartilage is present [9]

Achilles tendonitis is an inflammation of the Achilles tendon caused by contracted gastrocnemius/soleus or hyperpronation. The Achilles tendon can also rupture with trauma or overuse in which case patients will complain of a sudden pain in the calf after attempting a push-off movement, accompanied by an audible pop. Those with Achilles rupture have a positive Thompson test in which a squeeze to the calf of a prone patient with knee bent at 90 degrees does not result in plantar flexion [9, 11].

Retrocalcaneal and Achilles bursitis is inflammation of the bursa between the calcaneus and distal Achilles tendon or between the Achilles tendon and skin. It is caused by exercising, particularly on uneven ground, and exacerbated by poorly fitted shoes, direct trauma, infection, rheumatoid arthritis, and gout. Patients will complain of heel pain and exhibit localized edema [11].

Treatment and Rehabilitation of Musculoskeletal Pain/Disability

There are three main treatment categories for musculoskeletal joint pain of the lower extremities: physical therapy and exercise, medication, and invasive procedures.

Activity-Related Treatment

Essentially all musculoskeletal disorders benefit from physical therapy, an appropriate level of exercise, and stretching to strengthen musculature surrounding the joint. Activity-related treatments in combination with medication are classified as "conservative therapy." Physical therapy has been shown to restore range of motion, increase strength, and decrease pain [11]. For obese patients, weight loss combined with activity can be very effective [9]. Physical activity such as aquatic exercise is also effective for pain reduction and improving quality of life in those with knee and hip osteoarthritis [15].

Ligamentous injury of the knee or ankle significantly decreases stability of the corresponding joint. The general treatment plan for a Grade 1–2 injury is immobilization during the acute phase before appropriate activity and weight-bearing as tolerated with the assistance of a cast or brace [9]. For ligamentous injury of the ankle, even Grade 3 injuries respond well to conservative treatment [9].

Footwear must fit properly and offer adequate support, as poor kinetics of the foot and ankle negatively impact the knee and hip [4]. Clinical assessments of torsional flexibility, toe break flexibility, and wear patterns indicate whether footwear should be changed or if special orthotics are needed to restore appropriate alignment and prevent injury to all three joints of the lower extremity [4]. This assessment is particularly important in elderly patients as they develop a more pronated posture [6].

Medication

Non-opioid analgesics such as acetaminophen and NSAIDS are the mainstay for medical treatment of pain from osteoarthritis and other musculoskeletal disorders [2, 11]. Other non-opioid analgesics including local anesthetics and gabapentinoids are often part of the medical treatment. Medications targeting protein kinases, NGF, CGPR, and Nav1.7 are in various stages of development. Opioid analgesics, if prescribed, are recommended for the shortest course possible during the acute phase only. There is anecdotal evidence that glucosamine and chondroitin relieve the pain of osteoarthritis [11].

Invasive Procedures

Several compounds including steroids, preparations of hyaluronic acid, and platelet-rich plasma (discussed elsewhere in this text), among others, can be injected into the joints and bursae of the lower extremities. Nerve blocks and ablations can also be performed.

Hip

Steroids may be injected into the hip to treat pain associated with osteoarthritis, trauma, or acute capsulitis. Contraindications are local or systemic infection, coagulopathy, unstable joint, or intra-articular hip fracture. Injections can be repeated every 3–4 months without significant increase in cartilage compromise [2]. Procedures can be performed using landmarks or with imaging guidance (ultrasound or fluoroscopic) [16]. Figure 34.16a depicts a hip injection performed with fluoroscopic guidance, while Fig. 34.16b depicts a trochanteric bursa injection.

Patients with chronic hip pain, for which routine injections are unhelpful and surgery is not indicated, may benefit from blocks and radiofrequency ablation of the articular branches of the obturator and femoral nerves [18] as depicted in Fig. 34.17. Radiofrequency ablation of peripheral branches of the hip was first studied in 1997. Several prospective studies showed sig-

nificant improvement of chronic hip pain after 6 months [18]. Two independent diagnostic nerve blocks with local anesthetics are usually necessary before radiofrequency ablation (RFA) is attempted. Pain relief after diagnostic blocks should be at least 50% for RFA to be considered. Figure 34.18 shows needle placement during blocks and radiofrequency ablation in a patient with hip pain related to osteoarthritis.

Knee

Intra-articular (IA) steroid injections in the knee can be performed for cases of osteoarthritis, trauma, and degenerative and inflammatory conditions in a patient who has no local or systemic infection or coagulopathy [17]. Generally a solution of 5 mL of 1% lidocaine, a steroid medication, and/or 2 mL of hyaluronic acid is injected at the midpoint of the medial edge of the patella between the tibia and medial femoral condyle [17]. IA corticosteroid has been shown to provide short-term (<3 weeks) pain relief, but there is little evidence of efficacy in function improvement [19]. Viscosupplementation (VS) is generally ineffective in cases of complete collapse of joint space, but in some studies it is efficacious and more long-lasting than corticosteroid [19]. There is support for improvement in function with VS, although the benefits of function improvement between intra-articular corticosteroid and VS remain controversial [19]. Intra-articular knee injections can be performed based on anatomic landmarks or with ultrasound or fluoroscopic image guidance. Figure 34.19 depicts a fluoroscopically guided knee injection.

Fig. 34.16 (**a**) Fluoroscopic guided hip injection and trochanteric bursa injection. First image (*A*) shows 1 mL of contrast dye spreading in the left joint; second picture (*B*) taken at the completion of the injection of 5 mL of local anesthetic/steroid mixture. (**b**) (*C*) shows right left hip intra-articular injection (personal library) and (*D*) shows fluoroscopic guided left trochanteric bursa injection

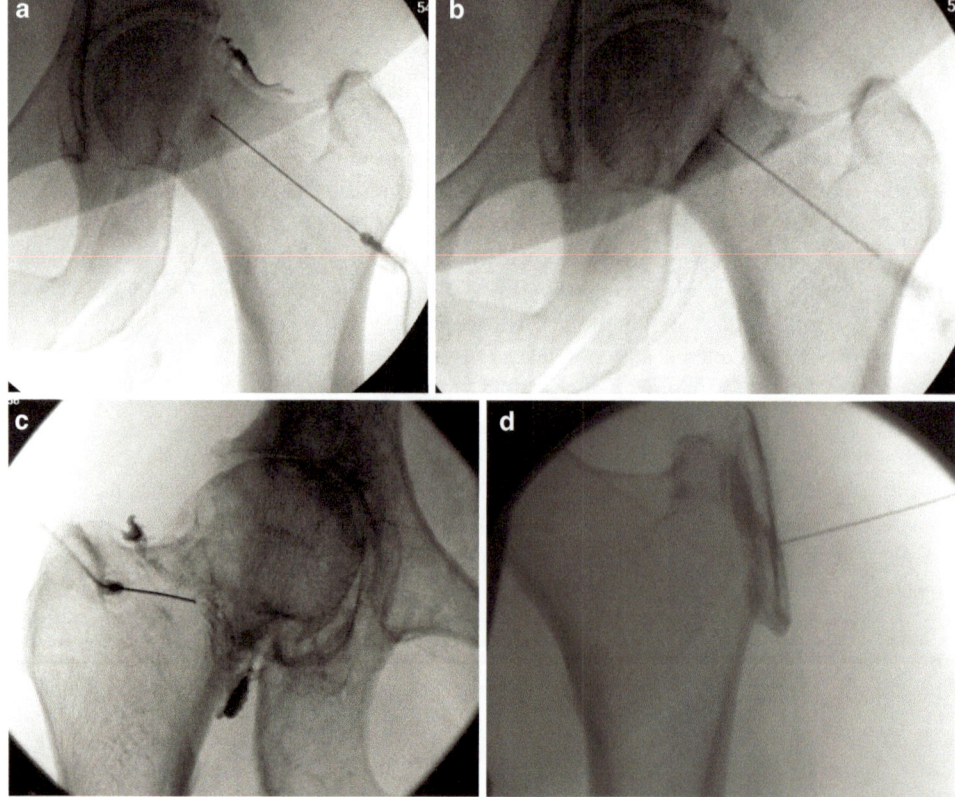

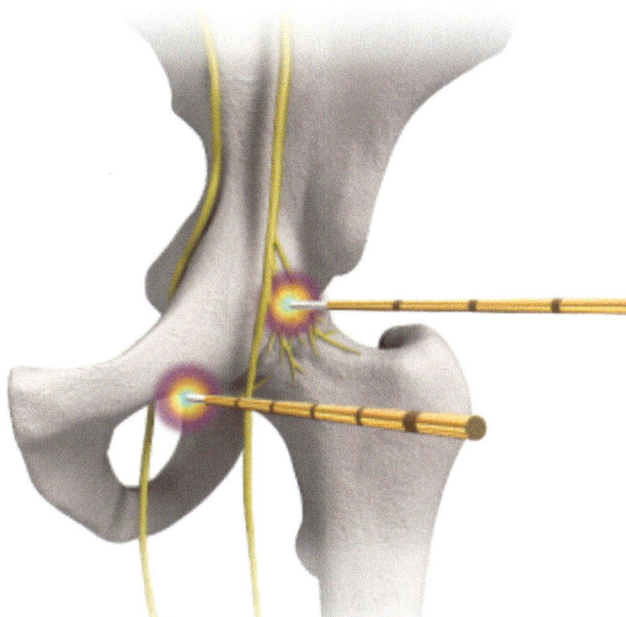

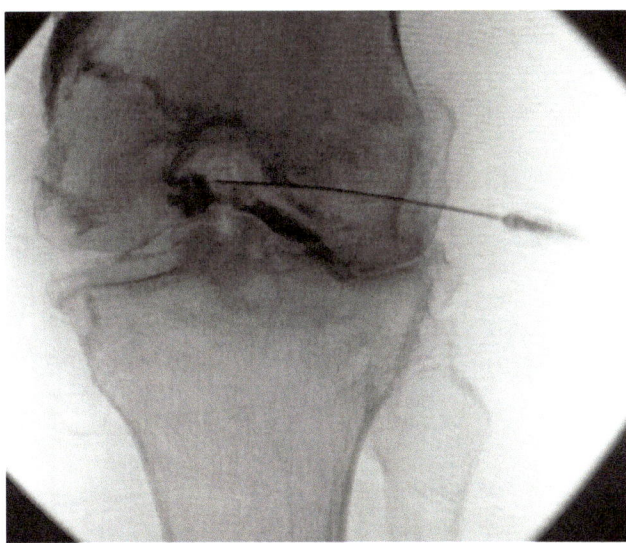

Fig. 34.19 Fluoroscopic guided knee injection showing spread of the medication (Synvisc) medial and lateral aspects of the knee

Fig. 34.17 Image of the peripheral articular branches of the obturator and femoral nerve that supply the hip joint (form Halyard); radiofrequency ablation of those branches provides pain relief in patients suffering from hip pain

Fig. 34.18 Diagnostic blocks and RFA of hip intra-articular branches. (**a**) A diagnostic block of the intra-articular branches of the obturator and femoral in a patient with continuous pain after total hip arthroplasty. (**b**) and (**c**) Diagnostic blocks of the intra-articular branches and spread of 1 cc of Omnipaque around those structures, while (**d**) shows the RFA of the articular branches of obturator and femoral

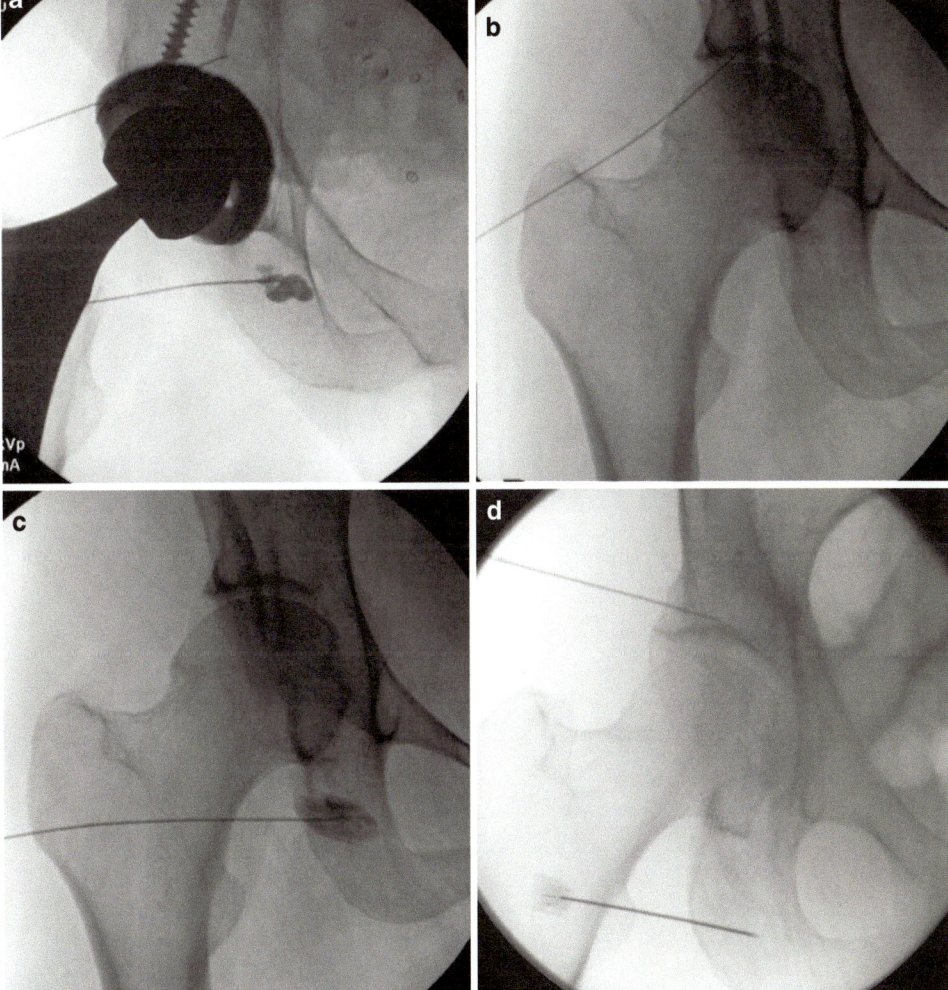

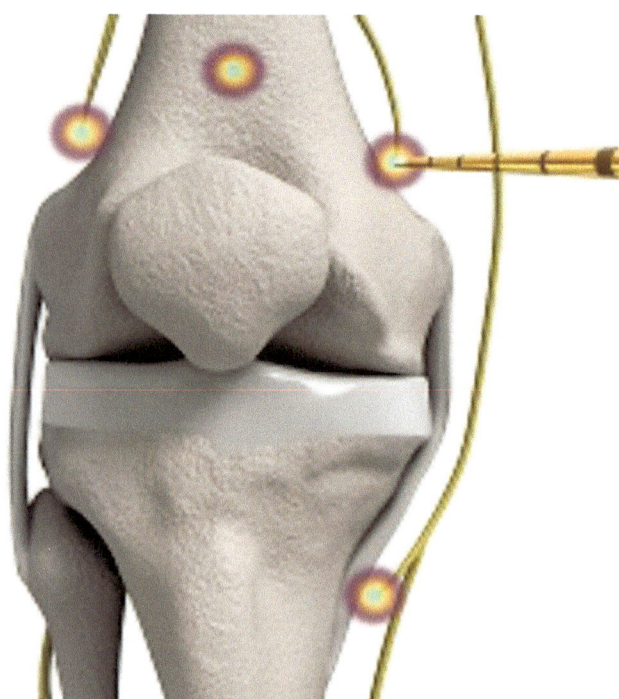

Fig. 34.20 Image of the peripheral branches of the genicular nerve of the knee (Halyard image); radiofrequency ablation of those branches produces significant pain relief in patients with chronic knee pain, no longer responsive to other treatment modalities of not surgical candidates

Patients with significant osteoarthritis of the knee and/or continued pain after surgery may benefit from radiofrequency ablation of the genicular nerves. The use of radiofrequency for the treatment of knee pain was first described in 2011. Since then several prospective studies have shown improvement at 4, 8, and 12 weeks after the procedure. Two diagnostic blocks with local anesthetic that reduce pain by 50% are needed before radiofrequency ablation of the genicular nerves is considered. Target areas for needle placement are depicted in Fig. 34.20. Figure 34.21 shows appropriate needle placement under fluoroscopic visualization.

Ankle Procedures

For acute capsulitis, chronic capsulitis, and traumatic injuries to the ankle, steroid joint injection is performed. Contraindications are local or systemic infection and coagulopathy. The injection may be placed into the tibio-talar joint at the junction of the tibia and fibula, just above talus [5, 17]. Several studies show the short-term benefit of the injections, but only a few studies have assessed long-term efficacy [5]. Viscosupplementation can be performed in the ankle to treat pain although results for pain and disability outcomes are conflicting [5].

Fig. 34.21 Genicular nerve diagnostic block (**a** and **b**) and RFA (**c** and **d**) in patient with severe OA of knee. Personal library

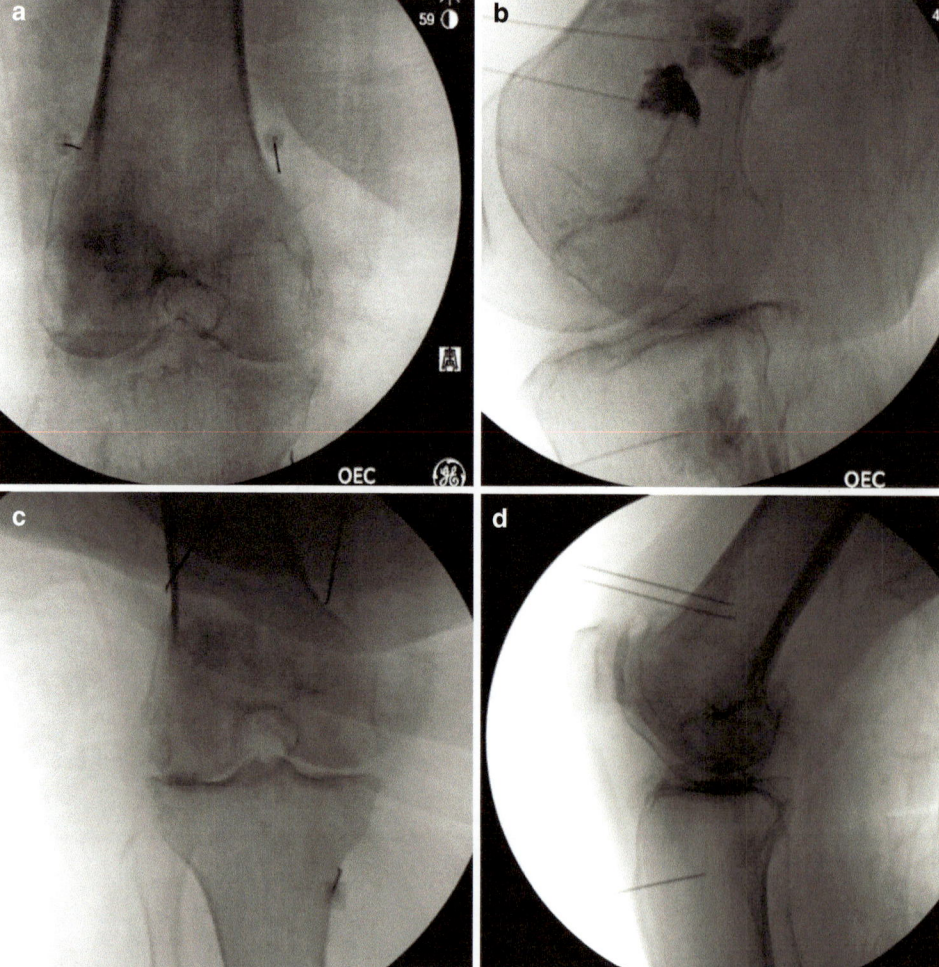

Surgical Procedures

Should conservative or minimally invasive treatments fail to provide adequate pain relief, patients progress to surgical procedures such as hip [11] or knee arthroplasty for osteoarthritis. Arthroscopic procedures on the knee are performed for meniscus or ligamentous injury [9]. As a rule, tendon rupture must be repaired surgically to prevent retraction of the tendon that is beyond repair [9]. For ligamentous injuries of the ankle, surgical treatment is reserved for the elite athlete. [9]

References

1. United States Bone and Joint Initiative. BMUS: the burden of musculoskeletal diseases in the United States. Available at: http://www.boneandjointburden.org/. Accessed 2 Oct 2016.
2. Karrasch C, Lynch S. Practical approach to hip pain. Med Clin N Am. 2014;98(4):737–54.
3. Thomas MJ, Roddy E, Zhang W, Menz HB, Hannan MT, Peat GM. The population prevalence of foot and ankle pain in middle and old age: a systematic review. Pain. 2011;152(12):2870–80.
4. Rao S, Riskowski JL, Hannan MT. Musculoskeletal conditions of the foot and ankle: assessments and treatment options. Best Pract Res Clin Rheumatol. 2012;26(3):345–68.
5. Soneji N, Peng P. Ultrasound-guided interventional procedures in pain medicine: a review of anatomy, sonoanatomy, and procedures: part VI: ankle joint. Reg Anesth Pain Med. 2015;41(1):99–116.
6. Menz HB. Biomechanics of the ageing foot and ankle: a mini-review. Gerontology. 2015;61(4):381–8.
7. Gatchel RJ, Schultz IZ, editors. Handbook of musculoskeletal pain and disability disorders in the workplace. New York: Springer; 2014.
8. Prather H, Colorado B, Hunt D. Managing hip pain in the athlete. Phys Med Rehabil Clin N Am. 2014;25(4):789–812.
9. Skinner HB, McMahon PJ, editors. Current diagnosis & treatment in orthopedics. 5th ed. New York: McGraw-Hill Education; 2014.
10. Agaliotis M, Mackey M, Jan S, Fransen M. Burden of reduced work productivity among people with chronic knee pain: a systematic review. Occup Environ Med. 2014;71(9):651–9.
11. Pobre T, Weiss J, Weiss LD. Oxford American handbook of physical medicine & rehabilitation. Oxford: Oxford University Press; 2010.
12. Wilson JJ, Furukawa M. Evaluation of the patient with hip pain. Am Family Phys. 2014;89(1):27–34.
13. Ward D, Parvizi J. Management of hip pain in young adults. Orthop Clin North Am. 2016;47(3):485–96.
14. Petersen W, Ellermann A, Gösele-Koppenburg A, et al. Patellofemoral pain syndrome. Knee Surg Sports Traumatol Arthrosc. 2013;22(10):2264–74.
15. Bartels EM, Lund H, Hagen KB, Dagfinrud H, Christensen R, Danneskiold-Samsøe B. Aquatic exercise for the treatment of knee and hip osteoarthritis. Cochrane Database Syst Rev. 2007;(4):CD005523.
16. Peng P. Ultrasound-guided interventional procedures in pain medicine: a review of anatomy, sonoanatomy, and procedures. Part IV: hip. Reg Anesth Pain Med. 2013;38(4):264–73.
17. Raj PP, Erdine S. Pain-relieving procedures: the illustrated guide. Hoboken: Wiley-Blackwell; 2012.
18. Salmasi V, Chaiban G, Eissa H, Tolba R, Lirette L, Guirguis MN. Application of cooled radiofrequency ablation in management of chronic joint pain. Tech Reg Anesth Pain Manage. 2014;18:137–44.
19. Peng P, Shankar H. Ultrasound-guided interventional procedures in pain medicine: a review of anatomy, sonoanatomy, and procedures. Part V: knee joint. Reg Anesth Pain Med. 2014;39(5):368–80.

Muscle and Myofascial Pain

35

Rene Przkora, Pavel Balduyeu, and Andrea Trescot

Introduction

Myalgia is a general term for pain in a muscle or muscles [1]. *Myofascial pain* has been defined as "pain associated with inflammation or irritation of muscle or of the fascia surrounding the muscle" [2]. *Myofascial pain syndrome* (MPS) describes a soft tissue pain syndrome where the pain is present primarily in a single region or quadrant of the body, as compared to other soft tissue pain syndromes, such as chronic fatigue syndrome, hypermobility syndrome, or fibromyalgia, where the pain is generalized. It can be acute or chronic; it can also be posttraumatic, persisting beyond the "normal" time of healing, usually beyond 3 or 6 months [1, 3].

Pain associated with MPS is thought to be of muscular origin, arising from *muscular trigger points* (MTrPs) in taut muscle bands. The central feature of MPS is the MTrP [1]. MTrPs can be active or latent. Characteristic of an active MTrP is the finding of a tender spot during deep palpation of an affected skeletal muscle corresponding to the patient's usual pain, with referral of pain to a specific area within the muscle or to an entirely different area. A latent MTrP does not cause passive spontaneous pain, but pain can be caused by manual pressure over the MTrP. Both active and passive MTrP should cause a pain in a reference zone.

MTrPs can be activated indirectly by other existing MTrPs, visceral disease, arthritic joints, joint dysfunctions, and emotional distress [3]. MPS can occur alone or in combination with other medical conditions such as spinal pain [3], and it is differentiated from inflammatory myositis and from fibromyalgia, both of which are defined as chronic, widespread pain associated with muscle tenderness, but without MTrPs. The prevalence of myofascial pain is estimated to be 8% in academic general internal clinics among all visits and 30% among visits with a primary complain of pain [4].

Anatomy and Pathophysiology

The pathophysiology of MPS is complex and not completely understood, but significant progress has been made to explain, at least in part, the findings and clinical course of patients with MPS.

Muscle Fibers and Sensation

Muscle fibers contain nociceptors and non-nociceptors. *Nociception* is the activity induced in neural pathways by potentially tissue-damaging stimuli (e.g., mechanical, chemical, thermal) [5]. Nociceptors are free nerve endings connected to the CNS by thin myelinated or unmyelinated afferent fibers [1], but their exact structure is not defined, and they are indistinguishable from thermoreceptive or mechanoreceptive receptors under electron microscopy. However, the presence of differing morphological types of free nerve ending in muscle supports the assumption that these receptors do not form a homogeneous group, but consist of functionally different types [1]. Non-nociceptors represent a separate class termed "ergoreceptors"; these mediate circulatory and respiratory adjustments during muscle work.

Trigger Point "Triggers"

Development of myofascial pain depends on multiple predisposing and causative factors [6]:

- Genetics (temperament, intelligence, cognitive/emotional characteristics, gender)

R. Przkora · P. Balduyeu
Department of Anesthesiology, College of Medicine, University of Florida, Gainesville, FL, USA

A. Trescot (✉)
Pain and Headache Center, Eagle River, AK, USA

© Springer Nature Switzerland AG 2019
Y. Khelemsky et al. (eds.), *Academic Pain Medicine*, https://doi.org/10.1007/978-3-030-18005-8_35

- Environment (trauma, chronic repetitive muscle strain, physical/sexual/emotional status, poor posture, diet, education, income, coping skills)
- Stochastic (hormonal, systemic disease, neuromuscular lesions, age of trauma)
- Nutritional (vitamin D, B complex, iron)

These triggering and predisposing factors can cause the development of latent MTrPs, which subsequently can be activated.

Trigger Points and Biochemical Changes

Trigger points are areas of discrete palpable tenderness and spasm, potentially caused by excessive acetylcholine (ACh) release [1]. They are reproducible in location and pattern and are thought to represent areas of ischemia within the muscle. When ischemic muscle goes into spasm, it causes decreased blood flow, which causes a shift to anaerobic metabolism, resulting in accumulation of lactic acid, which causes more spasm [1]. This theory is supported by research analyzing the fluid content of human skeletal MTrP, demonstrating elevated concentrations of proteins, bradykinin, calcitonin, calcitonin gene-related peptide, substance P, tumor necrosis factor-a, interleukin-1b, serotonin, norepinephrine, and lower pH [7]. These conditions are potentially responsible for nociceptor activation and further increase of ACh release, leading to more spasms and taut bands [1]. The observation of spontaneous electrical activity measured via needle electromyography in MTrPs supports this hypothesis [8]. Interestingly, the injection of phentolamine, a vasodilator and alpha 1 blocker, eliminates this spontaneous electrical activity, supporting the theory of an ischemic role in MPS [9].

Peripheral and Central Sensitization and Referred Pain

The activation of peripheral receptors in the muscle is primarily detected by group III (thinly myelinated) and group IV (unmyelinated) nerve fibers that transmit the signal to the spinal cord via the dorsal horn. The sensory input then expands in the dorsal horn of the spinal cord, resulting in the patterns of referred pain (pain "felt" in an area different of its origin) that has been observed in patients with MPS [1].

It is important to understand that referred pain is not specific to MPS. Referred pain is a common symptom in intervertebral disc disease, facet joint syndrome, and diseases of internal organs, such as myocardial infarction or pancreatitis [10]. As an example, cervical trigger points can frequently resemble pain caused by cervical facet joint syndrome, since both syndromes have referred pain to the occipital, temporal, and frontal areas of the head [11].

Peripheral sensitization is described as a reduction in the pain threshold and an increase in responsiveness of the peripheral nociceptors which could be caused by a variety of endogenous substances, including neuropeptides and inflammatory mediators [2]. In contrast, *central sensitization* occurs when there has been chronic stimulation at the spinal cord level because of persistent myofascial pain, changes occur at the dorsal horn neurons that produce long-lasting increases in the excitability of the spinal pathways. Active trigger points by nociceptive stimulation from the muscle can initiate peripheral sensitization which could further sensitize dorsal horn neurons causing central sensitization. Similarly, central sensitization can also promote trigger point activity.

Clinical Presentation and Diagnosis

Pain Complaints

Patients with active myofascial MTrPs usually complain of localized, deep, aching pain in the tissues, including the muscles and joints. They rarely complain of sharp, cutaneous-type pain. The myofascial pain may be referred to a site distant from the MTrP, often in a pattern that is characteristic for each muscle. Sometimes, the patient is aware of numbness or paresthesia rather than, or in addition to, pain [12]. MPS can be difficult to diagnose because the MTrP may be in a different place than the pain site.

Autonomic, Motor, and Sleep Dysfunction

Autonomic dysfunction caused by MTrPs includes abnormal sweating, persistent lacrimation, persistent coryza, excessive salivation, and pilomotor activities. Related proprioceptive disturbances caused by MTrPs include imbalance, dizziness, tinnitus, tension headaches [3, 12], and distorted weight perception of lifted objects.

Dysfunction of motor units caused by MTrPs includes spasm of other muscles, weakness, loss of coordination, and decreased work tolerance [3, 12].

Sleep can be affected by MTrPs pain. This, in turn, can increase pain sensitivity the next day [3].

Clinical Assessment

Common findings in MPS include pain migration, pain with movement, sudden onset ("I just woke up with it"), and non-radicular patterns of pain. There are often traumatic triggers, such as chronic repetitive motions or motor vehicle acci-

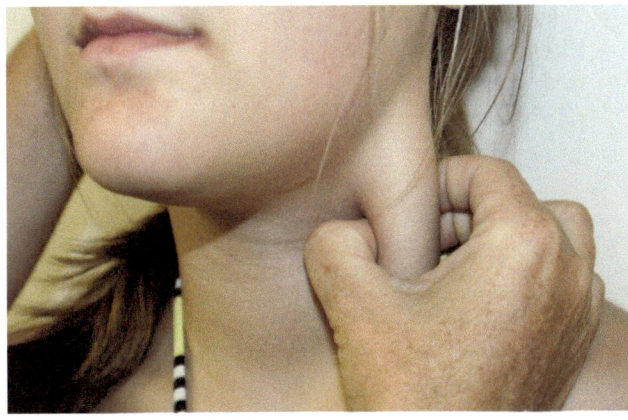

Fig. 35.1 Physical examination of trigger points. (Image courtesy of Andrea Trescot, MD)

dents. Manual palpation is considered to be subjective and unreliable [13, 14], but together with clinical presentation, it remains a mainstay to the diagnosis. Generally, by gentle rubbing across the direction of the muscle fibers of a superficial muscle (tangentially, "like strumming a guitar string") (Fig. 35.1), the examiner can feel a nodule at the MTrP and a rope-like induration that extends from this nodule to the attachment of the taut muscle fibers at each end of the muscle. Alternatively, a taut band can be snapped or rolled under the finger in accessible muscles. Palpation along the taut band reveals a nodule exhibiting a highly localized, exquisitely tender spot that is characteristic of an MTrP [3, 13]. Application of digital pressure on either an active or latent MTrP can elicit a referred pain pattern characteristic of that muscle, though injection of the MTrP may be more effective in eliciting the referral pattern [15]. If the patient "recognizes" the elicited sensation as a familiar experience, this establishes the MTrPs as being active and is one of the most important diagnostic criteria available. In addition to referred pain, MTrPs may elicit other sensory changes such as tenderness and dysesthesias. Snapping palpation of the MTrP frequently evokes a transient twitch response of the taut band fibers, called a "jump sign" [12]. The same twitch response can be elicit by needle penetration and is thought to be due to the transient reflex contraction of a group of tense muscle fibers that traverse the MTrP. As a consequence, muscles with active MTrPs have a restricted passive (stretch) range of motion because of pain, and when strongly contracted against fixed resistance, they elicit further pain [12].

EMG

MTrPs can be identified by needle electromyography (EMG) as there is a presence of spontaneous low-voltage motor end-plate activity as well as high-voltage spike activity that is highly characteristic of, but not pathognomonic for, MTrPs [8, 16, 17].

Imaging

Trigger points can be visualized by *ultrasound* but generally for guidance in injection rather than diagnostically (Fig. 35.2) [18]. *Magnetic resonance elastography* (MRE) can quantitate asymmetries in muscle tone that could previously only be identified subjectively by examination [19]. *Thermography* has been used to identify trigger points, but is difficult to translate into useful intervention [20]. An *algometer*, *pressure dolorimeter*, or electrical stimulation may be used to assess the response to stimulation of the trigger point when compared to the surrounding muscle tissue. But, despite emerging imaging techniques, MPS remains predominantly a clinical diagnosis.

Travell and Simons proposed the following criteria for the diagnosis of MTrPs [3]:

Essential criteria:

1. Taut band palpable (muscle accessible to palpation)
2. Exquisite spot tenderness of a nodule in a taut band
3. Patient's recognition of current pain complaint by pressure on the tender nodule (identification of an active trigger point)
4. Painful limit to full stretch range of motion

Confirmatory observations:

1. Visual or tactile identification of local twitch response
2. Ultrasound imaging of local twitch response induced by needle penetration of tender nodule
3. Pain or altered sensation (in the distribution expected from a trigger point in the muscle) on compression of the tender nodule
4. Electromyographic demonstration of spontaneous electrical activity characteristic of active loci in the tender nodule of a taut band

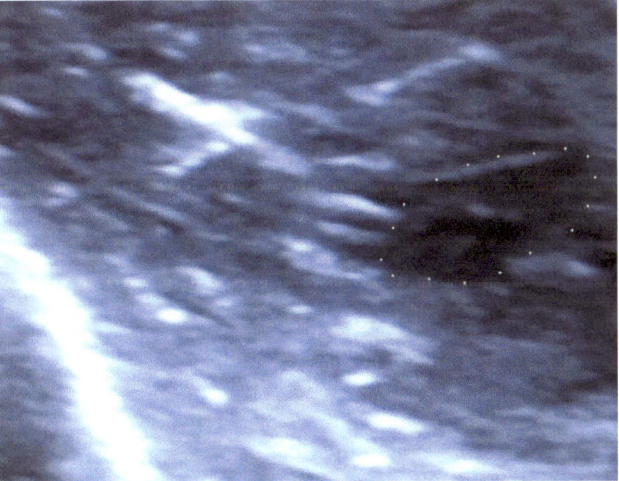

Fig. 35.2 Ultrasound evaluation of trigger point. (Image courtesy of Rene Przkora, MD, PhD)

Treatment

When treating MPS, it is important to identify and treat predisposing and perpetuating factors. If the underlying pathology is not given the appropriate treatment, the MTrP cannot be completely and permanently inactivated. Treatment of active MTrPs may be necessary in situations in which active MTrPs persist even after the underlying etiologic lesion has been treated appropriately [21].

The goal is to eliminate the trigger points, reverse trigger point-induced weakness, restore normal muscle function, and decrease pain. It should be a systematic and multidisciplinary effort. Conservative or less invasive modalities should be considered first before advancing to more invasive treatment options.

Patient Education

One first step is patient education about the underlying pathophysiology and possible central sensitization. Studies have shown that patients who have insight into their conditions are able to make better treatment choices [22].

Physical Modalities

Several physical modalities have been shown to be beneficial in MPS. Lifestyle and ergonomic adjustments are recommended. Stretching appears to correlate well with the proposed pathophysiology of shortened muscle sarcomeres in MPS. The use of Kinesio tape has also been found useful [23]. Based on observations by Travell and Simons [3], passive stretching after the application of vapocoolant spray to reduce pain ("spray and stretch") was termed the "single most effective treatment" for patients suffering from MPS. Transcutaneous electric nerve stimulation (TENS) has been studied using different modes of stimulation and intensity, and results are promising, with a reduction in pain and increase in pain threshold. However, as improvements usually cease soon after therapy, TENS should not be used as monotherapy in MPS [24]. A newer intervention, magnetic stimulation, may have beneficial effects in MPS based on limited studies [24].

Summary of physical modalities

- Ischemic compression [25]
- Stretching exercises, medicine ball exercises [26]
- Spray and stretch technique [3]
- Myofascial therapy or myofascial release therapy [27]
- Massage therapy: "Milk" the lactic acid out of the muscles [28]
- Transcutaneous electrical nerve stimulation (TENS) [29]

- Iontophoresis [30]
- Ultrasound therapy [29, 31, 32]
- Laser therapy [33, 34]
- Hyperbaric oxygen therapy [35]

Pharmacologic Interventions

Currently, there are no FDA-approved medications for the treatment of MPS. Several medication classes have been used to treat patients with MPS, but there is a paucity of randomized controlled trials (RCTs) addressing the effectiveness of systemic medications in MPS. Most recommendations are drawn from the treatment of similar syndromes such as fibromyalgia.

Among the systemic medications studied in MPS, nonsteroidal anti-inflammatory drugs (NSAIDs) have been used most successfully, including during the acute phase. Unfortunately, there is concern about the side effects of long-term use of NSAIDs with regard to cardiac, gastrointestinal, and renal complications [36]. Data regarding the effectiveness of "muscle relaxants" are limited; some evidence supports efficacy of the alpha-2 adrenergic agonist tizanidine [24]. Opioids have been used for MPS, but the current evidence is so limited that this type of therapy is usually not recommended [24], especially with the additional risks of opioid therapy such as tolerance, immunosuppression, hormonal imbalance, addiction, overdose, and diversion [37]. Although there is evidence that tricyclic antidepressants (i.e., amitriptyline), serotonin-norepinephrine reuptake inhibitors (i.e., duloxetine), and membrane stabilizers (i.e., gabapentin, pregabalin) are beneficial in other soft tissue pain syndromes such as fibromyalgia or temporomandibular pain, their effectiveness in patients with MPS has not been clearly demonstrated and other interventions should be tried first [24]. In contrast, topical anesthetics/analgesics, such as patches containing lidocaine or diclofenac, can be considered since studies have shown a decrease in pain and improved range of motion of affected body areas in the limited studies available [24, 38–40].

Summary of pharmacologic interventions

- NSAIDs
- Muscle relaxants
- Topical anesthetic/NSAID patches

Injection/Needle Therapy

Trigger point injections (TPIs) (Fig. 35.3) are part of the comprehensive treatment plan of patients with MPS;

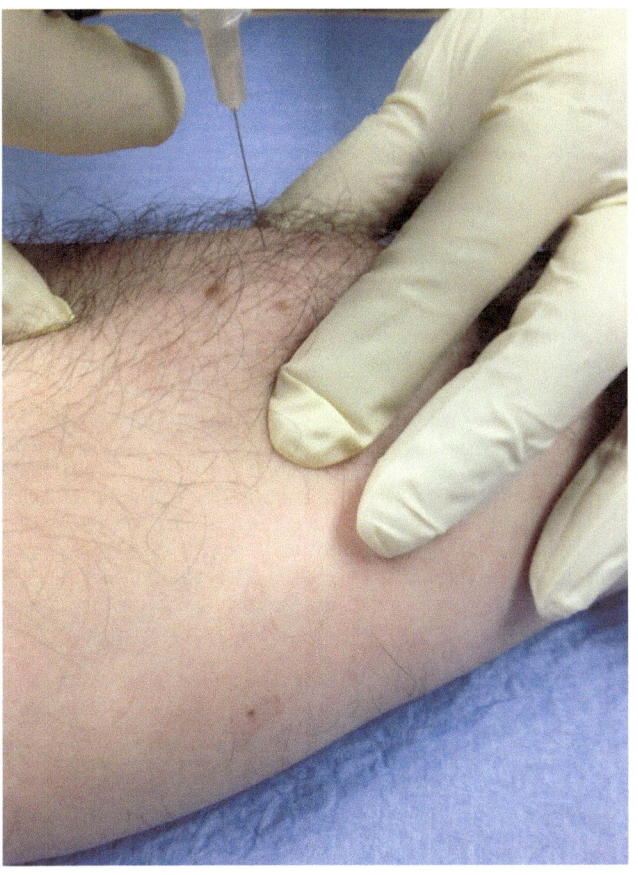

Fig. 35.3 Trigger point injection. (Image courtesy of Rene Przkora, MD, PhD)

details, such as one versus many needles, site of the needle placement (the center of the MTrP instead of the acupuncture site), movement of the needle, the depth of needle insertion, the force of stimulation, and the elicitation of a "local twitch response" (LTR) [46]. Though there are many variations in techniques, the use of multiple rapid needle insertions seems to be the most effective [47].

Dry needling and local anesthetic injections appear to be similarly effective; however, the addition of a local anesthetic helps to avoid postinjection soreness that develops in up to 100% cases after dry needling, depending on the needle size [41].

Use of botulinum toxin type A for MTrP injections remains controversial, although a growing number of studies demonstrate clinical benefit for MTrPs and related pain conditions such as tension-type headaches and dystonia [48]. Botulinum toxin works by preventing ACh release from the presynaptic nerve terminal and decreasing spasm and may also have a direct antinociceptive effect [49].

Summary of injection/needle therapy

- Acupuncture
- Dry needling
- Local anesthetic injections
- Botulinum toxin type A injections

however, they should not be the only treatment approach given the underlying pathophysiology. Elicitation of a local muscle twitch response during TPIs appears to correlate with the best result [41]. TPIs are commonly performed by pain physicians and primary care providers and are the second most common pain procedure after epidural steroid injections in Canada [42]. There is no difference clinically if the injectate contains local anesthetics alone or the addition of nonsteroidal anti-inflammatory drugs, vitamins, or steroids. Ultrasound may be considered in order to better visualize the surrounding anatomy (i.e., blood vessels, nerves, pleura) and selectively inject desired muscles and fascial planes.

Acupuncture has also been used for MPS. Practiced for thousands of years, acupuncture relies on a series of meridians to locate needle locations. These acupuncture sites are very close to common trigger point injection sites. Although there can be demonstrable pain relief, it is often short-lived [43]. One randomized trial noted no improvement of acupuncture over lidocaine injections for myofascial pain [44].

Dry needling, also known as *intramuscular stimulation* (IMS), is a technique popularized by Gunn [45]. Acupuncture and dry needling are different techniques, differing not just in underlying philosophies but also in many of the technical

References

1. Mense S, Gerwin RD. Muscle pain: understanding the mechanisms. New York: Springer; 2010.
2. Mosby's Dictionary of Medicine, Nursing & Health Professions. St. Louis: Mosby; 2009.
3. Travell J, Simons D. Travell & Simons' myofascial pain and dysfunction: the trigger point manual. Philadelphia: Lippincott Williams & Wilkins; 1992.
4. Skootsky SA, Jaeger B, Oye RK. Prevalence of myofascial pain in general internal medicine practice. West J Med. 1989;151(2):157–60.
5. Portenoy RK, Kanner RM. Pain management: theory and practice. Philadelphia: F. A. Davis; 1996.
6. Gerwin RD. Classification, epidemiology, and natural history of myofascial pain syndrome. Curr Pain Headache Rep. 2001;5(5):412–20.
7. Shah JP, Phillips TM, Danoff JV, Gerber LH. An in vivo microanalytical technique for measuring the local biochemical milieu of human skeletal muscle. J Appl Physiol. 2005;99(5):1977–84.
8. Hubbard DR, Berkoff GM. Myofascial trigger points show spontaneous needle EMG activity. Spine. 1993;18(13):1803–7.
9. Hubbard DR. Chronic and recurrent muscle pain. J Musculoskel Pain. 1996;4(1–2):123–44.
10. Vecchiet L, Vecchiet J, Giamberardino MA. Referred muscle pain: clinical and pathophysiologic aspects. Curr Rev Pain. 1999;3(6):489–98.
11. Bogduk N, Simons DG. Neck pain: joint pain or trigger points. In: Vaeroy H, Merskey H, editors. Progress in fibromyalgia and myofascial pain. Pain research and clinical management. Amsterdam: Elsevier; 1993.

12. Mense S, Gerwin R. Muscle pain: diagnosis and treatment. New York: Springer; 2010.

13. Myburgh C, Larsen AH, Hartvigsen J. A systematic, critical review of manual palpation for identifying myofascial trigger points: evidence and clinical significance. Arch Phys Med Rehabil. 2008;89(6):1169–76.

14. Gerwin RD, Shannon S, Hong CZ, Hubbard D, Gevirtz R. Interrater reliability in myofascial trigger point examination. Pain. 1997;69(1–2):65–73.

15. Hong CZ, Kuan TS, Chen JT, Chen SM. Referred pain elicited by palpation and by needling of myofascial trigger points: a comparison. Arch Phys Med Rehabil. 1997;78(9):957–60.

16. Ojala TA, Arokoski JPA, Partanen JV. Needle-electromyography findings of trigger points in neck-shoulder area before and after injection treatment. J Musculoskel Pain. 2006;14(1):5–14.

17. Simons DG, Hong C-Z, Simons LS. Prevalence of spontaneous electrical activity at trigger spots and at control sites in rabbit skeletal muscle. J Musculoskel Pain. 1995;3(1):35–48.

18. Sikdar S, Shah JP, Gilliams E, Gebreab T, Gerber LH, editors. Assessment of myofascial trigger points (MTrPs): a new application of ultrasound imaging and vibration sonoelastography. 30th Annual International IEEE EMBS Conference; Vancouver, BC, Canada; 2008.

19. Chen Q, Bensamoun S, Basford JR, Thompson JM, An KN. Identification and quantification of myofascial taut bands with magnetic resonance elastography. Arch Phys Med Rehabil. 2007;88(12):1658–61.

20. Dibai-Filho AV, Guirro RR. Evaluation of myofascial trigger points using infrared thermography: a critical review of the literature. J Manipulative Physiol Ther. 2015;38(1):86–92.

21. Hong CZ. Treatment of myofascial pain syndrome. Curr Pain Headache Rep. 2006;10(5):345–9.

22. Bandura A. Self-efficacy mechanism in physiological activation and health-promoting behavior. In: Madden JL, Matthysse S, Barchas S, editors. Adaption, learning, and affect. New York: Raven Press; 1986.

23. Wu WT, Hong CZ, Chou LW. The Kinesio Taping method for myofascial pain control. Evid Based Complement Alternat Med. 2015;2015:950519.

24. Desai MJ, Saini V, Saini S. Myofascial pain syndrome: a treatment review. Pain Ther. 2013;2(1):21–36.

25. Cagnie B, Castelein B, Pollie F, Steelant L, Verhoeyen H, Cools A. Evidence for the use of ischemic compression and dry needling in the management of trigger points of the opper trapezius in patients with neck pain: a systematic review. Am J Phys Med Rehabil. 2015;94(7):573–83.

26. Quinn SL, Olivier B, Wood WA. The short-term effects of trigger point therapy, stretching and medicine ball exercises on accuracy and back swing hip turn in elite, male golfers – a randomised controlled trial. Phys Ther Sport. 2016;22:16–22.

27. Ajimsha MS, Al-Mudahka NR, Al-Madzhar JA. Effectiveness of myofascial release: systematic review of randomized controlled trials. J Bodyw Mov Ther. 2015;19(1):102–12.

28. Menard MB. Immediate effect of therapeutic massage on pain sensation and unpleasantness: a consecutive case series. Glob Adv Health Med. 2015;4(5):56–60.

29. Rai S, Ranjan V, Misra D, Panjwani S. Management of myofascial pain by therapeutic ultrasound and transcutaneous electrical nerve stimulation: a comparative study. Eur J Dent. 2016;10(1):46–53.

30. Kaya A, Kamanli A, Ardicoglu O, Ozgocmen S, Ozkurt-Zengin F, Bayik Y. Direct current therapy with/without lidocaine iontophoresis in myofascial pain syndrome. Bratisl Lek Listy. 2009;110(3):185–91.

31. Srbely JZ, Dickey JP. Randomized controlled study of the antinociceptive effect of ultrasound on trigger point sensitivity: novel applications in myofascial therapy? Clin Rehabil. 2007;21(5):411–7.

32. Kavadar G, Caglar N, Ozen S, Tutun S, Demircioglu D. Efficacy of conventional ultrasound therapy on myofascial pain syndrome: a placebo controlled study. Agri. 2015;27(4):190–6.

33. Carrasco TG, Guerisoli LD, Guerisoli DM, Mazzetto MO. Evaluation of low intensity laser therapy in myofascial pain syndrome. Cranio. 2009;27(4):243–7.

34. Snyder-Mackler L, Bork C, Bourbon B, Trumbore D. Effect of helium-neon laser on musculoskeletal trigger points. Phys Ther. 1986;66(7):1087–90.

35. Kiralp MZ, Uzun G, Dincer O, Sen A, Yildiz S, Tekin L, et al. A novel treatment modality for myofascial pain syndrome: hyperbaric oxygen therapy. J Natl Med Assoc. 2009;101(1):77–80.

36. Lacey PH, Dodd GD, Shannon DJ. A double blind, placebo controlled study of piroxicam in the management of acute musculoskeletal disorders. Eur J Rheumatol Inflamm. 1984;7(3):95–104.

37. Benyamin R, Trescot AM, Datta S, Buenaventura R, Adlaka R, Sehgal N, et al. Opioid complications and side effects. Pain Physician. 2008;11(2 Suppl):S105–20.

38. Hsieh LF, Hong CZ, Chern SH, Chen CC. Efficacy and side effects of diclofenac patch in treatment of patients with myofascial pain syndrome of the upper trapezius. J Pain Symptom Manage. 2010;39(1):116–25.

39. Affaitati G, Fabrizio A, Savini A, Lerza R, Tafuri E, Costantini R, et al. A randomized, controlled study comparing a lidocaine patch, a placebo patch, and anesthetic injection for treatment of trigger points in patients with myofascial pain syndrome: evaluation of pain and somatic pain thresholds. Clin Ther. 2009;31(4):705–20.

40. Firmani M, Miralles R, Casassus R. Effect of lidocaine patches on upper trapezius EMG activity and pain intensity in patients with myofascial trigger points: a randomized clinical study. Acta Odontol Scand. 2015;73(3):210–8.

41. Hong CZ. Lidocaine injection versus dry needling to myofascial trigger point. The importance of the local twitch response. Am J Phys Med Rehabil. 1994;73(4):256–63.

42. Peng PW, Castano ED. Survey of chronic pain practice by anesthesiologists in Canada. Can J Anaesth. 2005;52(4):383–9.

43. Kung YY, Chen FP, Chaung HL, Chou CT, Tsai YY, Hwang SJ. Evaluation of acupuncture effect to chronic myofascial pain syndrome in the cervical and upper back regions by the concept of Meridians. Acupunct Electrother Res. 2001;26(3):195–202.

44. Ga H, Choi JH, Park CH, Yoon HJ. Acupuncture needling versus lidocaine injection of trigger points in myofascial pain syndrome in elderly patients – a randomised trial. Acupunct Med. 2007;25(4):130–6.

45. Gunn CC. Neuropathic myofascial pain syndromes. In: Loeser JD, Butler SH, Chapman CR, Turk DC, editors. Bonica's managment of pain. 3rd ed. Philadelphia: Lippincott Williams & Wilkins; 2001.

46. Cagnie B, Dewitte V, Barbe T, Timmermans F, Delrue N, Meeus M. Physiologic effects of dry needling. Curr Pain Headache Rep. 2013;17(8):348.

47. Chou LW, Hsieh YL, Kuan TS, Hong CZ. Needling therapy for myofascial pain: recommended technique with multiple rapid needle insertion. Biomedicine. 2014;4:13.

48. Khalifeh M, Mehta K, Varguise N, Suarez-Durall P, Enciso R. Botulinum toxin type A for the treatment of head and neck chronic myofascial pain syndrome: a systematic review and meta-analysis. J Am Dent Assoc. 2016;147(12):959–73.e1.

49. Hackett R, Kam PC. Botulinum toxin: pharmacology and clinical developments: a literature review. Med Chem. 2007;3(4):333–45.

Regenerative Medicine

Jonathan Snitzer, Sunny Patel, Xiao Zheng,
Houman Danesh, and Yury Khelemsky

Introduction

Regenerative medicine encompasses approaches to treat pain by using mostly biologic compounds with the goal of repairing damaged tissues. This chapter will address two main implements of this branch of pain medicine: platelet-rich plasma (PRP) and stem cells.

Platelet-Rich Plasma (PRP)

History

The concept of regenerative medicine existed long before stem cells or platelet-rich plasma (PRP). In Aristotle's time, observations of salamander tail regeneration started to inform the concepts of the body's regenerative capacity. PRP was used as early as the 1950s for dermatologic conditions [1]. In 1987, PRP was used during open-heart surgery to augment healing and to avoid homologous blood product transfusion [2]. In the 1990s, PRP use gradually increased, especially in oral maxillofacial surgery, where it was associated with improved graft success [3]. In the 2000s, PRP grew in popularity in the fields of orthopedics and sports medicine, given its promise of augmenting the body's natural bone-healing mechanisms [4]. Mishra and Pavelko in 2006 integrated PRP into the specialty of pain management by showing a significant reduc-

tion in pain after PRP injection for chronic lateral epicondylitis [5]. The use of PRP by athletes such as Hines Ward and Tiger Woods has accelerated the interest in PRP for musculoskeletal conditions in both the medical and public world.

Definition

Platelet-rich plasma (PRP) is defined as plasma with supraphysiologic concentrations of platelets and other cellular components. The normal range for platelets in whole blood is 150,000–450,000 platelets per microliter. While there is no standardized concentration of platelets and other cell types that is required for PRP, in general the range is between 3 and 9× baseline concentration. Greater than four times baseline platelet concentration or 1–1.5 million/microL of platelets is thought to be therapeutic [6–8]. Additionally, there are no standardized mechanisms for collecting and preparing PRP. As a result, there are qualitative and quantitative differences between injectates, making research and evaluation of efficacy extremely difficult.

Platelets contain a plethora of growth factors, enzymes, and other bioactive compounds within alpha-granules that are involved in wound and tissue healing [1]. The main growth factors associated with tissue healing are platelet-derived growth factor (PDGF), transforming growth factor beta (TGF-B), vascular endothelial growth factor (VEGF), insulin-like growth factor (IGF-1), hepatocyte growth factor (HGH), fibroblast growth factor (FGF), and epidermal growth factor (EGF) [9]. Appropriate concentrations and presence of white blood cells (WBC) are currently under debate. The concern regarding WBC and neutrophils is that their activating role in the inflammatory process could further exacerbate and delay healing [10, 11].

Currently, there are a variety of PRP classification systems. The revised system formed by Dohan Ehrenfest consists of four groups: pure platelet-rich plasma (P-PRP),

J. Snitzer
Pain Management Specialist, Fairview Clinics, Blaine, MN, USA

S. Patel · X. Zheng
Icahn School of Medicine at Mount Sinai, New York, NY, USA

H. Danesh
Department of Anesthesiology, Perioperative and Pain Medicine, Mount Sinai Hospital, New York, NY, USA

Y. Khelemsky (✉)
Department of Anesthesiology, Mount Sinai Medical Center, New York, NY, USA

© Springer Nature Switzerland AG 2019
Y. Khelemsky et al. (eds.), *Academic Pain Medicine*, https://doi.org/10.1007/978-3-030-18005-8_36

Table 36.1 PLRA Classification

PLRA classification		Criteria	Final score
P	Platelet count	Volume injected	Cells/µL
L	Leukocyte content	>1%	+
		<1%	−
R	Red blood cell content	>1%	+
		<1%	−
A	Activation	Yes	+
		No	−

leukocyte- and platelet-rich plasma (L-PRP), pure platelet-rich fibrin (P-PRF), and leukocyte- and platelet-rich fibrin (L-PRF) [12]. Another sports medicine-centered classification system focuses on the concentration of platelets and leukocytes and whether the sample is activated. There are four groups: L-PRP solution, L-PRP gel, P-PRP solution, and P-PRP gel [13]. The PLRA classification system (Table 36.1) proposed by Mautner attempts to include the critical components from the other classification systems: platelet concentration, leukocyte concentration, red blood cells, activation agent, and volume of injectate. The PLRA system's goal is to standardize the important aspects of the injectate in order to make evaluation of treatment outcomes more meaningful [14].

Derivation

PRP is derived from a sample of autologous whole blood drawn from the patient. Sterile precautions are extremely important when collecting the patient's blood in order to prevent infection [4]. Additionally, care should be used to avoid unnecessary trauma to prevent premature activation of platelets and the clotting cascade. Currently, there are a variety of different systems and processes used for PRP preparation. These vary in initial volume of the whole blood, final volume, final concentration of leukocytes, platelets, and other growth factors, rate and number of cycles, spin time of centrifuge, and the addition of an activating agent. In general, once the blood is drawn, an anticoagulant (citrate-dextrose) is added to prevent activation of the clotting cascade. The sample is then prepared using one of two general methods: PRP or buffy-coat. In the PRP method, two cycles of centrifugation are performed: the first cycle, termed the soft spin (1200–1500 RPM), separates the RBCs from the remaining whole blood and the second cycle, termed the hard spin (4000–7000), separates PRP from the platelet-poor plasma (PPP). In the buffy-coat method, high-speed centrifugation is performed, separating the sample into three layers: red blood cells, buffy-coat (platelets/white blood cells), and PPP [15]. The buffy-coat layer is then centrifuged again resulting in a higher concentration of platelets.

Indications/Uses

Tendon Pathology

Overuse injuries are common and can affect tendons throughout the body, and ultimately lead to tendinosis. In general, tendon healing is slower than other tissues due to poor vascular supply. PRP has been used to treat a variety of different tendon pathologies. Some of the best data for PRP use is in the treatment of lateral epicondylitis, also known as tennis elbow. The incidence of lateral epicondylitis can be as high as 2% [16]. Mishra and Pavelko first illustrated the promise of PRP in their sentinel unblinded study of 20 patients with lateral epicondylitis. They showed significant improvement in VAS scores following PRP injection at up to 3 years post-injection [5]. In a randomized double-blinded controlled trial of 100 patients comparing steroid and PRP injections for lateral epicondylitis, there was significant improvement in both VAS and DASH scores at 26 and 52 weeks in the PRP group [17]. Additionally, at 2-year follow-up, 81% of the PRP group had >25% reduction in their VAS scores compared to only 40% of those in the steroid group [17]. Conversely, in a randomized double-blinded study comparing steroid, saline, and PRP injection for lateral epicondylitis, there was no statistical difference between the groups [18].

PRP has also been shown to be an effective treatment for other tendinopathies such as plantar fasciitis and Achilles tendinosis [19]. Jain and colleagues in a randomized trial of 60 patients comparing PRP and steroid injections for plantar fasciitis demonstrated a significant improvement in VAS, range of motion, and American Orthopaedic Foot and Ankle Surgery (AOFAS) scores at 1 year [20]. Of note, there was no statistical difference at either 3 or 6 months. In a randomized study of 40 patients comparing steroids to PRP injections for chronic plantar fasciitis, PRP was shown to be more effective, with improved AOFAS scores at 3, 6, 12, and 24 months [21].

Intra-articular Pathology

As with tendinous pathologies, intra-articular cartilage injuries and degeneration exhibit slow and poor healing. Knee osteoarthritis (OA) is extremely common and has a tremendous economic burden on our society. As of 2012, approximately 46 million Americans suffer from knee OA, with nearly 50% of people over the age of 85 having symptomatic knee OA [22]. OA is thought to be secondary to an imbalance of pro-inflammatory and anti-inflammatory cytokines ultimately leading to cartilage destruction [23]. PRP has been shown to not only mediate the inflammatory response and improve vascular supply but also to stimulate chondrogenesis [24]. In a large meta-analysis and systemic review of PRP for knee OA, PRP injections demonstrated efficacy at 6–12 months [25, 26]. Additionally, there was a trend toward superiority over viscosupplementation in both duration of action and reduction in pain [25]. Interestingly, the reduction in pain scores was significantly greater in patients with mild to moderate OA compared to more severe cases [26]. Conversely, in a large randomized controlled trial of 443 patients, PRP was shown to be no more effective than viscosupplementation [27]. Of note, both interventions showed improvement in pain scores and functionality. PRP injections have been used to treat arthritis in other joints. A randomized controlled trial comparing PRP alone to PRP and hyaluronic acid (HA) and HA alone for hip OA revealed that the PRP group had lower VAS scores at 2, 6, and 12 months post-injection, but the results were only clinically significant at 6 months [28].

Ligament Pathology

Current randomized trials are limited for PRP use for ligament injuries, although interest of using PRP for partial tears as an alternative to surgery is increasing. Avoiding surgery while expediting and optimizing healing is of extreme interest especially in the world of athletics. In a retrospective study of 44 pitchers receiving one to three PRP injection following partial ulnar collateral ligament tears, the patients had significantly better outcomes compared to prior conservative therapy standards [29, 30]. Using the modified Conway scale, 15 patients had excellent results, 17 had good results, 2 had fair results, and 10 had poor outcomes. Of note, 4 out of 6 of the professional pitchers in the study were able to return to pitch in Major League Baseball. PRP has also been used to improve healing following anterior cruciate ligament (ACL) injuries. A large systematic review did not show any clinically significant benefit of using PRP during ACL repair surgery [31].

Disc and Spine Pathology

Presently, there is growing interest in the application of PRP to the treatment of low back pain, although current research is still limited. Facet joints are synovial joints, and like peripheral synovial joints may develop degenerative changes secondary to injury or overuse. As a result, the use of PRP may be an effective treatment to both decrease inflammation and stimulate healing. In a small prospective study, 19 patients with facet joint syndrome received intra-articular facet joint injections with PRP [32]. Patients were followed up for 3 months, and 15 of the 19 patients had either good or

excellent relief [32]. These results are encouraging, but this study is significantly limited secondary to the absence of a control group.

PRP is also being explored as a treatment option for symptomatic degenerative disc disease. A recent double-blind randomized controlled study demonstrated significant improvement at 8 weeks in the Numeric Rating Scale (NRS), Functional Rating Index (FRI), and North American Spine Society (NASS) Outcome Questionnaire compared to the control group after patients received an intradiscal PRP injection [33]. Additionally, patients in the treatment group maintained significant improvement in their FRI score at 1 year [33].

PRP has also been used to treat sacroiliac (SI) joint pain. In a small case series of four patients with SI joint instability and chronic severe back pain, PRP was injected into the SI joint and patients were followed up at 12 and 48 months [34]. At 12 months, all patients reported significant improvement in their joint stability, back pain, and quality of life. These results were maintained at 48 months.

Complications and Contraindications

In general, if the sample is prepared appropriately using sterile technique and the procedure is performed with image guidance, the risk of complications is limited. As with any injection, there is a risk of bleeding or infection. Additionally, surrounding structures such nerves and vasculature can be injured. Although it is common to have an initial increase in pain following the injection, persistent worsening of pain is also possible [17]. Of note, for the initial increase in a pain following the procedure, it is preferred to avoid NSAIDs secondary to their inhibitory effects on platelets. There are a variety of absolute and relative contraindications to PRP injection, including but not limited to thrombocytopenia, platelet dysfunction, infection (systemic or local), anticoagulant therapy, metastatic cancer, and pregnancy.

Future Directions

The future of PRP for musculoskeletal pathology is promising. PRP injections are minimally invasive and have an excellent safety profile, making PRP a desirable treatment option. Currently, PRP research lacks standardization and in order to truly elucidate and demonstrate its effects, we will need to develop more consistent research models. Presently, the exact composition of different cell types and growth factors needed to optimize tissue healing is unknown.

Stem Cells

Terminology

Stem cells refer to lines of cells capable of proliferating and subsequently differentiating into the many tissues of an organism. This has sparked much ethical debate especially since the capability of harvesting them from human embryos became a reality in 1998. Given that disease processes that result in chronic pain are often result from an inability to regenerate damaged tissue, stem cell research has the potential to revolutionize the management of many chronic pain syndromes such as osteoarthritis, neuropathies, and tendinopathies [35]. Prior to reviewing this complex topic, key definitions are listed in Table 36.2.

Derivation and Techniques

Embryonic stem cells (ES) are collected from pre-implantation blastocysts. In the past, stem cells were removed from embryos fertilized in vitro or created from somatic cell nuclear transfer. Somatic cell nuclear transfer (SCNT) is the process of cloning in which a nuclear material from a somatic cell is transplanted into an enucleated egg cell. This ultimately produces an embryo genetically identical to the somatic donor. Embryos were allowed to form an inner cell mass which was abundant in stem cells. Harvesting the cells at this level of development led to the destruction of the embryo. Consequently, this process was the center of much of the ethical debate surrounding embryonic stem cell research. A newer process called altered nuclear transfer (ANT) proceeds much in the same manner as SCNT; however, the nuclear contents are modified to prevent the formation of a human embryo and still produce stem cells. Another new technique called blastomere extraction removed one of the eight blastomeres formed from a 2-day-old embryo, in which the remaining seven blastomeres were capable of being re-implanted into the mother and subsequently allowed to develop into healthy human embryos, assuming no defects were detected in genetic testing.

Adult stem cells (AS) are present in most tissues to maintain tissue and repair injuries. Hematopoietic stem cells differentiate into the various blood cell lines and are collected from bone marrow and peripheral blood. Bone marrow and blood is typically extracted from the hip using a large specialized needle. The aspirate undergoes a process called apheresis using a special machine in which stem cells were separated out from bone fragments, fat, and other components. Peripheral blood can also be used to obtain hematopoietic stem cells, although they are much fewer in number than in the bone marrow. Much of the interest in stem cells relating to pain management involves mesenchymal cells (MSCs) which give rise to fat, bone, cartilage, and connective tissue. Though they have classically been isolated from bone marrow, new techniques allow them to be obtained from fat using a less invasive liposuction procedure. The removed tissue then undergoes further filtration processes to isolate MSCs. The cells can then be grown in standard culture with different media, matrixes, cytokines, and growth factors to achieve desired differentiation.

Induced pluripotent stem cells (IPS) are obtained by a process of introducing genes present in pluripotent stem cells into mature cells when those genes are not typically expressed. This results in a few of those cells reverting back to a more immature, less differentiated state [36].

Therapeutic Targets

Discogenic Pain

The treatment of chronic lower back pain has been one of the most common uses of human mesenchymal stem cells in pain management. The process entails integration of cultured MSCs derived from bone marrow with nucleus pulposus cells to stimulate chondrogenic differentiation. These cells are then injected into degenerative discs in which they would serve to regenerate and buttress collagen matrices. Multiple small nonrandomized, uncontrolled studies have reported improvement in pain scores during a 1–2-year follow-up. One study following 10 patients with injection of BMSCs into the annulus fibrosis showed improvement in pain scores for low back and radicular pain [37].

The largest randomized controlled trial was initiated in 2007 in which 28 canine subjects were randomized to have percutaneous injection of damaged disc-derived chondrocytes injected into the annulus fibrosis 12 weeks after microdiscectomy or have microdiscectomy alone. MRI was used to confirm decreased reduction in disc height in the experimental group, with decreased pain scores, and decreased disability. It was also found that the experimental group had evidence of new proteoglycan and collagen formation in degenerative

Table 36.2 Key Definitions

Type of cells	Definition
Stem	Cells capable of self-renewal and differentiation
Totipotent	Capacity to differentiate into embryonic and extra-embryonic tissues (placental)
Pluripotent	Capacity to differentiate into tissue of the body derived from the embryonic germ layers that form the inner mass in the blastocyst (endoderm, mesoderm, ectoderm)
Multipotent	Capacity to differentiate into any cells of a particular germ layer
Unipotent	Capacity to differentiate into only one cell type

areas the level of injection [38]. Other studies have shown that injection of stem cells within intervertebral discs result in no improvement in lower back pain [39]. There is no consensus on this novel use of MSCs, though many studies are encouraging. Larger blinded RTCs are needed to further investigate intradiscal stem cell therapy to help elucidate its utility.

Osteoarthritis

There are no current FDA treatments approved for the use of stem cell injections to repair or regenerate damaged cartilage in osteoarthritis; however, research is ongoing. Mechanisms behind improvement in cartilage have been hypothesized to be due to secretion and promotion of growth factors/cytokines to repair damaged tissue and inhibition of MMP-13, a protein produced by chondrocytes that damages cartilage in OA. Several research projects are attempting to discern the efficacy of cartilage repair using injected autologous chondrocytes in comparison to mesenchymal stem cells. Most researchers speculate that MSCs should provide significant advantages over autologous chondrocytes due to abundance in all tissues, improved responsiveness to biologic and artificial manipulation, broad range of expression, and capacity to differentiate into regenerative tissue [40]. Studies have demonstrated that although the capacity to differentiate does not change with age, shear cell number and proliferative potential do decline. A small cohort study showed marked improvement in pain scores on the Western Ontario and McMaster Universities Osteoarthritis Index (WOMAC) after intra-articular injection of MSCs in a total of 12 patients who previously failed conservative management. T2 MRI showed improvement in knee cartilage quality and no adverse outcomes were reported [41]. Another randomized trial compared intra-articular knee injections of hyaluronic acid and MSCs and found that both groups reported improved pain, but cartilage quality appeared superior in the stem cell group [42]. Numerous other studies have been undertaken concluding that stem cell injections into joints have contributed to the healing of native cartilage [43]. Joint injection procedures have had a low incidence of adverse events, but do include pulmonary embolism, tumor formation, and joint infection [44]. Mechanisms behind improved cartilage profiles have been hypothesized to be due to secretion and promotion of growth factors/cytokines to repair damaged tissue and inhibition of MMP-13, a protein produced by chondrocytes that damages cartilage in OA [45]. Many more clinical trials need to be undertaken with greater number of patients to make a more definitive statement regarding likely benefits of intra-articular stem cell injections in the treatment of OA.

Neuropathic Pain

Target diseases of most neuropathic pain studies involving stem cells include trigeminal neuralgia and diabetic neuropathy. Various mechanisms have been theorized including immunomodulation resulting in decreased inflammatory response to injured tissue, angiogenic stimulation resulting in improved vascularity and oxygen delivery to affected sites. A study using spinal cord injury in a rat model showed that neuropathic pain may be reduced with transplantation of BM-MSCs or UC-MSCs, but motor function recovery, hyperalgesia, and allodynia appear to be unchanged [46]. A recent study with eight patients with trigeminal neuralgia that failed pharmacotherapy showed that majority of patients reported improved pain and decreased gabapentin requirements after intraneural injections of adipose MSCs. In another small study, 10 out of 15 patients reported improvement in pudendal neuropathy after injection [47]. Studies on stem cells targeting diabetic neuropathy have not yet been conducted in human model, although animal studies have shown promise [48].

Tendinopathies

Tendon injury remains a common cause of discomfort, pain, and limitation in population typically stemming from inflammation and overuse injury. Stem cells are currently being researched to aid in tendon repair due to their capacity to differentiate into tenocytes, perform proliferative and synthetic function, and secrete growth factors to aid in regeneration of tendon tissue. MSCs are preferred over ECs and iPSCs for their decreased likelihood of teratoma formation given their restricted self-renewal and lineage differentiation potential. BMSCs do still have the potential to form ectopic bone in transplant injection sites. Pretreatment of MSCs with specific growth factors to drive tenogenic differentiation prior to treatment has largely shown success in improved healing. Delivery of stem cells via intralesional injection or direct transplantation has shown the greatest likelihood of stem cells taking residence in target tissue. Two studies assessing the injection of allogeneic ADSCs cells for treatment of chronic lateral epicondylitis have yielded positive results [49]. As stated previously, the majority of these studies are in animal models and have short follow-up periods of 4–12 weeks. Most studies in human are small and uncontrolled, and as such, there is no FDA-approved stem cell treatment of tendinopathies in humans at this time.

References

1. Sprugel KH, McPherson JM, Clowes AW, Ross R. Effects of growth factors in vivo. I. Cell ingrowth into porous subcutaneous chambers. Am J Pathol. 1987;129(3):601–13.

2. Ferrari M, Zia S, Valbonesi M, Henriquet F, Venere G, Spagnolo S, et al. A new technique for hemodilution, preparation of autologous platelet-rich plasma and intraoperative blood salvage in cardiac surgery. Int J Artif Organs. 1987;10(1):47–50.

3. Marx RE, Carlson ER, Eichstaedt RM, Schimmele SR, Strauss JE, Georgeff KR. Platelet-rich plasma: growth factor enhancement for bone grafts. Oral Surg Oral Med Oral Pathol Oral Radiol Endod. 1998;85(6):638–46.

4. Hall MP, Band PA, Meislin RJ, Jazrawi LM, Cardone DA. Platelet-rich plasma: current concepts and application in sports medicine. J Am Acad Orthop Surg. 2009;17(10):602–8.

5. Mishra A, Pavelko T. Treatment of chronic elbow tendinosis with buffered platelet-rich plasma. Am J Sports Med. 2006;34(11):1774–8.

6. Marx RE. Platelet-rich plasma: evidence to support its use. J Oral Maxillofac Surg. 2004;62(4):489–96.

7. Dhurat R, Sukesh M. Principles and methods of preparation of platelet-rich plasma: a review and author's perspective. J Cutan Aesthet Surg. 2014;7(4):189–97.

8. Giusti I, Rughetti A, D'Ascenzo S, Millimaggi D, Pavan A, Dell'Orso L, et al. Identification of an optimal concentration of platelet gel for promoting angiogenesis in human endothelial cells. Transfusion. 2009;49(4):771–8.

9. Anitua E, Andia I, Ardanza B, Nurden P, Nurden AT. Autologous platelets as a source of proteins for healing and tissue regeneration. Thromb Haemost. 2004;91(1):4–15.

10. Scott A, Khan KM, Roberts CR, Cook JL, Duronio V. What do we mean by the term "inflammation"? A contemporary basic science update for sports medicine. Br J Sports Med. 2004;38(3):372–80.

11. Tidball JG. Inflammatory processes in muscle injury and repair. Am J Physiol Regul Integr Comp Physiol. 2005;288(2):R345–53.

12. Dohan Ehrenfest DM, Andia I, Zumstein MA, Zhang CQ, Pinto NR, Bielecki T. Classification of platelet concentrates (Platelet-Rich Plasma-PRP, Platelet-Rich Fibrin-PRF) for topical and infiltrative use in orthopedic and sports medicine: current consensus, clinical implications and perspectives. Muscles Ligaments Tendons J. 2014;4(1):3–9.

13. Mishra A, Harmon K, Woodall J, Vieira A. Sports medicine applications of platelet rich plasma. Curr Pharm Biotechnol. 2012;13(7):1185–95.

14. Mautner K, Malanga GA, Smith J, Shiple B, Ibrahim V, Sampson S, et al. A call for a standard classification system for future biologic research: the rationale for new PRP nomenclature. PM R. 2015;7(4 Suppl):S53–9.

15. Fitzpatrick J, Bulsara MK, McCrory PR, Richardson MD, Zheng MH. Analysis of platelet-rich plasma extraction: variations in platelet and blood components between 4 common commercial kits. Orthop J Sports Med. 2017;5(1):2325967116675272.

16. Verhaar JA. Tennis elbow. Anatomical, epidemiological and therapeutic aspects. Int Orthop. 1994;18(5):263–7.

17. Peerbooms JC, Sluimer J, Bruijn DJ, Gosens T. Positive effect of an autologous platelet concentrate in lateral epicondylitis in a double-blind randomized controlled trial: platelet-rich plasma versus corticosteroid injection with a 1-year follow-up. Am J Sports Med. 2010;38(2):255–62.

18. Krogh TP, Fredberg U, Stengaard-Pedersen K, Christensen R, Jensen P, Ellingsen T. Treatment of lateral epicondylitis with platelet-rich plasma, glucocorticoid, or saline: a randomized, double-blind, placebo-controlled trial. Am J Sports Med. 2013;41(3):625–35.

19. Monto RR. Platelet rich plasma treatment for chronic Achilles tendinosis. Foot Ankle Int. 2012;33(5):379–85.

20. Jain K, Murphy PN, Clough TM. Platelet rich plasma versus corticosteroid injection for plantar fasciitis: a comparative study. Foot. 2015;25(4):235–7.

21. Monto RR. Platelet-rich plasma efficacy versus corticosteroid injection treatment for chronic severe plantar fasciitis. Foot Ankle Int. 2014;35(4):313–8.

22. Cheng OT, Souzdalnitski D, Vrooman B, Cheng J. Evidence-based knee injections for the management of arthritis. Pain Med. 2012;13(6):740–53.

23. Goldring MB. The role of the chondrocyte in osteoarthritis. Arthritis Rheum. 2000;43(9):1916–26.

24. Sampson S, Gerhardt M, Mandelbaum B. Platelet rich plasma injection grafts for musculoskeletal injuries: a review. Curr Rev Musculoskelet Med. 2008;1(3–4):165–74.

25. Khoshbin A, Leroux T, Wasserstein D, Marks P, Theodoropoulos J, Ogilvie-Harris D, et al. The efficacy of platelet-rich plasma in the treatment of symptomatic knee osteoarthritis: a systematic review with quantitative synthesis. Arthroscopy. 2013;29(12):2037–48.

26. Chang KV, Hung CY, Aliwarga F, Wang TG, Han DS, Chen WS. Comparative effectiveness of platelet-rich plasma injections for treating knee joint cartilage degenerative pathology: a systematic review and meta-analysis. Arch Phys Med Rehabil. 2014;95(3):562–75.

27. Filardo G, Di Matteo B, Di Martino A, Merli ML, Cenacchi A, Fornasari P, et al. Platelet-rich plasma intra-articular knee injections show no superiority versus viscosupplementation: a randomized controlled trial. Am J Sports Med. 2015;43(7):1575–82.

28. Dallari D, Stagni C, Rani N, Sabbioni G, Pelotti P, Torricelli P, et al. Ultrasound-guided injection of platelet-rich plasma and hyaluronic acid, separately and in combination, for hip osteoarthritis: a randomized controlled study. Am J Sports Med. 2016;44(3):664–71.

29. Dines JS, Williams PN, ElAttrache N, Conte S, Tomczyk T, Osbahr DC, et al. Platelet-rich plasma can be used to successfully treat elbow ulnar collateral ligament insufficiency in high-level throwers. Am J Orthop. 2016;45(5):296–300.

30. Rettig AC, Sherrill C, Snead DS, Mendler JC, Mieling P. Nonoperative treatment of ulnar collateral ligament injuries in throwing athletes. Am J Sports Med. 2001;29(1):15–7.

31. Figueroa D, Figueroa F, Calvo R, Vaisman A, Ahumada X, Arellano S. Platelet-rich plasma use in anterior cruciate ligament surgery: systematic review of the literature. Arthroscopy. 2015;31(5):981–8.

32. Wu J, Du Z, Lv Y, Zhang J, Xiong W, Wang R, et al. A new technique for the treatment of lumbar facet joint syndrome using intra-articular injection with autologous platelet rich plasma. Pain Physician. 2016;19(8):617–25.

33. Tuakli-Wosornu YA, Terry A, Boachie-Adjei K, Harrison JR, Gribbin CK, LaSalle EE, et al. Lumbar intradiskal platelet-rich plasma (PRP) injections: a prospective, double-blind, randomized controlled study. PM R. 2016;8(1):1–10; quiz

34. Ko GD, Mindra S, Lawson GE, Whitmore S, Arseneau L. Case series of ultrasound-guided platelet-rich plasma injections for sacroiliac joint dysfunction. J Back Musculoskelet Rehabil. 2017;30(2):363–70.

35. Chakravarthy K, Chen Y, He C, Christo PJ. Stem cell therapy for chronic pain management: review of uses, advances, and adverse effects. Pain Physician. 2017;20(4):293–305.

36. Hospital BCs. About stem cells 2017. Available from: http://stemcell.childrenshospital.org/about-stem-cells/.

37. Orozco L, Soler R, Morera C, Alberca M, Sanchez A, Garcia-Sancho J. Intervertebral disc repair by autologous mesenchymal bone marrow cells: a pilot study. Transplantation. 2011;92(7):822–8.

38. Meisel HJ, Siodla V, Ganey T, Minkus Y, Hutton WC, Alasevic OJ. Clinical experience in cell-based therapeutics: disc chondrocyte transplantation, a treatment for degenerated or damaged intervertebral disc. Biomol Eng. 2007;24(1):5–21.

39. Haufe SM, Mork AR. Intradiscal injection of hematopoietic stem cells in an attempt to rejuvenate the intervertebral discs. Stem Cells Dev. 2006;15(1):136–7.

40. Wyles CC, Houdek MT, Behfar A, Sierra RJ. Mesenchymal stem cell therapy for osteoarthritis: current perspectives. Stem Cells Cloning. 2015;8:117–24.

41. Orozco L, Munar A, Soler R, Alberca M, Soler F, Huguet M, et al. Treatment of knee osteoarthritis with autologous mesenchymal stem cells: a pilot study. Transplantation. 2013;95(12):1535–41.

42. Saw KY, Anz A, Siew-Yoke Jee C, Merican S, Ching-Soong Ng R, Roohi SA, et al. Articular cartilage regeneration with autologous peripheral blood stem cells versus hyaluronic acid: a randomized controlled trial. Arthroscopy. 2013;29(4):684–94.

43. Wong KL, Lee KB, Tai BC, Law P, Lee EH, Hui JH. Injectable cultured bone marrow-derived mesenchymal stem cells in varus knees with cartilage defects undergoing high tibial osteotomy: a prospective, randomized controlled clinical trial with 2 years' follow-up. Arthroscopy. 2013;29(12):2020–8.

44. Peeters CM, Leijs MJ, Reijman M, van Osch GJ, Bos PK. Safety of intra-articular cell-therapy with culture-expanded stem cells in humans: a systematic literature review. Osteoarthr Cartil. 2013;21(10):1465–73.

45. Kuroda K, Kabata T, Hayashi K, Maeda T, Kajino Y, Iwai S, et al. The paracrine effect of adipose-derived stem cells inhibits osteoarthritis progression. BMC Musculoskelet Disord. 2015;16:236.

46. Yousefifard M, Nasirinezhad F, Shardi Manaheji H, Janzadeh A, Hosseini M, Keshavarz M. Human bone marrow-derived and umbilical cord-derived mesenchymal stem cells for alleviating neuropathic pain in a spinal cord injury model. Stem Cell Res Ther. 2016;7:36.

47. Venturi M, Boccasanta P, Lombardi B, Brambilla M, Contessini Avesani E, Vergani C. Pudendal neuralgia: a new option for treatment? Preliminary results on feasibility and efficacy. Pain Med. 2015;16(8):1475–81.

48. Waterman RS, Morgenweck J, Nossaman BD, Scandurro AE, Scandurro SA, Betancourt AM. Anti-inflammatory mesenchymal stem cells (MSC2) attenuate symptoms of painful diabetic peripheral neuropathy. Stem Cells Transl Med. 2012;1(7):557–65.

49. Lui PP. Stem cell technology for tendon regeneration: current status, challenges, and future research directions. Stem Cells Cloning. 2015;8:163–74.

Visceral Pain

Leonardo Kapural and Jeremy Naber

Mechanisms of Chronic Abdominal Pain

Chronic abdominal pain is affected by physical, emotional, and perceptual individual responses. Maladaptive neuroplastic changes in the setting of hyperalgesia and allodynia can result in increased perception and exaggerated response to any type of noxious stimulus or a pain response to normally non-noxious stimuli. Such neuroplastic adaptations often involve both neurons and glial cells and are referred to as peripheral and central sensitization [1]. In some instances of chronic abdominal pain, there is no obvious tissue injury or structural disease discovered. These characteristics, namely, the presence of visceral hypersensitivity through central and peripheral mechanisms without evidence of structural change, are the hallmark of dysmotility disorders such as irritable bowel syndrome (IBS).

Gastrointestinal inflammation has been implicated in the evolution of acute or chronic pain in a variety of disease including inflammatory bowel disease, celiac disease, and acute infectious gastroenteritis [2]. Heightened expression of transient receptor potential vanilloid type 1 (TRPV1) may be found in both intestinal inflammation and other non-visceral chronic pain syndromes. [3]. Often, a neuropathic pain component is present in chronic abdominal pain syndromes such as chronic pancreatitis. This is thought to be produced through direct alterations of the dorsal root ganglia of neurons that innervate the pancreas [4]. The visceral hyperalgesic reaction observed in chronic pancreatitis perpetuates ongoing neuropathic pain [5].

Prevalence and Etiology

Generalized chronic abdominal pain is a frequent complaint. At least 25% of adults have had it at least once in their lifetime [6, 7]. The prevalence of abdominal pain is similar in different ages, ethnicities, or geographic regions [7, 8]. Women report abdominal pain with a greater frequency than men [7].

Inflammatory bowel disease (IBD) is considered a disease of adolescents and young adults as evidenced by peak incidence from ages 15 to 35 years [9, 10]. For those in clinical remission of IBD, about 20% have chronic abdominal pain treated with opioids. The utility of opioid medication in this population, as with other patient populations, has been recently called into question. Preexisting psychiatric disease, smoking, female gender, and longer duration of the disease are all risk factors for persistent chronic abdominal pain.

Another common cause of chronic abdominal pain is chronic pancreatitis, which has seen a worldwide incidence increase. The most likely cause is alcohol abuse; however, other etiologies should be investigated. Of the patients requiring medications and interventions, chronic intermittent pain persists in about 80–90% [11].

The development of postsurgical adhesions causing chronic abdominal pain has an incidence of 45–90% in some studies. Open procedures, use of implants such as mesh, and a contaminated surgical field (i.e., gallbladder, bowel contents, etc.) carry higher risk for adhesion formation. Chronic abdominal pain is also linked to common surgical procedures such as cholecystectomy, herniorrhaphy, and adhesiolysis. Risk factors for the development of this pain include the duration and type of surgery, preexisting psychiatric illness, female sex, and younger age [12].

Chronic abdominal pain is often present in association with chronic abdominal wall pain (CAWP) as well as chronic visceral disease. About 10–30% of those afflicted by chronic abdominal pain are due to chronic abdominal wall pain (CAWP). Anterior cutaneous nerve entrapment syndrome (ACNES) may be responsible for up to 30% of cases of chronic abdominal wall pain [13, 14].

L. Kapural (✉) · J. Naber
Carolinas Pain Institute & Center for Clinical Research,
Winston-Salem, NC, USA

© Springer Nature Switzerland AG 2019
Y. Khelemsky et al. (eds.), *Academic Pain Medicine*, https://doi.org/10.1007/978-3-030-18005-8_37

Clinical Presentation

The abdomen should first be inspected to provide a clue of the chronic pain source. Surgical scars from should be noted. If the patient has localized allodynia or hyperalgesia, the possibility of nerve damage or a neuroma should be considered. Chronic abdominal wall pain (CAWP) is diagnosed from a thorough physical examination and a detailed patient history. The pain is most often well localized to a tender point while palpating. Visceral pain, however, is difficult to localize [15, 16]. The key physical examination for diagnosing abdominal wall pain is Carnett's test [15]. An increase in pain when palpating during abdominal muscle contraction is considered a positive Carnett's test. Intra-abdominal pain may be somewhat reduced when abdominal muscles are contracted. The physical examination should also include sensory and sympathetic assessment, especially if abdominal cutaneous nerve entrapment syndrome (ACNES), neuroma, or severe neuralgia is suspected. ACNES at the lateral border of the rectus muscle is the most common cause of abdominal wall pain [17]. Injections of the abdominal wall, preferably with ultrasound guidance, may have both diagnostic and therapeutic utility in these cases [17, 18]. Functional motility disorders can mimic chronic abdominal pain through viscerosomatic referral. When the cause of the abdominal pain is unclear, actively listening and addressing the patient's concerns is paramount. In order to better direct treatment, psychosocial assessment should be performed, including objective tests such as depression inventories.

Establishing the Diagnosis

Organic disease must be excluded, but repetitive diagnostic testing should be avoided. Patients are frequently subjected to extensive workups to determine the root cause of their chronic abdominal pain, but most causes of visceral pain remain idiopathic. Physical examination sometimes provides additional information. Nerve blocks can be therapeutic and diagnostic or have prognostic value. Most often, nerve blocks in chronic abdominal pain are used to help establish a diagnosis. Through anatomic or pharmacologic approaches, one can elucidate the likely progressions involved in the ongoing abdominal pain.

Frequently used diagnostic and or therapeutic block techniques are listed below:

1. Sympathetic blocks: splanchnic nerve block, celiac nerve block, superior hypogastric nerve block, and ganglion impar block.
2. Somatosensory blocks: paravertebral nerve blocks, intercostal nerve blocks, transversus abdominis plane (TAP) blocks, and blocks of the ilioinguinal, iliohypogastric, and genitofemoral nerves.

Differential retrograde epidural block can be used as an invasive diagnostic tool to distinguish visceral vs non-visceral sources of pain [19, 20]. In order to perform this block, an epidural catheter is first placed under fluoroscopy. Injection of saline twice (placebo), followed by additional doses of fast onset/fast offset local anesthetic, is then performed. The diagnostic value of performing a differential blockade is based on the sensitivity of nerve fibers of various sizes, myelination, and function to local anesthetics. Local anesthetic blockade has a more pronounced effect on sympathetic fibers and visceral afferent nerves. This is in contrast to large sensory or motor fibers, mostly because of the higher visceral C vs A δ fiber ratio (10:1) [19, 20].

Transversus abdominis plane (TAP) blocks may be both diagnostic and therapeutic as it may confirm somatosensory pain origin. The TAP block provides analgesia across the anterolateral abdominal wall from the costal margin to the inguinal ligament. The use of ultrasound guidance to perform the block allows placement of local anesthetic around the anterior branches of the thoracolumbar ventral rami, creating a blockade of the somatics of the anterior abdominal wall. Ultrasound-guided approach for the TAP block allows visualization of the three muscular layers of the lateral abdominal wall, namely, the external oblique (most superficial), internal oblique (IO), and transverse abdominus (TA) muscle (deepest). The tip of the needle is advanced until between the IO and TA muscles, and then local anesthetic is deposited in this plane. Though the initial data is positive, the utility of a single TAP block for determining the source of abdominal pain from the abdominal wall is debatable [17]. For those patients with CAWP, a single guided injection TAP block, or continuous infusion, can be used for treatment [17, 20].

Treatment

The treatment of severe abdominal pain is complex. It requires the integration of multiple specialties to evaluate, diagnose, and create an effective treatment plan.

Conservative Treatment

Lifestyle changes may be necessary, including abstinence from alcohol and smoking cessation. In pharmacological management, mild pains can warrant the use of acetaminophen or nonsteroidal anti-inflammatory drugs, with consideration of the possible side effects. The use of short-acting opioids can be added for acute pain. Side effects such as nausea and vomiting can be minimized with low-dose antiemetics, and constipation can be controlled with laxatives or medications that block intestinal mu opioid receptors [21]. Antidepressants and membrane stabilizers frequently prescribed for neuropathic pain can be used for chronic abdominal pain as well [22, 23]. Ketamine is another medication utilized in the treatment of chronic pain. Specifically, S-ketamine infusion has been used to reduce visceral hyperalgesia [24].

Psychological Interventions

For patients with persistent chronic abdominal pain, psychological treatments should be considered early in the treatment process [25–34]. One such therapeutic approach is biofeedback. Current clinical studies on conventional biofeedback are promising, but more definitive clinical evidence is lacking [25]. Thermal biofeedback seems to be appropriate for chronic abdominal pain [26]. Electromyography (EMG) biofeedback techniques demonstrate a reduction in constipation and pain [27, 28]. Other useful therapies for IBS include relaxation techniques, cognitive therapy, thermal biofeedback, and psychological education [29, 30].

In order to suspend peripheral awareness, analgesic hypnosis is utilized to induce a relaxed state with focused attention and inner absorption. Hypnotherapy is frequently utilized in the treatment of patients with chronic pain from IBS. Studies have found the reduction in IBS symptoms with improvement in the quality of life, as well as increased pain perception threshold in patients with IBS [31].

Cognitive behavior therapy (CBT) is another method that includes relaxation, coping skills, and training in order to help reduce pain [34]. However, when utilized in IBS patients, CBT had ambiguous results [32].

In order to provide short- and long-term benefits for control of chronic abdominal pain, patients should be enrolled in a multidisciplinary chronic pain rehabilitation program. This program should include patient education, physical therapy, occupational therapy, medication management, psychotherapy for the individual or a group, cognitive therapy, biofeedback techniques, weaning of opioids, or other habitually used substances and muscle relaxation techniques [33].

Interventional Approaches

The use of nerve blocks, ablative procedure, and neuromodulation techniques all have the goal of interrupting or modifying the pain pathways. Multiple mechanisms have been proposed for use in abdominal pain relief.

The splanchnic nerves and celiac plexus are the most common targets. Abdominal organ sympathetic innervation is derived from preganglionic fibers of T5 to T12 that combine with the ventral rami. Along with the communicating rami, they run along the sympathetic chain and then synapse at the level of the celiac, aortic, renal, and superior mesenteric ganglia. The splanchnic nerves, along with the vagal preganglionic parasympathetic fibers, sensory fibers of the phrenic nerve, and postganglionic sympathetic fibers, combine to form the celiac plexus. The plexus is found anterior to the abdominal aorta at the origin of the celiac artery. The splanchnic nerves are located in a narrow space between the lateral border of the vertebra and pleura [34].

Both splanchnic and celiac plexus blocks are accomplished percutaneously under the guidance of fluoroscopy (Figs. 37.1 and 37.2). There exist several approaches to block the celiac plexus, including transaortic, retrocrural, and transdiscal. Neither has been shown to have a distinct advantage over another. The celiac plexus block is classically

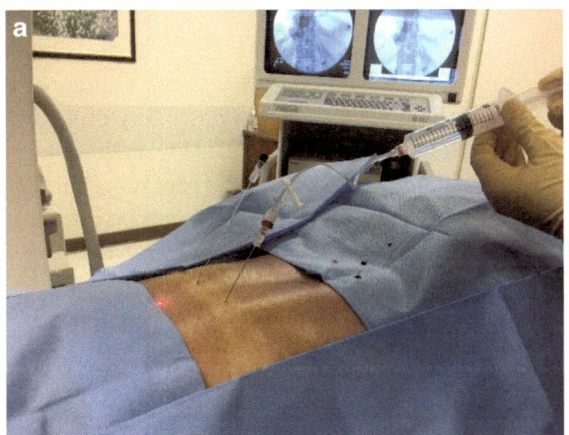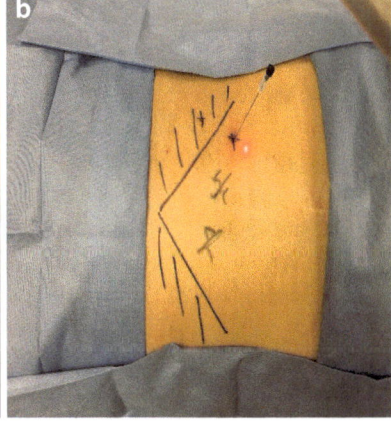

Fig. 37.1 Photographs of an injection of local anesthetic after the proper needle positioning during the splanchnic nerve block (**a**) and proper drawing to delineate location of 12th rib for the celiac plexus block (**b**). Note in (**a**) that an injection of contrast and local anesthetic on one side (in this picture left) is followed by an advancement of spinal needle and injection to the right. Obvious reason for this stepwise approach is to prevent needle advancement on the opposite side if pleural spread of contrast is shown ipsilaterally. (**b**) Safety triangle is shown at the lower edge of 12th rib bilaterally, area lined above triangle is "no-needle placement area." An oblique fluoroscopy angle with a slight tilt caudally will then allow a safe needle advancement to the landmark at mid-concavity of the L1 vertebral body (1B)

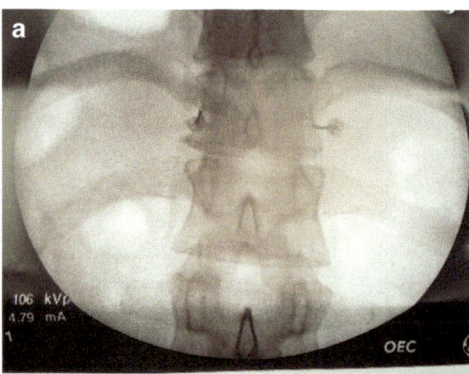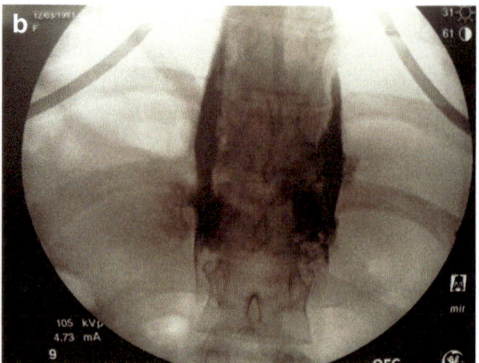

Fig. 37.2 near here. Splanchnic block at T11 level. 22 G spinal needle is advanced in AP view (**a**). Caudal fluoroscopy angle and tunnel view needle placement in a close proximity to T11 vertebral body. One needle at the time is advanced to avoid bilateral pneumothorax.

(**b**) Confirmation of bilateral spread of the local anesthetic after confirmation of proper location of the contrast. Paravertebral spread of 10–15 cc of bupivacaine is shown

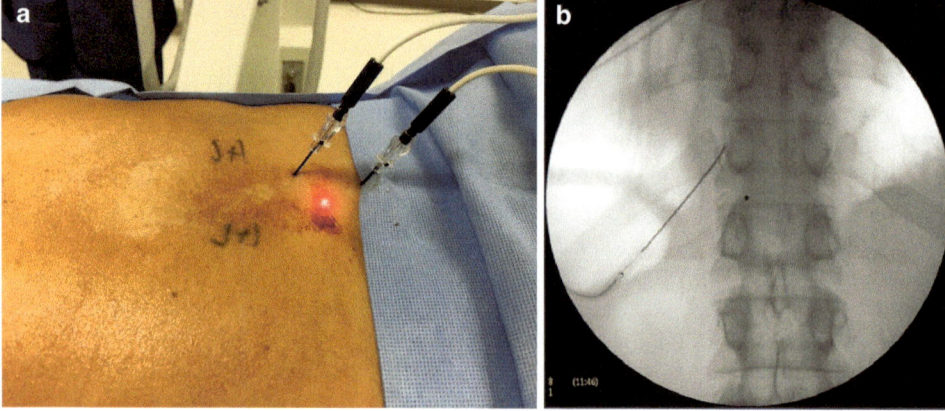

Fig. 37.3 Radiofrequency (RF) denervation of splanchnic nerves. Curved electrodes are positioned under 60 degrees caudal angle at T11 and T12 vertebral level (**a**). Photograph illustrates a proper positioning of radiofrequency electrodes. (**b**) RF electrodes shown in lateral fluoroscopic view. Active tip is located between the posterior and middle third

vertebral body width at T11 level and middle and anterior third at T12 level. Sensory stimulation at 0.5 V and 50 Hz is conducted to confirm concordant pain, and nonionic contrast is injected before denervation, to rule out intravascular placement of the electrodes (not shown)

described by placing a needle through paraspinal area of the middle back around the L1 vertebrae (Fig. 37.1b).

A less common approach is the T11 bilateral splanchnic block (Fig. 37.1a). This method is performed in the paravertebral compartment medial to the pleural cavity, next to the greater and lesser splanchnic nerves located in the posterior third of the T11 vertebral body (Figs. 37.1 and 37.2; [11]). Fluoroscopically guided T11 bilateral splanchnic blocks have been found recently to afford significantly longer pain relief from those patients who suffer from chronic nonmalignant abdominal pain as compared to those who had a celiac plexus block. We found that patients had similar decreases in their pain scores in celiac blocks and splanchnic blocks, but longer pain relief after the splanchnic block [35].

The use of endoscopic ultrasound guidance when performing a celiac plexus block or celiac plexus neurolysis resulted in pain relief in only 55% of the patients at 4- and

8-week follow-up. The complications of this approach are about 1.8%, with the possibility of more serious complications such as paraplegia [11]. Following successful splanchnic nerve block (>50% pain relief), a radiofrequency (RF) denervation (Fig. 37.3a, b) can be considered. Advantages of splanchnic RF include long-term pain relief with rare complications.

A larger cases series on the use of the RF ablative technique suggested significant long-term improvements in pain scores [36, 37], opioid use, and frequency of acute hospitalizations [36–38]. Common complications include hypotension, diarrhea, and post-procedural neuritis [36–38].

Thoracoscopic splanchnicectomy may provide pain relief over 6 months in about 25% of the patients. Due to low success rate, extensive dissection of the parietal pleura, risk of anesthesia with endotracheal double lumen tube, as well as prone positioning, neurotomy of splanchnic nerves at the thoracic level is rarely performed [39].

Fig. 37.4 Thoracic placement of the spinal cord stimulation leads to control of chronic abdominal pain. T9–T10 interspace is accessed using Tuohy needle and loss of resistance technique (**a**). Lead arrays over the midline of T4 and T5 vertebral bodies to achieve relief from chronic abdominal pain (**b**)

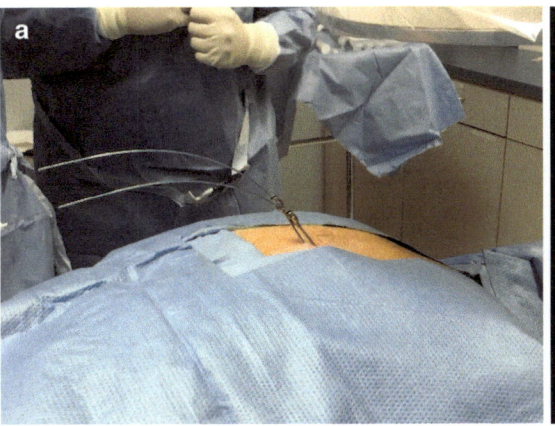
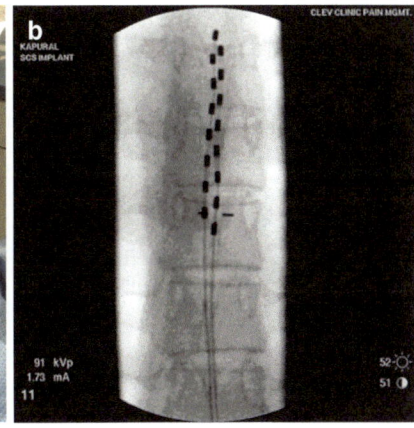

Spinal cord stimulation (SCS) appears to be an effective longer-term therapeutic solution for patients suffering from chronic abdominal pain ([40–44]; Fig. 37.4). Patients with visceral hyperalgesia from dysmotility disorder, postsurgical visceral adhesions, and chronic pancreatitis have all been treated with SCS. The first case series found trial conversion rate of about 86%. Following a permanent implantation with minimal attrition, about 50% of pain relief was maintained long term [42].

A few studies documented placement of the standard octrode lead tip near the fifth thoracic vertebral body height in the posterior epidural space [42, 43]. In the subgroup of patients with chronic pancreatitis, VAS pain scores were similarly reduced by approximately half with long-term opioid reduction by more than 60% [40–44].

Surgical Approaches

Published surgical interventions for control of chronic abdominal pain pertain mainly to relief from chronic pain resulting from pancreatitis. The surgeries include pancreatic duct decompression with or without a resection [45, 46]. One method of providing persistent ductal drainage includes a lateral pancreaticojejunostomy known as the Partington-Rochelle modification of the Puestow procedure. Other drainage procedures include the Frey and Duval method. The Frey procedure involves resecting the head of the pancreas in addition to a lateral longitudinal drain of the duct, as seen in the Puestow procedure. More extensive approaches include distal or subtotal pancreatectomies, Whipple, Berger, and Berne procedures. The most extreme form of resection is the total pancreatectomy and is sometimes indicated in patients with severe chronic abdominal pain from chronic pancreatitis [45, 46].

Preoperative opioid use has been found to be a negative predictor of long-term pain relief from surgical or endoscopic interventions. This may be due to central sensitization or opioid dependence [47, 48]. Despite carrying similar complication rates, surgical procedures seem to provide superior pain relief compared to endoscopic interventions [49, 50].

Conclusion

An in-depth understanding of clinical, physical, and psychosocial features surrounding chronic abdominal pain is required, and treatment options should be tailored to the needs of the patient. Pharmacological treatment plan for chronic abdominal pain should include non-opioids. Drugs such as membrane stabilizer and antidepressants have shown some efficacy. Other potential analgesics include NGF inhibitors and TRPV1 antagonists. NMDA receptor antagonists may be useful. Celiac plexus and splanchnic nerve blocks and splanchnic radiofrequency ablation for the treatment of nonmalignant chronic abdominal pain need to be further studied. Spinal cord stimulation appears to be an efficacious minimally invasive approach. Surgical interventions are reserved for most resistant cases of severe pain.

References

1. Anaparthy R, Pasricha PJ. Pain and chronic pancreatitis: is it the plumbing or the wiring? Curr Gastroenterol Rep. 2008;10:101–6.
2. Azpiroz F, Bouin M, Camilleri M, et al. Mechanisms of hypersensitivity in IBS and functional disorders. Neurogastroenterol Motil. 2007;19(1 Suppl):62–88.
3. Jones RC 3rd, Xu L, Gebhart GF. The mechanosensitivity of mouse colon afferent fibers and their sensitization by inflammatory mediators require transient receptor potential vanilloid 1 and acid-sensing ion channel 3. J Neurosci. 2005;25(47):10981–9.
4. DiMagno MJ, DiMagno EP. Chronic pancreatitis. Curr Opin Gastroenterol. 2012;28:523–31.
5. Pasricha PJ. Unraveling the mystery of pain in chronic pancreatitis. Nat Rev Gastroenterol Hepatol. 2012;9:140–51.
6. Wallander MA, Johansson S, Ruigomez A, García Rodriguez LA. Unspecified abdominal pain in primary care: The role of gastrointestinal morbidity. Int J Clin Pract. 2007;61(10):1663–70.
7. Sandler RS, Stewart WF, Liberman JN, Ricci JA, Zorich NL. Abdominal pain, bloating, and diarrhea in the united states: Prevalence and impact. Dig Dis Sci. 2000;45(6):1166–71.
8. Heading RC. Prevalence of upper gastrointestinal symptoms in the general population: a systematic review. Scand J Gastroenterol Suppl. 1999;231:3–8.
9. Calkins BM, Mendeloff AI. Epidemiology of inflammatory bowel disease. Epidemiol Rev. 1986;8:60–91.

10. Calkins BM, Lilienfeld AM, Garland CF, Mendeloff AI. Trends in incidence rates of ulcerative colitis and Crohn's disease. Dig Dis Sci. 1984;29(10):913–20.

11. Puylaert M, Kapural L, van Zundert J, Peek D, Lataster A, Mekhail N, van Kleef M, Keulemans Y. Pain in chronic pancreatitis (Chapter 26). In: van Zundert J, Patjin J, Hartrick C, Lataster A, Huygen F, Mekhail N, van Kleff M, editors. Evidence-based interventional pain practice: according to clinical diagnoses. Oxford: Wiley Blackwell; 2012. p. 202–12.

12. Tolba R. Rizk. The epidemiology of chronic abdominal pain. In: Kapural L, editor. Chronic abdominal pain, an evidence-based comprehensive guide to clinical management. New York: Springer; 2015. p. 195–201.

13. Chrona E, Kostopanagiotou G, Damigos D, Batistaki C. Anterior cutaneous nerve entrapment syndrome: management challenges, vol. 97; 2002. p. 824–30.

14. Lindsetmo R, Stulberg J. Chronic abdominal wall pain—a diagnostic challenge for the surgeon. Am J Surg. 2009;198:129–34.

15. Carnett JB. Intercostal neuralgia as a cause of abdominal pain and tenderness. Surg Gynecol Obstet. 1926;42:625–32.

16. Sharpstone D, Colin-Jones DG. Chronic, non-visceral abdominal pain. Gut. 1994;35:833–6.

17. Narouze S. Chronic abdominal wall pain: diagnosis and interventional treatment. In: Kapural L, editor. Chronic abdominal pain: an evidence-based, comprehensive guide to clinical management. New York: Springer; 2015. p. 189–95.

18. Gray DWR, Seabrook G, Dixon JM, et al. Is abdominal wall tenderness a useful sign in the diagnosis of non-specific abdominal pain? Ann R Coll Surg Engl. 1988;70:233–4.

19. Rizk MK, Tolba R, Kapural L, Mitchell J, Lopez R, Mahboobi R, Vrooman B, Mekhail N. Differential epidural block predicts the success of visceral block in patients with chronic visceral abdominal pain. Pain Pract. 2012;12:595–601.

20. Veizi IE, Hajek S. Establishing diagnosis of chronic abdominal pain: pain medicine view. In: Kapural L, editor. Chronic abdominal pain: an evidence-based, comprehensive guide to clinical management. New York: Springer; 2015. p. 33–45.

21. Gachago C, Draganov PV. Pain management in chronic pancreatitis. World J Gastroenterol. 2008;14:3137–48.

22. Olesen SS, Bouwense SA, Wilder-Smith OH, van Goor H, Drewes AM. Pregabalin reduces pain in patients with chronic pancreatitis in a randomized, controlled trial. Gastroenterology. 2011;141:536–43.

23. Olesen SS, Graversen C, Olesen AE, et al. Randomised clinical trial: pregabalin attenuates experimental visceral pain through subcortical mechanisms in patients with painful chronic pancreatitis. Aliment Pharmacol Ther. 2011;34:878–87.

24. Bouwense SA, Buscher HC, van Goor H, Wilder-Smith OH. S-ketamine modulates hyperalgesia in patients with chronic pancreatitis pain. Reg Anesth Pain Med. 2011;36:303–7.

25. Palsson OS, Whitehead WE. Psychological treatments in functional gastrointestinal disorders: a primer for the gastroenterologist. Clin Gastroenterol Hepatol. 2013;11(3):208–16.

26. Coulter ID, Favreau JT, Hardy ML, Morton SC, Roth EA, Shekelle P. Biofeedback interventions for gastrointestinal conditions: a systematic review. Altern Ther Health Med. 2002;8(3):76–83.

27. Humphreys P, Gevirtz R. Treatment of recurrent abdominal pain: components analysis of four treatment protocols. J Pediatr Gastroenterol Nutr. 2000;31:47–51.

28. Bassotti G, Chistolini F, Sietchiping-Nzepa F, De Roberto G, Morelli A, Chiarioni G. Biofeedback for pelvic floor dysfunction in constipation. Br Med J. 2004;328(7436):393–6.

29. Blanchard EB, Schwarz SP, Suls JM, Gerardi MA, Scharff L, Greene B, et al. Two controlled evaluations of multicomponent psychological treatment of irritable bowel syndrome. Behav Res Ther. 1992;30(2):175–89.

30. Schwarz SP, Blanchard EB, Neff DF. Behavioral treatment of irritable bowel syndrome: a 1 year follow-up study. Biofeedback Self Regul. 1986;11(3):189–98.

31. Kupers R, Faymonville ME, Laureys S. The cognitive modulation of pain: hypnosis and placebo induced analgesia. Prog Brain Res. 2005;150:251–69.

32. Drossman DA, Toner BB, Whitehead WE. Cognitive-behavioral therapy versus education and desipramine versus placebo for moderate to severe functional disorders. Gastroenterology. 2003;125:19–31.

33. Sweiss G. In: Kapural L, editor. Chronic abdominal pain, an evidence-based comprehensive guide to clinical management. New York: Springer; 2015. p. 195–201.

34. Rathmell JP, Gallant JM, Brown DL. Computed tomography and the anatomy of celiac plexus block. Reg Anesth Pain Med. 2000;25:411–6.

35. Badhey H, Jolly S, Kapural L. Bilateral splanchnic block at T11 provides longer pain relief than celiac plexus block from nonmalignant abdominal pain. 2015 RAMP Supplement Abstr 145.

36. Prithvi Raj P, Sahinder B, Lowe M. Radiofrequency lesioning of splanchnic nerves. Pain Pract. 2002;2:241–7.

37. Garcea G, Thomasset S, Berry DP, Tordoff S. Percutaneous splanchnic nerve radiofrequency ablation for chronic abdominal pain. ANZ J Surg. 2005;75:640–4.

38. Verhaegh BP, van Kleef M, Geurts JW, et al. Percutaneous radiofrequency ablation of the splanchnic nerves in patients with chronic pancreatitis: results of single and repeated procedures in 11 patients. Pain Pract. 2013;13(8):621–6.

39. Buscher HC, Jansen JB, van Dongen R, Bleichrodt RP, van Goor H. Long-term results of bilateral thoracoscopic splanchnicectomy in patients with chronic pancreatitis. Br J Surg. 2002;89:158–62.

40. Khan I, Raza S, Khan E. Application of spinal cord stimulation for the treatment of abdominal visceral pain syndromes: case reports. Neuromodulation. 2005;8:14–27.

41. Kapural L. Neuromodulation for chronic visceral abdominal pain. In: Kapural L, editor. Chronic abdominal pain, an evidence-based comprehensive guide to clinical management. New York: Springer; 2015. p. 195–201.

42. Kapural L, Nagem H, Tlucek H, Sessler DI. Spinal cord stimulation for chronic visceral abdominal pain. Pain Med. 2010;11:347–55.

43. Kapural L, Deer T, Yakovlev A, et al. Technical aspects of spinal cord stimulation for managing chronic visceral abdominal pain: the results from the national survey. Pain Med. 2010;11:685–91.

44. Kapural L, Cywinski JB, Sparks DA. Spinal cord stimulation for visceral pain from chronic pancreatitis. Neuromodulation. 2011;14:423–6.

45. Tea S. Resection vs drainage in treatment of chronic pancreatitis: long-term results of a randomized trial. Gastroenterology. 2008;134:1406–11.

46. Mullhaupt B, Ammann RW. Total pancreatectomy for intractable pain in chronic pancreatitis? Pancreas. 2010;39:111–2.

47. Ahmed Ali U, Nieuwenhuijs VB, van Eijck CH, et al. Clinical outcome in relation to timing of surgery in chronic pancreatitis: a nomogram to predict pain relief. Arch Surg. 2012;147:925–32.

48. Negi S, Singh A, Chaudhary A. Pain relief after Frey's procedure for chronic pancreatitis. Br J Surg. 2010;97:1087–95.

49. Dite P, Ruzicka M, Zboril V, Novotny I. A prospective, randomized trial comparing endoscopic and surgical therapy for chronic pancreatitis. Endoscopy. 2003;35:553–8.

50. Cahen DL, Gouma DJ, Nio Y, et al. Endoscopic versus surgical drainage of the pancreatic duct in chronic pancreatitis. N Engl J Med. 2007;356:676–84.

Chronic Urogenital and Pelvic Pain

Zakari A. Suleiman and Corey W. Hunter

Introduction

Chronic pelvic pain (CPP) is a complex, debilitating disorder defined as "a non-malignant pain perceived in the pelvis in either men or women that must have been continuous for at least 6 months." [1] CPP (also known as chronic urogenital pain) is considered a "catch all" term that includes a variety of diagnoses ranging from pudendal neuralgia and coccydynia to vulvodynia and painful bladder syndrome [2].

In general terms, the symptoms of CPP include:

- Neuropathic symptoms such as paresthesias, numbness, burning, and/or lancinating pain in the pelvis, anus, and/ or genitals
- Pain with sitting
- Pain on urination and/or defecating
- Pain associated with coitus and ejaculation

The pelvis is supplied by somatic, sympathetic, and parasympathetic nervous system which makes isolation of pain-generating structures in the region challenging. Thus, painful stimuli and/or reversible causes of pelvic pain are difficult to identify, resulting in delayed diagnosis and treatment and resultant progression to a chronic pain state. Behavioral, sexual, and emotional comorbidities are common in this population [3, 4].

CPP is typically a diagnosis of exclusion that, in addition to the aforementioned pathologies, also involves other pathologic states such as prostatitis, interstitial cystitis, pelvic inflammatory disease (PID), or vestibulitis. CPP typically results after an insult or injury to the somatosensory nervous system (peripheral or central), often characterized by dysesthesias, allodynia, and hyperesthesia [1]. It may also include a localized neuralgia-like penile pain from pudendal neuralgia or scrotal pain from genitofemoral neuralgia subsequent to a vascular aneurysm. All causes of CPP should be distinguished from "pelvic pain syndromes" which may mimic the presentation of a neuralgia but without obvious pathology (i.e., pudendal neuralgia, etc.).

Conservative management is usually effective in early cases of pelvic pain; however, many patients who develop chronic pain require more aggressive treatments such as injections (i.e., hypogastric plexus block, ganglion impar block, pudendal nerve block, etc.), neurostimulation, and surgery.

Anatomy

The sympathetic nerve fibers that mediate visceral pain from the pelvic region often travel with somatic fibers though gray rami communicans (GRC) from the adjacent ganglion. This input is transmitted to the spinal cord through white rami communicans (WRC) from T1 to L1/2 and emerges as myelinated, preganglionic fibers [5]. Nociceptive input from pelvic region (below L2) is contained within sympathetic fibers.

Sympathetic Innervation

Superior hypogastric plexus contains sympathetic innervation of the pelvic viscera at the T12-L2 spinal cord levels (Fig. 38.1).

Parasympathetic Innervation

The parasympathetic innervations to the pelvic viscera are mediated through the splanchnic nerves, S2 through S4 nerve roots.

Z. A. Suleiman
Department of Anaesthesia, University of Ilorin Teaching Hospital, Ilorin, Nigeria

C. W. Hunter (✉)
Ainsworth Institute of Pain Management, New York, NY, USA
e-mail: corey.hunter@nyumc.org

© Springer Nature Switzerland AG 2019
Y. Khelemsky et al. (eds.), *Academic Pain Medicine*, https://doi.org/10.1007/978-3-030-18005-8_38

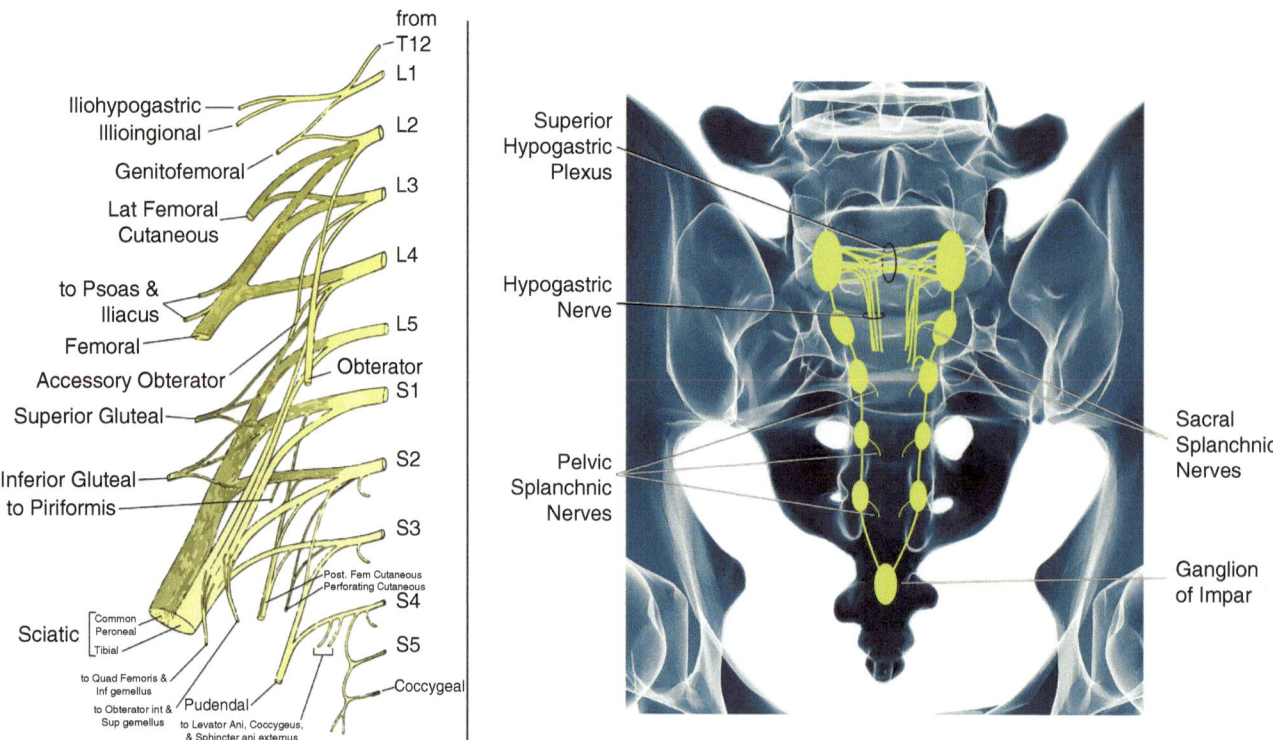

Fig. 38.1 Illustration of the lumbosacral plexus and relevant nerves of the pelvic region (left). Illustration of the sympathetic innervation of the pelvic region (right)

Pelvic Splanchnic Nerves

Nervi erigentes are splanchnic nerves that arise from the S2, S3, and S4 spinal nerves and provide parasympathetic innervation to the hindgut (the distal portion of the gastrointestinal system starting at the distal third of the transverse colon) (Fig. 38.1).

Sacral Splanchnic Nerves

These paired visceral nerves connect the inferior hypogastric plexus to the sympathetic trunk in the pelvis. The efferent preganglionic and postganglionic fibers emerge anterior to the ganglia of the sympathetic trunk (Fig. 38.1).

Superior Hypogastric Plexus

The superior hypogastric plexus is located in the retroperitoneal space at the bifurcation of the aorta anterior to the L5/S1 intervertebral disc. The plexus contains afferent and efferent fibers from the sympathetic nervous system (SNS), as well as some parasympathetics. It innervates the bladder, urethra, vagina, vulva, ovaries, prostate, penis, testicles, uterus, ureter, pelvic floor (perineum), descending colon, and rectum (Fig. 38.1).

Inferior Hypogastric Plexus

The inferior hypogastric plexus, also known as the hypogastric nerve, is the continuation of superior hypogastric plexus. It is located on both sides of the rectum in the male, or vagina in females, and contributes to the innervations of uterovaginal plexus, prostatic plexus, visceral plexus, and middle rectal plexus.

Ganglion Impar

The ganglion impar is a retroperitoneal structure located at the level of the sacrococcygeal junction (SCJ). It is the most caudal segment of the confluence of the sacral sympathetic chain as it passes anteromedially over the sacrum. It is the terminal fusion of the two sacral sympathetic chains, located between the SCJ and the lower segment of the first coccyx. The fusion of the two chains typically positions the ganglion midline, which makes it relatively accessible to intervention [6]. The ganglion impar carries innervation from the perineum, distal rectum, anus, distal urethra, distal vagina, vulva, coccyx, and scrotum (Fig. 38.1).

Pudendal Nerve

The pudendal nerve contains sensory, motor, somatic and sympathetic fibers and acts as the main nerve supply to the perineum and the external genitalia [7]. It is formed from the anterior divisions of the S2, S3, and S4 nerves of the sacral plexus. It coils around the ischial spine and sacrospinous ligament and enters the perineum through the lesser sciatic foramen before exiting the pelvis through the greater sciatic notch between the piriformis and coccygeus muscles. After giving off inferior rectal nerves and perineal nerve, it terminates as the posterior scrotal/labial nerves and dorsal nerve of the penis/clitoris. The pudendal nerve innervates the external genitalia in both males and females as well as the bladder, rectum, pelvic floor muscles, the skin and muscles of the perineum, the external urethral sphincter and external anal sphincter. It also contains sympathetic fibers which innervate penile erectile tissue (Figs. 38.1 and 38.2).

Obturator Nerve

The obturator nerve is formed by the lumbar plexus (L2–4) and supplies the hip joint and adductor muscles of the hip. The anterior, medial, and posterior proximal thigh is supplied, with the saphenous nerve, by obturator nerve.

Genitofemoral Nerve

The genitofemoral nerve is derived from the fibers of L1 and L2 nerve roots. The nerve descends on the anterior surface of psoas major muscle and terminates as genital and femoral branches. Femoral branch provides innervations to the skin over femoral triangle; and the skin over scrotum, cremasteric muscle and labia majora, is supplied by the genital branch. The genital branch, responsible for the cremasteric reflex, passes through the inguinal canal in males. In females, it terminates in the skin of the mons pubis and labia majora in females.

Ilioinguinal Nerve

The ilioinguinal nerve is formed by the ventral ramus of L1 and occasionally T12. It runs between the second and third layers of abdominal muscles and passes in the inguinal canal. It enters the abdomen posterior to the medial arcuate ligaments and passes inferolaterally, running through the transverse abdominal muscle, while its branches pierce the external oblique aponeurosis. In both sexes, the nerve together with blood/lymphatic vessels and the spermatic cord/round ligament enter the inguinal canal before providing cutaneous innervation of the scrotum/labium majora, the root of the penis, mons pubis, and adjacent medial aspect of the thigh. Internal oblique and transversus abdominis muscles receive their motor supply from the ilioinguinal nerve.

Iliohypogastric Nerve

The ventral ramus of L1 spinal nerve forms the iliohypogastric nerve. It runs through the transverse abdominal muscle, and along with the ilioinguinal nerve its branches pierce the external oblique aponeurosis before running deep to the internal oblique. It provides cutaneous innervations to the hypogastric region, superolateral quadrant of the buttock and over the iliac crest; and supplies motor innervation to the internal oblique and transverse abdominal muscles (overlapping with the ilioinguinal nerve).

Nerve	T12	L1	L2	L3	L4	S1	S2	S3	S4	S5
Iliohypogastric	■	■								
Ilioinguinal		■								
Genitofemoral		■	■							
Obturator			■	■	■					
Posterior Femoral Cutaneous						■	■	■		
Inferior Rectal							■	■		
Pudendal							■	■	■	
Coccygeal								■	■	■

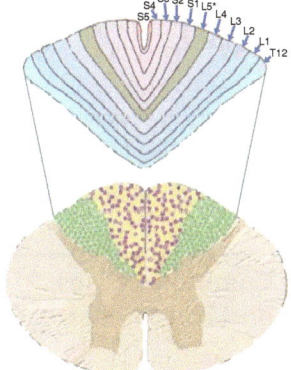

Fig. 38.2 Innervation of the relevant nerves of the pelvis are listed in the table to the left along with an illustration (right) of where the nerve roots are positioned within the dorsal columns of the spine cord in the lower thorax

Epidemiology

The prevalence of CPP in the United States and United Kingdom is reported to be as high as 14.7% and 24%, respectively, in women of reproductive age [8, 9]. CPP is more common in the female population (affecting over 9 million women in the United States) and has often initially been labeled as interstitial cystitis/painful bladder syndrome (IC/PBS) [10]. In as many as 61% of women, the cause of their CPP was unknown [11]. In men, CPP is typically caused by chronic prostatitis, accounting for 90–95% of all cases (CP) [8, 12]. Predisposing and/or associated factors in the female population include a history of multiple laparoscopies, endometriosis, sexual or physical abuse, vulvar vestibulitis, fibromyalgia, and irritable bowel syndrome [9, 13–17].

Clinical Differentiation of Gastrointestinal, Urologic, Gynecologic, and Musculoskeletal Pain

Differentiation of pain emanating from gastrointestinal, urologic, gynecologic, and musculoskeletal structure from chronic pelvic pain requires comprehensive assessment but is often quite difficult. Conditions such as malignancy and inflammatory bowel disease should be ruled out. Identification of an underlying pathology may be absent in one-third to one-half of the cases [18], and at times, the diagnosed pathologic condition may insufficiently explain the severity of pain being experienced by the patient [19].

Psychological Principles in Clinical Assessment, Explanation, and Treatment

Anxiety and depression are common psychiatric comorbidities in patients with chronic pelvic pain. Psychological assessment will reveal patient's mood, pain-coping mechanisms, functionality, social milieu, patient-provider interactions, and secondary gain status. Coexistence of anxiety or depression with chronic pain disorders such as endometriosis can determine the severity of the symptoms and effectiveness of the treatments [20]. Successful management of CPP can be achieved only when biological, psychological, and social factors are appropriately addressed.

Common Causes, Diagnostic Evaluation, and Treatment in Men

Chronic Prostatitis (CP)/Prostadynia (PD)

CP/PD still makes up a large portion of all cases of CPP in men [21]. In the United States alone, approximately 25% of men presenting with genitourinary tract problems are diagnosed with prostatitis, and up to 30% of those are ultimately diagnosed with CP/PD [22, 23].

PD has been considered a diagnosis of exclusion and a possible variant of IC, as it may represent different manifestations of the same disease process [24].

Historically, it was thought that CP/PD was simply the result of inflammation; a hypothesis supported by the fact that symptomatic relief was often obtained with the administration of anti-inflammatory medications [27]. With further investigation, however, the disease process was also found to be associated with hypertrophy of smooth muscle, periurethral edema, and pelvic floor dysfunction resulting from increased tone in local musculature [28]. These phenomena have led to the supposition that the disease may actually also be due to an imbalance of the inflammatory cascade, proliferation of neurotrophin nerve growth factor (implicated in neurogenic inflammation), autoimmune processes, and central sensitization that result in the development of a neuropathic pain state.

Common Causes, Diagnostic Evaluation, and Treatment in Women

Interstitial Cystitis (IC)/Painful Bladder Syndrome (PBS)

IC has a prevalence of 3–6% in the general population [29]. IC/PBS is characterized by frequency, urgency, dyspareunia, nocturia, and often pelvic and/or abdominal pain [30]. In 2002, the International Continence Society defined IC/PBS as suprapubic pain related to bladder filling (along with increased frequency) – without a proven urinary tract infection [31].

In 2007, the European Society for the Study of Interstitial Cystitis (ESSIC) proposed that the term "bladder pain syndrome" be used in parallel with or instead of IC in accordance with the following criteria:

- Chronic (>6 months) pelvic pain
- Pressure or discomfort perceived to be related to the urinary bladder
- Accompanied by at least one other urinary symptom like persistent urge to void or frequency [32]

While the exact etiology of IC/PBS is still unknown, many possible mechanisms have been proposed including autoimmune disorders, infection, pelvic floor dysfunction, toxins, and bladder wall defects. Many experts agree that a defect in the urothelial lining or glycosaminoglycan layer is most likely the primary cause [10]. When the urothelium is exposed to a particular noxious stimulus, mast cell activation occurs within the bladder wall, an influx of potassium ions up-regulates afferent nerves, which in turn activate more mast cells.

This positive-feedback loop leads to increased sensory nerve fiber activity in the bladder, chronic inflammation, and ultimately a neuropathic pain state involving the innervation of the bladder in which pain is manifested as visceral allodynia and hyperalgesia of the bladder and the adjacent pelvic organs [33].

Cystoscopy and hydro-distention is used to diagnose IC/PBS, and visualized tissue can be biopsied when other probable causes of pain have been excluded. In symptomatic patients, small petechial hemorrhages called "glomerulations" on bladder distention can be indicative of the disease state [34]. Hunter's ulcer can be seen on cystoscopy in 10% of patients with IC/PBS. In patients with long-standing IC/PBS, histological examination yields marked edema and injury to the blood vessels and nerves in the muscularis layer (consistent with neurogenic inflammation) [34]. IC/PBS, deafferentation of bladder and vasomotor injury to the bladder bear a striking similarity to CRPS [35–37]. IC/PBS in a female patient can be mistaken for vaginitis, vestibulodynia, or pelvic floor dysfunction [38].

Coccydynia

Coccydynia (coccygodynia) is a painful condition in or around the area of the coccyx. It is often related to trauma, infection, tumor, or osteoarthritis of the sacrococcygeal joint which is typically aggravated by sitting. However, the cause of pain in certain cases of coccydynia is unknown and may be referred pain from surrounding visceral structures such as the rectum, sigmoid colon, the urogenital system or spasm of the pelvic floor [39]. The idiopathic form comprises <1% of all non-traumatic disorders of the spinal column [40]. There is a documented correlation between weight and incidence of coccydynia; and its female-to-male ratio, like IC/PBS, is 5:1 [41, 42].

Vulvodynia

Vulvodynia, first described in 1984, is defined as vulvar discomfort in the absence of either objective physical exam findings or a diagnosed neurological disorder [26, 27]. Patients usually complain of a constant, intermittent, or contact-provoked sharp or burning pain that occurs in the vulva. Provoked vestibulodynia, or vulvar vestibulitis, is the most common variant and is defined by pain triggered from a stimulus, which is normally painless (i.e., wearing tight clothing, inserting tampons, etc.) [28]. An incidence of 15–16% has been reported; however, the true incidence may be higher [9, 43].

The exact cause of the vulvodynia is a subject of controversy; however, the most strongly favored explanation is the "muscular hypothesis" that suggests an increase in muscular tone in the superficial area of perineum [29]. Neurogenic inflammation has also been implicated, as biopsies of afflicted patients showed chronic inflammation of the mucosa along with neural hyperplasia [32].

Treatment

Pharmacologic

Medication is rarely effective in this particular cohort of patients. While it is not completely understood as to why this is the case, it may be the result of a frequent failure to recognize the cause and/or mechanism of the pain. Nonetheless, pharmacologic therapies should be trialed. Opioids and other potentially habit-forming substances should be avoided if at all possible in patients with CPP. The medications that may be prescribed for this condition:

- Non-steroidal anti-inflammatories.
- Cox-2 inhibitors (meloxicam and celecoxib).
- Topical lidocaine.
- Membrane stabilizers (gabapentin and pregabalin).
- Anti-depressants (SSRIs, SNRIs, and TCAs).
- Tramadol or tapentadol – these should be attempted before opioids if safe and there is no potential cross-reaction with any other medications currently being taken.
- Tizanidine or baclofen – these two drugs have a centralized mechanism of action as compared to other more commonly used muscle relaxers (i.e., cyclobenzaprine) that tend to be more sedating in nature and could potentially become habit forming.
- Opioids should be avoided.

Psychological

Psychosocial elements are extremely prevalent in CPP and may play an important role in one's ability to respond to treatment. Additionally, sexual assault and/or emotional trauma may manifest as pain – consequently, it is of the utmost importance to make sure these patients have ready access to psychological treatment protocols such as cognitive behavioral therapy (CBT) [31].

Physical Therapy(PT)

Physical therapy, including pelvic floor PT, is absolutely mandatory for the management of chronic pelvic pain. When used as part of a multimodal, multidisciplinary approach, patients have been shown to report significant benefit [32, 33]. Exercises typically focus on pelvic floor muscle relaxation, ultrasound, and stretching.

Interventional

As with most chronic pain conditions, interventional pain management techniques can be introduced if the patient does not respond to more conservative methods. There are a number of different therapies to choose from and that should be attempted starting with the least invasive first. Examples of interventional pain procedures include:

- Trigger point injections
- Chemodenervation using botulinum toxin
- Ganglion impar blocks
- Inferior hypogastric plexus blocks
- Superior hypogastric plexus blocks
- Peripheral nerve blocks
  - Pudendal
  - Ilioinguinal/iliohypogastric
  - Genitofemoral
  - Lateral femoral cutaneous
- Chemodenervation using dehydrated alcohol or phenol
- Pulsed radiofrequency ablation

Neuromodulation

In 1997, FDA approved epidural sacral nerve root stimulation for the treatment of urinary urgency, frequency, urge incontinence, and retention [34–36]. The mechanism behind sacral nerve stimulation's (SNS) ability to modulate micturition is still being investigated. It may activate or reset the somatic afferents involved in sensory processing and the micturition reflex pathways in the spinal cord [34]. Other researchers have proposed that SNS may interfere with sympathetic signals to the bladder involved in the guarding and vesicosympathetic reflex, which control continence and filling, respectively [34, 35] More recent studies with PET have revealed an increased activity in the paraventricular gray of the brain which is involved in activation or inhibition of the micturition reflex [34, 37].

Apart from its promising ability to relief pain of IC/PBS, SNS has shown efficacy in the treatment of bladder dysfunction, incontinence, urinary retention/frequency, and fecal incontinence [34, 36, 38–41]. As use of the technology evolved, SNS had been expanded from a traditionally unilateral approach to a more aggressive bilateral one, as pain with IC/PBS is seldom unilateral [42]. Many subsequent smaller studies were able to demonstrate reductions in both pain and

opioid requirements with the more aggressive approach to SNS [43–46].

In addition to IC/PBS, SNS is also an effective intervention for treating CP/PD, coccydynia, vulvodynia, anorectal pain, and pelvic pain from general pelvic floor dysfunction and spinal cord infarction [1, 10, 25, 40, 47–50]. Despite the availability of data supporting the use of SNS, some patterns of pain remain unresponsive to the intervention, level of pain control varies greatly from one study to the next, and studies have failed to consistently demonstrate an overall improvement in quality of life for patients [43, 49] Furthermore, some authors posit that general complication rates with SNS have been unacceptably high [51].

Alternative sites for stimulation have been suggested, including the dorsal columns at T11–L1 levels, at T5–7 levels, and at the level of the conus [1, 52]. While the exact mechanism of pelvic analgesia secondary to spinal cord stimulation (e.g., dorsal column stimulation) remains unclear, it may have to do with the anatomy of the dorsal columns.

Traditional spinal cord stimulation, while effective and well documented in the literature, has presented neuromodulators with a difficulty [2, 5]. This cohort of patients has the highest rate of explants among all the diagnoses treated with SCS with the two most commonly cited reasons being loss of therapeutic effect and/or collateral paresthesias in unaffected area(s) of pain. Dorsal root ganglion stimulation (DRGS) is a relatively new innovation in neuromodulation that may potentially mitigate some of the deficiencies with tradition SCS for CPP. In 2018, Hunter and Yang published on a novel target array for treating CPP with DRGS by stimulating the L1 and S2 levels [52].

If neurostimulation is ineffective, targeted drug delivery could also be considered as a final and last resort. The catheter should be placed either at the level of the conus or near the sacral nerve region. If this therapy is to be utilized, one should abide by the latest, up-to-date PACC (Polyanalgesic Consensus Council) guidelines with regard to choosing which drug(s) to employ as well as how to titrate due to the potential for side effects known to occur.

References

1. Kothari S. Neuromodulation approaches to chronic pelvic pain and coccydynia. Acta Neurochir Suppl. 2007;97:365–71.
2. Hunter C, et al. Neuromodulation of pelvic visceral pain: Review of the literature and case series of potential novel targets for treatment. Pain Pract. 2013;13(1):3–17.
3. Fall M, Baranowski AP, Fowler CJ, et al. EAU guidelines on chronic pelvic pain. Eur Urol. 2004;46(6):681–9.
4. Fall M, Baranowski AP, Elneil S, et al. Guidelines on chronic pelvic pain. In: EAU guidelines. Edition presented at the 23rd EAU annual congress, Milan; 2008.

5. Hunter CW, Stovall B, Chen G, Carlson J, Levy R. Anatomy, pathophysiology and interventional therapies for chronic pelvic pain: a review. Pain Physician. 2018;21(2):147–67.
6. Chang-seok O, et al. Clinical implications of topographic anatomy on ganglion impar. Anesthesiology. 2004;101:249–50.
7. Grant's atlas of anatomy, 11th ed. Lipincot Wiliams & Wilkins, Philadelphia, Pennsylvania (2005) p. 221.
8. Zondervan KT, Yudkin PL, Vessey MP, et al. The community prevalence of chronic pelvic pain in women and associated illness behavior. Br J Gen Pract. 2001;51:541–7.
9. Mathias SD, Kupperman M, Liberman RF, et al. Chronic pelvic pain: prevalence, health related quality of life, and economic correlates. Obstet Gynecol. 1996;87:838–41.
10. Fariello JY, Whitmore K. Sacral neuromodulation for IC/PBS, chronic pelvic pain, and sexual dysfunction. Int Urogynecol J. 2010;21:1553–8.
11. Mathias SC, Kupperman M, Liberman RF, et al. Prevalence, health-related quality of life, and economic correlates. J Obstet Gynaecol. 1999;106:1149–55.
12. De la Rosette JJ, Hubregste MR, Meuleman EJ, et al. Diagnosis and treatment of 409 patients with prostatitis syndromes. Urology. 1993;41:301–7.
13. Janicki TI. Chronic pelvic pain as a form of complex regional pain syndrome. Clin Obstet Gynecol. 2003;46:797–803.
14. Heim C, Ehlert U, Hanker JP, et al. Abuse related posttraumatic stress disorder and alterations of the hypothalamic-pituitary adrenal axis in women with chronic pelvic pain. Psychosom Med. 1998;60:309–18.
15. Aaron LA, Herrell R, Ashton S, et al. Comorbid clinical conditions in chronic fatigue: a co-twin control study. J Gen Intern Med. 2001;16:24–31.
16. Martinez-Lavin M. Is fibromyalgia a generalized reflex sympathetic dystrophy? Clin Exp Rheumatol. 2001;19:1–3.
17. Longstreth GF. Irritable bowel syndrome and chronic pelvic pain. Obstet Gynecol Surv. 1994;49:505–7.
18. Reiter RC. Nongynecologic somatic pathology in women with chronic pelvic pain and negative laparoscopy. J Reprod Med. 1991;36:253.
19. Stout AL. Relationship of laparoscopic findings to self report of pelvic pain. Am J Gynecol. 1991;164:73.
20. Laganà AS, La Rosa VL, Rapisarda AMC, et al. Anxiety and depression in patients with endometriosis: impact and management challenges. Int J Womens Health. 2017;9:323–30. https://doi.org/10.2147/IJWH.S119729.
21. Abrams P, Cardozo L, Fall M, et al. Reports from the standardization subcommittee of the International Continence Society. Am J Obstet Gynecol. 2002;187:116–26.
22. Schaeffer AJ. Classification (traditional and National Institutes of Health) and demographics of prostatitis. Urology. 2002;60:5–6.
23. Anothaisintawee T, Attia J, Nickel JC, et al. Management of chronic prostatitis/chronic pelvic pain syndrome: a systematic review and network meta-analysis. JAMA. 2011;305:78–86.
24. Moldwin RM. Similarities between interstitial cystitis and male chronic pelvic pain syndrome. Curr Urol Rep. 2002;3:313–8.
25. Parker J, Buga S, Sarria JE, et al. Advancements in the management of urologic chronic pelvic pain: what is new and what do we know? Curr Urol Rep. 2010;11:286–91.
26. Wehbe SA, Fariello JY, Whitmore K. Minimally invasive therapies for chronic pelvic pain syndrome. Curr Urol Rep. 2010;11:276–85.
27. Forrest JB, Nickel JC, Moldwin RM. Chronic prostatitis/chronic pelvic pain and male interstitial cystitis: enigmas and opportunities. Urology. 2007;69:60–3.
28. Schaeffer AJ. Classification (traditional and National Institutes of Health) and demographics of prostatitis. Urology. 2002;60:5–6.
29. Berry SH, Stoto MA, Elliott W, et al. Prevalence of interstitial cystitis/painful bladder syndrome in the United States. The Rand Interstitial Cystitis Epidemiology (RICE) study. Poster presented at the annual meeting of the American Urological Association. Chicago, IL; April 25–30, 2009.
30. Comiter CV. Sacral neuromodulation for the symptomatic treatment of refractory cystitis: a prospective study. J Urol. 2003;169:1369–73.
31. Nickel JC, Mullins C, Tripp DA. Development of an evidence-based cognitive behavioral treatment program for men with chronic prostatitis/chronic pelvic pain syndrome. World J Urol. 2008;26(2):167–72.
32. Markwell SJ. Physical therapy management of pelvi/perineal and perianal pain syndromes. World J Urol. 2001;19(3):194–9.
33. Rosenbaum TY, Owens A. The role of pelvic floor physical therapy in the treatment of pelvic and genital pain-related sexual dysfunction (CME). J Sex Med. 2008;5(3):513–23; quiz 524–5
34. Van Kerrebroeck PE. Advances in the role of sacral nerve neuromodulation in lower urinary tract symptoms. Int Urogynecol J. 2010;21:S467–74.
35. Mayer RD, Howard FM. Sacral nerve stimulation: neuromodulation for voiding dysfunction and pain. Neurotherapeutics. 2008;5:107–13.
36. Powell CR, Kredert KJ. Long-term outcomes of urgency-frequency syndrome due to painful bladder syndrome treated with sacral neuromodulation and analysis of failures. J Urol. 2010;183:173–6.
37. Das Gupta R, Critchley HD, Dolan RJ, et al. Changes in brain activity following sacral neuromodulation for urinary retention. J Urol. 2005;174:2268–72.
38. Jonas U, Fowler CJ, Chancellor MB. Efficacy of sacral nerve stimulation for urinary retention: results 18 months after implantation. J Urol. 2001;165:15–9.
39. Van Balken MR, Vergust H, Bemelmans BLH. The use of electrical devices for the treatment of bladder dysfunction: a review of methods. J Urol. 2004;172:846–51.
40. Pettit PDM, Thompson JR, Chen AH. Sacral neuromodulation: new applications in the treatment of female pelvic floor dysfunction. Curr Opin Obstet Gynecol. 2002;14:521–5.
41. Michelsen HB, Christensen P, Krogh K, et al. Sacral nerve stimulation for faecal incontinence alters colorectal transport. Br J Surg. 2008;95:779–84.
42. Zabihi N, Mourtzinos A, Maher MG, et al. Short term results of bilateral S2-S4 sacral neuromodulation for the treatment of refractory interstitial cystitis, painful bladder syndrome, and pelvic pain. Int Urogynecol J Pelvic Floor Dysfunct. 2008;19:553–7.
43. Maher CF, Carey MP, Pl D, et al. Percutaneous sacral nerve root neuromodulation for intractable interstitial cystitis. J Urol. 2001;165:884–6.
44. Seigel S, Paszkiewicz E, Kirkpatrick C, et al. Sacral nerve stimulation in patients with chronic intractable pelvic pain. J Urol. 2001;166:1742–5.
45. Everaert K, Devulder J, De Muynck M, et al. The pain cycle: implications for the diagnosis and treatment of pelvic pain syndromes. Int Urogynecol J. 2001;12:9–14.
46. Yang KS, Kim YH, Park HJ, et al. Sacral nerve stimulation for the treatment of chronic intractable anorectal pain – a case report. Korean J Pain. 2010;23(1):60–4.
47. Govaert B, Melehorst J, van Kleef M, et al. Sacral neuromodulation for the treatment of chronic functional anorectal pain: a single center experience. Pain Pract. 2009;10:49–53.
48. Kim SH, Kim SH, Kim SW, et al. Sacral nerve and spinal cord stimulation for intractable neuropathic pain caused by spinal cord infarction. Neuromodulation. 2007;10:369–72.
49. Brookoff D, Bennett DS. Neuromodulation in intractable interstitial cystitis and related pelvic pain syndromes. Pain Med. 2006;7:S166–84.

50. Feler CA, Whitworth LA, Fernandez J. Sacral modulation for chronic pain conditions. Anesthesiol Clin North America. 2003;21:785–95.

51. Seigel SW, Catanzaro F, Dijkema HE, et al. Long term results of a multicenter study on sacral nerve stimulation for treatment of uri-nary urge incontinence, urgency-frequency, and retention. Urology. 2000;5:87–91.

52. Hunter CW, Yang A. Dorsal root ganglion stimulation for chronic pelvic pain: a case series technical report on a novel lead configura-tion. Neuromodulation. 2019;22(1):87–95.

Pain in Pregnancy and Labor

Demetri Koutsospyros and Lawrence Epstein

Introduction

Factors Influencing the Perception of Pain in Pregnancy Compared with the Nonpregnant State

Estrogens

- Highly lipophilic and have low molecular weight thus easily penetrating CNS and affecting multiple CNS receptors and nerves in both the spinal cord and brain.
- Influence receptive field properties of primary afferents in the trigeminal and pudendal nerves [1].
- Increase GABA release.
- Up-regulate GABA-A receptors.
- Up-regulate serotonin.
- Estrogen receptors are present in lumbosacral spinal cord, especially in the substantia gelatinosa.
- Estrogen receptors present in the dorsal horn of the lumbosacral region increase in density when estrogen levels are high [2].

Behavioral, Psychological, and Social Factors

There is increased susceptibility to pain during pregnancy due to anxiety. Specific causes of anxiety include:

- Fear of pregnancy itself
- Implications on the future of the mother
- Stress about future motherhood

D. Koutsospyros
Department of Anesthesiology, Montefiore Medical Center, Bronx, NY, USA

L. Epstein (✉)
Department of Anesthesiology, James J Peters Veterans Affairs Medical Center, Bronx, NY, USA

Positive attitudes toward pregnancy may decrease pain or increase tolerance to pain.

Cultural views of pregnancy and childbirth cannot be overlooked as factors in either decreasing or increasing pain due to preconceived notions as to what pain signifies, as well as ideas on how one should behave during pregnancy [3].

Causes of Pain in Pregnancy

Presence and Growth of the Gravid Uterus

- Increase in lumbar lordosis.
- Stretching of anterior and posterior longitudinal ligaments of the lumbar spine causes spreading of symphysis pubis and SIJ leading to pelvic pain.
- New spondylolisthesis or worsening of current spondylolisthesis (secondary to increased lordosis and laxity).
- Resultant increase in anterior pelvic tilt causing altered lower extremity mechanics.
- Increased joint stress especially in the lumbar facets, hips, sacroiliac joints, and knees.
- Weakness and separation of abdominal muscles.
- Pressure in abdomen can cause visceral pain and cramping.
- Stretching of the round ligament leading to lower pelvic pain.
- Radicular symptoms can be common and are usually due to direct compression of lumbosacral nerves from uterus/fetal head [4].

Nerve Entrapment Syndromes and Neuropathic Pain

- Cutaneous branches of thoracic nerves which pierce the abdominal wall muscles can be stretched or become entrapped as the abdominal wall is stretched. This will usually cause a unilateral pain, although bilateral pain can occur [5].

© Springer Nature Switzerland AG 2019
Y. Khelemsky et al. (eds.), *Academic Pain Medicine*, https://doi.org/10.1007/978-3-030-18005-8_39

- Similarly, the iliohypogastric, genitofemoral, and lateral femoral cutaneous nerves can become entrapped. This can lead to pain in the groin, labia, and thighs [6].
- Carpal tunnel syndrome and tarsal tunnel syndrome are more common in pregnancy due to increased fluid retention and peripheral edema [7].
- Cesarean section scars can become painful as they become stretched.

Headaches

- Unlikely to begin during pregnancy [8].
- If preexisting, they tend to improve during pregnancy [9].
- Headaches often go untreated or undertreated due to fears regarding the safety of commonly used medications.

Joint Pain

- New joint pains are very common in pregnancy. Causes include hormonal changes (higher levels of relaxin leading to increased joint laxity, increased fluid retention, and tissue swelling secondary to higher levels of cortisol, progesterone, and estrogen) and anatomic changes (as listed previously) [10].
- Pregnancy can alter the course of preexisting inflammatory conditions, but the effects are not uniform (i.e., there is increased disease activity in systemic lupus erythematosus, but decreased disease activity in rheumatoid arthritis, etc.) [11].

Principles of Pain Management in Pregnancy

Risks to the growing fetus from treatment modalities are of primary concern. It is important to make the patient an active participant in her care and to be transparent about all treatment options and what is known about their effect on the fetus, as well as what is not known.

Generally speaking, a multidisciplinary approach, closely coordinated with the obstetric team, is widely considered to be the best and safest for the pregnant patient. This will provide maximal benefit while minimizing risk to the fetus by avoiding using medications which may have unsafe for the fetus. The Federal Drug Administration (FDA) has developed categories describing the safety of medications used in pregnancy (Table 39.1). Commonly used analgesics are listed in Table 39.2, according to the FDA pregnancy classification. Of note, avoiding NSAIDS not just in the third trimester but in the first trimester should be considered.

Table 39.1 FDA pregnancy categories

Category	Description
A	Well-controlled studies in humans show no risk to the fetus
B	No well-controlled studies have been conducted in humans Animal studies show no risk to the fetus
C	No well-controlled studies have been conducted in humans Animal studies have shown an adverse effect on the fetus
D	Evidence of human risk to the fetus exists; however, benefits may outweigh the risks in certain situations
X	Controlled studies in animals or humans demonstrate fetal abnormalities; the risk in pregnant women clearly outweighs any possible benefit

Table 39.2 FDA pregnancy categories of common pain medications

Category	Description
A	
B	Acetaminophen, oxycodone, lidocaine, and ibuprofen (first and second trimester), naproxen (first and second trimester)
C	All opioids except oxycodone, gabapentin, topiramate, tricyclic antidepressants, SNRIs, muscle relaxants, benzodiazepines (temazepam is X), steroids, ketorolac, nabumetone, and etodolac
D	Aspirin, NSAIDS (third trimester)
X	

Common Conditions

Low Back Pain

Low back pain is extremely common in pregnancy due to the changes mentioned earlier. Recommended treatments include:

- Prophylactic strengthening and exercise therapies.
- Education: Posture education, ergonomics, braces to help teach correct posture, and ergonomics. Bracing should only be used temporarily for teaching purposes.
- Scheduled rest for spasms and acute pain [12].
- Physical therapy: Especially postural modifications, back strengthening, stretching, and self-mobilization techniques.
  - Lumbar spine flexion exercises help strengthen abdominal muscles and decrease lordosis which is accentuated in pregnancy.
  - Extension exercises help improve paraspinal muscle strength/function providing more lumbar support.
  - Other popular PT exercises which have been shown to help women during pregnancy include pelvic tilt, knee pull, straight leg raising, curl up, lateral straight leg raises, and Kegel exercises [13].

- Acupuncture has been shown to be superior to physical therapy with no significant adverse effects. It is recommended that acupuncture points which stimulate the cervix and uterus are avoided as they may stimulate labor [14].
- Manual therapy has also been shown to be effective, especially osteopathic manipulative treatment [15].
- Water therapy, which occasionally gets grouped with physical therapy, has been shown to improve pain while decreasing demand for sick leave for back pain [16].
- TENS has been shown by small studies to be more effective than exercise and acetaminophen with no noted adverse effects. The recommendation is to keep the current density low [17].
- Medication should be used judiciously and with risks for both the patient and the fetus weighed against the potential benefit.
  - Acetaminophen is considered a first-line analgesic.
  - Opioids should be used for severe pain with the understanding that when they are given chronically in the perinatal period, they can cause a withdrawal syndrome in the newborn. NSAIDs should generally be avoided throughout pregnancy, especially during the first and third trimesters. In the third trimester, they can cause uterine artery vasoconstriction and premature closing of the ductus arteriosus in the fetus.
  - Gabapentin is associated with craniofacial abnormalities, neural tube defects, and mental deficiency.
  - When taken in the third trimester, amitriptyline causes withdrawal symptoms in neonates which presents with cardiac problems, irritability, respiratory distress, muscle spasms, urinary retention, and seizures. When taken earlier in pregnancy, developmental delay and limb abnormalities have been reported.
  - Steroids have been studied in patients with chronic conditions which require daily steroid use throughout pregnancy. These studies are mostly inconclusive. An earlier study, which was slightly underpowered, showed an increase in cleft lip/palate incidence from 1/1000 in the general population to 3–6/1000 in patients with chronic steroid use. Later, better powered studies either failed to show a correlation or showed an even smaller increase of cleft lip/palate in chronic steroid users. Studies on these patients have also showed a higher likelihood of preterm birth and low birth weight. However, due to concomitant rheumatic or autoimmune diseases in these patients, it was unclear if the steroids were the causative agents. There have also been studies showing that the use of prednisone or prednisolone may help improve pregnancy outcomes.
  - Local anesthetics can be given intravenously, epidurally, or intramuscularly for the treatment of different types of pain in pregnancy. There is theoretical local anesthetic ion trapping in the fetus due to the lower pH of fetal blood as well as higher free (nonprotein bound) concentration of local anesthetic making it more likely to cross the placenta. However, fetuses have been shown to be more resistant to local anesthetic toxicity than adults, so it is more likely to see toxic side effects in the mother prior to the fetus being affected.
- Interventional procedures are always an option in the pregnant patient but with certain precautions. While it is well known and repeatedly proven that fluoroscopically guided injections are superior to blind injections, the use of fluoroscopy in early pregnancy should be avoided.
  - Blind injections such as interlaminar epidural steroid injections or trigger point injections are safe options when performed by experienced providers.
  - Ultrasound-guided injections have been shown to be both safe and effective.
  - For radicular pain, ultrasound-guided selective nerve root blocks have been shown to be superior to a caudal approach.
  - Ultrasound-guided sacroiliac joint injections have been shown to be very effective for sacroiliitis which is very common in pregnancy [4].
  - Ultrasound-guided joint injections are considered safe and effective.

Neuropathic Pain

- Carpal tunnel syndrome can be treated with activity modification, day or night splinting, and ultrasound-guided steroid injections [18].
- Meralgia paresthetica usually does not require treatment and improves spontaneously after delivery. If pain becomes too severe during pregnancy or persists after delivery, steroid/local anesthetic infiltration at the site of maximal tenderness and lateral femoral cutaneous nerve block are both safe and effective options. Stretching exercises can be safe and effective as an alternative to interventional techniques [19].
- Nerve entrapment syndromes can be safely injected with local anesthetic +/− steroid under ultrasound guidance [5].
- Intercostal neuralgia can be safely treated with topical lidocaine, intercostal nerve blocks, and/or epidural steroid injections [20]. If long-lasting relief cannot be achieved with these measures, intercostal nerve radiofrequency ablation is likely safe as cardiac RFA has been shown to be safe in multiple small studies and intrauterine RFA is frequently performed for twin reversed arterial perfusion sequence (TRAP) and has been shown to be safe for the surviving twin.

Pelvic and Abdominal Pain

- Patient education is the easiest and arguably most effective treatment for the management of pelvic pain. Information on ergonomics, appropriate physical activity, and avoidance of maladaptive movements/poor posture can also be very helpful and a good introduction to physical therapy if needed in the future [4].
- Massage, water gymnastics, acupuncture, pelvic belts, and exercise are all effective and safe treatments for pelvic pain. They are all preferred over medical management. Of note, pelvic belts should only be used for short periods of time [21].

Mechanisms and Characteristics of Labor Pain

Labor is divided into three stages.

- The first stage of labor consists of the beginning of labor until the cervix is fully dilated. Pain is due to dilation, distension, and stretching of the cervix.
  - This pain is typically visceral and is described as dull, crampy, achy, poorly localized, and often referred to other areas.
  - Pain impulses travel through sensory nerves and adjacent sympathetic fibers of T10–L1. Additional neighboring levels may occasionally be implicated as well, as sympathetics can synapse at multiple levels.
- The second stage of labor begins immediately after full dilation of the cervix and ends with delivery of the fetus.
  - Pain in this stage of labor is due to the passage of the baby through the vaginal canal causing stretching and tearing of multiple tissues including fascia, subcutaneous tissues, and skin.
  - This pain is typically somatic and is described as sharp and localized in the perineum.
  - This somatic pain is transmitted through the pudendal nerve to sacral nerve roots S2–S4.
- The third stage of labor begins after delivery of the baby and ends with the delivery of the placenta.
  - Typically less painful than the first two stages, but is described as dull visceral pain from continued uterine contractions.

Benefits and Potential Adverse Consequences of Labor Pain

The vast majority of study with regard to labor pain deals with different methods of treating it safely and effectively. There has been little research into adverse effects of labor pain on the parturient or baby and even less into the benefits of labor pain.

Pain has several physiologic and psychological effects on the laboring parturient.

- Most negative physiologic effects of labor pain manifest themselves via alterations in the respiratory patterns of the parturient as well as her body's catecholamine-mediated stress response [22].
- The respiratory effects include increased oxygen consumption and hyperventilation with resulting respiratory alkalosis secondary to hypocarbia.
- The stress response effects include increased gastric acidity, decreased gastric emptying, increased cardiac output, increased peripheral vascular resistance leading to elevated blood pressures, decreased placental perfusion, and at times paradoxical or incoordinate uterine activity potentially leading to changes in fetal heart rate.
- It is hypothesized that these responses, at their extremes, can produce maternal acidemia, fetal acidosis, and dysfunctional labor. However, to date there is no data proving that increased labor pain has any measurable negative outcomes on labor or delivery [23].
- It has been found that parturients, especially primiparas, who receive better labor analgesia have higher arterial oxygen saturations [24] and better neonatal acid base status [25] with an inverse correlation to their scores on the visual pain analog scale.
- Psychologically, it has been found that parturients who had good labor analgesia subjectively had an overall more positive childbirth experience and memory of that experience [26].
- Long after delivery, memories of labor pain can invoke negative reactions in some patients, while in others it can lead to feelings of increased self-esteem and self-efficacy [27]. This is largely due to preexisting cultural and psychosocial conditioning and does not appear to correlate to pain scores.

One possible benefit of labor pain which has been studied and measured is the increased concentration of beta-endorphin in the colostrum of lactating mothers who have gone through the labor process and vaginal delivery as opposed to those who have undergone cesarean section [28]. The predominant theory is that there are increased endorphin levels in the parturient during painful labor which leads to concomitant increase in beta-endorphin concentrations in colostrum. The increased beta-endorphin helps decrease newborns' stress response in the perinatal period.

Management of Labor Pain

Management of the laboring patient is typically not performed by a pain management specialist. Usually, in this acute situation, pain is managed by an anesthesiologist, obstetrician, or midwife via various methods with varying levels of evidence.

- The highest quality evidence for efficacy exists for combined spinal epidural, epidural, and inhaled analgesia.
  - Combined spinal epidural relieves pain faster than epidural, although with higher frequency of pruritus and with less nausea/vomiting/dizziness than inhaled analgesia.
  - Epidural, while very effective for treating labor pain, is associated with more instrumental vaginal births and increased rate of cesarean section for fetal distress, although overall section rate was unchanged from placebo or alternate therapy (e.g., parenteral opioids or inhaled analgesia).
  - Inhaled analgesia (nitrous oxide), though not available at many centers, can be highly effective, but is associated with adverse effects including nausea, vomiting, and dizziness.
- There is moderate evidence that acupuncture, massage, relaxation, local anesthetic nerve blocks, non-opioid drugs, or water immersion therapy may improve labor pain with few adverse effects. Studies on the above are usually limited to single trials and most require further study, but they remain as alternatives.
  - Acupuncture was associated with a lower rate of assisted vaginal birth and c-section.
  - Relaxation was associated with a lower rate of assisted vaginal birth.
- There is currently not enough evidence to support hypnosis, TENS, aromatherapy, parenteral opioids, or biofeedback as being more effective than placebo [29].

References

1. Hapidou EG. Perception of pain during pregnancy and labor. In: Stefan Lautenbacher RBF, editor. Pathophysiology of pain perception. New York: Springer Science & Business Media; 2012.
2. Aloisi A. Gonadal hormones and sex differences in pain reactivity. Clin J Pain. 2003;19(3):168–74.
3. Ebirim LN, Buowari OY, Ghosh S. Physical and psychological aspects of pain in obstetrics. In: Pain in perspective. London: InTech; 2012. p. 219–36.
4. Shah S, Banh ET, Koury K, Bhatia G, Nandi R, Gulur P. Pain Management in Pregnancy: multimodal approaches. Pain Res Treat. 2015;2015:1 15.
5. Peleg R, Gohar J, Koretz M, Peleg A. Abdominal wall pain in pregnant women caused by thoracic lateral cutaneous nerve entrapment. Eur J Obstet Gynecol Reprod Biol. 1997;74(2):169–71.
6. Deal CL, Canoso JJ. Meralgia paresthetica and large abdomens. Ann Intern Med. 1982;96(6):787–8.
7. Padua L, Aprile I, Caliandro P, Carboni T, Meloni A, Massi S, Mazza O, Mondelli M, Morini A, Murasecco D, Romano M, Tonali P. Symptoms and neurophysiological picture of carpal tunnel syndrome in pregnancy. Clin Neurophysiol. 2001;112(10):1946–51.
8. Ertresvåg JM, Zwart JA, Helde G, Johnsen HJ, Bovim G. Headache and transient focal neurological symptoms during pregnancy, a prospective cohort. Acta Neurol Scand. 2005;111(4):233–7.
9. Nappi RE, Albani F, Sances G, Terreno E, Brambilla E, Polatti F. Headaches during pregnancy. Curr Pain Headache Rep. 2011;15(4):289–94.
10. Choi HJ, Lee JC, Lee YJ, Lee EB, Shim SS, Park JS, Jun JK, Song YW. Prevalence and clinical features of arthralgia/arthritis in healthy pregnant women. Rheumatol Int. 2008;28(11):1111–5.
11. Silman A, Kay A, Brennan P. Timing of pregnancy in relation to the onset of rheumatoid arthritis. Arthritis Rheum. 1992;35(2): 152–5.
12. Borg-Stein J, Dugan SA. Musculoskeletal disorders of pregnancy, delivery and postpartum. Phys Med Rehabil Clin N Am. 2007;18(3):459–76.
13. Sabino J, Grauer JN. Pregnancy and low back pain. Curr Rev Musculoskelet Med. 2008;1(2):137–41.
14. Pennick VE, Young G. Interventions for preventing and treating pelvic and back pain in pregnancy. Cochrane Database Syst Rev. 2013;(8)
15. Licciardone JC, Buchanan S, Hensel KL, King HH, Fulda KG, Stoll ST. Osteopathic manipulative treatment of back pain and related symptoms during pregnancy: a randomized controlled trial. Am J Obstet Gynecol. 2010;202(1):43–8.
16. Granath AB, Hellgren MS, Gunnarsson RK. Water aerobics reduces sick leave due to low back pain during pregnancy. J Obstet Gynecol Neonatal Nurs. 2006;35(4):465–71.
17. Keskin EA, Onur O, Keskin HL, Gumus II, Kafali H, Turhan N. Transcutaneous electrical nerve stimulation improves low back pain during pregnancy. Gynecol Obstet Invest. 2012;74(1): 76–83.
18. Seror P. Pregnancy-related carpal tunnel syndrome. J Hand Surg. 1998;23(1):98–101.
19. Mabie WC. Peripheral neuropathies during pregnancy. Clin Obstet Gynecol. 2005;48(1):57–66.
20. Sax TW, Rosenbaum RB. Neuromuscular disorders in pregnancy. Muscle Nerve. 2006;34(5):559–71.
21. Vleeming A, Albert HB, Ostgaard HC, Sturesson B, Stuge B. European guidelines for the diagnosis and treatment of pelvic girdle pain. Eur Spine J. 2008;17(6):794–819.
22. Walls JD, Gaiser R. Chronic pain in the obstetric patient. Anesthesiol Clin. 2013;31(3):505–15.
23. Lowe NK. The nature of labor pain. Am J Obstet Gynecol. 2002;186(5):S16–24.
24. Brownridge P. The nature and consequences of childbirth pain. Eur J Obstet Gynecol Reprod Biol. 1995;59:S9–15.
25. Deckardt R, Fembacher PM, Schneider KT, Graeff H. Maternal arterial oxygen saturation during labor and delivery: pain-dependent alterations and effects on the newborn. Obstet Gynecol. 1987;70(1):21–5.
26. Hur MH. Effects of one-to-one labor support on labor pain, labor stress response, childbirth experience and neonatal status for primipara. Korean J Women Health Nurs. 2001;7(2):188–202.
27. Niven CA, Murphy-Black T. Memory for labor pain: a review of the literature. Birth. 2000;27.244–53.
28. Zanardo V, Nicolussi S, Giacomin C, Faggian D, Favaro F, Plebani M. Labor pain effects on Colostral Milk Beta-endorphin concentrations of lactating mothers. Biol Neonate. 2001;79:87–90.
29. Jones L, Othman M, Dowswell T, Alfirevic Z, Gates S, Newburn M, Jordan S, Lavender T, Neilson J. Pain management for women in labour: an overview of systematic reviews. Cochrane Database Syst Rev. 2012;3:CD009234.

Headache

Dmitri Souza, Irena Kiliptch, and Alex Feoktistov

Introduction

Some of the earliest records describing headaches can be found in the ancient texts more than five thousand years ago [1, 2]. Hippocrates was the first to describe what we today know as headache disorder [2–4]. Our understanding and ability to diagnose and treat continues to grow [5–8]. Headache disorders are among the most prevalent global health issues involving the nervous system [9]. Headache is the most common cause of absenteeism from school and from work [10]. The World Health Organization (WHO) estimates that nearly 50% of adults worldwide have had one or more symptomatic headaches within the past year [11]. Tension headaches make up the largest majority, and are the most common form of headache [12]. Chronic headaches affect around 15% of the general population, causing various levels of disability and social dysfunction [13]. The role of pain medicine specialists in the diagnosis and treatment of headaches is significant. This chapter will provide a basic introduction to the classification and treatment of select headache disorders.

Headache Classification

Recent understanding of headache disorders has markedly increased and continues to expand. Since the first classifications, we have been able to distinguish migraine headaches, tension-type headaches, cluster headaches, paroxysmal hemicranias, and chronic versus episodic headaches, among many other forms. Naturally, a new, more detailed clinical characterization has emerged. In 1988 the International Headache Society provided the first official headache disorder classification that included presentation, etiology, and pathogenesis. The first classification lacked supporting research and was written based on expert opinion of the time [14]. The need for an updated text was answered in 2004 when the 2nd edition, and in 2013, when the 3rd edition of the International Classification of Headache Disorders were created [15]. It included medication overuse headache, and some other newly described headache disorders [16].

Migraine Headache

Migraine headache, the second most common type of headache (after tension), affects 15% of women and 5% of men worldwide [17]. Migraine headaches can occur at any age, however onset is most common prior to the third decade of life. Migraines predominantly present with unilateral throbbing, pulsating sensation with significant pain [16]. This headache can be accompanied by nausea/vomiting, photophobia, sensitivity to smells and sounds [10]. Migraines can often be triggered by both exogenous and endogenous factors including, but not limited to: hormonal changes, certain foods, disordered sleep, weather conditions, alcohol, and caffeine. The typical length of the headache can range from 4 to 72 hours with fast onset occurring from 20 minutes to 1 hour [2, 10, 14, 16, 17].

Migraines are often associated with prodrome and/or aura. Patients with migraines that present with aura experience painless and reversible visual disturbances. These disturbances include but are not limited to scotomas, flashing lights, and distortions. Patients may also experience abnormalities with hearing or smell, weakness of extremities, aphasia, blindness, confusion, vertigo, or hemiplegia [10, 17].

Considering this wide variety of symptoms migraines are further subcategorized into episodic and chronic. There are also basilar-type migraines, hemiplegic migraine, and other, less common types [6, 9, 10, 17].

D. Souza (✉)
Western Reserve Hospital, Heritage College of Osteopathic Medicine, Ohio University, Cuyahoga Falls, OH, USA

I. Kiliptch
Avalon University School of Medicine, Toronto, ON, Canada

A. Feoktistov
Clinical Research, Diamond Health Clinic, Glenview, IL, USA

© Springer Nature Switzerland AG 2019
Y. Khelemsky et al. (eds.), *Academic Pain Medicine*, https://doi.org/10.1007/978-3-030-18005-8_40

Cluster Headache

Cluster headaches are the third most common type of primary headaches [18]. They are classified under the main category of trigeminal autonomic cephalalgias (TACs). Cluster headaches are frequently described to be the worst pain and most severe pain ever suffered [19]. These headaches are often a true pain emergency. This form of headaches occurs almost exclusively in males [20]. Cluster headaches most often present in the third to fourth decade of life. This episodic headache usually occurs in clusters followed by remission periods. Cluster headaches present with severe unilateral pain, usually retro- or supraorbital that occur between 2–8 times per day and last between 15 minutes and 3 hours. The onset of cluster headaches is rapid. The exact duration of each cluster may vary, but typically lasts 8–12 weeks with spontaneous recovery and remission lasting for many months or years [20]. Cluster headaches can occur at the night, shortly after onset of sleep, causing patient to wake up with pain. Exact triggers are variable and poorly understood; some possible triggers are alcohol, histamines, and smoking [18, 19]. Patients often experience trigeminal autonomic symptoms, which include burning, boring sensation, rhinorrhea, ptosis, contracted pupil, facial flushing, ipsilateral lacrimation, conjunctival injection, among others [19].

Cluster headaches are subcategorized into episodic and chronic. Episodic cluster headaches occur from 1 week to 1 year of the episode and have remission periods that last greater than 1 month. Chronic cluster headache is defined by regularly occurring clusters with remission periods lasting less than 1 month [18–20].

Other Trigeminal Autonomic Cephalalgias

Trigeminal autonomic cephalalgias (TAC) are brief in nature and are associated with various autonomic symptoms. The exact duration of the headache is a key component in diagnosis [21]. Trigeminal autonomic cephalalgias include chronic and episodic paroxysmal hemicranias and SUNCT syndrome (short-lasting unilateral neuralgiform headache attack with conjunctival injection and tearing) [22].

Refractory Headache

Refractory headaches are poorly understood, as a result many cases are overlooked, and patients continue to suffer. As of today, there is no unified standard for diagnosing refractory headaches. However, multiple sources agree that for patients to qualify as having refractory headaches, they need to have failed some combination of acute and/or prophylactic therapies, as well and suffer some degree of headache induced

Table 40.1 Refractory headache classification [26]

Class I	Mild	Patients who have failed two broad-spectrum forms of abortive treatments (NSAIDS, other analgesics)
Class II	Moderate	Patients who have failed more specialized medication such as triptans and ergotamine-containing therapies
Class III	Severe	Patients who have failed the above therapies in addition to opioids, dopamine agonists, and corticosteroids
Class IV	Very severe	Abovementioned, in addition to a high degree of disability

disability [23, 24]. This publication suggests that a patient is considered as having refractory headache if they have failed at least two of the following preventative therapies: beta-blockers, calcium channel blockers, antidepressants, and anticonvulsants. Another publication suggests that a patient who has failed to respond to triptan and ergotamine-containing medication, in addition to NSAIDs or other analgesics, be considered as having failed abortive therapy [25]. In 2010, criteria were developed, which subcategorized refractory headache patients into various classes (Table 40.1) [26, 27].

Similar ideas regarding the failure of prophylactic therapies were supported by other researchers [24–27]. Class III and Class IV were considered to be ideal candidates for advanced interventional techniques [28]. Although these criteria were originally developed for refractory migraines, they may be applied to other subcategories of refractory headaches. Various studies over the years have tried to find the exact cause of refractory headaches, looking into possible structural, functional changes, and genetic changes in patients who have refractory headaches. A group of researchers hypothesized that periaqueductal gray (PAG) matter dysfunction may play a role in migraine headaches [29]. PAG activation was later found responsible for pain modulation in individuals with refractory headaches [30]. In addition, several genes involved in the pathogenesis of refractory migraine have been identified [31].

Medication Overuse Headache

Overuse of drug therapies as a means of stopping acute headache attacks can be problematic as it has the tendency to cause a different form of headache. This headache is known as medication overuse headache (MOH). This form of headache may superimpose onto the primary headache and can lead to the development of refractory headaches [32]. Many sources have shown that overuse of drug therapies can lead to a change in the characteristic of the headache from episodic to a chronic form [32]. As a patient continues to overuse a drug, the prophylactic success drastically decreases and the only effective treatment is to withdraw from the particular treatment. Contradictory to the abovementioned, some cases have shown no clinical significance when discontinuing overused drug therapies [33]. Topiramate was shown, by a random double-bind placebo-controlled study, to be effective in patients who have chronic migraines with superimposed medication overuse headaches [34, 35]. Before making a definitive clinical diagnosis of refractory or intractable headache, all overused therapies must be tapered and discontinued. It is interesting to note that patients with overuse headaches often present with higher rates of depression, anxiety, and lower pain tolerance [35].

Treatment

Headache treatment depends on type of headache, intensity, chronicity (episodic versus chronic), and patient characteristics, including comorbidities, liver and kidney function, previous exposure to pharmacological agents or interventions, and many others.

Pharmacological Treatment

Migraine headache treatment is a science and an art that is constantly adapting, developing, and progressing. Ergotamine was first introduced and proven effective in 1916, with the first placebo-controlled trial completed in 1928 [36]. Several decades later the use of triptans as an abortive medication changed the world of migraines. Many prophylactic methods were also originally put forth in the twentieth century [37]. One of the recent discoveries in the treatment of migraine is the development of calcitonin gene-related peptide (CGRP) receptor antagonist [38]. CGRP receptor was found to play an important role in the activation of central and peripheral nervous systems. There are two classes of drugs have been in development: receptor antagonists (CGRP-RAs) and monoclonal antibodies (CGRP mAbs). One of the most important features of this type of treatment, compared to other drugs, used for migraine prophylaxis, is a favorable safety profile, at least in the short term [38]. Specifically, a recently FDA-approved CGRP-RA has no contraindications [39].

The severity and type of a headache often dictates treatment. Abortive medications are used to provide rapid pain relief. These medications include NSAIDS, triptans, ergotamine-containing medications, as well as multitude of other adjuncts. Acetaminophen, barbiturates, and caffeine have limited value because of a significant risk of medication overuse headache. Prophylactic medications are used as a preventative treatment. These include Federal Drug Administration (FDA)-approved topiramate, botulinum toxin, and one of the CGRP mAbs, erenumab [10, 37–39]. There are a number of antidepressants, anticonvulsants, calcium channel blockers, beta-blockers, and antiemetics, including metoclopramide, among others, which are used off label [10]. There are reports of successful use of nutritional supplements for migraine prophylaxis. These include magnesium and CoQ-10 [40, 41] (Table 40.2).

Table 40.2 Migraine management [37, 39–50]

Pharmacological	Abortive	NSAIDs
		Triptans
		Ergotamine and related medications
		Antiemetics
		Membrane stabilizers
		Antipsychotics
		Steroids
		Magnesium
	Prophylactic	Topiramate
		Botulinum toxin
		Erenumab
		Other membrane stabilizers
		SSRI
		SNRI
		TCA
		Calcium channel blockers
		Beta-blockers
		Magnesium
		CoQ-10
Interventional	Invasive	Occipital nerve block
		Occipital nerve pulsed RF
		Occipital nerve cryoablation
		Sphenopalatine ganglion block
		Trigger point injections
		Cervical medial branch blocks
		Cervical medial branch RFA
		Botulinum toxin injections
		Branches of trigeminal nerve blocks (i.e., supraorbital, auriculotemporal, etc.) and pulsed RF/cryoablation
		Occipital Nerve Stimulation
	Noninvasive	Cephaly
		GammaCore
Comprehensive		Lifestyle modification
		Dietary modification
		Cognitive behavioral therapy
		Biofeedback
		Hypnosis
		Mindfulness
		Other psychological therapies
		Occupational therapy
		Chiropractic manipulation
		Acupuncture

NSADs nonsteroidal anti-inflammatory drugs, *SSRI* selective serotonin reuptake inhibitors, *SNRI* serotonin-norepinephrine reuptake inhibitors, *TCA* tricyclic antidepressants, *RFA* radiofrequency ablation

Interventional Treatment

There are a number of interventional procedures which can be utilized in headache management. Seven randomized controlled trials, as well as three high-quality systematic reviews, showed the usefulness of occipital nerve block in the treatment of severe migraine headache [51–54]. Sphenopalatine ganglion blocks can be utilized as well [42]. There is a role for trigger point injections [51]. Cervicogenic headaches or nociceptive input from the upper cervical spine that triggers or potentiates primary headaches may be amenable to cervical medial branch blocks [43]. If significant, but temporary relief is achieved with medial branch blocks, a radiofrequency ablation procedure of the same medial branches may provide mid- to long-term relief of neck pain and headache. Botulinum toxin injections are FDA approved for chronic migraine prophylaxis [44]. Advanced interventional treatment options, including occipital nerve stimulation and spinal cord stimulation, have shown to be effective in some patients with severe persistent migraine headaches [45]. There are some reports indicating that ablative procedures can be utilized [55]. There are also noninvasive neuromodulation options available, including transcutaneous vagal nerve stimulation, as well as supraorbital nerve stimulation [46].

Comprehensive Headache Management

New techniques and treatments are always being developed, yet there is still a large population of patients who cannot find effective treatment. The best chance of success in these patients is a collaborative multidisciplinary approach involving combinations of lifestyle and diet modification, psychological support, physical therapy, and complementary and alternative therapies, along with pharmacological and interventional therapies [47–50].

References

1. Friedman AP. The headache in history, literature, and legend. Bull N Y Acad Med. 1972;48(4):661–81.
2. Guerrero-Peral AL, de Frutos Gonzalez V, Pedraza-Hueso MI. Galeata: chronic migraine independently considered in a medieval headache classification. J Headache Pain. 2014;15:16.
3. Green D. New cure for headache found in old Greek manuscript. N Y State J Med. 1974;74(9):1671–5.
4. Huppert D, Brandt T. Descriptions of vestibular migraine and Meniere's disease in Greek and Chinese antiquity. Cephalalgia. 2017;37(4):385–90.
5. Magiorkinis E, Diamantis A, Mitsikostas DD, Androutsos G. Headaches in antiquity and during the early scientific era. J Neurol. 2009;256(8):1215–20.
6. Rose FC. The history of migraine from Mesopotamian to Medieval times. Cephalalgia. 1995;15(Suppl 15):1–3.
7. Rosner F. Neurology in the Bible and Talmud. Isr J Med Sci. 1975;11(4):385–97.
8. Albers L, von Kries R, Heinen F, Straube A. Headache in school children: is the prevalence increasing? Curr Pain Headache Rep. 2015;19(3):4.

9. Burch RC, Loder S, Loder E, Smitherman TA. The prevalence and burden of migraine and severe headache in the United States: updated statistics from government health surveillance studies. Headache. 2015;55(1):21–34.
10. Smitherman TA, Burch R, Sheikh H, Loder E. The prevalence, impact, and treatment of migraine and severe headaches in the United States: a review of statistics from national surveillance studies. Headache. 2013;53(3):427–36.
11. Steiner TJ, Birbeck GL, Jensen R, Katsarava Z, Martelletti P, Stovner LJ. The Global Campaign, World Health Organization and Lifting The Burden: collaboration in action. J Headache Pain. 2011;12(3):273–4.
12. Ferrante T, Manzoni GC, Russo M, Camarda C, Taga A, Veronesi L, et al. Prevalence of tension-type headache in adult general population: the PACE study and review of the literature. Neurol Sci. 2013;34(Suppl 1):S137–8.
13. Stovner LJ, Andree C. Prevalence of headache in Europe: a review for the Eurolight project. J Headache Pain. 2010;11(4):289–99.
14. Olesen J. International Classification of Headache Disorders, Second Edition (ICHD-2): current status and future revisions. Cephalalgia. 2006;26(12):1409–10.
15. Olesen J. ICHD-3 beta is published. Use it immediately. Cephalalgia. 2013;33(9):627–8.
16. Headache Classification Committee of the International Headache Society (IHS) The International Classification of Headache Disorders, 3rd edition. Cephalalgia. 2018;38(1):1–211.
17. Loder S, Sheikh HU, Loder E. The prevalence, burden, and treatment of severe, frequent, and migraine headaches in US minority populations: statistics from National Survey studies. Headache. 2015;55(2):214–28.
18. Snoer A, Lund N, Beske R, Jensen R, Barloese M. Pre-attack signs and symptoms in cluster headache: characteristics and time profile. Cephalalgia. 2018;38(6):1128–37.
19. Fischera M, Marziniak M, Gralow I, Evers S. The incidence and prevalence of cluster headache: a meta-analysis of population-based studies. Cephalalgia. 2008;28(6):614–8.
20. Alstadhaug KB, Ofte HK. Cluster headache. Tidsskr Nor Laegeforen. 2015;135(15):1361–4.
21. May A. Diagnosis and clinical features of trigemino-autonomic headaches. Headache. 2013;53(9):1470–8.
22. Bussone G. Strictly unilateral headaches: considerations of a clinician. Neurol Sci. 2014;35(Suppl 1):71–5.
23. Robbins L. Refractory headache definition. Headache. 2011;51(2):310–1.
24. Schulman EA, Lake AE 3rd, Goadsby PJ, Peterlin BL, Siegel SE, Markley HG, et al. Defining refractory migraine and refractory chronic migraine: proposed criteria from the Refractory Headache Special Interest Section of the American Headache Society. Headache. 2008;48(6):778–82.
25. Levin M. Refractory headache: classification and nomenclature. Headache. 2008;48(6):783–90.
26. Silberstein SD, Dodick DW, Pearlman S. Defining the pharmacologically intractable headache for clinical trials and clinical practice. Headache. 2010;50(9):1499–506.
27. Schwedt TJ, Silberstein SD. 14th International Headache Congress: clinical highlights. Headache. 2010;50(3):509–19.
28. Nizard J, Raoul S, Nguyen JP, Lefaucheur JP. Invasive stimulation therapies for the treatment of refractory pain. Discov Med. 2012;14(77):237–46.
29. Welch KM, Nagesh V, Aurora SK, Gelman N. Periaqueductal gray matter dysfunction in migraine: cause or the burden of illness? Headache. 2001;41(7):629–37.
30. Maizels M, Aurora S, Heinricher M. Beyond neurovascular: migraine as a dysfunctional neurolimbic pain network. Headache. 2012;52(10):1553–65.

31. Dichgans M, Freilinger T, Eckstein G, Babini E, Lorenz-Depiereux B, Biskup S, et al. Mutation in the neuronal voltage-gated sodium channel SCN1A in familial hemiplegic migraine. Lancet. 2005;366(9483):371–7.

32. Westergaard ML, Hansen EH, Glumer C, Olesen J, Jensen RH. Definitions of medication-overuse headache in population-based studies and their implications on prevalence estimates: a systematic review. Cephalalgia. 2014;34(6):409–25.

33. Rossi P, Faroni JV, Tassorelli C, Nappi G. Advice alone versus structured detoxification programmes for complicated medication overuse headache (MOH): a prospective, randomized, open-label trial. J Headache Pain. 2013;14:10.

34. Chiang CC, Schwedt TJ, Wang SJ, Dodick DW. Treatment of medication-overuse headache: a systematic review. Cephalalgia. 2016;36(4):371–86.

35. Limmroth V, Biondi D, Pfeil J, Schwalen S. Topiramate in patients with episodic migraine: reducing the risk for chronic forms of headache. Headache. 2007;47(1):13–21.

36. Zanchin G. Chapter 25: headache: an historical outline. Handb Clin Neurol. 2010;95:375–86.

37. Rapoport AM. The therapeutic future in headache. Neurol Sci. 2012;33(Suppl 1):S119–25.

38. Wrobel Goldberg S, Silberstein SD. Targeting CGRP: a new era for migraine treatment. CNS Drugs. 2015;29(6):443–52.

39. Edvinsson L. The CGRP pathway in migraine as a viable target for therapies. Headache. 2018;58 Suppl 1:33–47.

40. Hoffmann J, Charles A. Glutamate and its receptors as therapeutic targets for migraine. Neurotherapeutics. 2018;15(2):361–70.

41. Nattagh-Eshtivani E, Sani MA, Dahri M, Ghalichi F, Ghavami A, Arjang P, et al. The role of nutrients in the pathogenesis and treatment of migraine headaches: review. Biomed Pharmacother. 2018;102:317–25.

42. Mojica J, Mo B, Ng A. Sphenopalatine ganglion block in the management of chronic headaches. Curr Pain Headache Rep. 2017;21(6):27.

43. Castien RF, van der Wouden JC, De Hertogh W. Pressure pain thresholds over the cranio-cervical region in headache: a systematic review and meta-analysis. J Headache Pain. 2018;19(1):9.

44. Simpson DM, Hallett M, Ashman EJ, Comella CL, Green MW, Gronseth GS, et al. Practice guideline update summary: botulinum neurotoxin for the treatment of blepharospasm, cervical dystonia, adult spasticity, and headache: report of the Guideline Development Subcommittee of the American Academy of Neurology. Neurology. 2016;86(19):1818–26.

45. Cadalso RT Jr, Daugherty J, Holmes C, Ram S, Enciso R. Efficacy of electrical stimulation of the occipital nerve in intractable primary headache disorders: a systematic review with meta-analyses. J Oral Facial Pain Headache. 2018;32(1):40–52.

46. Starling A. Noninvasive neuromodulation in migraine and cluster headache. Curr Opin Neurol. 2018;31(3):268–73.

47. Hedborg K, Muhr C. The influence of multimodal behavioral treatment on the consumption of acute migraine drugs: a randomized, controlled study. Cephalalgia. 2012;32(4):297–307.

48. Foroughipour M, Golchian AR, Kalhor M, Akhlaghi S, Farzadfard MT, Azizi H. A sham-controlled trial of acupuncture as an adjunct in migraine prophylaxis. Acupunct Med. 2014;32(1):12–6.

49. Ernst MM, O'Brien HL, Powers SW. Cognitive-behavioral therapy: how medical providers can increase patient and family openness and access to evidence-based multimodal therapy for pediatric migraine. Headache. 2015;55(10):1382–96.

50. Seng EK, Holroyd KA. Behavioral migraine management modifies behavioral and cognitive coping in people with migraine. Headache. 2014;54(9):1470–83.

51. Ashkenazi A, Blumenfeld A, Napchan U, Narouze S, Grosberg B, Nett R, et al. Peripheral nerve blocks and trigger point injections in headache management – a systematic review and suggestions for future research. Headache. 2010;50(6):943–52.

52. Palamar D, Uluduz D, Saip S, Erden G, Unalan H, Akarirmak U. Ultrasound-guided greater occipital nerve block: an efficient technique in chronic refractory migraine without aura? Pain Physician. 2015;18(2):153–62.

53. Tang Y, Kang J, Zhang Y, Zhang X. Influence of greater occipital nerve block on pain severity in migraine patients: a systematic review and meta-analysis. Am J Emerg Med. 2017;35(11):1750–4.

54. Zhang H, Yang X, Lin Y, Chen L, Ye H. The efficacy of greater occipital nerve block for the treatment of migraine: a systematic review and meta-analysis. Clin Neurol Neurosurg. 2018;165:129–33.

55. Abd-Elsayed A, Kreuger L, Wheeler S, Robillard J, Seeger S, Dulli D. Radiofrequency ablation of pericranial nerves for treating headache conditions: a promising option for patients. Ochsner J. 2018;18(1):59–62.

Orofacial Pain

Miles Day, Kathryn Glynn, Ryan McKenna,
Bhargav Mudda, and Katrina von-Kriegenbergh

Anatomy

The anatomic structures of the face that can serve as pain generators in orofacial pain can be categorized as the oral cavity, bony structures, muscles, nerves, and neighboring structures (Table 41.1). This chapter will focus on pain originating from the muscles and nerves of the face.

Muscles of Mastication (Fig. 41.1a, b)

The four muscles of mastication (Table 41.2) are mostly present in the temporal and infratemporal fossae and control mandibular movement during speech and mastication. Being derivatives of the first pharyngeal arch, they are supplied by terminal branches of the mandibular division of the trigeminal nerve [1–3].

Table 41.1 Potential pain generators

Oral cavity	Muscles
Dental pain	Myalgia
Periodontal disease	Oral parafunction
Oral mucous membrane disorders	Myofascial pain disorder
Salivary gland disorders	
Bony structures	**Nerves**
Disorders of the maxilla and mandible	Trigeminal neuralgia
Temporomandibular disorders	Glossopharyngeal neuralgia
Neighboring structures	Sphenopalatine neuralgia
Sinus disorders	
Disorders of the eye and ear	

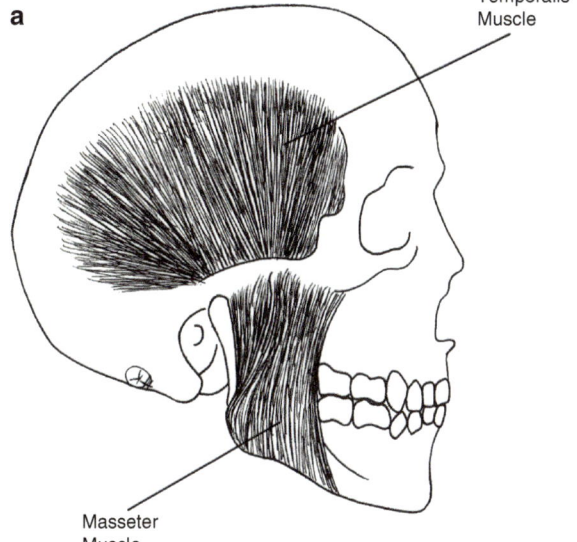

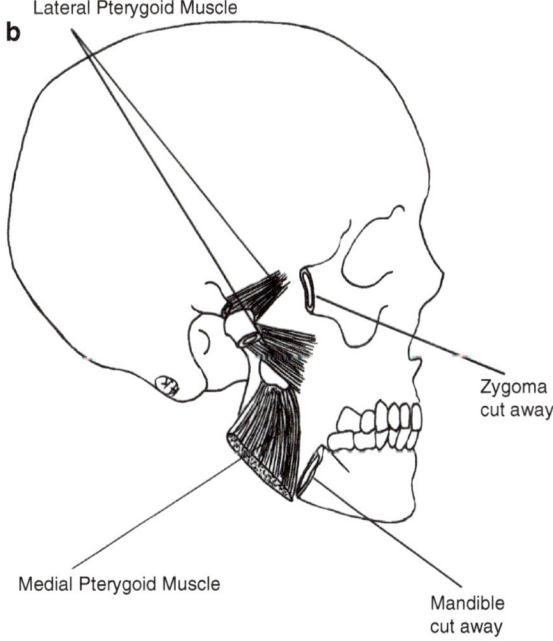

Fig. 41.1 (**a**) Muscles of mastication: temporalis and masseter muscles. (**b**) Muscles of mastication: lateral and medial pterygoid muscles

M. Day (✉) · K. Glynn · R. McKenna · K. von-Kriegenbergh
Department of Anesthesiology and Pain Medicine, Texas Tech
University Health Sciences Center, Lubbock, TX, USA
e-mail: miles.day@ttuhsc.edu

B. Mudda
Department of Anesthesiology, Texas Tech University Health
Sciences Center, Lubbock, TX, USA

© Springer Nature Switzerland AG 2019
Y. Khelemsky et al. (eds.), *Academic Pain Medicine*, https://doi.org/10.1007/978-3-030-18005-8_41

Table 41.2 Muscles of mastication

Muscle	Innervation	Function
Masseter	Masseteric nerve from the anterior trunk of the mandibular nerve	Elevation of mandible
Temporalis	Deep temporal nerves from the anterior trunk of the mandibular nerve	Elevation and retraction of mandible
Medial pterygoid	Nerve to medial pterygoid from the mandibular nerve	Elevation and side-to-side movements of the mandible
Lateral pterygoid	Nerve to lateral pterygoid directly from the anterior trunk of the mandibular nerve or from the buccal branch	Protrusion and side-to-side movements of the mandible

Temporalis

The temporalis is a fan-shaped muscle that fills much of the temporal fossa. It originates from the bony floor of the fossa superiorly to the inferior temporal line and is attached laterally to the surface of the temporal fascia [1–3]. The anterior fibers are arranged in a vertical fashion and the posterior fibers are oriented horizontally [2]. These fibers converge inferiorly to form a tendon that passes between the zygomatic arch and the infratemporal crest of the greater wing of the sphenoid. The temporalis muscle attaches to the anterior surface of the coronoid process and along the anterior margin of the ramus of the mandible, almost to the last molar. The temporalis is a powerful elevator of the mandible that also performs mandibular retraction and side-to-side movements. The temporalis is innervated by branches of the mandibular nerve called the deep temporal nerves that originate in the infratemporal fossa and then pass into the temporal fossa [3].

Masseter

The masseter is a quadrilateral-shaped muscle that overlies the lateral surface of the ramus of the mandible [1–3]. It is anchored superiorly to the zygomatic arch and inferiorly to most of the lateral surface of the ramus of the mandible. The superficial part of the masseter originates from the maxillary process of the zygomatic bone and the anterior two-thirds of the zygomatic process of the maxilla [2]. It inserts into the angle of the mandible and related posterior part of the lateral surface of the ramus of the mandible. The deep part of the masseter originates from the medial aspect of the zygomatic arch and the posterior part of its inferior margin and inserts into the central and upper part of the ramus of the mandible as high as the coronoid process [1–3]. Like the temporalis, the masseter muscle is a powerful elevator of the mandible. The masseter is innervated by the masseteric nerve from the mandibular nerve and supplied by the masseteric artery from the maxillary artery.

Medial Pterygoid

The medial pterygoid is a quadrangular muscle with deep and superficial heads. The deep head attaches superiorly to the medial surface of the lateral plate of the pterygoid and pyramidal processes of the palatine bone [1–3]. It descends obliquely downward, medial to the sphenomandibular ligament, to attach to the medial surface of the ramus of the mandible near the angle of the mandible. The superficial head originates from the tuberosity of the maxilla and adjacent pyramidal process of the palatine bone [2]. It joins the deep head to insert on the mandible. The vertical orientation of the fibers allows the medial pterygoid to elevate the mandible. It also assists the lateral pterygoid muscle in protruding the lower jaw. The nerve to the medial pterygoid from the mandibular nerve innervates the medial pterygoid [2].

Lateral Pterygoid

The lateral pterygoid is a thick triangular muscle with upper and lower heads. The upper head originates from the roof of the infratemporal fossa, lateral to the foramen ovale and foramen spinosum. The larger lower head originates from the lateral surface of the lateral plate of the pterygoid process and the inferior portion is positioned between the two heads of the medial pterygoid where they attach to the ramus of the mandible [1–3]. Fibers from both heads converge to insert into the capsule of the temporomandibular joint where the capsule is attached internally to the articular disk. Contraction of the lateral pterygoid fibers pulls the articular disk and head of the mandible forward onto the articular tubercle. The horizontal orientation of the fibers allows protrusion of the lower jaw. Unilateral contraction of the lateral and medial pterygoids moves the chin to the contralateral side [2]. However, when opposite movements at the two temporomandibular joints are coordinated, a chewing movement results. The lateral pterygoid nerve from the mandibular nerve provides innervation [3].

Nerves

The rich sensory innervation of the face and oral cavity is derived from the trigeminal system, the lower cranial nerves, and cervical nerves. With acute pain, there is usually close correlation with other signs and symptoms of the disease. The correlation is not as evident when dealing with chronic pain syndromes.

Sphenopalatine Ganglion

The sphenopalatine ganglion is a small triangular structure located in the pterygopalatine fossa. This fossa contains the internal maxillary artery and its branches, the maxillary nerve, and the sphenopalatine ganglion with its afferent and efferent branches. The sphenopalatine ganglion is located posterior to the middle turbinate and inferior to the maxillary nerve. Efferent branches of the ganglion form the posterior lateral nasal and pharyngeal nerves [3]. It contains parasympathetic fibers which originate in the superior salivatory nucleus and sympathetic fibers from the lower cervical sympathetic chain.

Stellate Ganglion

The stellate ganglion is irregular in shape and is likely formed by a fusion of the lower two cervical and first thoracic segmental ganglia (can also include the second and even third and fourth thoracic ganglia). The ganglion lies on the lateral border of longus coli, between the base of the seventh cervical transverse process and the neck of the first rib [3]. The vascular structures surrounding the ganglion include vertebral vessels anteriorly, the costocervical trunk of the subclavian artery branches near the lower pole of the ganglion, and the superior intercostal artery is lateral. The stellate ganglion sends grey rami communicantes to the seventh and eighth cervical and first thoracic spinal nerves. It also

gives off a cardiac branch, branches to nearby vessels, and a branch to the vagus nerve. The branches to blood vessels form plexuses on the subclavian artery and its branches [3].

Major Cranial Nerves

Cranial Nerve V: Trigeminal Nerve (Fig. 41.2)
The trigeminal nerve consists of afferent sensory, efferent motor, and parasympathetic fibers. The ophthalmic (V1), maxillary (V2), and mandibular (V3) trigeminal sensory nerve branches emerge from the anterior surface of the trigeminal (Gasserian) ganglion in Meckel's cave and innervate the facial skin, mucous membranes of the nose and mouth, teeth, orbital contents, and supratentorial meninges [1]. The ophthalmic division courses in the lateral wall of the cavernous sinus inferior to the trochlear nerve and exits the skull via the superior orbital fissure. The maxillary division also courses in the lateral wall of the cavernous sinus, exiting the skull via the foramen rotundum to enter the sphenopalatine fossa and the inferior orbital fissure. The mandibular

Fig. 41.2 Branches of the trigeminal nerve

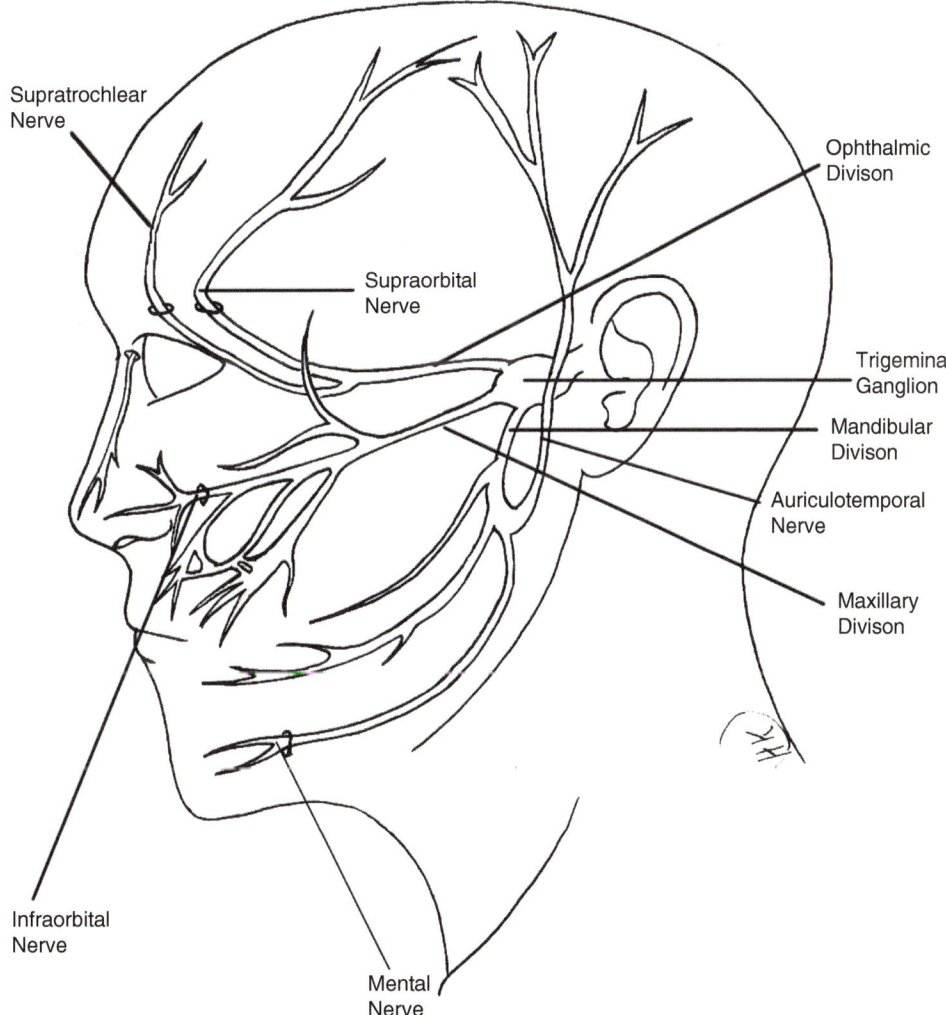

division exits the skull through the foramen ovale. Sensory input from these three branches travel centrally from the trigeminal ganglion via the trigeminal sensory root in the prepontine subarachnoid cistern to the trigeminal sensory nucleus, which is composed of mesencephalic, principal sensory, and descending spinal nuclei (nucleus caudalis) that descend to the cervical spinal cord. Sensory information ultimately ascends to the contralateral thalamus [4].

The motor efferents originate in the motor trigeminal nucleus in the pons, medial to the principal sensory nucleus, emerge from the ventral pons as the motor root, and travel inferior to the trigeminal ganglion and then alongside the mandibular sensory division to innervate the muscles of mastication (masseter, temporalis, pterygoids), the mylohyoid, tensors tympani and palatini, and anterior belly of the digastric [3].

Trigeminal nerve branches carry efferent postganglionic parasympathetic innervation from the pterygopalatine ganglia to the lacrimal gland and from the submandibular ganglia to the salivary glands. Preganglionic parasympathetic fibers travel in the facial nerve [4].

Cranial Nerve VII: Facial Nerve

The facial nerve comprises afferent gustatory, afferent sensory, efferent motor, and parasympathetic fibers. It innervates taste buds in the anterior two-thirds of the tongue. Unipolar neurons with cell bodies in the geniculate ganglion within the temporal bone carry taste information from the taste buds via the chorda tympani facial nerve branch, which is joined by the lingual branch of the trigeminal nerve [4]. The chorda tympani nerve branch joins the main trunk of the facial nerve just proximal to the stylomastoid foramen. From the geniculate ganglion, taste information travels proximally to enter the solitary tract and ultimately the rostral solitary (or gustatory) nucleus in the rostral medulla via the nervus intermedius, which passes through the internal auditory canal. Afferent sensory information from the soft palate, middle ear, tympanic membrane, and external auditory canal travels in the facial nerve.

Cranial Nerve IX: Glossopharyngeal Nerve

The glossopharyngeal nerve contains afferent gustatory, afferent sensory, efferent motor, and parasympathetic fibers and innervates taste buds in the posterior one-third of the tongue [1, 3]. Unipolar glossopharyngeal neurons with cell bodies in the superior and inferior (petrosal) ganglia of the glossopharyngeal nerve at the jugular foramen in the base of the temporal bone carry taste information from the taste buds to the ganglia, and then proximally into the brainstem solitary tract and rostral solitary (or gustatory) nucleus in the rostral medulla [3]. Afferent sensory information from the uvula, tonsil, pharynx, auditory canal, middle ear, and carotid sinus and bulb travels in the glossopharyngeal nerve via the

petrosal ganglion. Within the brainstem, sensory information is carried to the solitary nucleus and pain information to the spinal nucleus of the trigeminal nerve [3].

The motor efferents originate in the rostral nucleus ambiguus in the medulla, exit the brainstem dorsolateral to the inferior olive, and exit the skull via the jugular foramen in the temporal bone, while traversing the petrosal ganglion without synapsing. After exiting the jugular foramen, glossopharyngeal branches innervate the stylopharyngeus muscle and the superior pharyngeal constrictors [5].

The glossopharyngeal nerve carries efferent preganglionic fibers from the brainstem inferior salivatory nucleus via the main glossopharyngeal trunk. The tympanic nerve branch (Jacobson nerve) comes off of the main trunk at the jugular foramen and carries parasympathetic information to the otic ganglion via the lesser superficial petrosal nerve. Postganglionic fibers travel from the otic ganglion in the auriculotemporal nerve, a branch of the trigeminal nerve, to reach the parotid gland [5].

Vascular

Maxillary Artery

The maxillary artery is the largest branch of the external carotid artery in the neck and is a major source of blood supply for the nasal cavity, the lateral wall and roof of the oral cavity, all teeth, and the dura mater in the cranial cavity. It originates within the substance of the parotid gland and then passes forward into the infratemporal fossa [1–3].

The first part of the maxillary artery gives origin to two major branches (the middle meningeal and inferior alveolar arteries) and a number of smaller branches (deep auricular, anterior tympanic, and accessory meningeal). The second part of the maxillary artery gives origin to deep temporal, masseteric, buccal, and pterygoid branches, which course with branches of the mandibular nerve. The third part of the maxillary artery is in the pterygopalatine fossa [1, 3].

Middle Meningeal Artery

The middle meningeal artery is the largest of the meningeal vessels and supplies much of the dura mater, bone, and related bone marrow of the cranial cavity walls [1, 3]. Within the cranial cavity, the middle meningeal artery and its branches travel in the periosteal layer of dura mater, which is tightly adherent to the bony walls.

Inferior Alveolar Artery

The inferior alveolar artery descends from the maxillary artery to enter the mandibular foramen and canal with the inferior alveolar nerve [1, 3]. It is distributed with the inferior alveolar nerve and supplies all lower teeth, and contributes to the supply of the buccal gingivae, chin, and lower lip.

Pterygoid Plexus of Veins

Veins that drain regions supplied by arteries branching from the maxillary artery in the infratemporal fossa and pterygopalatine fossa connect with the pterygoid plexus. These tributary veins include those that drain the nasal cavity, roof and lateral wall of the oral cavity, all teeth, muscles of the infratemporal fossa, paranasal sinuses, and nasopharynx [1, 3]. Also, because there are no valves in veins of the head and neck, anesthetic inadvertently injected under pressure into veins of the pterygoid plexus can backflow into tissues or into the cranial cavity.

History Taking, Physical Examination and Diagnostic Studies

Perhaps the most crucial element to the workup of orofacial pain, or any chronic pain condition, is a thorough history and physical examination. By the time some patients with orofacial pain have reached a multidisciplinary pain practice, they have likely received different, often conflicting, views regarding their management. It is critical to listen to their narrative uninterrupted as this improves patient satisfaction thus leading to improved outcomes [6]. Key elements to elicit at the initial patient visit include the onset of their pain. It is important to obtain information regarding recent infections or trauma. It is also important to ask how the patient characterizes the pain. It may be described as sharp, dull, stabbing, burning or nagging or a combination thereof. One should ask whether the location of the pain is unilateral or bilateral and determine if it is in one particular distribution or is it widespread. One should also inquire about the severity of the pain: mild, moderate, and severe. Ask about associated symptoms that occur with the pain such as tinnitus, vertigo, diplopia, depression, and headaches. Determine if there is associated nausea, photophobia, or aura [7]. Ask if the pain refers anywhere and if there is pain with chewing or swallowing or pain with innocuous stimuli like applying makeup, shaving, or even smiling [8]. Obtain information regarding autonomic symptoms the patient may experience such as nasal congestion, lacrimation, and flushing. Ask the patient if their eyes or mouth are dry or if he/she loses taste in any part of the tongue. Find out if the pain is accompanied by loss of sensation and, if so, where. Asking the aforementioned questions will go a long way in ferreting out the diagnosis. Other information to obtain is the length of time the painful attacks last? Do they occur frequently, constantly, or intermittently? Are there any exacerbating factors such as chewing, swallowing, or stress? Are there any factors that relieve the pain such as rest, analgesics, heat, or ice? It is also important to know if the patient has tried any previous treatments for the pain and what kind of results they have had. Ask if the pain is the same as when it started or is it different since the initia-

tion of treatment. It is not uncommon that the patient presents to a pain medicine practitioner with a pain different from the one for which the patient initially sought treatment.

As with all physical examinations, the initial workup of a patient with orofacial pain should begin with vital signs. General observations such as facial symmetry and posture, particularly of the cervical spine, can be of value. Cranial nerve testing is essential when examining a patient with orofacial pain. Trigeminal nerve (CN V) lesions will demonstrate loss of sensation in one or more of the three distributions of the nerve. The examining physician should pay particular attention to where the pain extends and where it does not [8]. The temporomandibular joint (TMJ) should be palpated while the patient is asked to open and close the jaw. Palpation of the masseter and temporalis musculature should be conducted to further evaluate pain elicited by myofascial pain of the head and neck and to assess the integrity of the motor component of CN V [9]. These muscles should be palpated for firmness and tenderness using 2–3 pounds of pressure. Other muscles of mastication, the medial and lateral pterygoids, should also be palpated on physical exam as these are also innervated by CN V_3. CN VII palsies can be elicited by having the patient close their eyes against resistance, smile and wrinkle the forehead. CN IX function can be assessed by checking a gag reflex. Examination of the bony structures of the face such as the sinuses and temporomandibular joint should be included in the initial patient workup. The maxillary and frontal sinuses can be palpated and transilluminated. Pain originating from the upper neck can present as pain in the face. Upper cervical exam should include assessing range of motion of cervical spine, mobility testing of upper cervical facets, and upper cervical musculature, such as splenius, sternocleidomastoid, and upper trapezius muscles. The oral cavity should be properly assessed as dental pain is a common cause of oral pain. A thorough evaluation for decay, fracture, or signs of infection (i.e., edema, drainage, etc.) must be included in the physical exam. Furthermore, other causes of oral pain related to pulp inflammation, periapical inflammation, and disorders of the periodontium should be properly screened via physical exam. Diseases of the oral mucous membranes are present due to various causes, and proper integrity of the mucous membranes is vital determination. Examination for oral mucosal lesions, erosions, erythema, and vesicles plays a key role in making this determination [10]. Furthermore, it is possible for pain, stuffiness, and tinnitus found on routine examination to have a musculoskeletal etiology. An ear exam can help rule out potential structural abnormalities that can be contributing to the whole spectrum of orofacial pain. For instance, internal derangement of the TMJ can often cause ear pain that is sharp and jabbing when the mandible is manipulated.

Diagnostic Studies

Initial diagnostic imaging with the help of x-rays should be considered in all acute traumatic conditions and in conditions that are suspicious for possible bony derangement. Dedicated plain x-ray films such as dental radiographs are important when considering cracked teeth, periodontitis, oral mucous membrane disorders, among others, within the differential [11]. Salivary gland diseases are best investigated using ultrasound [11]. Primary osteoarthritis is frequently seen in patients with a long history of missing teeth. Screening imaging obtained via dental panoramic image, a tomograph, or dental CT scan can aid in identifying underlying primary osteoarthritis. It is not uncommon for intracranial and extracranial tumors to cause pain in the head and face region. Headache and facial pain of unknown origin should necessitate a need for ruling out underlying occult tumor. Tumors must be ruled out with the use of appropriate imaging such as computed tomography (CT) and magnetic resonance imaging (MRI), and magnetic resonance angiography [11]. It is important to note the value of magnetic resonance imaging (MRI) in the overall management of facial pain. MRI is usually necessary to sufficiently deduce most initial differential diagnosis plans. Most commonly, MRI of the brain, brainstem, and base of the skull is performed to evaluate for and to rule out lesions, demyelinating plaques and vascular abnormalities. MRI of the TMJ is the "gold standard" to evaluate for any displacements of the articular cartilage or to assess soft tissue details [11]. In order to assess other chronic osteoarthritic or bony changes, CT scans are preferred. Effusions are commonly seen on T2-weighted signal in patients who present with the inability to bring the teeth together accompanied by pain in the ear. Further diagnostic studies are indicated when MRI findings or physical examination are abnormal.

Evidence-Based Treatment Options

Trigger Point Injections

Myofascial pain (MFP) can often present as a dull, continuous aching pain. This pain can be localized via trigger points, typically manifested as a taut band of muscle [12]. This pain can be reproduced by palpation of the musculature affected and when palpated, should duplicate the patient's complaint. This can also occur within the muscles of mastication which along with other musculature of the head and neck can tend to cause tension-type headaches [9]. Pain of the eyes, ears, TMJ, and teeth can arise from trigger points

of the masticatory musculature [9]. Due to relatively high incidence of being affected by trigger points within these muscles, injection of such identified trigger points with local anesthetic and/or steroid can prove to be efficacious. Some studies have also shown the value of botulinum toxin (Botox) injections in conjunction with anesthetic in treatment of trigger points. For instance, bruxism which refers to both clenching and grinding of the teeth and often related to masseter hypertrophy can lead to destruction of otherwise healthy teeth, potentially exacerbate periodontal disease and is a known cause of headaches and facial pain [9]. Botox injection can help eliminate facial pain, decrease symptoms related to temporomandibular disorder (TMD), and potentially aid in treatment of associated symptoms related to periodontal disease [10].

Another indication for Botox in the head and neck region is as treatment of sialorrhea. Botox is injected into the parotid and submaxillary salivary glands to inhibit the stimulation of the cholinergic receptors. Common side effects during excessive use of Botox include chewing difficulties, dysphagia, and xerostomia. The efficacy of targeted trigger point injections is highly variable and dependent on patient compliance with a strict physical therapy regimen. This regimen can include modalities such as myofascial release as well as use of occlusal appliances, dental guards, etc. [10].

Stellate Ganglion Block

The stellate ganglion block is a sympathetic block used to treat multiple pain etiologies including CRPS of the face and upper limb, phantom tongue pain, cluster headaches, vasospastic disorders, cancer-associated pain, phantom limb pain, central pain, ischemic pain, dentition pain, atypical facial pain, post-herpetic neuralgia, glaucoma, optic nerve neuritis, hyperhidrosis, atypical chest pain, pulmonary embolism, intractable angina pectoris, Meniere's syndrome, Scleroderma, and Raynaud's disease [13]. There is also literature describing its utility for vasospasm, hot flashes, and post-traumatic stress disorder [14–16]. Contraindications include local or systemic infection, coagulopathy, medication allergy, severe alteration of local anatomy, and patient refusal – similar to all pain procedures [13, 17].

While the majority of studies do show some patient improvement utilizing this block technique, there is no proven long-lasting benefit with LA injection. Steroids and other adjuncts such as clonidine may be added to enhance patient response. To get longer-lasting relief, treating the stellate ganglion with radiofrequency thermocoagulation (RFTC), pulsed radiofrequency (pRF), and neurolytic solutions may be effective. As mentioned earlier, large-scale placebo-controlled double-blinded studies have not been performed on this procedure; however, in the hands of a properly trained interventional pain physician, this block can be a valuable treatment option [18].

Sphenopalatine Ganglion Block

The Sphenopalatine Ganglion (SPG) lies deep within the pterygopalatine fossa [19]. Blocking this ganglion is considered a sympathetic block, even though it contains sympathetic, parasympathetic, sensory, and sensorimotor fibers. The ganglion can be blocked by a variety of both invasive and noninvasive procedures and lysis can be performed with neurolytic solutions, RFTC and pRF [20–23].

Unfortunately, as with other sympathetic procedures, evidence in the literature supporting its use is limited. Common indications for the block include trigeminal neuralgia, posttraumatic headache, cluster headache, cancer-associated pain, tooth pain, sphenopalatine neuralgia, atypical facial pain, and migraine [19]. Its use has also been applied to low back pain, myofascial pain, and fibromyalgia. The evidence of efficacy for this procedure appears to be stronger than for the stellate ganglion block [19].

The SPG can be blocked topically by applying viscous lidocaine to the inside of the nares using pledgets; however, some studies have indicated that this approach is not superior to placebo. The infrazygomatic approach can be a challenging procedure but allows for visualization of the blockade and the ability to diagnostically test the approach for future neurolytic procedures. After a positive SPG block, a longer-lasting interventional pain procedure may be indicated, and both radiofrequency ablation and pRF approaches have been described [20–23]. These procedures can cause bradycardia also known as the Konen reflex, which can be treated with administration of glycopyrrolate or atropine [24].

Glossopharyngeal Ganglion Block

The fibers arising from the glossopharyngeal ganglion perform both motor and sensory functions. This intervention should be considered for tongue, hypopharynx, and palatine tonsil pain. In addition, the nerve receives input from carotid sinus and is important in hemostasis of blood pressure, pulse, and respiration. Neurolytic techniques can be used, and a diagnostic nerve block should be performed to determine what motor and sensory deficits the patient will have after destruction of the nerve. Neurolytic techniques may be helpful to manage pain arising for tumors of posterior tongues, hypopharynx, and tonsils. Another important indication for this block is glossopharyngeal neuralgia in patients who have failed conservative therapy and are not candidates for surgical decompression [25].

Trigeminal Ganglion Block

The trigeminal nerve is the major sensory nerve of the head and is implicated in a variety of pain syndromes. The trigeminal system is composed of three major divisions, which originate at a single branching point, the Gasserian Ganglion, located in Meckel's Cave. Distally the trigeminal nerve divides further into terminal branches including the supraorbital, supratrochlear, infraorbital, lacrimal, zygomaticotemporal, inferior alveolar, mental, and auriculotemporal, among others. These branches are all amendable to nerve blocks. Neurolytic techniques have been described for these structures. Cryoneurolysis is the favored technique for the peripheral nerves while pRF or traditional RFTC has commonly been used for the Gasserian Ganglion. Other methods of ablation include balloon compression and glycerol gangliolysis [26]. A review article by Guo et al. indicated that traditional radiofrequency was more effective than pRF with respect to analgesia, and recurring pain was more common with pRF [27].

There is no large RCT comparing the variety of treatments for trigeminal neuralgia. Some smaller studies have shown good relief from ablation of the ganglion [26]. Complete pain relief in 97% of patient with true trigeminal neuralgia with a median time to recurrence at 24 months has been reported. At Texas Tech, the rate of pain-free outcomes at 6 years (with repeat procedures) is 78%.

Fang et al. compared high-voltage with standard-voltage pulsed radiofrequency of the Gasserian ganglion in the treatment of idiopathic trigeminal neuralgia in a randomized controlled trial. At 1 year post procedure, the effective rate of the procedure was 19% in the standard-voltage group compared to 69% in the high-voltage group [28].

Thapa et al. reported on two cases of refractory classic trigeminal neuralgia successfully treated using extended duration pulsed radiofrequency [29]. The group theorized that the extension of the pulsing to 8 minutes produced the results.

Eissa and his group performed a retrospective study on the efficacy and safety of combined pulsed and conventional radiofrequency treatment of refractory cases of idiopathic trigeminal neuralgia [30]. Their results indicated excellent analgesia and reduced consumption of analgesics for more than 6 months in patients who received pulsed radiofrequency combined with conventional radiofrequency to the Gasserian ganglion for treatment of idiopathic trigeminal neuralgia.

Other Considerations for Procedures

As mentioned earlier in this chapter, pain in the upper cervical spine can refer and present as pain in the face. For instance, the primary indication for performing an atlantoaxial (A-A) nerve block is usually suboccipital pain. The pain can occasionally radiate to TMJ exacerbated by head rotation and cause pain in the inner ear as well. The A-A joint is responsible for significant stability and mobility to the head and neck and can commonly be affected in whiplash injuries and cervicogenic headaches [31]. Careful consideration must be undertaken when performing these injections due to the danger of aiming toward interlaminar space, foramen magnum, as well as for uptake in this highly vascular region. Vascular uptake of local anesthetic with these injections commonly results in ataxia and in adverse situations even small volumes of anesthetic uptake into the vertebral artery can cause grand mal seizures. Injections targeted toward the medial branch of C2 and C3 and the third occipital nerve (TON) may be effective for the relief of facial pain that is either directly referred or triggered/potentiated by input from these structures via the trigeminocervical complex (Figs. 41.3 and 41.4).

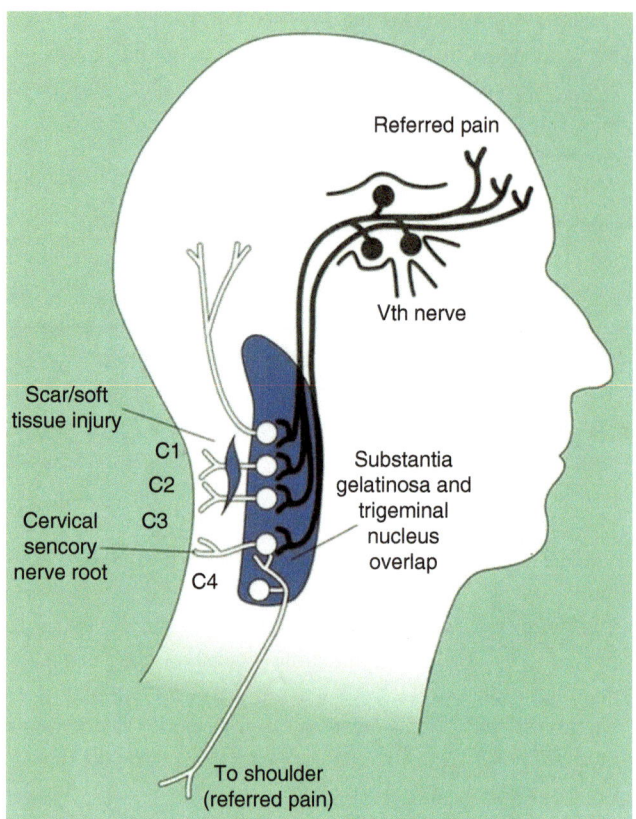

Fig. 41.4 Trigeminocephalic relay

Conclusion

As with any pain complaint, a proper history and physical examination is the initial step to establishing a differential diagnosis. Radiological studies can be helpful and should be ordered only when necessary to establish a diagnosis. Interventional procedures should be considered if conservative therapy has been partly effective or ineffective in managing the pain.

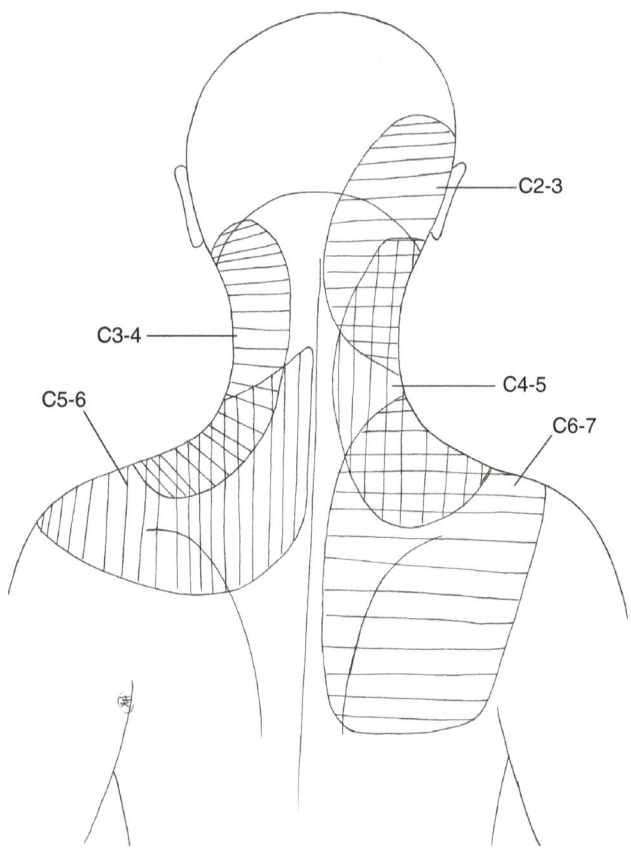

Fig. 41.3 Referral patterns of the cervical facet joints (medial branches)

References

1. Ellis H, Feldman S, Harrop-Griffiths W, Lawson A. Anatomy for anaesthetists. 8th ed. Oxford: Blackwell 8th Science; 2004.
2. Standring S. Head and neck: overview and surface anatomy. In: Stranding S, editor in chief. Gray's anatomy. Amsterdam:Elsevier; 2016. p. 399–415.
3. Standring S. Infratemporal and pterygopalatine fossae and temporomandibular joint. In: Stranding S, editor in chief. Gray's anatomy. Amsterdam: Elsevier; 2016. p. 534–55.
4. Shoja MM, Nelson OM, Grissenaur CJ, et al. Anastomoses between lower cranial and upper cervical nerves: a comprehensive review with potential significance during skull base and neck operations. Part 1: trigeminal, facial and vestibulocochlear nerves. Clin Anat. 2014;27:118–3.
5. Shoja MM, Oyesiku NM, Griessenauer CJ, et al. A comprehensive review with potential significance during skull base and

neck operations, part II: glossopharyngeal, vagus, accessory, and hypoglossal nerves and cervical spinal nerves 1–4. Clin Anat. 2014;27:131–44.

6. Zakrzewska J. Multi-dimensionality of chronic pain of the oral cavity and face. J Headache Pain. 2013;14:37.

7. Obermann M, Mueller D, Yoon MS, et al. Migraine with isolated facial pain: a diagnostic challenge. Cephalgia. 2007;27:1278–82.

8. Cruccu G, Finnerup N, Jensen T, et al. Trigeminal neuralgia: new classification and diagnostic grading for practice and research. Neurology. 2016;87:220–2.

9. Kim N, Park R, Park J. Botulinum toxin type A for the treatment of hypertrophy of the masseter muscle. Plast Reconstr Surg. 2010;125:1693–705.

10. Ihde S, Konstantinovic V. The therapeutic use of botulinum toxin in cervical and maxillofacial conditions: an evidence-based review. Oral Surg Oral Med Oral Pathol Oral Radiol Endod. 2007;104:e1–e11.2.

11. Benzon H. Practical management of pain. 1st ed. Philadelphia: Elsevier/Mosby; 2014. p. 424–9.

12. Wong C, Wong S. A new look at trigger point injections. Anesthesiol Res Pract. 2012;2012:492452.

13. Elias M. Cervical sympathetic and stellate ganglion blocks. Pain Physician. 2000;3:294–304.

14. Prabhakar H, Jain V, Rath G, et al. Stellate ganglion block as alternative to intrathecal papaverine in relieving vasospasm due to subarachnoid hemorrhage. Anesth Analg. 2007;104:1311–2.

15. Lipov E, Joshi J, Sanders S, et al. Effects of stellate-ganglion block on hot flushes and night awakenings in survivors of breast cancer: a pilot study. Lancet Oncol. 2008;9:523–32.

16. Lipov E, Navaie M, Stedje-Larsen E, et al. A novel application of stellate ganglion block: preliminary observations for the treatment of post-traumatic stress disorder. Mil Med. 2012;177:125–7.

17. Diwan S, Staats P. Atlas of pain medicine procedures. 1st ed. Amsterdam: McGraw-Hill; 2015. p. 336–42.

18. Racz G, Noe CE. Techniques of neurolysis. Basel: Springer; 2016. p. 101–2.

19. Day M. Sympathetic blocks: the evidence. Pain Pract. 2008;8:98–109.

20. Shah R, Racz G. Long-term relief of posttraumatic headache sphenopalatine ganglion pulse radiofrequency lesioning: a case report. Arch Phys Med Rehabil. 2004;85:1013–6.

21. Waldman SD. Atlas of interventional pain management, Fourth Edition. 1st ed. Amsterdam: Elsevier; 2015. p. 11–4.

22. Ferrante F, Kaufman A, Dunbar S, et al. Sphenopalatine ganglion block for the treatment of myofascial pain of the head, neck and shoulders. Reg Anesth Pain Med. 1998;23:30–6.

23. Sanders M, Zuurmond W. Efficacy of sphenopalatine ganglion blockade in 66 patients suffering from cluster headache: a 12- to 70-month follow-up evaluation. J Neurosurg. 1997;87:876–80.

24. Konen A. Unexpected effects due to radiofrequency thermocoagulation of the sphenopalatine ganglion: two case reports. Curr Rev Pain. 2000;10:30–3.

25. Benzon H, Raja S, Liu S, Fishman S, Cohen S. Essentials of pain medicine. 4th ed. Philadelphia: Elsevier; 2018. p. 763–77.

26. Racz G, Noe C. Techniques of neurolysis. 2nd ed. Basel: Springer; 2016. p. 75–83.

27. Guo J, Dong X, Zhao X. Treatment of trigeminal neuralgia by radiofrequency of the Gasserian ganglion. Rev Neurosci. 2016;27(7):739–43.

28. Fang L, Tao W, Jingjing L, Nan J. Comparison of high-voltage with standard voltage pulsed radiofrequency of Gasserian ganglion in the treatment of idiopathic trigeminal neuralgia. Pain Pract. 2015;15:595–603.

29. Thapa D, Ahuja V, Dass C, Verma P. Management of refractory trigeminal neuralgia using extended duration pulsed radiofrequency application. Pain Physician. 2015;18:E433–5.

30. Eissa A, Reyad R, Saleh E, El-Saman A. The efficacy and safety of combined pulsed and conventional radiofrequency treatment of refractory cases of idiopathic trigeminal neuralgia: a retrospective study. J Anesth. 2015;29(5):728–33.

31. Racz G, Sanel H, Diede J. Atlanto-occipital and atlanto axial injections in the treatment of headache and neck pain. In: Waldman S, Winnie A, editors. Interventional pain management. Philadelphia: WB Saunders; 1996. p. 220–2.

Neuropathic Pain

42

Theodore Eckman and Jianguo Cheng

Definition

Neuropathic pain occurs when there is spontaneous activity of the nervous system or an aberrant response to otherwise "normal" sensory stimulation, such as fine touch. This includes pain that arises "as a direct consequence of a lesion or disease affecting the somatosensory system" [1]. This is in contrast to nociceptive pain that is a physiological, adaptive response to tissue disease or damage that results from activation of nociceptors. There are numerous etiologies that can cause neuropathic pain (i.e., systemic diseases, physical injury, genetic diseases, infection, autoimmune, etc.). Neuropathic pain can further be divided into central versus peripheral, depending on where the predominant lesion or disease process is occurring in the nervous system. It is common for neuropathic pain syndromes to display elements of both peripheral and central neuropathic pain.

A related term, neuropathy, is used to describe a general disease of nerve function and structures. Neuropathies can be isolated to a single nerve (e.g., mononeuropathy), discreet nerves (e.g., mononeuropathy multiplex), or diffuse, multiple nerves (e.g., polyneuropathy). Despite the variety of locations and the multitude of differing etiologies, patients with neuropathic pain syndromes and painful neuropathies often share similar sensations, including parasthesias, dysesthesias, hyperpathia, allodynia, hyperalgesia, and spontaneous pain [2].

Epidemiology

Neuropathic pain is very common in the outpatient pain management setting and is second only to musculoskeletal pain in terms of prevalence [3]. It has been estimated that

neuropathic pain afflicts approximately 2–3% of the general population [4]. Therefore, the physical and societal burden associated with neuropathic pain is substantial. The estimated direct cost related to treatment of neuropathic pain is at least $40 billion annually in the United States, and this is most likely an underestimate [5]. There are also substantial indirect costs of neuropathic pain, and in total neuropathic pain patients generate healthcare costs that are three times higher than matched controls [6].

Diabetic Neuropathy

Diabetic neuropathy is the most common type of neuropathic pain. The 2011 Diabetes fact sheet, published by the Centers for Disease Control and Prevention (CDC), reports that 25 million Americans have diabetes. The likelihood of neuropathy increases with the duration of disease, and it is estimated that 60% of diabetic patients will develop diabetic neuropathy over their lifetime [7, 8]. Approximately 8 million people in the United States suffer with symptomatic diabetic neuropathy and account for more than 50 billion in annual spending [8].

Post-herpetic Neuralgia

Post-herpetic neuralgia (PHN) is a complication seen in patients following reactivation of the varicella-zoster virus (VZV), commonly referred to as shingles. Shingles occurs in approximately 1 million people annually in the United States, thereby making shingles the neurological disease with the highest incidence in the United States [9]. The lifetime incidence in the general population of developing shingles is 1:3, and there is increasing incidence in the elderly. Ultimately, approximately 15% of people who have shingles develop PHN, and this amounts to approximately 150,000 new cases annually in the United States [10].

T. Eckman
Allegheny Health Network, Erie, PA, USA

J. Cheng (✉)
Departments of Pain Management and Neurosciences, Cleveland Clinic, Cleveland, OH, USA
e-mail: chengj@ccf.org

© Springer Nature Switzerland AG 2019
Y. Khelemsky et al. (eds.), *Academic Pain Medicine*, https://doi.org/10.1007/978-3-030-18005-8_42

Trigeminal Neuralgia

Trigeminal neuralgia (TN), also known as tic douloureux, is a disabling condition and a common cause of facial pain. It was first described as early as the seventeenth and eighteenth centuries [11], and the pain is capable of causing such suffering that TN has been referred to as the suicide disease [12]. The disease has an incidence of approximately 4.5 cases per 100,000 people and increases in occurrence in the 6th to 8th decades of life [13]. This amounts to approximately 10,000 new diagnoses each year, and there is a slight female predominance of 1.7:1.

Central Post-stroke Pain

Central post-stroke pain (CPSP) can be a devastating and intractable central neuropathic pain condition that is seen in stroke patients. Approximately 795,000 people in the United States suffer a stroke annually [14]. Among these patients, 19–74% will develop post-stroke pain, which amounts to at least 150,000 new cases of post-stroke pain per year [15].

Clinical Characteristics

Patients with neuropathic pain often present with symptoms of allodynia, hyperalgesia, and paresthesias, such that the combination of words used to describe their pain includes the following: tingling, pins and needles, burning, stabbing, and aching. The first useful distinction to be made includes identifying the pattern of involvement. For instance, peripheral nerve lesions that are focal are often the result of processes that produce localized damage and include nerve entrapment, mechanical injuries, thermal injuries, electrical injuries, radiation injuries, and vascular or neoplastic processes [2]. In contrast, polyneuropathies often present with bilateral and symmetric distribution and occur secondarily to metabolic disorders (such as diabetic neuropathy), toxic substances (such as chemotherapy-induced peripheral neuropathy), vitamin deficiencies, and immune reactions [2]. While pain is often the presenting symptom for neuropathic pain states and painful polyneuropathies, there are often other sensory abnormalities present. In patients who are suspected of having a polyneuropathy, a detailed neurological examination is necessary. In addition to standard sensory examinations (i.e., vibration, proprioception, light touch, etc.), it is also useful to employ special stimuli including light-touch rubbing, ice, single pinprick, and multiple pinpricks [2]. The purpose of these sensory tests is to better isolate the fibers involved in the disease process. For instance, light-touch rubbing or stroking of the affected area can reveal allodynia – a state when a usually non-noxious stimulus produces pain.

Moreover, ice application can assess for temperature sensation, single pinprick testing may elicit a sensory deficit or hyperpathia, and repeated pinprick may elicit summation or lingering after sensations, all of which are common in polyneuropathy [2]. As the disease process does not have to be isolated to sensory nerves alone, a full motor exam should also be performed.

Pathologic Mechanisms in the Nervous System

There is no single and completely accepted theory for the development of neuropathic pain, although numerous mechanisms have been proposed. As there are different etiologies for neuropathic pain, it is probable that there are different mechanisms that can cause similar symptomatology. Often there are concomitant changes in both the peripheral and central nervous systems that have differing predominance depending on the condition. Some common mechanisms include changes in ion channel number and density resulting in central and peripheral sensitization, cortical reorganization, disinhibition of neuronal circuitry, and cellular and molecular changes as a result of the immune response following nerve damage and sympathetic dysfunction [2].

After an injury to a peripheral nerve, the density and number of ion channels (particularly sodium) increase along the entire exon. This increased concentration of channels then results in hypersensitivity and ectopic foci, and it also provides the theoretical basis for the use of sodium channel blockers and membrane stabilizers for the treatment of neuropathic pain [16]. Additionally, sprouting of sympathetic fibers into the affected nerve's dorsal root ganglia can occur [17]. This is accompanied by an increased expression of alpha-adrenoreceptors, and these changes form the theoretical basis for the utility of sympathetic blocks for attenuating sympathetically maintained pain [17]. There are numerous other changes that occur following a peripheral nerve injury, including neurogenic inflammation, alteration in the peripheral immune system [17, 18], and ephaptic transmission resulting in cross-circuiting of peripheral nerve fibers [19]. In summary, there are numerous changes that occur in the periphery following nerve injury, and it is most likely a complex interplay of these events that leads to the development of neuropathic pain.

Central nervous system (CNS) changes may accompany peripheral nerve injury. Certain neuropathic pain states, such as PHN and diabetic neuropathy, exhibit altered CNS input, and this might be the primary mechanism of pain. In diabetic neuropathy, there appears to be little or no evidence of peripheral sensitization or ephaptic transmission [20]. Pain likely arises from the loss of large fiber (A-beta) mediated sensory input leading to a decrease in "gating," which skews the balance toward increased nociceptive transmission from A-delta and C fibers [21]. Furthermore, A-beta fibers begin to aberrantly activate second-order pain pathways, which results in the perception of typically non-noxious stimuli as painful [2]. This is far from a complete description of the role of the CNS in neuropathic pain, and there are likely additional changes in the spinal cord, midbrain, and cerebral cortex.

Diagnostic Studies

As already discussed, the clinical history, medical comorbidities, and neurological exam are often enough to establish a diagnosis and initiate treatment. There are numerous other diagnostic studies that can be considered including electromyography (EMG), nerve conduction studies (NCS), quantitative sensory testing (QST), thermography, and skin biopsies. The biggest criticism of these studies is that they often do not change management. For example, EMGs and NCVs are often employed to differentiate whether a disease process is demyelinating (reduction in nerve conduction velocities) or axonal (reduction in amplitudes of evoked responses) [2]. However, these studies are better at identifying large fiber involvement, whereas most neuropathic pain conditions predominantly involve small fibers [22]. Furthermore, there is little data to support the routine use of thermography, QST, or skin biopsy in patients with neuropathic pain [23].

Common Neuropathic Pain Syndromes

Painful Diabetic Polyneuropathy (PDPN)

Diabetic neuropathy with its severe manifestation known as painful diabetic polyneuropathy (PDPN) is a length-dependent disorder of peripheral nerve fibers. It is characterized by distal-to-proximal loss of peripheral nerve axons and their associated function [24]. A typical presentation involves pain in the extremities that is described as tingling/burning and often associated with numbness. The most common presentation is that of a generalized, symmetrical polyneuropathy – therefore, multiple nerve fibers (e.g., sensory, motor, autonomic) can be affected. The differential diagnosis can be quite broad on initial presentation and can include infectious causes (i.e., HIV/AIDS, hepatitis, syphilis, etc.), medication/toxin exposure (i.e., chemotherapy, alcohol, radiation, isoniazid, uremia, etc.), and mechanical causes (i.e., intervertebral disc herniation, spinal cord tumors, etc.).

Diabetic neuropathy typically presents with loss of sensation to monofilament examination (Semmes Weinstein

monofilament examination (SWME)) [25]. Typically, there are no other tests that are needed, aside from basic laboratory tests pertinent to the management of diabetes mellitus, to establish a diagnosis. EMG/NCV can be used, but they are often of little value as polyneuropathies predominantly affect small fibers. If there is accompanying motor weakness, changes in gait, or concern for other mechanical causes, then it would be warranted to obtain neuroimaging. The prevalence of diabetic neuropathy and specifically PDPN increases with age, duration of diabetes, and with worsening glucose control [26]. Numerous treatment plans and algorithms have been proposed including the well-known Toronto Expert Panel on Diabetic Neuropathy. A multimodal approach focusing on tighter glycemic control, lifestyle modifications (diet and exercise), medications, and advanced therapies is essential for a positive treatment outcome [27].

The mechanisms that contribute to the pathophysiology of diabetic neuropathy have not been completely elucidated, and there are likely multiple factors involved. The pathophysiology does appear to involve the toxic effects of high glucose levels, nonenzymatic glycosylation of different enzymes and other molecules, generation of reactive oxygen species, and the accumulation of advanced glycation end products (AGEs) [24]. All of these changes may contribute to peripheral nerve ischemia [28].

Post-herpetic Neuralgia (PHN)

PHN is a chronic neuropathic pain syndrome that results as a complication following an episode of acute herpes zoster viral infection (e.g., shingles), which is caused by a reactivation of dormant varicella-zoster virus (VZV). Following primary infection (e.g., chicken pox), the virus remains dormant in the dorsal root ganglia until reactivated during a period of relative immunosuppression, which can happen as one ages due to normal waning T-cell immunity or during a period of frank immunosuppression, as may be seen with chemotherapy or HIV/AIDS [9]. Pain resulting from shingles typically follows a dermatomal distribution of the affected nerve(s). Risk factors that increase the probability of the development of PHN include the following: advanced age, female gender, presence of a painful VZV prodrome prior to rash formation, greater VZV rash severity, significant pain during the acute phase, elevated fever in the acute phase, and sensory dysfunction in the affected dermatome [9]. While it is often stated that a course of steroids or antivirals during the acute shingles phase decreases the incidence of PHN, conclusive data is lacking to support this assertion [29, 30]. Vaccination of older adults with the goal of preventing outbreak of acute herpes zoster is the most effective means of preventing PHN.

Trigeminal Neuralgia (TN)

TN is characterized by paroxysmal attacks of unilateral, electric-like, lancinating, or stabbing facial pain in the distribution of the trigeminal nerve, typically V2 or V3 [31]. Less commonly, multiple divisions are involved simultaneously. There is growing evidence that the majority of cases (90%) of TN are secondary to compression of the trigeminal ganglion by an aberrant loop of an artery or vein [32]. The anomalous vascular compression of the trigeminal nerve as it courses in the subarachnoid space from the pons to the gasserian ganglion in Meckel's cave [12] is thought to lead to demyelination resulting in spontaneous, ectopic firing of the nerve. An MRI/MRA should be performed to evaluate for this vascular anomaly or other causes of nerve compression.

In addition to the classically described electric-like paroxysmal facial pain, patients often complain of weight loss secondary to an inability to chew, as well as general feelings of isolation. It is not uncommon for patients to have undergone numerous dental procedures for "jaw pain" prior to an accurate diagnosis. It is also worth noting that the primary form of TN does not have any identifiable neurological abnormalities on exam. If neurologic deficits are seen on exam, prompt neurosurgical consultation should be sought to evaluate for tumor compression, saccular aneurysm, or arteriovenous malformation [32]. Tension headaches, migraines, hemicrania continua, atypical facial pain, and other less common headache disorders should be considered as well. The anticonvulsant carbamazepine has become the initial medication of choice for treatment of TN. Studies have demonstrated 58–100% of patients achieving complete or near complete pain control with this medication [33]. Other medications in the anticonvulsant class, gabapentinoids, tricyclic antidepressants, NSAIDS, and opioids, among others, have been used with varying degrees of success. Trigeminal nerve and ganglia blocks/ablations, radiosurgery (e.g., gamma knife), and surgery are reserved for refractory cases.

Central Post-stroke Pain (CPSP)

CPSP presentation depends on the location of the CNS lesion. Central post-stroke pain of thalamic origin is generally considered to be one of the most severe pain syndromes and is characterized with a severe burning of parts of or the entire body contralateral to the side of the thalamic lesion [34]. Additional descriptions that patients suffering from CPSP often use include burning and freezing. As can be expected, this condition is often misdiagnosed and underdiagnosed as a substantial number of post-stroke patients are left with residual cognitive and expressive difficulties that preclude an accurate description of their symptoms [35]. Furthermore, there are other pain syndromes that develop in post-stroke patients such as headaches, hemiplegic shoulder pain, contractures, spasticity, and other musculoskeletal pain generators that confound the overall clinical picture. Nonetheless, CPSP should be considered in any post-stroke patient when their affected side (corresponding to a lesion seen on MRI or CT scan) demonstrates allodynia, hyperalgesia, or stimulus-evoked dysesthesia [34].

Proposed pathophysiological mechanisms include attenuation of central inhibition, imbalance of chemical stimuli, and central sensitization [36]. While central sensitization is an incompletely understood phenomenon, changes in firing threshold, receptor density, and acquired channelopathies appear to be involved [37, 38]. Treatment commonly involves a combination of medications typically used for the treatment of other neuropathic pain syndromes.

Treatment

The treatment of neuropathic pain remains quite challenging. This is in large part because the collection of conditions that causes neuropathic pain represents a heterogeneous group where the pain is probably caused by different mechanisms. There are, in some cases, more specific treatments for a neuropathic pain syndrome (such as carbamazepine or oxcarbazepine as the first-line treatment for TN and the maintenance of tight glycemic control for diabetic neuropathy). The Neuropathic Pain Special Interest Group (NeuPSIG), which is part of the International Association for the Study of Pain (IASP), has published guidelines and recently updated their treatment algorithm in 2015 [39]. In the algorithm, NeuPSIG organized medications according to level of evidence and then suggested the order in which they should be trialed.

According to the NeuPSIG recommendations, first-line treatments for neuropathic pain syndromes include gabapentin, pregabalin, and antidepressants (selective serotonin-norepinephrine reuptake inhibitors (SNRIs) and tricyclic antidepressants). Out of these medications, the number needed to treat (NNT) is lowest for tricyclic antidepressants (3.6) and then followed by SNRIs (6.4), gabapentin (7.2), and pregabalin (7.7) [39]. The decision to choose one of the medications over another is often dictated by which side effect(s) of a particular medications is either less or more desirable, such as using TCAs for comorbid depression or difficulties with sleeping. Second-line treatments include capsaicin and lidocaine patches for peripheral neuropathic pain because while the evidence is comparatively weak for these interventions, they are very well tolerated. Opioids are currently considered second- or third-line agents. Previously, opioids were considered first- or second-line agents, but the downgrade parallels decreased enthusiasm about their use as more data emerges demonstrating poor efficacy and the risks of opioid-associated overdose, mortality, diversion, and misuse [39].

There is data that supports the use of combined medications for the treatment of neuropathic pain. A review of the literature, evaluating studies on the efficacy of adding an additional medication from different drug classes to gabapentin therapy, revealed significantly better pain reduction with the addition of another medication class [40]. A more recent study of fibromyalgia patients, a condition that likely involves a substantial neuropathic element, determined that the combination of pregabalin and duloxetine provided a greater decrease in pain ratings with combination therapy as opposed to each medication used individually [41].

In addition to pharmacotherapy, there are a multitude of procedures available for the treatment of neuropathic pain states. An exhaustive list and discussion of these interventions is beyond the scope of this chapter. However, a brief discussion is warranted. For example, sympathetic nerve blocks have been used for a variety of pain conditions thought to have a sympathetically maintained component. Complex regional pain syndrome (CRPS) and post-herpetic neuralgia have both been studied with the use of sympathetic nerve blocks, and while the relief is often short-lived, it can result in better participation with physical therapy and may have predictive utility for the use of neuromodulation [42, 43]. Additional examples of interventions include trigeminal ganglion nerve blocks for TN and paravertebral blocks or intercostal nerve blocks for post-thoracotomy pain syndrome. If the duration of analgesia needs to be extended, radiofrequency ablation, pulsed radiofrequency ablation, cryoablation, or chemical neurolysis may be indicated.

Lastly, an exciting area of research and recent advancement has been in the area of neuromodulation, specifically spinal cord stimulation (SCS). There are two particularly difficult to treat patient populations that have received substantial benefit from SCS: CRPS and post-laminectomy pain syndrome. For example, the use of SCS for the treatment of CRPS has been extensively studied [44, 45] and is superior when added to conventional medical management with physical therapy as opposed to the use of those therapies without SCS [46]. It has also been shown to be a cost-effective treatment [47]. There are also emerging new targets for neuromodulation, namely, dorsal root ganglion (DRG) stimulation, which has been shown to be superior to conventional SCS for patients with CRPS [48]. There is a comparable amount of research for post-laminectomy pain syndrome, and more recent attention has been given to novel stimulation patterns (burst stimulation vs. tonic stimulation) and the use of kilohertz stimulation, with superior outcomes. SCS has also been shown to be efficacious and cost-effective in patients with refractory diabetic neuropathy [49–51].

References

1. Treede R-D, Jensen TS, Campbell JN, et al. Neuropathic pain: redefinition and a grading system for clinical and research purposes. Neurology. 2008;70:1630–5.
2. Hurley RW, Goldstein HV, Rathmell JP. Chapter 55: painful peripheral neuropathies. In: Benzon HT, Raja SN, Liu SS, et al., editors. Essential of pain medicine. 3rd ed. St. Louis: Elsevier/Saunders; 2011. p. 386–94.
3. Geber C, Baumgartner U, Schwab R, et al. Revised definition of neuropathic pain and its grading system: an open case series illustrating its use in clinical practice. Am J Med. 2009;122:S3–S12.
4. Hall GC, Carroll D, Parry D, et al. Epidemiology and treatment of neuropathic pain: the UK primary care perspective. Pain. 2006;122:156–2.
5. Turk DC. Clinical effectiveness and cost-effectiveness of treatments for patients with chronic pain. Clin J Pain. 2002;18:355–65.
6. Berger A, Dukes EM, Oster G. Clinical characteristics and economic costs of patients with painful neuropathic disorders. J Pain. 2004;5:143–9.
7. Dyck PJ, Kratz KM, Karnes JL, et al. The prevalence by staged severity of various types of diabetic neuropathy, retinopathy, and nephropathy in a population-based cohort: the Rochester Diabetic Neuropathy Study. Neurology. 1993;43:817–24.
8. Callaghan BC, Hur J, Feldman EL. Diabetic neuropathy: one disease or two? Curr Opin Neurol. 2012;25(2):536–41.
9. Kaye AD, Argoff CE. Chapter 1: Postherpetic neuralgia. In: Kaye AD, Shah RV, editors. Case studies in pain management. Cambridge, UK: Cambridge University Press; 2015. p. 1–15.
10. Berger A, Dukes EM, Oster G. Clinical characteristics and economic costs of patients with painful neuropathic disorders. J Pain. 2004;5:143–9.
11. Stookey B, Ransohoff J. Trigeminal neuralgia: its history and treatment. Springfield: Charles C. Thomas; 1959.
12. Eboli P, Stone JL, Audin S, et al. Historical characterization of trigeminal neuralgia. Neurosurgery. 2009;64:1183–7.
13. Tenser R. Trigeminal neuralgia: mechanisms of treatment. Neurology. 1998;51:17–9.
14. Internet Stroke Center. 2006. Stroke statistics http://www.strokecenter.org/patients/about-stroke/stroke-statistics/. Accessed 7 Jan 2017.
15. Kim JS. Post-stroke pain. Expert Rev Neurother. 2009;9(5):711–21.
16. Woolf CJ, Mannion RJ. Neuropathic pain: aetiology, symptoms, mechanisms, and management. Lancet. 1999;353:1959–64.
17. Fields H, Rowbotham M. Multiple mechanisms of neuropathic pain: a clinical perspective. Seattle: IASP Press; 1994.
18. Scholz J, Woolf CJ. The neuropathic pain triad: neurons, immune cells and glia. Nat Neurosci. 2007;10:1361–8.
19. Galer BS. Neuropathic pain of peripheral origin: advances in pharmacologic treatment. Neurology. 1995;45:S17–25; discussion S35–6
20. Calcutt NA. Potential mechanisms of neuropathic pain in diabetes. Int Rev Neurobiol. 2002;50:205–28.
21. Fields HL, Basbaum AI. Central nervous system mechanisms of pain modulation. In: Wall PD, Melzack R, editors. Textbook of pain. Edinburgh, UK: Churchill-Livingstone; 1994. p. 243–57.
22. Horowitz SH. The diagnostic workup of patients with neuropathic pain. Med Clin North Am. 2007;91:21–30.
23. Haanpaa ML, Backonja MM, Bennett MI, et al. Assessment of neuropathic pain in primary care. Am J Med. 2009;122:S13–21.
24. Doulatram G, Raj T. Chapter 8: Diabetic neuropathy. In: Kaye AD, Shah RV, editors. Case studies in pain management. Cambridge, UK: Cambridge University Press; 2015. p. 52–63.
25. Feng Y, Schlosser FJ, Supio BE. The Semmes Weinstein monofilament examination as a screen tool for diabetic peripheral neuropathy. J Vasc Surg. 2009;50(3):675–82.

26. Centers for Disease Control and Prevention. National diabetes fact sheet: national estimates and general information on diabetes and prediabetes in the United States. Atlanta: Centers for Disease Control and Prevention; 2011.

27. Tesfaye S, Vileikyte L, Rayman G, et al. Painful diabetic peripheral neuropathy: consensus recommendations on diagnosis, assessment and management. Diabetes Metab Res Rev. 2011;27(7):629–38.

28. Shakher J, Stevens MJ. Update on the management of diabetic polyneuropathies. Diabetes Metab Syndr Obes. 2011;4:289–305.

29. Chen N, Li Q, Yang J, et al. Antiviral treatment for preventing postherpetic neuralgia. Cochrane Database Syst Rev. 2014. http://onlinelibrary.wiley.com/doi/10.1002/14651858.CD006866.pub3/abstract;jsessionid=E37027B3628E2E1AFF4793F715A78032.f04t03.

30. Han Y, Zhang J, Chen N, et al. Corticosteroids for preventing postherpetic neuralgia. Cochrane Database Syst Rev. 2013. http://onlinelibrary.wiley.com/doi/10.1002/14651858.CD005582.pub4/abstract

31. Gronseth G, Cruccu G, Alksne J, et al. Practice parameter: the diagnostic evaluation and treatment of trigeminal neuralgia: an evidence-based review. Neurology. 2008;71:1183–90.

32. Maury J, Kaye AD, Gould HJ. Chapter 44: Pain management in trigeminal neuralgia. In: Kaye AD, Shah RV, editors. Case studies in pain management. Cambridge, UK: Cambridge University Press; 2015. p. 316–23.

33. Sindrup S, Jensen T. Pharmacotherapy of trigeminal neuralgia. Clin J Pain. 2002;18:22–7.

34. Klit H, Finnerup NB, Jensen TS. Central post-stroke pain: clinical characteristics, pathophysiology, and management. Lancet Neurol. 2009;8(9):857–68.

35. Leijon G, Boivie J. Central post-stroke pain: a controlled trial of amitriptyline and carbamazepine. Pain. 1989;36(1):27–36.

36. Kumar B, Kalita J, Kumar G, et al. Central poststroke pain: a review of the pathophysiology and treatment. Anesth Analg. 2009;108(5):1645–57.

37. Woolf CJ. Central sensitization: implications for the diagnosis and treatment of pain. Pain. 2011;152(3):S2–S15.

38. McMahon SB, Lewin GR, Wall PD. Central hyperexcitability triggered by noxious inputs. Curr Opin Neurobiol. 1993;3(4):602–10.

39. Finnerup NB, Attal N, Haroutounian S, et al. Pharmacotherapy for neuropathic pain in adults: a systematic review and meta-analysis. Lancet Neurol. 2015;14(2):162–73.

40. Jongen JL, Hans G, Benzon HT, et al. Neuropathic pain and pharmacological treatment. Pain Pract. 2014;14(3):283–95.

41. Gilron I, Chapparro LE, Tu D, et al. Combination of pregabalin with duloxetine for fibromyalgia: a randomized controlled trial. Pain. 2016;157:1532–40.

42. Becker WJ, Ablett DP, Harris CJ, et al. Long term treatment of intractable reflex sympathetic dystrophy with intrathecal morphine. Can J Neurol Sci. 1995;22:153–9.

43. Wu CL, Marsh A, Dworkin RH. The role of sympathetic nerve blocks in herpes zoster and postherpetic neuralgia. Pain. 2000;87:121–9.

44. Simpson EL, Duenas A, Holmes MW, et al. Spinal cord stimulation for chronic pain of neuropathic or ischaemic origin: systematic review and economic evaluation. Health Technol Assess. 2009;13:1–154.

45. Grabow TSM, Tella PKM, Raja SNM. Spinal cord stimulation for complex regional pain syndrome: an evidence-based medicine review of the literature. Clin J Pain. 2003;19:371–83.

46. Kemler M, de Vet C, Barendse G, et al. Effect of spinal cord stimulation for chronic complex regional pain syndrome Type I: five-year final follow-up of patients in a randomized controlled trial. J Neurosurg. 2008;108:292–8.

47. Taylor RS, Buyten JPV, Buchser E. Spinal cord stimulation for complex regional pain syndrome: a systematic review of the clinical and cost-effectiveness literature and assessment of prognostic factors. Eur J Pain. 2006;10:91–101.

48. Liem L, Russo M, Huygen F, et al. One-year outcomes of spinal cord stimulation of the dorsal root ganglion in the treatment of chronic neuropathic pain. Neuromodulation. 2014;18:41–9.

49. Slangen R, Schaper NC, Faber CG, et al. Spinal cord stimulation and pain relief in painful diabetic peripheral neuropathy: a prospective two-center randomized controlled trial. Diabetes Care. 2014;37(11):3016–24.

50. de Vos CC, Meier K, Zaalberg PB, et al. Spinal cord stimulation in patients with painful diabetic neuropathy: a multicentre randomized clinical trial. Pain. 2014;155(11):2426–31.

51. Slangen R, Faber CG, Schaper NC, et al. A trial-based economic evaluation comparing spinal cord stimulation with best medical treatment in painful diabetic peripheral neuropathy. J Pain. 2017;18(4):405–14.

Complex Regional Pain Syndrome

Nancy S. Lee, Sean Li, and Peter Staats

Definition

Complex regional pain syndromes (CRPS) I and II, formerly known as reflex sympathetic dystrophy (RSD) or causalgia, respectively, are characterized by pain of the upper or lower extremity, usually after injury or trauma to the limb. The head and face may also be affected. Systemic and neurogenic inflammation, as well as exaggerated and dysfunctional responses by the central and peripheral nervous systems, contribute to severe neuropathic pain which can lead to immobility, atrophy, and loss of functionality of the affected limb [1, 2]. The degree of pain is often disproportionately greater than the inciting injury. Signs of neurogenic inflammation such as edema, erythema, temperature asymmetry, and skin discolorations of the affected extremity may be observed on physical exam. CRPS can affect patients of all ages and more commonly affects females [3].

Common Clinical Characteristics

Diagnosis of CRPS is clinical after excluding other causes of pain. There are no specific lab tests or imaging that can confirm CRPS. The Budapest Clinical Diagnostic Criteria for CRPS (Table 43.1) is helpful in differentiating CRPS from other types of neuropathic pain and making the diagnosis [1]. Figure 43.1 illustrates some of the clinical characteristics of CRPS of the lower extremity.

CRPS is divided into three subcategories. In CRPS Type 1, there is no specific identified nerve lesion as the inciting

N. S. Lee (✉)
Department of Anesthesiology, Montefiore Medical Center, Bronx, NY, USA
e-mail: nalee@montefiore.org

S. Li · P. Staats
Premier Pain Centers, Shrewsbury, NJ, USA

cause of the pain. CRPS Type 2 is associated with a lesion to a nerve. CRPS-NOS (not otherwise specified) is a subtype that was added to include patients who do not meet the criteria for CRPS but whose presentation cannot be explained by another disease process [1].

Pathophysiologic Mechanisms

The pathophysiology of CRPS is multidimensional: systemic and neurogenic inflammation, dysregulation of the central and peripheral nervous systems, as well as psychosocial factors are thought to be key elements. Inflammation and dysregulation begin when injury or trauma to the limb stimulates peripheral nerve tracts conducting nociceptive signals [1]. Constant stimulation can lead to sensitization of the peripheral nervous system, and also of the spinal cord causing central sensitization [2]. In these early stages of CRPS, hyperalgesia occurs as a result of increased inflammation and sensitization. As the disease progresses to the later stages of CRPS, severe pain prevents patients from using the affected limb, leading to atrophy of the nerves and muscles.

Diagnostic Procedures and Therapeutic Interventions

The course of CRPS is variable as it can resolve spontaneously or cause chronic pain and severe debility wherein the patient permanently loses function of the affected limb. Early, aggressive treatment is encouraged to prevent progression of the disease. Multimodal therapy is advocated to restore function of the affected limb; this may consist of pharmacotherapy, interventional pain management physical therapy, occupational therapy, and psychotherapy (Table 43.2).

Table 43.1 Budapest diagnostic criteria for CRPS

Budapest clinical diagnostic criteria			
1. Continuing pain, disproportionate to any inciting event			
2. Must report at least one symptom in three of the four following categories			
Sensory	Vasomotor	Sudomotor/edema	Motor/trophic
Reports of hyperesthesia and/or allodynia	Reports of temperature asymmetry and/or skin color changes and/or skin color asymmetry	Reports of edema and/or sweating changes and/or sweating asymmetry	Reports of decreased range of motion and/or motor dysfunction (weakness, tremor, dystonia) and/or trophic changes (hair, nail, skin)
3. Must display at least one sign at time of evaluation in *two or more* of the following categories			
Sensory	Vasomotor	Sudomotor/edema	Motor/trophic
Evidence of hyperalgesia (to pinprick) and/or allodynia (to light touch and/or deep somatic pressure and/or joint movement)	Evidence of temperature asymmetry and/or skin color changes and/or asymmetry	Evidence of edema and/or sweating changes and/or sweating asymmetry	Evidence of decreased range of motion and/or motor dysfunction (weakness, tremor, dystonia) and/or trophic changes (hair, nail, skin)
4. There is no other diagnosis that better explains the signs and symptoms			

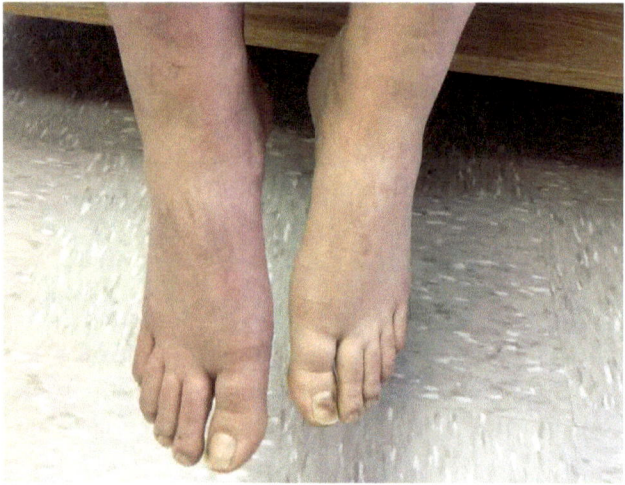

Fig. 43.1 This image illustrates edema and color change of the right lower extremity common in CRPS. (Image courtesy of Dr. Sean Li)

Medical Therapy

Upregulation of pro-inflammatory cytokines (tumor necrosis factor alpha (TNF-α), interleukin (IL)-2, IL-1 beta, and IL-6) and downregulation of anti-inflammatory cytokines (IL-4 and IL-10) have been found in the early stages of CRPS [2]. One study found that levels of most pro-inflammatory cytokines normalized after 6 months with analgesic treatment [4], while another study found that elevated levels of pro-inflammatory cytokines remained in the blood, blister fluid, and CSF [5]. Nonsteroidal anti-inflammatory drugs (NSAIDs) and TNF-alpha inhibitors have been used to treat the inflammation and pain associated with CRPS, but neither have been found to be effective at long-term pain reduction [6, 7]. A single clinical trial supports the use of oral corticosteroids for up to 12 weeks in acute CRPS [8]. Lack of evidence and the adverse effects of chronic steroid administration limit the use of oral corticosteroids in chronic CRPS [1].

Antioxidants, with their ability to scavenge reactive oxygen metabolites associated with inflammation, may have an important role in both preventing and treating CRPS. Prophylaxis with a daily 500 mg dose of vitamin C has been found to reduce the incidence of CRPS after wrist fractures [9], but not in distal radius fractures [10]. Evidence is currently limited for Vitamin C prophylaxis in CRPS of the lower extremities. Dimethyl sulfoxide (DMSO), another free radical scavenger, has been found to improve pain when applied topically to the affected limb [11, 12].

Bisphosphonates, traditionally used to treat diseases of the bone such as osteoporosis, not only reduce bone resorption and remodeling found in CRPS, but demonstrate inhibitory effects on the nociceptive neurons of bone [13]. Trials with oral alendronate [13], IV pamidronate [14], and IV neridronate infusion [15] have all shown improvements in pain. Active international trials for neridronate and other bisphosphonates are ongoing. Of note, one study found that bisphosphonates, along with NMDA antagonists and vasodilators, provided longer pain relief than other medications used to treat CRPS [16]. Bone scans are often used to detect neovascularization and bone resorption, and thus may be especially helpful when prescribing bisphosphonates for CRPS.

Ketamine, an NMDA antagonist, has also shown promise in treating CRPS. Intravenous infusion of ketamine (with a maximum dose of 0.35 mg/kg/h, not exceeding 25 mg/h over 4 hours) for 10 days provided significant pain relief compared to placebo [17]. Furthermore, ketamine infusions improved pain in patients whose pain had been refractory to other treatments [18, 19]. Ketamine also reduced swelling and improved pain when applied topically in patients with acute CRPS-1 [20]. However, it should be noted that improvements are temporary; abuse potential, psychomimetic and autonomic side effects, as well as poor per oral (PO) absorption limit regular use for this chronic pain condition. Despite also functioning as an NMDA antagonist, intra-

Table 43.2 Treatment options for CRPS

Multimodal treatment for CRPS					
Medical therapy		*Interventional therapy*		*Psychotherapy*	*Physiological*
Anti-inflammatory	NS AIDS TNF-a inhibitors Oral corticosteroids	IV regional blocks with local anesthetics		Family intervention	Occupational therapy
Antioxidants	**Vitamin C topical** **DMSO**	Nerve blocks	**Stellate ganglion block** **Thoracic or lumbar sympathetic nerve block**	Relaxation training	Physical therapy
Bisphosphonates	**Alendronate** **Pamidronate** **Neridronate**	**Spinal cord stimulation**		Cognitive pain coping skills	
NMDA Antagonists	**Ketamine** Magnesium	**Dorsal root ganglion stimulation**			
Anticonvulsants	Gabapentin Pregabalin	Surgical sympathectomy			
Antidepressants Opioids	SSRI, SNRI, TCA				
Muscle relaxants	**Baclofen**				

Treatments in bold indicate pain relief and therapeutic effectiveness supported by literature

venous (IV) magnesium has not been shown to improve pain in CRPS patients [21].

Medications traditionally effective in treating neuropathic pain, such as gabapentin and pregabalin, have had limited success in treating CRPS. In one randomized clinical trial, gabapentin significantly reduced sensory deficits, but did not provide pain relief compared to placebo [22]. There may, however, be an indication for gabapentinoids to be used when other treatment options have been exhausted. Gabapentin was effective in treating recurrent CRPS-1 in one case study when patients stopped responding to physiotherapy and regional sympathetic blockade [23]. Compelling evidence is once again limited regarding the efficacy of antiepileptic drugs in treating CRPS, although carbamazepine was found to provide significant pain relief in one randomized clinical trial [24].

Antidepressants are also widely used in treating chronic pain. Although the association between chronic pain and psychological disorders such as depression is undeniable, there are no studies that suggest a psychogenic component of CRPS specifically and there is insufficient evidence to support the use of selective serotonin reuptake inhibitors (SSRIs), serotonin-norepinephrine reuptake inhibitors (SNRIs), and tricyclic antidepressants (TCAs) for the treatment of CRPS. Instead, psychological interventions such as involving family members and training patients in relaxation and cognitive pain coping skills are recommended [1].

The role of opioids in CRPS has mirrored the evolving treatment paradigm of opioids for chronic pain. The limited supporting evidence for opioids and overwhelming concerns for opioid abuse make opioids an unappealing long-term treatment option for CRPS management.

For CRPS patients presenting with dystonia, baclofen is recommended orally or via an intrathecal pump in severe cases [1].

Physical Therapy

Physical therapy constitutes one of the most important components of treatment. Desensitization focuses on reversing the central sensitization that occurs in CRPS. Methods include introducing a progression of sensory stimuli, such as fabrics ranging from silk to those that are more textured like towels [1], as well as motor stimuli through graded exercise with increasing weight and intensity. Contrast baths, where two baths are set at different temperature and the difference in temperatures are slowly increased, help patients to reset their altered perception of temperature.

Interventional Therapy

Several interventional treatment methods have been effective for CRPS, either as a supplement to pharmacotherapy or as the therapy sought when symptoms are refractory to medical management.

Currently, there are conflicting results for intravenous regional blocks with local anesthetics. Some studies have concluded that IV regional anesthesia (Bier block) with lidocaine and additional agents such as guanethidine reduces pain, improves dexterity, and decreases edema [25, 26]. However, the fourth edition CRPS Diagnostic and Treatment Guidelines highlight a high-quality meta-analysis that reports lack of proven effect of IV regional anesthesia, as well as some studies with negative outcomes [27].

The pain fibers within the sympathetic chain can be targeted based on the affected limb. Stellate ganglion and thoracic sympathetic nerve blocks are utilized in CRPS of the upper extremity, while lumbar sympathetic nerve blocks target the lower extremities. Thoracic and lumbar sympathetic nerve blocks have both shown positive results [28, 29], providing significant pain relief and lower depression scores for up to 12 months [29]. Stellate ganglion blocks have also been found to effectively reduce pain [30] and increase range of motion in the wrist [31].

Spinal cord stimulation (SCS) modulates pain signaling at the dorsal column and dorsal horn with a low-voltage current in the epidural space. It may also have an effect on the sympathetic nervous system of the affected limb. SCS therapy was proven to reduce pain and improve quality of life for 2–3 years in Kemler's landmark study in 2004 [32] as well as a follow-up trial in 2008 [33]. These positive results in improvement of pain and quality of life have been reproduced in other studies [34, 35]. In addition to pain relief, patients report improvements in dystonia and ability to perform daily living activities [36]. Interventional treatment methods such as SCS often tend to be used after medical management has been exhausted. However, some practitioners recommend starting SCS earlier in the course of CRPS, as opposed to later, due to its initial efficacy and possible ability to stop further progression of the disease [37].

More recently, dorsal root ganglion (DRG) stimulation has been shown to be effective in treating CRPS of the lower extremity in the ACCURATE trial [38]. Patients naïve to stimulation with chronic, intractable pain for at least 6 months were randomized to dorsal root ganglion stimulation or traditional spinal cord stimulation. Treatment success was superior in the DRG group at the primary end point of 3 months and also at 12 month follow-up. These patients reported significant pain relief and improvement in quality of life, functional status, and psychological deposition. The superior results of DRG may be due to the ability to specifically target affected dermatomes.

The most invasive treatment option, surgical sympathectomy, involves resection or clamping of the sympathetic chain in an open or minimally invasive surgical procedure. Alcohol or phenol injections along the sympathetic chain are sometimes supplemented to provide additional, albeit less permanent, chemical sympathectomy [39]. The lack of high quality studies supporting surgical or chemical sympathectomy for CRPS, and serious complications such as worsening pain and hyperhidrosis preclude sympathectomies from being a viable standard treatment options [39].

Summary

Complex regional pain syndrome, as indicated by its name, is indeed a multifaceted constellation of symptoms that requires further study of pathology and treatment. Managing CRPS may be overwhelming for the provider, as there is no clear first-line treatment and pain is often severe. It is important to discuss the prognosis of the disease with the patient and patient's family in order to establish realistic expectations for treatment and progression of the syndrome. Medical therapy will need to be targeted to the patient and their specific symptoms. Discussions regarding interventional therapies should take place early on as evidence is best for prompt treatment and should start immediately upon diagnosis once other causes have been excluded. Treatment should be multidisciplinary and include a significant component of specialized physical and occupational therapies.

References

1. Harden RN, Oaklander AL, Burton AW, Perez RS, Richardson K, Swan M, et al. Complex regional pain syndrome: practical diagnostic and treatment guidelines, 4th edition. Pain Med. 2013;14(2):180–229.
2. Schlereth T, Drummond P, Birklein F. Inflammation in CRPS: role of the sympathetic supply. Auton Neurosci. 2014;182:102–7.
3. Pardo MC Jr., Miller RD. Basics of anesthesia. 7 ed. Philadelphia, PA: Elsevier; 2017.
4. Lenz M, Uceyler N, Frettloh J, Hoffken O, Krumova EK, Lissek S, et al. Local cytokine changes in complex regional pain syndrome type I (CRPS I) resolve after 6 months. Pain. 2013;154(10):2142–9.
5. Parkitny L, McAuley JH, Pietro FD, Stanton TR, O'Connell NE, Marinus J, et al. Inflammation in complex regional pain syndrome: a systematic review and meta-analysis. Neurology. 2013;80(1):106–17.
6. Breuer AJ, Mainka T, Hansel N, Maier C, Krumova EK. Short-term treatment with parecoxib for complex regional pain syndrome: a randomized, placebo-controlled double-blind trial. Pain Physician. 2014;17(2):127–37.
7. Eckmann MS, Ramamurthy S, Griffin JG. Intravenous regional ketorolac and lidocaine in the treatment of complex regional pain syndrome of the lower extremity: a randomized, double-blinded, crossover study. Clin J Pain. 2011;27(3):203–6.
8. Christensen K, Jensen EM, Noer I. The reflex dystrophy syndrome response to treatment with systemic corticosteroids. Acta Chir Scand. 1982;148(8):653–5.
9. Zollinger PE, Tuinebreijer WE, Breederveld RS, Kreis RW. Can vitamin C prevent complex regional pain syndrome in patients with wrist fractures? A randomized, controlled, multicenter dose-response study. J Bone Joint Surg Am. 2007;89(7):1424–31.
10. Evanview N, McCarthy C, Kleinlugtenbelt YV, Ghert M, Bhandari M. Vitamin C to prevent complex regional pain syndrome in patients with distal radius fractures: a meta-analysis of randomized controlled trials. J Orthop Trauma. 2015;29(8):e235–41.
11. Gaspar M, Bovaira M, Carrera-Hueso FJ, Querol M, Jimenez A, Moreno L. Efficacy of a topical treatment protocol with dimethyl sulfoxide 50% in type 1 complex regional pain syndrome. Farm Hosp. 2012;36(5):385–91.

12. Perez RS, Zuurmond WW, Bezemer PD, Kuik DJ, ACv L, JJd L, et al. The treatment of complex regional pain syndrome type I with free radical scavengers: a randomized controlled study. Pain. 2003;102(3):297–307.

13. Manicourt DH, Brasseur JP, Boutsen Y, Depreseux G, Devogelaer JP. Role of alendronate in therapy for posttraumatic complex regional pain syndrome type I of the lower extremity. Arthritis Rheum. 2004;50(11):3690–7.

14. Robinson JN, Sandom J, Chapman PT. Efficacy of pamidronate in complex regional pain syndrome type I. Pain Med. 2004;5(3):276–80.

15. Varenna M, Adami S, Rossini M, Gatti D, Idolazzi L, Zucchi F, et al. Treatment of complex regional pain syndrome type I with neridronate: a randomized, double-blind, placebo-controlled study. Rheumatology. 2013;52(3):532–42.

16. Wertli MM, Kessels AG, Perez RS, Bachmann LM, Brunner F. Rational pain management in complex regional pain syndrome 1 (CRPS 1)--a network meta-analysis. Pain Med. 2014;15(9):1575–89.

17. Schwartzman RJ, Alexander GM, Grothusen JR, Paylor T, Reichenberger E, Perreault M. Outpatient intravenous ketamine for the treatment of complex regional pain syndrome: a double-blind placebo controlled study. Pain. 2009;147(1–3):107–15.

18. Nama S, Meenan DR, Fritz WT. The use of sub-anesthetic intravenous ketamine and adjuvant dexmedetomidine when treating acute pain from CRPS. Pain Physician. 2010;13(4):365–8.

19. Shirani P, Salamone AR, Schulz PE, Edmondson EA. Ketamine treatment for intractable pain in a patient with severe refractory complex regional pain syndrome: a case report. Pain Physician. 2008;11(3):339–42.

20. Ushida T, Tani T, Kanbara T, Zinchuk VS, Kawasaki M, Yamamoto H. Analgesic effects of ketamine ointment in patients with complex regional pain syndrome type 1. Reg Anesth Pain Med. 2002;27(5):524–8.

21. Fischer SG, Collins S, Boogaard S, Loer SA, Zuurmond WW, Perez RS. Intravenous magnesium for chronic complex regional pain syndrome type 1 (CRPS-1). Pain Med. 2013;14(9):1388–99.

22. ACvd V, SGS-vd B, Kessels AH, Weber WE. Randomised controlled trial of gabapentin in Complex Regional Pain Syndrome type 1. BMC Neurol. 2004;29(4):13.

23. Akkus S, Yorgancigil H, Yener M. A case of recurrent and migratory complex regional pain syndrome type I: prevention by gabapentin. Rheumatol Int. 2006;26(9):852–4.

24. Harke H, Gretenkort P, Ladleif HU, Rahman S, Harke O. The response of neuropathic pain and pain in complex regional pain syndrome I to carbamazepine and sustained-release morphine in patients pretreated with spinal cord stimulation: a double blinded randomized study. Anesth Analg. 2001;92:488–95.

25. Toda K, Muneshige H, Asou T. Intravenous regional block with lidocaine for treatment of complex regional pain syndrome. Clin J Pain. 2006;22(2):222–4.

26. Paraskevas KI, Michaloglou AA, Briana DD, Samara M. Treatment of complex regional pain syndrome type I of the hand with a series of intravenous regional sympathetic blocks with guanethidine and lidocaine. Clin Rheumatol. 2006;25(5):687–93.

27. Perez RS, Kwakkel G, Zuurmond WW, deLange JJ. Treatment of reflex sympathetic dystrophy (CRPS type I): a research synthesis of 21 randomized clinical trials. J Pain Symptom Manage. 2001;21(6):511–26.

28. Choi E, Cho CW, Kim HY, Lee PB, Nahm FS. Lumbar sympathetic block with botulinum toxin type B for complex regional pain syndrome: a case study. Pain Physician. 2015;18(5):E911–6.

29. Rde OR, Teixeira MJ, Yeng LT, Cantara MG, Faria VG, Liggieri V, et al. Thoracic sympathetic block for the treatment of complex regional pain syndrome type I: a double-blind randomized controlled study. Pain. 2014;155(11):2274–81.

30. Wei K, Feldmann RE Jr, Brascher AK, Benrath J. Ultrasound-guided stellate ganglion blocks combined with pharmacological and occupational therapy in Complex Regional Pain Syndrome (CRPS): a pilot case series ad interim. Pain Med. 2014;15(12):2120–7.

31. Yucel I, Demiraran Y, Ozturan K, Degirmenci E. Complex regional pain syndrome type I: efficacy of stellate ganglion blockade. J Orthop Traumatol. 2009;10(4):179–83.

32. Kemler MA, Vet HCWD, Barendse GAM, Wildenberg FAJMVD, Kleef MV. The effect of spinal cord stimulation in patients with chronic reflex sympathetic dystrophy: two years' follow-up of the randomized controlled trial. Ann Neurol. 2004;55(1):13–8.

33. Kemler MA, HCW d V, Barendse GAM, FAJMvd W, Mv K. Effect of spinal cord stimulation for chronic complex regional pain syndrome type I: five-year final follow-up of patients in a randomized controlled trial. J Neurosurg. 2008;108:292–8.

34. Sanders RA, Moeschler SM, Gazelka HM, Lamer TJ, Wang Z, Qu W, et al. Patient outcomes and spinal cord stimulation: a retrospective case series evaluating patient satisfaction, pain scores, and opioid requirements. Pain Pract. 2016;16(7):899–904.

35. Visnjevac O, Costandi S, Patel BA, Azer G, Agarwal P, Bolash R, et al. A comprehensive outcome-specific review of the use of spinal cord stimulation for complex regional pain syndrome. Pain Pract. 2017;17(4):533–45.

36. Harke H, Gretenkort P, Ladleif HU, Rahman S. Spinal cord stimulation in sympathetically maintained complex regional pain syndrome type I with severe disability. A prospective clinical study. Eur J Pain. 2005;9(4):363–73.

37. Poree L, Krames E, Pope J, Deer TR, Levy R, Schultz L. Spinal cord stimulation as treatment for complex regional pain syndrome should be considered earlier than last resort therapy. Neuromodulation. 2013;16(2):125–41.

38. Deer TR, Levy RM, Kramer J, Poree L, Amirdelfan K, Grigsby E, et al. Dorsal root ganglion stimulation yielded higher treatment success rate for complex regional pain syndrome and causalgia at 3 and 12 months: a randomized comparative trial. Pain. 2017;158(4):669–81.

39. Mailis A, Furlan A. Sympathectomy for neuropathic pain. Cochrane Database Syst Rev. 2003;(2):CD002918.

Pain in Infants, Children, and Adolescents

Veronica Carullo, Ellise Cappuccio, and Ingrid Fitz-James Antoine

Development

Noxious stimulation during early development (24–32 weeks) has a negative impact on intellectual outcome via reduction in white and grey matter volumes, thinner cortex (specifically in the frontal/parietal region), and altered pain processing in adulthood [1–4]. Pain transmission pathways are anatomically present at 22 weeks gestation, fully mature after birth, and consist of nociceptive pathways spatially located in the peripheral nervous system, the spinal cord, and supraspinal cortical regions. The integration of these systems produces the physiologic response to painful stimuli and individual pain perception. Maturation is bidirectional, proceeding from cortex to periphery and periphery to cortex. At 7 weeks of age, cutaneous peri-oral peripheral nociceptors appear, subsequently spread to face, palm and soles of feet at 11 weeks, to trunk and proximal leg and arm around 15 weeks, and finally to all mucocutaneous surfaces by week 20 of gestation. Simultaneously, ascending spinal cord pathways develop, and by week 12, peripheral nociceptive fibers extend into the dorsal horn of the spinal cord, with descent of corticospinal axons into the cervical spinal cord by 24 weeks, subsequently connecting to the grey matter of the spinal cord and to Group Ia inhibitory interneurons at term [5–8]. Cerebral cortical neurons from the periventricular zone migrate to the cortical zone as neuronal formation and migration occurs in waves, in a pattern of "deep-first, superficial-last." Once in their final laminar position, these cells undergo terminal differentiation under the influence of local environmental factors and three important translation factors (Pax6, Emx2, TLx), which regulate progenitor cell proliferation and cell differentiation from week 12 to term and beyond. This process is probably the most delicate and most profoundly disturbed during physiologic stress [9].

In preterm neonates, ascending pathways allow transmission of noxious stimuli to the brain while immature descending pathways cause incomplete modulation of pain, leading to hyperalgesia. This finding is compounded by a higher percentage of lower threshold receptors in the peripheral nervous system. Even before 30 weeks, mature limb withdrawal reflexes are evident and non-noxious stimuli may be perceived as painful because descending pathways responsible for integration and modulation mature after birth [10–13]. Gamma-amino-butyric acid (GABA) is important in the development of neuronal circuitry, connectivity, and modulation in the developing newborn and undergoes a switch from excitatory to inhibitory after term birth. GABA interneurons, which develop during the second and third trimester, are thought to be susceptible to stress and hypoxia, as well. GABA and glutamate concentration are decreased in in the right frontal region in non-sedated preterm infants during functional MRI, but show increased connectivity in the region that serves language, executive function, and cognition. At term, GABA concentration increases and connectivity decreases [14]. The plasticity of developing neurons makes them especially vulnerable. They have been shown to express long-term negative sequelae to noxious stimuli in the nervous system, even when these noxious stimuli appear to be adequately treated by physiologic parameters during the critical, neonatal period [15, 16]. Furthermore, exposure to repeated painful stimuli has been shown to have physiologic and behavioral implications in the neonatal period and into adulthood [17].

V. Carullo (✉)
Pediatric Pain Management, Pediatric Anesthesiology Fellowship Program, MontefioreMedical Center, The University Hospital for Albert Einstein College of Medicine, New York, NY, USA
e-mail: vcarullo@montefiore.org

E. Cappuccio · I. F.-J. Antoine
Montefiore Medical Center, Albert Einstein College of Medicine, Bronx, NY, USA

Pharmacokinetics/Dynamics

Adequately treating pain in the pediatric population requires an understanding of the differences in pharmacokinetics and pharmacodynamics between infants, children, and adults.

Y. Khelemsky et al. (eds.), *Academic Pain Medicine*, https://doi.org/10.1007/978-3-030-18005-8_44

When possible, oral administration of medications is preferred in the setting of chronic use. Gastric pH can affect the absorption of certain orally administered drugs. Infants have a relatively high or neutral gastric pH, which accounts for more rapid absorption of basic drugs and decreased absorption of weak acidic drugs. Additionally, gastric emptying affects the absorption. Neonates until around 6–8 months of life have a slow, linear pattern of gastric emptying versus the biphasic pattern of adults. While it may seem logical that slower gastric emptying would increase absorption, research suggests that certain medications are less bioavailable in neonates compared to older children and adults. Other factors affecting the absorption of orally administered drugs include decreased secretion and activity of bile salts and pancreatic fluid, underdeveloped intestinal mucosa and differences in intestinal bacterial colonization. Immaturity of neonatal bile salts is especially important if an infant is being treated with a fat-soluble drug [18].

Intramuscular injection of medications is conceptually important, for it is often the fastest way to administer an emergency drug to an infant or child. Because intramuscular injection relies on vascularity of the muscle in which the drug is injected, adequate systemic absorption may be unreliable in infants given the relative lack of muscle mass and amount of blood perfusion to the muscles [18], particularly if the drug is administered during a state of compromised perfusion. Alternatively, the subcutaneous route provides reliable absorption and is less painful.

Rectal administration of drugs is another useful alternative for selected agents in the absence of other options. The absorption of medications via this route varies among different age populations, likely secondary to differences in rectal pH and temperature. It is important to note that both location and depth of administration in the rectum affect the degree of first pass metabolism of the medication [18].

The differences in bioavailability, absorption, distribution and metabolism of drugs in infants are important to understand since this determines best practices in dosing and site of administration of medications under discussion [18, 19]. The most important determinants of drug distribution are total body water, plasma protein binding, and membrane permeability. Neonates have a proportionally higher percentage of total body water, leading to a significantly higher volume of distribution of water-soluble drugs. Once a drug is absorbed systemically, it exists in plasma in one of two forms: protein bound or as free drug. The proportion of these two states determines the drug efficacy and bioavailability.

Typically, neonates have a lower percentage of plasma proteins available, along with immature function of these proteins. An immature blood brain barrier may lead to a higher percentage of unbound drugs exerting central pharmacologic effect and mediating potential toxicity.

Drug metabolism, which occurs principally in the liver, facilitates excretion. This process is divided into phase I and phase II reactions. The enzymes involved in both of these processes are immature at birth and account for differences in plasma concentrations of metabolites in neonates versus older children or adults [19]. Additionally, decreased neonatal hepatic blood flow accounts for decreased hepatic clearance. The cytochrome p450 family constitutes the group of enzymes primarily responsible for phase I reactions. The aggregate functional activity in neonates is thought to be 30–60% of adult levels. This decreased function must be taken into account as it may necessitate a decreased medication dosing.

Phase II reactions, including glucuronidation, methylation, and acetylation, display important differences in neonates as well; morphine is a representative example. One of the metabolites of the glucuronidation of morphine, morphine-6-glucuronide (M6G), has potent analgesic properties. Studies in children and preterm neonates receiving morphine demonstrated higher concentrations of M6G, and thus increased dosing intervals are recommended for morphine in neonates to account for reduced metabolic clearance [19].

Excretion of drugs is dependent on glomerular filtration, tubular secretion, and reabsorption in the kidneys. The observed differences in these processes in the pediatric population are a result of alterations in renal blood and plasma flow, which reach adult levels around 2 years of age. Renal blood flow in neonates is approximately 20% that of adults, and must be considered to prevent accumulation of drugs in this age group [18, 19].

Perception

Pain is a subjective interpretation of a stimulus, real or expected, composed of cognitive, emotional, and physiologic factors. Pain perceived as severe can be overwhelming, leading to deep suffering. The perception of pain can vary based on several factors such as development level, prior experiences with pain, cultural differences, cognitive level, concomitant psychological comorbidities (i.e. anxiety, depression, etc.)and genetic variations. Catechol-O-methyltransferase (COMT), the enzyme mainly responsible for metabolism of noradrenaline, adrenaline, and dopamine, has been found to be an important regulator of pain perception, cognitive function, and mood in children. The understanding of this underlying genetic basis for why there is so much variability in children's pain experience may allow for future targeted approaches to analgesic therapy guided by pharmacogenomic testing [20].

Pharmacologic Treatment of Pain

Pharmacologic treatment depends on pathophysiology of pain, patient developmental level, allergies or sensitivities, route of administration, and dosing requirements. The etiology of the pain will determine which class of medication or combination of medications to use (i.e. local anesthetics, NSAIDs, opioids, neuropathic agents, muscle relaxants, etc.) Inpatient versus outpatient treatment, along with the severity of the pain affects the route of administration and modality of pain control (i.e. peripheral nerve block, neuraxial technique, IV patient-controlled (PCA) or nurse-controlled analgesia (NCA), etc).

Multimodal analgesia with utilization of opioid and non-opioid medications, as well as nonpharmacologic therapies effective in treating pain has become the recommended approach. The World Health Organization created an "analgesic ladder" to help guide management of pain in children and adults. These recommendations were updated in 2012 and recommend the use of a two-step ladder in children versus the traditional three-step ladder that is used in adults [21].

Anti-inflammatory medications such as acetaminophen and non-steroidal anti-inflammatory medicines are recommended in step one of the ladder for treatment of mild pain. For moderate to severe pain, opioids such as morphine are recommended in step two of the ladder. Anti-inflammatory drugs, such as acetaminophen, ibuprofen, naproxen, or ketorolac come in intravenous and oral formulations. The oral route remains the most common route of administration of these medications except in the perioperative period when intravenous administration is preferred. The benefits include high efficacy for mild to moderate (and sometimes severe) pain with a favorable side effect profile. The most commonly quoted side effects in children are gastrointestinal, which include but are not limited to GI upset and potential for increased bleeding. For infants and children without intravenous access and who are unable to take oral medications, rectally administered acetaminophen is an alternative option. Intravenous formulations of NSAIDs are relatively new and demonstrate efficacy, particularly in the perioperative setting. Ketorolac is a potent NSAID that may be administered intravenously or intramuscularly, and works exceptionally well for pain mediated by an inflammatory process. In addition, intravenous acetaminophen and intravenous ibuprofen are available in many institutions for perioperative analgesia or in situations where patients are unable to take oral medications (e.g. NPO).

If pain persists despite the use of the above-mentioned medications, or if pain is anticipated to be severe, opioids are commonly utilized. Codeine is an opioid that has traditionally been used in this setting but has recently fallen out of favor, especially in children. Codeine is a prodrug that is converted to morphine in the liver by the cytochrome p450 system, specifically CYP2D6. After several instances of respiratory depression and death in children prescribed codeine after surgery, evidence of ultra-rapid metabolism of codeine was discovered secondary to a CYP2D6 polymorphism, the frequency of which varies by ethnicity but seems to be the most common in patients of Ethiopian descent [22].

The potential for this fatal pharmacogenomic variant, combined with the fact that codeine is a weak and often ineffective analgesic particularly in individuals with the CYP2D6 polymorphism which renders them poor metabolizers of codeine, has virtually eliminated its use in the pediatric population. Instead, other medications such as tramadol, morphine or oxycodone should be considered for treatment of moderate to severe pain.

For severe, persistent pain, especially associated with serious systemic disease (i.e. sickle cell disease, cancer, etc.) or major surgery, other opioids such as fentanyl and hydromorphone are also frequently used. The choice of opioid is based on the overall care plan of the patient. Outpatient treatment requires oral opioids or other formulations, such as a fentanyl patch, whereas inpatient treatment may require intravenous injections, infusions, and/or nurse controlled/caregiver controlled analgesia (NCA/CCA) versus patient controlled analgesia (PCA) depending on the age, developmental level, and mental status of the pediatric patient. Depending on the severity and frequency of pain, longer acting opioids such as extended release morphine or methadone can be considered to ease the burden of frequent dosing and breakthrough pain.

The most common side effects of opioid medications are constipation, itchiness and nausea/vomiting, while the more serious side effect is respiratory depression leading to hypoxic tissue injury or death. Constipation leading to an ileus and bowel obstruction is a serious concern and a bowel regimen is suggested to accompany every opioid prescription. In the case of respiratory depression or obtundation from any of these medications, small doses of naloxone may be used to reverse the adverse effects of opioids, while taking into consideration that the analgesic effect may be reversed, as well.

While all of the above medications may be used for both chronic and acute pain, duration of treatment must be considered. While NSAIDs are extremely useful for acute pain, prolonged use can lead to gastrointestinal issues, such as ulcers, and potentially dangerous renal complications. In addition to the acute side of effects of opioids, propensity for addiction and misuse is significant, which should be seriously factored into decisions regarding use.

There are several systemic diseases in the pediatric population that commonly result in chronic pain. Sickle cell disease is of particular concern given the high doses of opioids commonly required to treat sickle cell pain during a crisis. Successfully treating acute vaso-occlusive crisis pain can be a challenge, often requiring hospital admission for administration of opioids intravenously, usually via patient-controlled analgesia. Methadone or ketamine can be useful adjuncts in these difficult situations.

Adjuvants such as steroids, anxiolytics, anti-depressants, hypnotics, anti-convulsants, gabapentinoids, membrane stabilizers, NMDA-receptor antagonists, or alpha-2-agonists can be also be of use, with the understanding that many of these uses are off-label in the pediatric (and adult) population. Particular care must be taken if starting a medication that may precipitate mood changes, as these are often more pronounced in children and adolescents.

The use of caudal catheters has been used with success in the neonatal intensive care unit to manage post-operative pain as an opioid sparing technique. One limiting factor for the use of caudal catheters is the ability for an institution to safely care for a patient with one in place. Education of all providers and staff caring for the patient is necessary, along with access to clinicians familiar with management and dosing considerations for this age-group. While peripheral nerve blocks and neuraxial blocks using local anesthetics with or without adjuvants are commonly used for acute pain in the adult and pediatric population, pediatric chronic pain is less commonly treated with these interventions. Reasons for this exclusion include lack of provider familiarity and frequent need for placement while deeply sedated or under general anesthesia, which differs from practice in adult patients. With regards to epidural steroid injections and many interventional procedures used in adult chronic pain, children often do not have the pathology treated with these modalities. There are exceptions, however, notably complex regional pain syndrome that is refractory to conventional, more conservative treatments and which often responds to sympathetic blocks for improvement of symptoms and restoration of function.

Non-pharmacologic Treatment of Pain

A multidisciplinary approach to pain management is the mainstay for treatment of pediatric chronic pain [23]. This approach includes the use of appropriate pharmacologic therapies combined with physical rehabilitation, psychological (i.e. cognitive behavioral therapy, biofeedback, etc.) and integrative therapies (i.e. acupuncture, guided imagery, music therapy, massage, yoga, etc.). Chronic pain and anxiety in children can affect behaviors and socialization, as well as perception of pain into adulthood. The ability of a provider to intervene therapeutically and educate both patients and parents may help avoid potentially detrimental, self-destructive behaviors and disability into adulthood. The impact of chronic pain places children at risk for school absence, limits educational performance, contributes to non-participation in extracurricular activities, and restricts social growth and psychosocial development. The comprehensive, multidisciplinary approach not only targets the nociceptive aspects of chronic pain, but also instills coping skills and mechanisms applicable to all aspects of the patient's life.

There are several pediatric hospitals across the United States that offer inpatient or day programs for rehabilitation

of children failing outpatient treatment and all employ this comprehensive, multidisciplinary model.

Pain Assessment Tools

A number of factors contribute to the challenges faced in both the understanding and the treatment of painful illnesses in the pediatric population. One such barrier is the need to accurately assess an individual's pain using the appropriate tool based on the patient's age and cognitive ability. Using validated self-report scales (i.e. Faces Scale, Visual Analogue Scale, Numerical Rating Scale, etc.), it is possible to obtain a pain assessment in school-aged children and adolescents who are otherwise neurologically intact. In neonates, infants, and toddlers, validated observational scales (i.e. Neonatal Infant Pain Scale, FLACC scale, etc.) are more commonly utilized. Additionally, it is important to assess if the child is competent to accurately self-report pain in situations compromised by disability (i.e. cognitive impairment, developmental delay, etc.) and language barriers.

When assessing pain, the provider must determine character, location, exacerbating and relieving factors, intensity, and tolerability. One should be cautious not to use personal bias to make assumptions about pain or the patient's tolerability, as this can lead to under-treatment or overtreatment. Behavioral observations, physiologic parameters, and self-reporting should all be considered. FLACC (face, legs, activity, crying, consolability) scale is typically used for infants and young children who are unable to communicate their pain. There are several scales available to help young children self-report pain, including the Wong Baker Faces and a graded color visual analogue scale [24]. Adolescents can typically use an adult NRS or VAS scales.

Special Considerations: Palliative Care and End-of-Life Issues

We know that for certain diseases such as cancer, pain at end-of-life may be particularly difficult to treat. In these situations an understanding of the patient and family's goals of care is crucial in providing an individualized approach to his/her pain. The four concepts as delineated in the WHO guidelines consist of "by the ladder," "by the clock," "by the mouth," and "by the child." Treatment should be aggressive and guided by an appropriate pain assessment. Opioids are typically the first-line pharmacologic agents in palliative care situations and at the end of life, although a multimodal approach also utilizing non-opioid analgesics, other adjuvants, and non-pharmacologic pain management strategies will provide the most comprehensive approach in addressing the multidimensional pain experience [25, 26].

Continuous opioid infusions have been commonly used for pain and sedation in this population. Institutional shifts have more recently trended towards nurse- or caregiver-controlled analgesia (NCA/CCA). A recent study found that patients who received opioids administered via NCA/CCA received significantly lower doses of opioids without a significant difference in pain scores [27]. While there are limitations to this practice, namely significant education of the surrogate provider, the results are promising and provide an alternative treatment option when making an individualized care plan. While the risks of undertreated pain in the neonatal population are known, more research is needed regarding the acute and long term effects of analgesics and efforts to provide the minimal effective dose are probably justified.

Ethics of Study and Treatment of Pain in Children

Premature births occur in 12% of newborns in the United States at a cost which approximates 28 billion United States dollars. The greatest economic burden is incurred in the immediate perinatal period. The practice of continuous morphine infusion in neonates has brought some issues to the forefront such as the potential impact on visually dependent intelligence quotient testing and the potential for decreased motor development [28, 29]. Anesthetic care and the management of acute and chronic pain to both the maternal-fetal and maternal-child unit has been linked to behavioral and psychosocial dysfunction in individuals subjected to the intensive care environment as newborns and children. Placebo administration is in most cases not an acceptable alternative for parents and many challenges and barriers still exist that limit the quantity and quality of successful pediatric research endeavors, particularly as it relates to drug development [30].

References

1. Grunau RE. Neonatal pain in very preterm infants: long term effects on brain neurodevelopment and pain reactivity. Rambam Maimonides Med J. 2013;4(4):e0025.
2. Volpe JJ. Neurobiology of periventricular leukomalacia in the premature infant. Pediatr Res. 2001;50(5):532–62.
3. Vinall J, Miller SP, Bjornson B, Fitzpatrick KPV, Poskitt KJ, Bryant R, Synnes AR, Cepeda IL, Grunau RE. Brain and cognitive development at school age. Pediatrics. 2014;133:412–21.
4. Brummelte S, Grunau RE, Chau V, Poskitt KJ, Brant R, Vinall J, Gover A, Synnes A, Miller SP. Procedural pain and brain development in premature newborns. Ann Neurol. 2012;71(3):385–96.
5. American Academy of Pediatrics & Canadian Paediatric Society Policy Statement. Prevention and management of pain in the neonate: an update. Pediatrics. 2006;118:2231–41.
6. Lee SJ, Ralston HJP, Drey E, Partridge JC, Rosen MA. Fetal pain: a systematic multidisciplinary review of the evidence. JAMA. 2005;294(8):947–54.
7. Lowery CL, Hardman MP, Manning N, Hall RW, Anand KJS, Clancy B. Neurodevelopmental changes of fetal pain. Semin Perinatol. 2007;31:275–82.
8. Schwaller F, Fitzgerald M. Consequences of pain in early life: injury induced plasticity in developing pain pathways. Eur J Neurosci. 2014;39(3):344–52.
9. Manuel MN, Mi D, Mason JO, Price DJ. Regulation of cerebral cortical neurogenesis by the Pax6 transcription factor. Front Cell Neurosci. 2015;9:70.
10. Slater R, Cantarella A, Gallella S, Worley A, Boyd S, Meek J, Fitzgerald M. Cortical pain responses in human infants. J Neurosci. 2006;26(14):3662–6.
11. Ranger M, Chau CM, Garg A, Woodward TS, Beg MF, Bjornson B, Poskitt K, Fitzpatrick K, Synnes AR, Miller SP, Grunau RE. Neonatal pain–related stress predictscortical thickness at age 7 years in children born very preterm. PLoS One. 2013;8:1–12. https://doi.org/10.1371/journal.pone.0076702.
12. Lee W, Morgan BR, Shroff MM, Sled JG, Taylor MJ. The development of regional functional connectivity in preterm infants into early childhood. Neuroradiology. 2013;55(S2):105–11.
13. Thomason ME, Scheinost D, Manning JH, Grove LE, Hect J, Marshall N, Hernandez-Andrade E, Berman S, Pappas A, Yeo L, Hassan SS, Constable T, Ment LR, Romero R. Weak functional connectivity in the human fetal brain prior to preterm birth. Nat Sci Rep. 2017;7:1–10. https://www.nature.com/articles/srep39286.
14. Kwon SH, Scheinost D, Lacadie C, Benjamin J, Myers EH, Rothman DL, Constable RT, Ment LR. GABA, resting state connectivity and the developing brain. Neonatology. 2014;106:149–55.
15. Penn AA, Gressens P, Fleiss B, Back SA, Gallo V. Controversies in preterm brain injury. Neurobiol Dis. 2015;92:90. https://doi.org/10.1016/j.nbd.2015.10.012.
16. Martinez-Biarge M, Groenendall F, Kersbergen KJ, Benders MJNL, Foti F, Cowan FM, deVries LS. MRI based preterm white matter injury classification, the importance of sequential imaging. In determining severity of injury. PLoS One. 2016;11(6):e0156245. https://doi.org/10.1371/journal.pone.0156245.
17. Hatfield LA. Neonatal pain: what's age got to do with it? Surg Neurol Int. 2014;5(Suppl 13):S479–89.
18. Fernandez E, et al. Factors and mechanisms for pharmacokinetic differences between pediatric population and adults. Pharmaceutics. 2011;3(1):53–72.
19. Berde CB, Sethna NF. Analgesics for the treatment of pain in children. NEJM. 2002;347(14):1094–103.
20. Sadhasivam S, Chidambaran V, Olbrecht VA, Esslinger HR, Zhang K, Zhang X, Martin LJ. Genetics of pain perception, COMT and postoperative pain management in children. Pharmacogenomics. 2014;15(3):277–84.
21. WHO Guidelines Approved by the Guidelines Review Committee. WHO guidelines on the pharmacological treatment of persisting pain in children with medical illnesses. Geneva: World Health Organization; 2012.
22. Chidambaran V, Sadhasivam S, Mahmoud M. Codeine and opioid metabolism: implications and alternatives for pediatric pain management. Curr Opin Anaesthesiol. 2017;30:349–56.
23. Odell S, Logan DE. Pediatric pain management: the multidisciplinary approach. J Pain Res. 2013;6:785–90.
24. Committee on Psychosocial Aspects of Child and Family Health. The assessment and management of acute pain in infants, children, and adolescents. Pediatrics. 2001;108(3):793–7.
25. Friedrichsdorf SJ, Kang TI. The Management of Pain in children with life-limiting illnesses. Pediatr Clin N Am. 2007;54:645–72.
26. Anghelescu DL, et al. Patient-controlled analgesia at the end of life at a pediatric oncology institution. Pediatr Blood Cancer. 2015;62(7):1237–44.
27. Czarnecki ML, et al. Is there an alternative to continuous opioid infusion for neonatal pain control? A preliminary report of

parent/nurse-controlled analgesia in the neonatal intensive care unit. Pediatr Anesth. 2014;24(4):377–85.

28. de Graaf J, van Lingen RA, Simons SH, Anand KJ, Duivenvoorden HJ, Weisglas-Kuperus N, Roofthooft DW, Groot Jebbink LJ, Veenstra RR, Tibboel D, van Dijk M. Long-term effects of routine morphine infusion in mechanically ventilated neonates on children's functioning: five-year follow-up of a randomized controlled trial. Pain. 2011;152(6):1391–7.

29. Simons SH, van Dijk M, van Lingen RA, Roofthooft D, Duivenvoorden HJ, Jongeneel N, Bunkers C, Smink E, Anand KJ, van den Anker JN, Tibboel D. Routine morphine infusion in pre-term newborns who reeceived ventilatory support: a randomized controlled trial. JAMA. 2003;290(18):2419–27.

30. Walker SM. Pain in children: recent advances and ongoing challenges. Br J Anaesth. 2008;101(1):101–10.

Pain in Older Adults (Geriatric)

David Vahedi and Vinoo Thomas

Epidemiology

Old age is commonly defined as an age of 65 years or older. The elderly population has risen from 4% of the total population in 1900 to 13% in 2010 and is expected to reach 20% of the total population by 2030 [1]. In 2008, the worldwide population of people 65 years and older was 506 million and expected to increase to 1.3 billion by 2040 [2]. However, due primarily to advancements in medicine, there has been a decrease in chronic disability in this population, from 72% identifying as non-disabled in 1982 to 81% in 2005. Much of the remaining disability relates to chronic pain issues, and addressing these appropriately can have a significant effect on an elderly patient's ability to maintain independence and quality of life.

Issues Related to Age Differences

Pain management in older adult can be difficult secondary to altered physiology, polypharmacy, and increases in comorbid disease prevalence. In adults 65 years-old or older, roughly 30–50% have two or more health problems and this increases in patients 85 years-old or older to 50–75% [1]. Polypharmacy naturally follows with the increase in medical conditions, introducing possible interactions with medicines used to treat pain. In addition to diseases seen with aging, there is a natural decline in physiologic status even in healthy elderly patients, which can lead to significant side effects of medications even at low doses.

Central Nervous System

In the central nervous system, there is a reduction in synthesis of neurotransmitters, opioid receptor density, and cerebral blood flow, as well as neuronal loss and atrophy, which together result in a decrease in inhibitory pain control and altered pain processing. The outcome is an increase in sensitivity to noxious stimuli and altered response to pain [1, 3].

Cardiovascular

In the cardiovascular system, there is a decrease in the cardiac index (CI), resulting higher drug peak levels, increasing the risk of toxicity [1].

Hepatobiliary

In the hepatic system, there is a reduction in liver mass, hepatic blood flow, hepatic enzymes, protein synthesis and regeneration rate, resulting in decreased serum albumin (less drug bound) and renal elimination (decreased conversion of lipophilic drug to hydrophilic metabolites) leading to higher toxicity risk. Dose adjustment may be required [1, 3, 4].

Renal

In the renal system, there is a reduction in kidney size, blood flow (RBF), and glomerular filtration rate (GFR, which decreases 1% per year after age 50) resulting in reduced renal elimination [1, 3, 4].

Gastrointestinal

In the gastrointestinal system, altered secretions, decreased blood flow, and changes in motility and absorptive surfaces,

D. Vahedi
Fellow in Pain Management, Mount Sinai Medical Center, New York, NY, USA

V. Thomas (✉)
Department of Anesthesiology/Pain Medicine, Mount Sinai Medical Center, New York, NY, USA

© Springer Nature Switzerland AG 2019
Y. Khelemsky et al. (eds.), *Academic Pain Medicine*, https://doi.org/10.1007/978-3-030-18005-8_45

cause variable alteration in drug absorption, bioavailability, and transit time [1, 3].

Body Composition

Changes in body composition, such as an increase in body fat and decrease in body water, lead to an increase in volume of distribution for lipophilic medications and an increase in plasma concentration of hydrophilic drugs. These changes result in delayed elimination and onset of action, as well as a higher frequency of side effects [1]. Sarcopenia, the loss of muscle mass as a result of aging, is a serious problem for the elderly, and when severe enough, can lead to accelerated deterioration with further weight loss, mental and physical decline, and increased mortality [5].

Integumentary

In the integumentary system, studies have shown that age-related changes in hydration and lipid structure result in increased barrier function of the stratum corneum for relatively hydrophilic compounds. However, in practice, there are no significant differences in the absorption of drugs from transdermal delivery systems between young and old individuals. The need for dose adaptation in elderly patients using transdermal drug delivery systems is therefore not related to differences in skin absorption but rather to age-related cardiovascular, cerebral, hepatic and/or renal compromise [6].

Vitamin Deficiency

Home-bound elderly, particularly those on anti-epileptic drugs or who do not absorb fat, are at high risk for vitamin D deficiency, which causes deep musculoskeletal and/or superficial light touch pain [7]. One-third of nursing home patients confined indoors for 6 months develop vitamin D deficiency, and as many as one-half of all community dwellers have reduced vitamin D levels [7, 8]. A single dose of 100,000 IU restores vitamin D levels and can reduce pain [7, 8].

Drug Pharmacology and Aging

Polypharmacy and drug interactions are significant problem for the elderly. Thirty percent of ambulatory older adults require medical care for adverse drug events and upward of 30% of hospitalizations in the elderly are causally related to drug effects. For opioids, the older brain appears to be more sensitive than that of young adults, whereas the pharmacokinetics of opioids are largely unaffected by age [5].

Pain Assessment: Limitations

Assessment of pain in the elderly can be challenging due to hearing impairment, visual impairment, functional and cognitive deterioration, and depression. These limitations can be addressed and/or circumvented using a variety of different tools.

Hearing Impairment

In the case of hearing impairment, pain can be assessed with the use of a visual pain scale or with the use of assistive hearing devices [3].

Visual Impairment

In the presence of visual impairment, use of larger print or verbal pain scales can assist in assessment [3].

Functional Impairment

In patients with functional impairment, validated tools for the evaluation of pain include Range of Motion Scale, performance of activities of daily living, Timed Up and Go Test, Katz Activities of Daily Living, and Functional Independence Measure [3].

Cognitive Impairment

In patients with mild-to-moderate cognitive impairment, use of the verbal descriptor scale (VDS) is a reliable and preferred method to assess pain. The numeric rating scale can also be used. For patients with severe cognitive impairment, validated tools to assess pain include the Pain Assessment Checklist for Seniors with Limited Ability to Communicate (PACSLAC), the Pain Assessment in Advanced Dementia, and the Doloplus-2 Scale [3]. Also, obtaining information from family members and caregivers can provide insight into the patient's condition [3].

Depression

With increasing age there is a higher prevalence of mood disorders [9]. Depression, in particular, can complicate the assessment of pain disorders by altering the perception of pain and leading to difficulty coping. Pain can also result in loss of function, which can worsen depression [1]. The Geriatric Depression Scale is a short self-report assessment used to identify depression in the elderly and can be helpful in pain assessment for the elderly.

The assessment should also evaluate quality of life using the Brief Pain Inventory or Geriatric Pain Measure [9].

Age-related Changes Relative to Pain Management

The elderly are sensitive to the effects and side effects of medications due to changes in physiology and accumulation of co-morbid conditions. They may also be at risk for additional barriers to care related to age, including personal beliefs, health practitioner beliefs, and loss or change of insurance.

Patient Related Barriers

A common misconception is that worsening pain is a normal part of the aging process and is therefore untreatable [1]. This belief can prevent the elderly patient from seeking treatment. Other patient related barriers include fear (of addiction, masking disease progression, loss of independence), as well as personal, cultural, and religious beliefs [1, 10].

Physician and Health Professional Related Barriers

Delayed referral to a pain specialist is common in the elderly as pain is often chronic and does not present urgently [1]. Time constraints also play a bigger role as comorbid conditions increase and the management of those conditions often takes precedence.

Health System Related Barriers

The health system as a whole can also fail the patient. Accessibility to treatment, distance to a specialist, transportation to and from the specialist, and insurance coverage are all barriers the elderly must overcome to obtain proper care [1].

Medication and Intervention Related Barriers

Insurance coverage can be a problem for medication or procedural approval, which can limit the tools available for the treatment of chronic pain. Polypharmacy, anticoagulant status, and complicated regimens can also limit treatment options [1].

Adverse Effects and Compliance

The incidence of adverse events from pain medications ranges from 6% to 30%, with a majority of these events being preventable [9]. The reason for the increased rate of adverse events in elderly patients is typically polypharmacy, multiple prescribers, inappropriate use, suboptimal monitoring, and changes in age-related pharmacodynamics and pharmacokinetics [1].

NSAID Usage

Given the increased risk of cardiovascular disease and heart failure with aging, caution is advised when prescribing NSAIDs for the elderly. Even in patients without known cardiovascular disease, NSAIDs have been associated with an increased risk of adverse cardiovascular events, including myocardial infarction, stroke, heart failure, atrial fibrillation and cardiovascular death [11]. However, the absolute increase in risk is small (one to two excess events per 1000 person-years) because the risk in patients without cardiovascular disease is low [11]. This is not the case in patients with known cardiovascular disease. A study, found that in an age (mean age 77) and sex matched cohort, the use of any NSAID (use in the preceding 14 days) was found to be associated with a 19% increased risk of hospital admission for heart failure compared with past use of any NSAID (use > 183 days prior) [12]. Specifically, the use of seven individual traditional NSAIDs (diclofenac, ibuprofen, indomethacin, ketorolac, naproxen, nimesulide, and piroxicam) and two individual COX-2 selective NSAIDs (etoricoxib and rofecoxib) were associated with an increased risk of hospital admission for heart failure [12]. The risk of heart failure doubled for diclofenac, etoricoxib, indomethacin, piroxicam and rofecoxib used at very high doses (≥ 2 defined daily dose equivalents) [12]. There was no evidence celecoxib increased the rate of admission for heart failure at commonly used doses [12]. In general, it is recommended to avoid NSAIDs in patients with established heart disease. However, if NSAID therapy is required, the lowest effective dose and shortest duration should be used.

Corticosteroid Usage

When NSAIDs are contraindicated, corticosteroids may serve as a useful short-term alternative in an acute pain episode. Corticosteroids may be helpful in the management of pain associated with polymyalgia rheumatica, rheumatoid arthritis, giant cell arteritis, cancer related pain, crystal-induced arthropathies, and compressive neuropathies [7, 13].

Acetaminophen Usage

Acetaminophen is metabolized by the liver and excreted by the kidneys, therefore doses should be adjusted in liver and renal impairment. Since the elderly have reduced function of these systems, it has been recommended that dosages be limited to 2000 mg/day [1].

Opioid Usage

Opioids should be used with caution in the elderly for several reasons. The CNS of the elderly has increased sensitivity to opioids, which can result in increased sedation, altered cognition, and increased risk of respiratory depression [5]. Reduced clearance of medications results in an increase in both drug and active metabolite concentrations [1]. Correspondingly, there is an increase in the side effect profile. It is recommended that meperidine, pentazocine, and high-dose tramadol (>200 mg/day) be avoided in the elderly because of the accumulation of neuroactive metabolites [1]. Chronic use of opioids can result in opioid-induced androgen deficiency (OPIAD) [14] and is significantly associated with various comorbidities such as obesity, type 2 diabetes, hypertension, osteoporosis and metabolic syndromes [15]. In addition, hypogonadism is associated with a decrease in muscle mass and presence of frailty. The use of androgen and/or growth hormone replacement therapy may be warranted in the elderly who require high-dose opioid therapy [1].

Fentanyl and Buprenorphine Patch Use in the Elderly

The use of a fentanyl patch in the elderly should be approached with caution due to increased CNS sensitivity to opioids and increased risk of life-threatening hypoventilation. The increased volume of distribution (Vd) seen in the elderly combined with the high Vd of fentanyl and reduced clearance of medications may result in an increased risk of adverse events. There is a common misconception among pain physicians that the fentanyl patch is safe in the treatment of pain in the elderly because of thinning of the skin and decreased uptake. However, it has been shown that despite skin changes, drug concentrations of transdermal medications are equal in the young and older adult [6].

If the use of continuous opioid therapy is deemed necessary in the setting of chronic moderate-to-severe pain, some have recommended the use of buprenorphine patch. Buprenorphine demonstrates a ceiling effect which may mitigate some of the risks of opioid use in this population. Caution should be used in renal failure, severe hepatic impairment, and hepatic failure [16].

Benzodiazepines and Non-benzodiazepine Sedatives/Hypnotics

The Center for Medicare and Medicaid Services performed an observational retrospective study on the concurrent use of opioids and benzodiazepine and non-benzodiazepine sedative/hypnotic medications. Roughly three million Medicare Part D members were found to be concurrent prescribed these medications and this practice was associated with an increased risk of overdose and death, primarily due to respiratory depression. It is not recommended to combine these treatment modalities in elderly patients.

Adjuvants/Co-analgesics

Tricyclic antidepressants (TCAs) are useful in treating neuropathic pain, however due to their anticholinergic effects/side-effect profile, this class of medication is often contraindicated [13]. TCAs can cause tachycardia, which in the older person with heart disease may result in an increased risk of angina and myocardial infraction. TCAs also increase the risk of falls due to orthostasis. In the treatment of neuropathic pain and fibromyalgia in the elderly, the use of mixed serotonin- and norepinephrine-uptake inhibitors (SNRIs) are associated with a better side-effect profile than TCAs [13]. Gabapentinoids (pregabalin and gabapentin) and other anticonvulsants with similar mechanism of action at voltage-gated calcium channels are effective in neuropathic pain conditions, however careful titration and frequent monitoring should be employed in the elderly patient [13].

Beers Criteria

Last updated in 2015, the Beers Criteria is a publication developed by an expert panel at the American Geriatrics Society which outlines medications to be avoided in older adults, select drugs that should have their dose adjusted based on the individual's kidney function, and select drug-drug interactions documented to be associated with harm in older adults [17]. This publication can be used to help guide medication management in the elderly and minimize the associated risks.

STOPP/START Criteria

A screening tool for current prescriptions (STOPP) and a screening tool to initiate the correct treatment (START) are advocated to minimize adverse drug events and improve medication appropriateness in older people during hospitalization for acute illnesses [18]. These tools may be of use to the pain management specialist in the outpatient setting as well, especially in the setting of polypharmacy.

Non-pharmacologic Treatments for Persistent Pain in Older Adults

I. Modalities in category IA (greatest safety and efficacy) include acupuncture and self-management education programs.
II. Modalities in category IB include mindful meditation, exercise, and massage.
III. Modalities in category IIB (other safe but less efficacious modalities) include cognitive behavioral therapy (CBT) and Tai-Chi.
IV. Modalities in category III include yoga [10].

Pharmacologic Treatments for Persistent Pain in Older Adults

I. Category IA recommendations include acetaminophen, oral NSAIDs, and opioids.
II. Category IB recommendations include the use of topical NSAIDs, tramadol, tricyclic antidepressants, anticonvulsants, and SNRIs.
III. Category IIB recommendations include the use of topical lidocaine [10].

These recommendations should be considered alongside the risks and caveats discussed earlier.

Interventional Pain Modalities

The use of interventional modalities can be both diagnostic and therapeutic, eliminating the need for medication use and sparing the patient from unwanted side effects [2]. Interventional modalities can also circumvent the issues associated with polypharmacy and compliance with medication regimens. For this reason interventional modalities should be considered early in the treatment of the elderly.

Chronologic Versus Physiologic Age

It is important to note that chronological age and physiologic age may not align in the elderly. One way to highlight differences among the elderly is to assess for frailty. Frailty is described as a state of decline and vulnerability in late life, characterized by weakness and decreased functional capacity. This increased vulnerability contributes to increased risk for multiple adverse outcomes, including procedural complications, falls,

institutionalization, disability, and death [19]. There is no gold standard for the diagnosis of frailty, however it is commonly diagnosed if three out of five criteria are met (FRAIL Scale):

1. weight loss
2. extreme fatigue
3. weakness in hand grip
4. slow walking speed
5. minimal physical activity [1].

Pain management becomes important in the prevention and management of frailty by improving functionality. Adequate analgesia enables the patient to participate fully and progress in a tailored exercise program [1]. A nutritional consult may prove to be beneficial in the elderly in order to prevent loss of muscle mass, osteoporosis and better control chronic conditions [1].

References

1. Rastogi R, Meek BD. Management of chronic pain in elderly, frail patients: finding a suitable, personalized method of control. Clin Interv Aging. 2013;8:37–46.
2. Kaye AD, Baluch A, Scott JT. Pain management in the elderly population: a review. Ochsner J. 2010;10(3):179–87.
3. Tracy B, Sean Morrison R. Pain management in older adults. Clin Ther. 2013;35(11):1659–68.
4. Fine PG. Chronic pain management in older adults: special considerations. J Pain Symptom Manag. 2009;38(2 Suppl):S4–s14.
5. Barash P, Cullen BF, Stoelting RK, Cahalan M, Stock MC, Ortega R. Clinical anesthesia, 7e: Ebook without multimedia. New York: Wolters Kluwer Health; 2013.
6. Kaestli LZ, Wasilewski-Rasca AF, Bonnabry P, Vogt-Ferrier N. Use of transdermal drug formulations in the elderly. Drugs Aging. 2008;25(4):269–80.
7. Davis MP, Srivastava M. Demographics, assessment and management of pain in the elderly. Drugs Aging. 2003;20(1):23–57.
8. Gloth F. Pain management in older adults: prevention and treatment. J Am Geriatr Soc. 2001;49(2):188–99.
9. Vadivelu N, Urman RD, Hines RL. Essentials of pain management. New York: Springer; 2011.
10. Makris UE, Abrams RC, Gurland B, Reid MC. Management of persistent pain in the older patient: a clinical review. JAMA. 2014;312(8):825–36.
11. Bhala N, Emberson J, Merhi A, Abramson S, Arber N, Baron JA, et al. Vascular and upper gastrointestinal effects of non-steroidal anti inflammatory drugs: meta analyses of individual partici pant data from randomised trials. Lancet (London, England). 2013;382(9894):769–79.
12. Arfe A, Scotti L, Varas-Lorenzo C, Nicotra F, Zambon A, Kollhorst B, et al. Non-steroidal anti-inflammatory drugs and risk of heart failure in four European countries: nested case-control study. Br Dent J. 2016;221(10):632.
13. Panel AGS. Pharmacological management of persistent pain in older persons. J Am Geriatr Soc. 2009;57(8):1331–46.
14. Smith HS, Elliott JA. Opioid-induced androgen deficiency (OPIAD). Pain Physician. 2012;15(3 Suppl):Es145–56.
15. Dandona P, Rosenberg MT. A practical guide to male hypogonadism in the primary care setting. Int J Clin Pract. 2010;64(6):682–96.

16. Vadivelu N, Hines RL. Management of chronic pain in the elderly: focus on transdermal buprenorphine. Clin Interv Aging. 2008;3(3):421–30.

17. Panel AGS. American Geriatrics Society 2015 updated beers criteria for potentially inappropriate medication use in older adults. J Am Geriatr Soc. 2015;63(11):2227–46.

18. O'Mahony D, O'Sullivan D, Byrne S, O'Connor MN, Ryan C, Gallagher P. STOPP/START criteria for potentially inappropriate prescribing in older people: version 2. Age Ageing. 2015;44(2):213–8.

19. Clegg A, Young J, Iliffe S, Rikkert MO, Rockwood K. Frailty in elderly people. Lancet. 2013;381(9868):752–62. https://doi.org/10.1016/S0140-6736(12)62167-9. Epub 2013 Feb 8.

Victor Tseng and William Caldwell

When assessing neurocognitively impaired patients, non-verbal pain indicators are often assessed first. Many bedside tools used in clinical practice are based upon these indicators. These nonverbal pain indicators can be broken down into three broad categories: facial expressions, vocal cues, and body language/movement. Common facial expressions include distinctive muscle movements such as grimacing, frowning, blinking, and twitching; vocal cues include grunting, crying, and shouting; body movements include withdrawing, fidgeting, limping, and tension.

Assessment of Pain in Children

It may not be intuitive to consider neonates/infants/toddlers/children as an impaired patient population given that they are neurologically appropriate for their given age. Nevertheless, when compared to a normal adult, assessment of pain can be difficult given limitations in language and other cognitive skills. Often, this population is not properly evaluated due to numerous factors such as lack of training in the practitioner, poor familiarity/comfort with pediatric medications and dosing, or frustration upon encountering a crying or otherwise uncooperative child. There are a number of pain scales in use for the pediatric population, the most common of which are discussed below.

PIPP Pain Scale

Originally developed in Canada, this scale is ideal for neonates around 36 weeks gestation. It is a 21 point scale where

Table 46.1 PIPP pain scale

	0	1	2	3
GA in weeks	≥36	32–35	28–31	<28
Alertness	Active Awake Opened eyes	Quiet Awake Opened eyes	Active Sleeping Closed eyes	Quiet Sleeping Closed eyes
	Facial movements +	Facial movements–	Facial movements +	Facial movements–
Maximal HR	Increased 0–4 bpm	Increased 5–14 bpm	Increased 15–24 bpm	Increased ≥25 bpm
Minimal O$_2$ saturation	Decreased 0–2.4%	Decreased 2.5–4.9%	Decreased 5–7.4%	Decreased ≥7.5%
Frowned forehead	Absent	Minimal	Moderate	Maximal
Eyes squeezing	Absent	Minimal	Moderate	Maximal
Nasolabial furrow	Absent	Minimal	Moderate	Maximal

GA gestational age, *HR* heart rate

a score of <=6 corresponds to minimum pain, 6–12 moderate pain, ≥12 significant pain. It is specifically used to gauge the intensity of a painful stimulus. The scoring is conducted by assessing a patient before and 30 seconds after a painful stimulus. It was recently revised to enhance validity and feasibility [1, 2] (Table 46.1).

Neonatal Infant Pain Scale (NIPS)

The NIPS pain scale is a 7 point pain scale which originated from CHEOPS (an older pain scale used for postop children) [3]. It is intended for use for neonates and children up to 1 year old. It is often used around the world for pain assessment (Table 46.2).

V. Tseng
Division of Regional Anesthesia & Acute Pain Management, Department of Anesthesiology, Westchester Medical Center, New York Medical College, Valhalla, NY, USA

W. Caldwell (✉)
Department of Anesthesiology, Pain Medicine, Stony Brook University Hospital, Stony Brook, NY, USA
e-mail: william.caldwell@stonybrookmedicine.edu

Table 46.2 NIPS pain scale

	0	1	2
Facial expression	Relaxed	Contracted	
Cry	Absent	Mumbling	Vigorous
Breathing	Relaxed	Altered from baseline	
Arms	Relaxed	Flexed or Stretched	
Legs	Relaxed	Flexed or Stretched	
Alertness	Sleeping or calm	Agitated	

Table 46.3 CRIES pain scale

	0	1	2
Crying	No cry or minimal cry	High pitched cry but consolable	High pitched cry that cannot be consoled
Requires O_2	No supplemental O_2	<30% supplemental O_2	>30% supplemental O_2
Increased VS Take last	Both HR and BP ≤ baseline	HR or BP > baseline but ≤20% of baseline	HR or BP > 20% of baseline
Expression	No grimace	Grimace alone	Grimace and non-cry vocalization
Sleepless	Continuously asleep	Awakened at frequent intervals	Constantly awake

CRIES Pain Scale

CRIES "is an acronym of five physiological and behavioural variables previously shown to be associated with neonatal pain," [4]. It is a 10 point scale based on C – Crying, R – Requires increased oxygen, I – Increased oxygen administration, E – Expression, S – Sleeplessness. When used to assess pain in the postop period, it was found to be both valid and reliable [5]. Its criteria are listed in Table 46.3. Of note, it is recommended to measure vital signs (VS) last given the confounding nature of response measurement on the other assessments.

FLACC Pain Scale

The FLACC (face, legs, activity, cry, consolability) pain scale is another pain assessment tool for minimally verbal patients. Like CRIES, it is also based on a 10 point scale (Table 46.4). It was originally developed using data from post-surgical patients 3 month–7 years old [6]. Currently, it is used across a broad range of patients for assessment of pain. A comprehensive review suggests that perhaps the best use of the FLACC pain scale remains for the population for which it was initially intended: neonates to children [7].

Table 46.4 FLACC pain scale

	0	1	2
Face	No particular expression or smile	Occasional grimace or frown, withdrawn, uninterested	Frequent to constant quivering chin, clenched jaw
Legs	Normal position or relaxed	Uneasy, restless, tense	Kicking, or legs drawn up
Activity	Lying quietly, normal position, moves easily	Squirming, shifting, back and forth, tense	Arched, rigid or jerking
Cry	No cry (awake or asleep)	Moans or whimpers; occasional complaint	Crying steadily, screams or sobs, frequent complaints
Consolability	Content, relaxed	Reassured by occasional touching, hugging or being talked to, distractible	Difficult to console or comfort

Assessment of Pain in Patients with Intellectual Disability and Developmental Delay

Identifying pain in this population depends on the particular disability of the patient, whether receptive, expressive, or cognitive. Often third-party inferences from caretakers and medical staff are substituted for patient input, with variable success. Longitudinal studies tracking pain in cognitively impaired children and adults reveals that chronic pain is common and undertreated [8, 9]. Of note, the majority of pain experienced by these patients appears to be unrelated to their underlying condition and is primarily due to accidents or other injuries that are not treated appropriately [10].

Facial Action Coding System (FACS)

For patients lacking verbal expression, one strategy is to use facial expressions or body language. Facial expressions, in particular have been shown to correlate well with pain across the entire spectrum of cognitive ability. In fact, research suggests that verbal report may actually underestimate pain in both verbal and poorly verbal populations [11]. One of the most prominent techniques which centers on facial expressions is the Facial Action Coding System (FACS) [12]. It is a system which objectively describes facial behaviors/expressions and categorizes them into 46 action units. The goal is to standardize facial expressions across the population and serves as a basis for comparing and interpreting observed facial expressions.

Evidence suggests that certain facial action units are associated with noxious stimuli. Four action units seem to be universal across the population when experiencing pain or discomfort [13]. These actions include: brow lowering, orbit tightening, upper-lip raising/nose wrinkling, and eye closure. Other actions were also noted, but did not seem to be consistent across different stimulations. As a result, when assessing for pain through the use of facial expressions, attention should be focused on these four likely universal signs of pain/discomfort.

Despite the usefulness of FACS for identification of pain in nonverbal patients, there are limitations in the clinical setting. Two major limitations are cost for training and the inherent subjectivity of the assessment. Training to become proficient in FACS requires an estimated 100 hours. Action units, while well characterized, still vary between different faces, especially in those with craniofacial abnormalities. Fortunately, research suggests that even untrained observers can reliably assess pain in others [14]. It's important to note that reliability may be impaired in patients with severe neurocognitive impairment [15].

Pain and Discomfort Scale (PADS)

The Pain and Discomfort Scale (PADS) was developed in order to characterize pain in neurocognitively impaired patient populations in a clinical setting [16]. Its creators sought to address some of the deficiencies of established modalities such as FACS for pain assessment. Its target population was specifically nonverbal adults. Research has shown that PADS is both sensitive and specific for multiple noxious sensory stimuli: pin-prick, heat, cold, deep pressure, and light touch [17]. It incorporates both facial expressions as well as trunk and limb movements.

Non-communicating Adult Pain Checklist (NCAPC)

The Non-Communicating Adult Pain Checklist (NCAPC) is another pain assessment scale designed for use in nonverbal patients [18]. Its items include a comprehensive assessment of the patient including vocal reaction, emotional reaction, facial expression, body language, protective reaction, and physiological reaction. It was found to be sensitive to pain in patients with neurocognitive disability regardless of severity [19].

PADS Versus NCAPC

Both the PADS and NCAPC were developed from the Non-Communicating Children Pain Checklist (NCCPC).

Both were proven to be sensitive for noxious stimuli in nonverbal patients, although research on their specificity is less robust. PADS and NCAPC were compared in a small scale study which found that both scales showed high interrater reliability, sensitivity, and high internal consistency [20]. For now, both are relatively easy scales to use for assessing pain in adults with limited ability to communicate and have evidence supporting their use. They do not require extensive training and are more practical when compared to FACS. It is noteworthy, however, that PADS may be easier and faster to use than NCAPC, but be less sensitive given that it has fewer items and is less comprehensive. No definitive data exists to recommend one over the other.

Assessment of Pain in Critically Ill Patients

Patients who are critically ill can be another special population where pain assessment is difficult. Even though most are normally able to express their pain and assist clinicians, critically ill patients are often too sick to participate meaningfully in this assessment. Furthermore, assessment is often complicated by airway management (intubation) requiring sedation and sometimes paralysis. Distressingly, poorly managed pain has been associated with increased morbidity and mortality [21]; conversely, well-managed pain has been associated with improved outcomes [22]. Two of the most prominent tools in use for ICU patients are described here.

Behavioral Pain Scale (BPS)

The BPS is a 3–12 point observational assessment tool for examining ICU patients [23]. The score the BPS yields does not, however, correspond to a standard definition. That is, no specific score correlates to mild, moderate), or severe pain in the patient. Even a minimum score of 3 does not exclude the possibility that the patient is in pain. It is a scale that helps the clinician look for and identify painful behavior, as well as track changes and response to therapy over time (Table 46.5).

Critical Care Pain Observation Tool (CPOT)

The CPOT was developed using Cardiac SICU patients in Canada [24]. It is also an observational assessment tool which has been judged to be easy to use in clinical practice [25]. It is a 0–8 point scale but similar to BPS in that no single score corresponds to a specific interpretation (Table 46.6).

Table 46.5 BPS pain scale

	1	2	3	4
Facial expression	Relaxed	Partially tightented	Fully tightened	Grimacing
Upper limb movements	No movement	Partially bent	Fully bent with finger flexion	Permanently retracted
Compliance with mechanical ventilation	Tolerating movement	Coughing but tolerating	Fighting ventilator	Unable to control ventilation

Table 46.6 CPOT

	0	1	2
Facial expression	Neutral/relaxed	Tense	Grimacing
Body movements	Absent	Protection	Restlessness/agitation
Compliance with ventilator or vocalization	Tolerating ventilator	Coughing	Fighting
	Or	Or	Or
	Normal talking	Sighing/moaning	Crying/sobbing
Muscle tension	Relaxed	Tense	Rigid

BPS Versus CPOT

Both BPS and are valuable in assessing ICU patients who cannot communicate. They are part of international guidelines for pain assessment in this population [26]. Each can be used to trend or guide pain assessment and response to treatment, but cannot definitively define pain during a single encounter. Both have been shown to be valid and reliable tools for pain assessment in the ICU population [27]. The CPOT, however, can accommodate both verbal and nonverbal patients. When compared head to head, research suggests the CPOT is superior to BPS in reliability and validity [28].

References

1. Hudson-Barr D, Capper-Michel B. Validation of the Pain Assessment in Neonates (PAIN) scale with the Neonatal Infant Pain Scale (NIPS). Neonatal Netw. 2002;21:15–21.
2. Stevens BJ, Gibbins S. The premature infant pain profile-revised (PIPP-R): initial validation and feasibility. Clin J Pain. 2014;30:238–43.
3. Lawrence J, Alcock D. The development of a tool to assess neonatal pain. Neonatal Netw. 1993;12:59–66.
4. Krechel SW, Bildner J. CRIES: a new neonatal postoperative pain measurement score. Initial testing of validity and reliability. Paediatr Anaesth. 1995;5:53–61.
5. McNair C, Ballantyne M. Postoperative pain assessment in the neonatal intensive care unit. Arch Dis Child Fetal Neonatal Ed. 2004;89:537–41.
6. Merkel S, Voepel-Lewis T. The FLACC: a behavioral scale for scoring postoperative pain in young children. Pediatr Nurs. 1997;23:293–7.
7. Crellin DJ, Harrison D. Systematic review of the Face, Legs, Activity, Cry and Consolability scale for assessing pain in infants and children: is it reliable, valid, and feasible for use? Pain. 2015;156:2132–51.
8. Stallard P, Williams L. Pain in cognitively impaired, non-communicating children. Arch Dis Child. 2001;85:460–2.
9. LaChapelle DL, Hadjistavropoulos T. Pain measurement in persons with intellectual disabilities. Clin J Pain. 1999;15:13–23.
10. Breau LM, Camfield CS, PJ MG, Finley GA. The incidence of pain in children with severe cognitive impairments. Arch Pediatr Adolesc Med. 2003;157:1219–26.
11. Kunz M, Scharmann S. The facial expression of pain in patients with dementia. Pain. 2007;133:221–8.
12. Ekman P, Friesen W. Manual for the facial action coding system. Palo Alto: Consulting Psychologists Press; 1978.
13. Prkachin K. The consistency of facial expressions of pain: a comparison across modalities. Pain. 1992;51:297–306.
14. Prkachin KM, Berzins S. Encoding and decoding of pain expressions: a judgement study. Pain. 1994;58:253–9.
15. Defrin R, Lotan M. The evaluation of acute pain in individuals with cognitive impairment: a differential effect of the level of impairment. Pain. 2006;124:312–20.
16. Bodfish JW. Identifying and measuring pain in persons with developmental disabilities: a manual for the Pain and Discomfort Scale (PADS). Western Carolina Center Research Reports. 2001.
17. Shinde SK, Danov S, Chen CC. Convergent validity evidence for the Pain and Discomfort Scale (PADS) for pain assessment among adults with intellectual disability. Clin J Pain. 2014;30:536–43.
18. Lotan M, Moe-Nilssen R. Reliability of the Non-Communicating Adult Patient Checklist (NCAPC), assessed by different groups of health workers. Res Dev Disabil. 2009;30:735–45.
19. Lotan M, Moe-Nilssen R. Measurement properties of the Non-Communicating Adult Pain Checklist (NCAPC): a pain scale for adults with Intellectual and Developmental Disabilities, scored in a clinical setting. Res Dev Disabil. 2010;31:367–75.
20. Meir Lotan AB. Comparing the non-communicating adult pain checklist (NCAPC) with the pain and discomfort scale (PADS) in evaluating pain in adults with intellectual disability. J Pain Manag. 2016;6:15–24.
21. Kastrup M, von Dossow V. Key performance indicators in intensive care medicine. A retrospective matched cohort study. J Int Med Res. 2009;37:1267–84.
22. Chanques G, Jaber S. Impact of systematic evaluation of pain and agitation in an intensive care unit. Crit Care Med. 2006;34:1691–9.
23. Payen JF, Bru O. Assessing pain in critically ill sedated patients by using a behavioral pain scale. Crit Care Med. 2001;29:2258–63.
24. Gélinas C, Fillion L. Validation of the critical-care pain observation tool in adult patients. Am J Crit Care. 2006;15:420–7.
25. Gélinas C. Nurses' evaluation of the feasibility and the clinical utility of the Critical-Care Pain Observation Tool. Pain Manag Nurs. 2010;11:115–25.

26. Barr J, Fraser GL. Clinical practice guidelines for the management of pain, agitation, and delirium in adult patients in the intensive care unit. Crit Care Med. 2013;41:262–306.

27. Rijkenberg S, Stilma W. Pain measurement in mechanically ventilated critically ill patients: behavioral pain scale versus critical-care pain observation tool. J Crit Care. 2015;30:167–72.

28. Stites M. Observational pain scales in critically ill adults. Crit Care Nurse. 2013;33:68–78.

Pain Relief in Persons with Substance Use and Addictive Disorders

Guensley R. Delva, Jacquelyn K. Francis, and Demetri Koutsospyros

Biopharmacologic and Neurophysiologic Basis of Addiction

According to the American Society of Addiction Medicine, addiction is defined as "continued use of a specific psychoactive substance despite physical, psychological, or social harm [1]." In 2013, the American Psychiatric Association released a memo highlighting revisions to the fifth edition of the Diagnostic and Statistical Manual of Mental Disorders (DSM-5) which referenced changes to the criteria of Substance use disorder by essentially combining the older categories of substance abuse and substance dependence into one disorder [2].

It is traditionally thought that the acute stimulation of dopaminergic mechanisms mediated by addictive drugs leads to changes in neuroadaptations and reward learning [3]. Information is uniquely thought to be processed via projections between the prefrontal cortex and the basal ganglia [3]. Adaptation to new behavior requires complex processing between both the limbic and motor circuitry [3]. At the initial step of processing new information, the limbic system is thought to yield influence over the motor circuitry in adapting the body to a new behavior [3]. This behavior is thought to stem from the result of dopamine, a neurotransmitter which heightens euphoria and pleasure, encouraging the continuation of a learned behavior [4]. If a behavior is not learned, the motor circuitry becomes malleable to adjustment if needed, however once a behavior is learned, over the course of repeated adjustments and attempts, the limbic sys-

tem is thought to disengage the motor circuitry and allow the neuronal adaptations to be organized around the new preferred task [3].

As it relates to drug addiction, it is believed that the essential relapse to drug seeking behaviors rests in one's limbic and motor circuitry's inability to process the negative responses to said behavior [3]. There is a reduced influence of the limbic circuitry in processing the negative environmental contingencies due to the imbalance of glutamate homeostasis along the limbic brain regions. This imbalance is responsible for addicts' inability to regulate drug seeking behavior regardless of this behavior's multiple negative effects [3]. Despite the molecular theory behind the brain's mechanism to addiction, twin studies suggest only a 31–40% genetic component to addiction, similar to many other systemic diseases [5].

Interactions Between Addiction and Pain

Full tissue recovery after an injury should result in the resolution of pain symptoms and the termination of the pain process. However, repetitive stimuli lead to pathological changes that can result in persistent pain in some patients. These repetitive signals result in prolonged stimulation and inflammation. Once the inflammation becomes chronic, it leads to a series of neurobiological changes, including reduction in pain threshold in primary afferent neurons, hyperexcitable states of receptors, phosphorylation of protein kinases, upregulation of sodium voltage gated channels, increased sensitization to substance P and upregulation of gene expression in the dorsal horn of neurons of the spinal cord leading to increases in production of receptors and ion channels [6]. Thus, chronic pain leads to phenotypic changes that become part of an individual's makeup.

In addition to these new sensory neurological pathways, evidence suggests that emotional and cognitive circuits in the brain also mediate chronic pain. The corticolimbic areas of the brain, including the mesolimbic dopamine system, the amygdala and the medial prefrontal cortex, have been shown to be particularly important in the transition from acute to

---

The original version of this chapter was revised. The correction to this chapter can be found at https://doi.org/10.1007/978-3-030-18005-8_49

G. R. Delva (✉)
Dartmouth Hitchcock Medical Center, Theodore Geisel School of Medicine, Lebanon, NH, USA

J. K. Francis
Hackensack University Medical Center, Hackensack, NJ, USA

D. Koutsospyros
Department of Anesthesiology, Montefiore Medical Center, Bronx, NY, USA

chronic pain states [7]. There is also evidence to suggest that chronic pain significantly physically alters this corticolimbic circuitry in a way that directly corresponds to the chronicity and intractability of certain pain conditions [8]. The mesolimbic dopamine circuitry, also known as the reward pathway, is important in motivated behavior and responsiveness to environmental stimuli. The pathway regulates motivation and desire and reinforces reward-related learning. In other words, the activation of the pathway informs the organism that the previous action should be repeated for a reward. It is therefore easy to understand why the mesolimbic system is also implicated in the modulation of the addiction liability of drugs of abuse. Converging evidence now suggests that understanding the interconnections of different components of the corticolimbic system is integral to understanding the link between chronic pain and addiction [9].

Drugs with abuse potential, such as opioids, cause high levels of dopamine to be released. These drugs override the homeostatic feedback native to the brain circuitry. The individual is therefore unresponsive to normal negative feedback mechanisms and continually seeks higher and higher doses of drug for relief [6]. The reward/motivation cycle is thus formed and reinforced, setting the stage for the primary problem of addiction.

Screening for Substance Use Disorder or Addiction in Patients with Pain

Addiction is a chronic disease wherein the brain's reward, motivation, memory, and related circuitry are dysfunctional, and the person continues to abuse a drug despite the harm it may cause them [10]. Of the 20.5 million Americans 12 or older that had a substance use disorder in 2015, two million had a substance use disorder involving prescription pain relievers [2]. Treatment admissions for opioid abuse has also increased by over 500% in the past 10 years, while the lifetime prevalence of any form of addiction, excluding tobacco, is estimated at 3–16% of the US population [11].

A 2008 study showed that an estimated 13.8 million people aged 12 or older had used oxycodone for non-medical reasons at least once during their lifetime [12] Inappropriate use of prescription opioids has reached epidemic proportions. Drug overdose is now the leading cause of accidental death in the US, with 52,404 lethal drug overdoses occurring in 2015. Opioid addiction is driving this epidemic, with 20,101 overdose deaths related to prescription pain relievers during this time period [13].

Given competing pressures faced by physicians to both diagnose and treat pain syndromes and identify individuals at risk for addictive disorders, the use of opioids in the treatment of pain poses a significant clinical challenge [14]. It is interesting to note that a review conducted by Weaver and Schnoll reported that rates of addiction in patient populations with chronic pain were no different from rates of addiction in the general population [15]. Although only a small minority of individuals prescribed opioids for chronic pain will subsequently develop abuse or addiction, increased rates of substance use disorders have been well documented in long-term opioid users [16]. The caveat is that opioids can be the most potent medications available to treat certain severe pain conditions and there is ever increasing pressure on physicians to adequately treat pain, minimize suffering and improve functioning.

Patients may have pain syndromes as well as concurrent opioid use disorder or may develop addictive behaviors while on long-term opioid therapy. There are no empirical guidelines for treating these patients. However, careful assessment of these patients to quantify their abuse potential is often recommended. In their 2008 landmark study, Passik and Kirsh set forth predictors, which have shown to have excellent discernment between high risk and low risk patients for opioid abuse [17].

The Opioid Risk Tool (ORT) and Screener and Opioid Assessment for Patients with Pain (SOAPP) are both tools available to prescribing physicians that enable them to assess for the risk of future inappropriate use of opioids in prospective patients. They both have been shown to have utility because of the quick method of administration and the important and useful data that they reveal.

ORT is a brief self-report screening tool that provides a simple way for physicians to categorize patients from low to high risk, with patients who score within the high risk results having 91% abuse potential. The tool has been shown to exhibit a high degree of sensitivity and specificity [18].

SOAPP has been updated since its initial publication [17] to Screener and Opioid Assessment for Patients with Pain-Revised (SOAPP-R). This screening tool also predicts possible future opioid abuse potential in chronic pain patients with a sensitivity of 80%. The tool is brief, and encompasses self-reported aberrant behaviors, laboratory toxicology reports and observations by the administering physician to determine a score.

Principles of Comprehensive Approach to Pain Management in Patients with Addiction, Either Active or in Recovery

Chronic pain is pain that lasts for duration longer than 3 months leading to prevention of normal functioning [19]. Unlike acute pain, which is an adaptation that evolved to alert the organism of an imminent threat or danger, chronic pain is not "useful" and should be minimized when possible. Access to pain control is an international human right and no patient should be denied access to appropriate analgesia regardless of the history of substance misuse or abuse. The challenge is coming up with a strategy for balancing this right without worsening or introducing possible drug abuse, misuse or addiction [20].

It is therefore imperative that physicians are aware of their treatment goals for patients so that they can supplement addiction treatment and not worsen the problem. Physicians need to increase their own awareness of the disease of addiction. There are clear differences between physical dependence, active addiction and addiction in remission and there are strategies for pain management for patients in each of these categories. Furthermore, physicians should not allow misconceptions and errors in defining the varying categories of individuals to cloud their judgment and their ability to provide treatment.

Maintenance or substitution medications, usually methadone or buprenorphine, which are designed to help these individuals to abstain from inappropriate drug use, are not a substitute for pain treatment. Many patients who are treated in traditional drug dependency programs without an active pain management component will leave prematurely because of lack of attention to their pain [21]. Pain specialists should use a comprehensive approach that considers all of their patients' comorbidities, their pain processes, as well as their addiction status, to provide an appropriate level of treatment.

Physicians should have general principles for dealing with all pain patients and these should be the same for patients in addiction programs with only a few minor changes. Incorporation of the use of medication agreements or contracts, setting and discussing appropriate goals with the patient prior to the initiation of treatment, giving appropriate amounts of medication, frequent monitoring with drug screens and pill counts, and careful and meticulous documentation have been shown to have success with these patients [22].

It is now recognized that depression, anxiety, poor coping, somatization, sleeplessness and hypochondriasis, among other comorbidities, are prevalent in the chronic pain population and, left untreated, are associated with greater risk for poor outcomes. A more holistic and multidisciplinary approach should be considered when treating these patients. It is unlikely that a single provider can adequately meet all of the needs of patients with chronic and intractable pain and chemical dependency. It is therefore necessary to involve interdisciplinary teams when feasible, including pain medicine physicians, psychologists, addiction specialists, and primary care physicians to carry out the complex and coordinated treatment plan necessary to treat this challenging population safely and appropriately.

If an opioid is indicated, it should be included as part of a multimodal approach including non-opioid modalities. NSAIDs, antineuropathic agents, muscle relaxants, and topical agents all warrant trials and have better safety and efficacy data for chronic use than opioids. Nerve blocks, joint injections, spinal injections, and other interventional procedures are also a good treatment option for this patient population as they can provide longer-term pain relief and decrease need for opioids. Additionally, chiropractic treatments, physical therapy, acupuncture, massage therapy, psychological and behavioral interventions can also be utilized.

In addition to active and multiple treatment modalities, it is recommended that routine drug screening of these patients be carried out. Opioid treatment guidelines from the Substance Abuse and Mental Health Services Administration (SAMHSA) state that opioid treatment programs must provide adequate testing or analysis for drugs of abuse, including at least 8 random drug abuse tests per year per patient in maintenance treatment. One published consensus recommendation for patients on chronic opioid therapy is that low risk patients should periodically be monitored with a minimum of 1 drug screen test every 6 months and medium or high risk patients, every 3 months (risk as determined by ORT or SOAPP-R) [23].

When an illicit drug appears in a urine toxicology screen, the lab results should be confirmed by GC/MS—the gold standard of drug testing—if point-of-care testing was used and a follow-up appointment should be scheduled with the patient. The patient should be interviewed in a non-judgmental, non-punitive fashion while reviewing the results of the test. Counseling should be provided, and another urine screen should be administered. Based on the results of the interview, the physician may decide to change therapy, discontinue opioids, or discharge the patient from the program, according to the initial established practice protocol. Risk stratification and continuous assessment will help to guide physicians to the level of care required for each patient.

Pharmacologic Treatment of Patients with Addiction

Effective drug addiction treatment aims to not only stop the compulsion and consequences which follow the patient's desire to have the drug at any cost, but additionally, to return these individuals to being productive and fully functioning members of their community.

Substitution or maintenance medications for patients addicted to opioid medication has evolved to be the standard of care since original studies on addiction and treatment of addiction began in the 1960s. This has been largely accomplished with the use of methadone, a μ opioid agonist, which is associated with success ranging from 60% to 90%. Buprenorphine, a partial μ opioid agonist and a κ receptor antagonist, has also had satisfactory results on par with those of methadone. The choice of incorporating either one of these drugs for treating patient addiction disorders is based on prescriber comfort and practice. A study of drug treatment outcomes in the 1980s documented that methadone saved taxpayers $12 for every $1 spent [24].

Methadone is a long acting full μ opioid receptor agonist with a highly variable half-life between 15 and 60 hours. The pharmacokinetics of the drug are such that it helps promote medication adherence due to once-a-day dosing and it provides a more consistent systemic medication level relative to short-acting opioids [25].

The use of buprenorphine for treatment has results similar to those of methadone treatment programs and physicians can prescribe the drug outside of the methadone maintenance program system. Buprenorphine has a greater safety profile than methadone due to the fact that it is a partial μ opioid receptor agonist, meaning there is a plateau on its dose-dependent euphoric effects and respiratory depression effects [26]. Most commonly dosed sublingually as a film or tablet, more recently buprenorphine has been approved for use as a long-acting subcutaneous injectable. This is in response to the concern of non-compliance, diversion and misuse of the oral formulation of the medication. For patients with pain as well as opioid dependence, buprenorphine may be a welcome choice of treatment given its safety profile, its ability to suppress opioid-seeking behavior, and the provision of analgesic effects [27]. It is important to recognize that while a patient is actively using buprenorphine, other opioid medications may not have any effect on pain control. It may be necessary to briefly stop buprenorphine and temporarily substitute it with a different type of opioid replacement therapy when the need for full opioid agonists for pain control is expected, such as the perioperative period.

When attempting to treat pain disorders in patients on concurrent opioid replacement therapy, many strongly advocate for non-opioid treatment modalities, including the use of tricyclic compounds, NSAIDs, anticonvulsants and topical agents. However, while detoxification and drug free modalities may seem appealing, this method has been shown to produce only a 5–10% success rate. The solution may lie somewhere in the middle. The FDA states that they "recognize the need to achieve balance between appropriate access and risk mitigation". In other words, treating professionals need to find a way to minimize potential adverse effects of unchecked and unsupervised access to opioid medications of patients known to have addictive disorder, while also respecting their right to access appropriate pain control [27].

Acute Pain Management of Patient with Active Addiction or in Recovery

The Joint Commission on Accreditation of Healthcare Organizations put forth various guidelines in their standards for pain management to assist healthcare providers with the task of providing appropriate pain treatment for patients who are actively addicted to opioids, or for those who are in recovery. A main point of these guidelines is the belief that acute pain should be managed with the same goals for all patients, regardless of addiction history [28]. It is recommended, however, that physicians have closer follow-up with patients who are in active addiction treatment or in recovery. To minimize abuse potential, it is important that physicians limit the opioid prescriber to one physician. Additionally, appropriate and adequate follow-up is warranted.

The Joint Commission on Accreditation of Healthcare Organization recommends an approach which includes prescribing the minimum effective dose of medications necessary to treat and manage the patient's pain, to wean periodically to reassess pain control, and to incorporate the use of non-psychotropic pain medications when possible. It is important to note that often individuals who have an opioid abuse history do not receive adequate pain control. This can produce a vicious cycle, wherein trying to control their pain, these individuals will self-medicate, thus increasing the risk of relapse.

Physicians can be most useful to their patients by being well-versed in the literature surrounding the treatment of patients with a history of opioid dependence. They should learn how to differentiate between *physical dependence*, *tolerance*, *substance abuse*, and *active* versus *recovering addiction*. Additionally, they should learn to recognize the difference between an individual seeking pain relief and drug-seeking behaviors, and to identify common physiologic adaptations that are seen with pain medications, including tolerance and dependence.

The goal of treating patients with acute pain who are in active addiction or recovery is to understand that adequate pain control is a priority. Appropriate history and physical examination should be performed to ensure that an effective multi-modal approach is employed. Furthermore, the lowest, most effective dose of an opioid (if indicated) should be utilized. Another useful recommendation by the Joint Commission on Accreditation of Healthcare Organizations is to aim for the provision of around the clock pain control. This is in contrast to providing pain medications on an "as-needed" basis only. This strategy aims to prevent the peaks and troughs that are common with as-needed pain medications and to reduce patient's overall discomfort and time spent seeking pain relief. The use of long-acting medications, with short acting medications for break-through pain, is encouraged and is the most commonly advocated regimen.

Historically, the choice of pain medication was based on the World Health Organization's stepladder approach for mild, moderate, and severe pain. Step 1, mild pain, can be treated with acetaminophen, non-steroidal anti-inflammatory drugs (NSAIDs), and cyclooxygenase-2 (COX-2) inhibitors. Step 2, moderate pain, can be treated with the same agents with the addition of a weak opioid such as codeine or hydrocodone. Step 3, severe pain, should be treated with strong opioids such as morphine, oxycodone, hydromorphone, or methadone. The caveat is that this ladder was originally created to treat patients with cancer-related pain, and it is becoming increasingly evident that a more multimodal approach that focuses specifically on each individual patient's needs is more effective.

Agonist-antagonist drugs such as pentazocine, nalbuphine, and butorphanol should be avoided in treating addicts who are actively abusing narcotics and those on opioid maintenance programs (i.e., methadone maintenance) because the agonist-antagonist drugs can precipitate an opioid withdrawal syndrome.

Additionally, it is important to note that patients with opioid addiction and tolerance may require larger opioid doses and more frequent dosing than opioid-naive patients. The best analgesia is achieved when withdrawal states and anxiety related to inadequate pain relief are prevented. For patients on methadone maintenance, methadone may be used at increased doses in addition to the daily methadone dose, however this must be arranged by the patient with their maintenance clinic to ensure single provider prescribing and dispensing. Methadone effectively provides pain relief between 4 and 6 hours, so inpatient treatment can be split into 3 or 4 doses daily, that is, dosing every 6 or 8 hours to take advantage of the analgesic window in addition to the maintenance component. Patients should also be encouraged to intensify support programs during the period of acute pain management to decrease risk of relapse [29].

Analgesic Response to Opioids in Patients with Addiction

Disproportionately high concentrations of all opioid receptors can be found in the amygdala, the nucleus accumbens and the caudate putamen in patients with addiction [4]. The predominant receptors most known for exerting analgesic effect are the μ opioid receptors [5]. Opioids are largely differentiated by their affinity for various opioid receptors – most notably μ, κ, and δ – and their ability to trigger varying neural responses as a result of their interaction. Opioid receptors belong to a class of G-protein receptors which activate inhibitory G proteins and in turn inhibit the cascade of signaling pathways that mediate pain signaling [30]. Newer studies allude to the idea that μ opioid receptors in the setting of repeated agonist interaction are essentially desensitized and uncoupled. This leads to a blunted analgesic effect and explains the phenomenon of tolerance to opioids in the setting of addiction or repeated use in general [31].

Observations of the cellular neuroadaptations to chronic opioids leading to tolerance, withdrawal, and addiction note the theory of receptor tolerance playing a huge role in diminishing analgesic response to opioids in patients with addiction. Contributions from both decreased cell surface expression of μ opioid receptors and decreased efficacy of agonist coupling to the receptors in chronic opioid users lead to decreased potency of agonist effect on receptors Christie et al. [52]. In essence, altered binding to and response of opioid receptors presents a dual challenge in patients battling addiction; the analgesic response is blunted requiring higher dosing which in turn reinforces the reward pathway. With continued chronic high dose use, efforts to ameliorate long term pain after a history opioid abuse can prove to be futile due to established systemic tolerance to opioids.

Another phenomenon that limits analgesic response to opioids in patients with addiction includes increased sensitivity to pain stimuli, known as opioid induced hyperalgesia (OIH). The molecular mechanisms behind OIH likely involve neuroplastic changes involving both the peripheral and central nervous system and activation of N-methyl-D-aspartate (NMDA) receptors in facilitating the nociceptive pathway [32]. Multiple observations confirm the hypothesis that OIH is caused by chronic opioid exposure with mixed support for the hypothesis of the development of OIH after acute perioperative opioid exposure [32]. There is no cure for OIH, and some debate as to its prevalence, though most recommendations focus on minimizing or stopping opioid exposure [33]. Unlike opioid tolerance, OIH cannot be overcome with increasing opioid doses as it is a complex sensitization of pain [34]. Options in minimizing the risk of OIH include using specific agents that are NMDA receptor antagonists, providing combination therapy with non-specific NSAIDs or COX-2 inhibitors if treating inflammatory pain, using non-opioid medications such as antidepressants and anticonvulsants when treating neuropathic pain, and utilizing a rotation to a different and longer-acting opioid if required to yield analgesia [32].

Risks and Benefits of Opioid Use in Treatment of Chronic/Cancer Pain in Patients with Substance Use Disorder or Addiction

As of 2010, the prevalence of chronic pain in adults in the United States is estimated to be above 40% [5]. As of 2013, more than a third of the 44,000 drug overdose deaths were the result of pharmaceutical opioids while heroin accounted for only 19% [5]. Opioids not only mediate the attenuation of cancer/chronic pain signals by exerting analgesic effects, they simultaneously trigger the reward pathway in the brain. This dual activity proves to be the biggest challenge in managing analgesic responses to opioids in patients with addiction. It is hypothesized that in individuals suffering from pain syndromes and addiction, the experience of pain is worsened in the setting of addiction [35]. In addition, there is strong suggestion that patients with history of addiction to other substances with exposure to opioids are at an increased risk for opioid abuse or relapse [11]. With this in mind, it is imperative that a multimodal approach be utilized to help tackle the challenges of managing their pain.

The tendency of health care professionals to "undermedicate" opioid analgesics in general was termed "opiophobia" [36]. Unfortunately, in the setting of addiction these fears can become exaggerated and inadequate treatment of pain, via opioids or otherwise, can lead to relapse [37]. A study published in 2004 observed the experience of chronic and severe pain in patients undergoing methadone therapy and noted that pain played a major role in relapsing into continued substance abuse [38]. In contrast, a 2001 study following 6 patients receiving methadone maintenance therapy for opioid abuse who were being treated for cancer related pain and found no evidence of relapse in those patients [39]. In part because of the concerns regarding opioid therapy in these patients, there is a paucity of randomized controlled studies looking at the use of opioids for chronic pain in patients with substance abuse/addiction.

With more attention focused on the adverse effects of chronic opioid use as a national health crisis, more efforts are being made to approach pain management from a multimodal approach [40]. Acute pain management should be initiated with non-opioid modalities including interventional techniques, NSAIDs and low dose short-acting opioids which can later be titrated down as the acute episodes of pain improve [41]. The benefits of leaning towards non-opioid modalities include fewer adverse side effects and a greater safety profile [42]. Furthermore, an interdisciplinary approach to pain management is often more effective in managing both the psychological and physiologic aspect of an addict's pain syndrome [43].

Needs of Special Populations or Treatment Groups of Patients with Addiction

A study of over 57 million births in the USA between 1998 and 2011 found a 127% increase in the rate of women diagnosed with opioid abuse or dependence at the time of delivery [44]. In light of the rise of opioid abuse in this population, the U.S. Congress passed the Protecting Our Infants Act of 2015 which mandates that the Department of Health and Human Services assess and offer recommendations on treatments for women who abuse opioids during pregnancy. Many of the varying needs and concerns of this subpopulation of opioid abusing parturients include, but are not limited to, managing opioid treatment of both non-obstetric and obstetric pain, and limiting potential for relapse to addiction for patients on opioid maintenance. There is no clear consensus from the American College of Obstetricians and Gynecologists (ACOG) regarding standard of care, however,

there is recognition of the utility for methadone, buprenorphine and buprenorphine/naloxone in managing addiction during pregnancy [45]. At no point has it been recommended that pregnant patients with addiction undergoing opioid-assisted therapy be denied opioids for adequate pain relief. Furthermore, according to a joint committee opinion by ACOG and the American Society of Addiction (ASAM), neuraxial modalities for anesthesia continue to remain appropriate for management of pain in labor or delivery, even in the setting of opioid abuse, dependence and addiction in pregnancy [46]. The other challenge to be mindful of is the titration of appropriate opioid analgesic dosages. A study observing post-cesarean delivery pain in the setting of patients with addiction using buprenorphine noted a 47% increase in opioid requirement versus patients not using buprenorphine [47]. Abstinence from maintenance opioids can prove to be more detrimental than beneficial, with possible relapse.

For patients receiving maintenance methadone or buprenorphine therapy who are admitted to a hospital, there are common provider concerns that alter care, including: (1). The idea that maintenance opioid agonist therapy (methadone or buprenorphine) provides adequate analgesia alone, (2). Belief that use of opioids in the acute setting leads to addiction relapse, (3). Fear that additive effects of opioid analgesics in conjunction with opioid replacement therapy will cause respiratory depression, and (4). Physician concern about being manipulated [37]. Patients should be treated with an understanding that their pain is separate from the addiction. Retrospective chart reviews allude to the difficulty in managing pain in patients on methadone maintenance therapy, with some requiring more medication than anticipated and others leaving the hospital against medical advice [48, 49]. For hospitalized patients undergoing methadone maintenance therapy, it is recommended that their respective programs be notified. The purpose of this is to confirm their daily methadone dose, and to also make them aware of any administration of opioid analgesics, when indicated, which may or may not be detectable by drug testing [37]. In addition, there should be no cessation of their daily opioid agonist therapy unless medically indicated. Furthermore, patients should be reassured that their pain will be managed with a clear discussion of goals between the provider and patient in order to eliminate any anxiety about their pain.

Legal, Regulatory, Reimbursement Issues Limiting Access to Care for Patients with Pain and Addiction

Legal concerns for the use of pain medications in addicted patients can be managed effectively with clear documentation of the indication for the medication, dose, dosing interval, and amount provided [50]. One major concern for providers is discerning patients in need of pain relief from those looking to satiate their addiction. The legal consequence for overprescribing opioids tends to be a major impedance in providing proper pain management for patients in need. The Uniform Controlled Substance Act of 1970 is a federal law which regulates the use of opioids when used for purposes of opioid detoxification and/or maintenance, but not for pain relief [50]. In addition, the Psychotropic Substances Act of 1978, an amendment to the Controlled Substances Act, limits restrictions on opioid prescriptions for pain relief. In 2015, President Obama aimed to address the public health crisis of prescription drug abuse and the heroin epidemic by issuing a memorandum to federal departments and agencies which mandated increased prescriber training. Additionally, to improve access to treatment for addiction in patients with opioid use disorders, President Obama instructed federal departments and agencies to review barriers to medication-assisted treatment for these conditions [51]. The U.S. Department of Health and Human Services separately issued an initiative to address the opioid abuse problem by focusing on decreasing opioid overdoses and decreasing mortality associated with abuse.

References

1. Benson H, Raja S, Liu S, Fishman S, Cohen S. Essentials of pain medicine. 3rd ed. Amsterdam: Elsevier Saunders; 2011.
2. American Psychiatric Association Substance Related and Addictive Disorders. 2013. https://dsm.psychiatryonline.org/doi/10.1176/appi.books.9780890425596.dsm16. Accesssed 8 May 2018.
3. Kalivas PW. The glutamate homeostasis hypothesis of addiction. Nat Rev Neurosci. 2009;10:561–72.
4. Mistry CJ, Bawor M, Desai D, Marsh DC, Samaan Z. Genetics of opioid dependence: a review of the genetic contribution to opioid dependence. Curr Psychiatr Rev. 2014;10(2):156–67.
5. Volkow ND, McLellan AT. Opioid abuse in chronic pain–misconceptions and mitigation strategies. N Engl J Med. 2016;374:1253–63.
6. Elman I, Borsook D. Common brain mechanisms of chronic pain and addiction. Neuron. 2016;89:11–36.
7. Chang L, Alicata D. Structural and metabolic brain changes in the striatum associated with methamphetamine abuse. Addiction. 2007;102(Supp 1):16–32.
8. Hashmi JA, Baliki MN. Shape-shifting pain: chronification of back pain shifts brain representation from nociceptive to emotional circuits. Brain. 2013;136(pt 9):2751–68.
9. Vasson-Presseau E, Tetrault E. Corticolimbic anatomic characteristics predetermine risk for chronic pain. Brain. 2016;139(pt 7):1958–70.
10. Saxon AJ, et al. Genetic determinants of addiction to opioids and cocaine. Harv Rev Psychiatry. 2005;13:218–46.
11. Savage SR, Horvath R. Opioid therapy of pain. In: Ries R, editor. Principles of addiction medicine. 4th ed. Philadelphia: Lippincott Williams & Wilkins; 2009. p. 1329–53.
12. Rockvill MD. Substance abuse and mental health administration office of applied studies. Results from the 2007 national survey on drug use and health: national findings. 2008. NSDUH series H-34, DHHS publication No. SMA 08-4343.
13. Rudd RA, Seth P, David F, Scholl L. Increases in drug and opioid-involved overdose deaths — United States, 2010–2015. MMWR Morb Mortal Wkly Rep. 2016;65:1445–52.
14. Ling W, et al. Prescription opiod abuse, pain and addiction: clinical issues and implications. Drug Alcohol Rev. 2011;30:300–5.
15. Weaver M, Schnoll S. Abuse liability in opioid therapy for pain treatment in patients with an addiction history. Clin J Pain. 2002;18:S61–9.
16. Edlund MH, et al. Do users of regularly prescribed opioids have higher rates of substance abuse problems than nonusers? Pain Med. 2007;8:647–56.
17. Passik SD, et al. The interface between pain and drug abuse and the evolution of strategies to optimize pain management while minimizing drug abuse. Exp Clin Psychopharmacol. 2008;16:400–4.
18. Webster LR, Webster RM. Predicting aberrant behaviors in opioid-treated patients: preliminary validation of the Opioid Risk Tool. Pain Med. 2005;6(6):432–42.
19. Seymour M, Pattersen S. Estimating the prevalence of chronic pain in a given geographical area. J Observational Pain Med. 2014;1(3):15–19.
20. Lohman D, Shleifer R, et al. Access to pain treatment as a human right. BMC Med. 2010;8:8.
21. Woods B. A comprehensive approach to pain management. Addiction Professional. 2011;9(1):14–6.
22. Gourlay DL, Heit HA, Almahrezi A. Universal precautions in pain medicine: a rational approach to the treatment of chronic pain. Pain Med. 2005;6(2):107–12.
23. Peppin JF, Passik SD, Couto JE. Recommendations for urine drug monitoring as a component of opioid therapy in the treatment of chronic pain. Pain Med. 2012;13(7):886–96.
24. Nadelmann E, LaSalle L. Two steps forward, one step back: current harm reduction policy and politics in the United States. Harm Reduct J. 2017;12(1):37.
25. Chou R. Clinical guidelines from the APS/AAPS on the use of chronic opioid therapy in chronic non-caner pain: what are the key messages for clinical practice? Pol Arch Med Wewn. 2009;119(7–8):469–77.
26. Heit HA. Buprenorphine: new tricks with an old molecule for pain management. Clin J Pain. 2008;24(2):93–7.
27. Ling W, Mooney L. Prescription opioid abuse, pain and addiction: clinical issues and implications. Drug Alcohol Rev. 2011;30(3):300–5.
28. Simmons JC. Pain management: new initiatives arise to provide quality care. Qual Lett Healthc Lead. 2001;13(6):2–11.
29. Prater CD, Zylstra RG. Successful pain management for the recovering addicted patient. Prim Care Companion J Clin Psychiatry. 2002;4(4):125–31.
30. Al-Hasani R, Bruchas MR. Molecular mechanisms of opioid receptor-dependent signaling and behavior. Anesthesiology. 2011;115:1363–81.
31. Waldhoer M, Bartlett SE, Whistler JL. Opioid receptors. Annu Rev Biochem. 2004;73:953–90.
32. Lee M, Silverman S, Hansen H, et al. A comprehensive review of opioid induced hyperalgesia. Pain Physician. 2011;14:145–61.
33. Arout CA, Edens E, Petrakis IL, et al. Targeting opioid-induced hyperalgesia in clinical treatment: neurobiological considerations. CNS Drugs. 2015;29:465.
34. Silverman SM. Opioid induced hyperalgesia: clinical implications for the pain practitioner. Pain Physician. 2009;12(3):679–84.
35. Savage SR, Schofferman J. Pharmacological therapies for drug and alcohol addictions. In: Miller N, Gold M, editors. Pharmacological therapies of pain in drug and alcohol addictions. New York: Dekker; 1995. p. 373–409.
36. Morgan JP. American opiophobia: customary underutilization of opioid analgesics. Adv Alcohol Subst Abuse. 1985 Fall–1986 Winter;5(1–2):163–73.

37. Alford DP, Compton P, Samet JH. Acute pain management for patients receiving maintenance methadone or buprenorphine therapy. Ann Intern Med. 2006;144(2):127–34.

38. Karasz A, Zallman L, Berg K, Gourevitch M, Selwyn P, Arnsten JH. The experience of chronic severe pain in patients undergoing methadone maintenance treatment. J Pain Symptom Manag. 2004;28(5):517–25.

39. Manfredi PL, Gonzales GR, Cheville AL, Kornick C, Payne R. Methadone analgesia in cancer pain patients on chronic methadone maintenance therapy. J Pain Symptom Manag. 2001;21(2):169–74.

40. Kelly MA. Addressing the opioid epidemic with multimodal pain management. Am J Orthop (Belle Mead NJ). 2016;45(7):S6–8.

41. Mehta V, Langford R. Acute pain management in opioid dependent patients. Rev Pain. 2009;3(2):10–4.

42. Savarese JJ, Tabler NG. Multimodal analgesia as an alternative to the risks of opioid monotherapy in surgical pain management. J Healthc Risk Manag. 2017;37:24–30.

43. Hampel C, Schenk M, Göbel H, et al. Pain therapy in addicted patients. Schmerz. 2006;20(5):445–59.

44. Arnaudo CL, Andraka-Christou B, Allgood K. Psychiatric comorbidities in pregnant women with opioid use disorders: prevalence, impact, and implications for treatment. Curr Addict Rep. 2017;4(1):1–13.

45. Laslo J, Brunner J-M, Burns D, et al. An overview of available drugs for management of opioid abuse during pregnancy. Matern Health Neonatol Perinatol. 2017;3:4.

46. The American College of Obstetricians and Gynecologists Women's Health Care Physician. Committee opinion. Number 524, May 2012.

47. Jones HE, Johnson RE, Milio L. Post-cesarean pain management of patients maintained on methadone or buprenorphine. Am J Addict. 2006;15:258–9.

48. Rowley D, McLean S, O'Gorman A, et al. Review of cancer pain management in patients receiving maintenance methadone therapy. Am J Hosp Palliat Care. 2011;28:183.

49. Hines S, Theodorou S, Williamson A, et al. Management of acute pain in methadone maintenance therapy in-patients. Drug Alcohol Rev. 2008;27:519.

50. Prater CD, Zylstra RG, Miller KE. Successful pain management for the recovering addicted patient. Prim Care Companion J Clin Psychiatry. 2002;4:125–31.

51. The White House: Office of the Press Secretary. Obama administration marks progress in substance use disorder prevention, treatment, recovery, and research. Nov 2016. Retrieved from https://obamawhitehouse.archives.gov/the-press-office/2016/11/30/fact-sheet-obama-administration-marks-progress-substance-use-disorder. 20 Aug 2017.

52. Christie MJ. Cellular neuroadaptations to chronic opioids: tolerance, withdrawal and addiction. Br J Pharmacol. 2008;154(2):384–96. https://doi.org/10.1038/bjp.2008.100.

Pain Relief in Areas of Deprivation and Conflict

Sam Nia and Jason H. Epstein

Introduction

Pain management is a subspecialty practice predicated on the use of medicines, physical therapy and interventional approaches, many of which require significant resources. In areas of deprivation and conflict, access to this care can be limited. This chapter seeks to elucidate the unique challenges facing pain management in the developing world and in areas plagued by conflict. Major causes of pain, barriers to the delivery of pain management, as well as insights into how pain management may be delivered in these areas are explored in the sections below. Additional considerations should be given to specific regional, cultural, and religious beliefs and how this factors into the delivery of healthcare.

Worldwide Causes of Pain

Causes of pain in the developing world are similar to those in the developed world, but with an increased prevalence of advanced cancer, HIV/AIDS, diet or exposure related neuropathy as well as pain related to trauma and torture. While these disease states are not restricted to the developing world, certain factors increase the risks for poorly controlled pain in these patient populations.

Cancer

New rates of cancer in developing nations are estimated at 14 million annually and projected to increase 70% by 2020. Of those patients, more than 60% are estimated to suffer from pain during the course of disease or treatment. Some causes of this disproportionately high level of pain are due to delays in diagnosis due to lack of cancer screening. In developing countries, it is observed that males most commonly succumb to liver and stomach cancers and females to cervical cancer [1]. The cancer burden in Africa has been growing, which constitutes about 17% of Africa's non-communicable disease (NCD) mortality rate. Many of these cancer deaths are attributed to preventable factors such as tobacco use, low hepatitis B vaccination rates and lack of physical activity in urban areas. As mortality rates improve, environmental influences such as carcinogen exposure have been increasingly implicated [2].

HIV/AIDS

HIV/AIDS continues to be a growing problem in the developing world and upwards of 60% of those diagnosed will experience pain during the course of their illness. The Joint United Nations Program on HIV/ AIDS (UNAIDS) has estimated 22.4 million HIV-infected people and 1.4 million deaths in 2008 [2, 3]. A separate study demonstrated that up to 94% of HIV programs in sub-Saharan Africa report challenges in managing pain in this patient population. The largest issues reported were drug availability and lack of providers [4]. Pain secondary to HIV/AIDS is often overlooked compared to other pain causes. A study of Uganda's palliative care programs describe a facility where the palliative care nurse only covers the cancer and gynecology wards, leaving HIV/AIDS patients with decreased access to services [5].

Neuropathic Pain

Associations also exist between individuals of lower socioeconomic standing, illiteracy, and chronic neuropathic pain symptoms, often leading to under-reporting. In 2013, Harifi

S. Nia
Department of Anesthesiology UMASS Memorial Healthcare, Worcester, MA, USA

J. H. Epstein (✉)
Department of Anesthesiology, James J Peters Veterans Affairs Medical Center, Bronx, NY, USA
e-mail: jhe2001@med.cornell.edu

© Springer Nature Switzerland AG 2019
Y. Khelemsky et al. (eds.), *Academic Pain Medicine*, https://doi.org/10.1007/978-3-030-18005-8_48

et al. conducted a telephone survey of over 5000 random individuals in Morocco and concluded that chronic pain with neuropathic symptoms was historically underestimated in that third-world country [6].

Trauma

In war-torn regions, conflict saps resources from economic, governmental and social infrastructure. Treatment for traumatic injuries along with loss of productivity that occurs can impose significant epidemiological and economic hardship. While very limited data exists for chronic pain complaints during armed conflict, Cohen et al. reported that of 162 US soldiers medically evacuated from the theater of combat, the most common diagnosis was lumbar herniated disc (24%) and only 17% were injured during battle [7]. This further highlights the fact that much of the chronic pain seen in areas of conflict is not necessarily caused by traumatic injury.

Torture

According to Amnesty International's 2009 findings, which document the state of civil rights in 157 separate countries, fully half of all countries surveyed carried out systematic torture. It is unfortunate to note that of those, the most universally advanced "G-20" countries continue to employ institutionalized physical torture. Nonetheless, exposure to torture is still most likely to be encountered in areas of conflict and deprivation. When considering the impact of torture on chronic pain worldwide, it is worth considering that recent figures suggest that there are in excess of 500,000 survivors currently living as refugees in the United States [8].

A Danish study noted a predominance of male victims, but this may not account for under-reporting due to stigmas surrounding forced sexual contact perpetrated against both males and females [8]. The sequelae of torture for survivors are numerous and often result in chronic pain ranging from specific inflicted wounds to more generalized headache syndromes and musculoskeletal pain. Physical symptoms are sadly only a portion of the burden these survivors must carry, as it has been shown that psychiatric complaints are also much higher amongst those individuals.

Torture is perpetrated against individuals for a variety of reasons including extracting information and establishing institutionalized fear and intimidation. Whatever the reason for carrying out torture, the victims often suffer on an emotional, cognitive and physical basis. Christo et al. reported that while the most common form of physical torture is blunt trauma, other injuries from torture methods such as penetrating injuries, suspension, electric shock, asphyxiation, removal of tissue, sensory deprivation, sexual torture, humiliation and genital mutilation are also carried out throughout the world [8]. Pain practitioners dealing with the results of torture must make every effort to be responsible and sensitive in uncovering the mechanism of torture a patient has experienced to better address the patient's specific pain syndrome. Furthermore, addressing co-morbid psychiatric issues of PTSD, depression and anxiety must also be included as part of the pain management plan.

Variability of Availability and Access to Adequate Pain Treatment Worldwide

The issue of addressing pain management on a global scale was initially addressed by the World Health Organization by way of their Cancer Pain Analgesia Ladder first published in 1986 [9]. In 2010, Lohman et al., characterized some of the barriers that lead to the variability and availability of pain management around the world. These include difficulties putting drug supply systems in place, failure to enact policies on pain and palliative treatment, poor training of healthcare workers, restrictive drug control regulations, fear of legal action against healthcare workers and unnecessarily high cost of treatment [10].

Failure of Governments to Create Functioning Drug Supply Systems

In 1961, the Single Convention on Narcotic Drugs put forth a system for regulating supply and demand of narcotics including pain medications. This is overseen by the International Narcotics Control Board (INCB). Individual governments must submit estimates for what controlled substances, such as morphine, that may be needed; however, many governments do not have adequate systems in place to accurately estimate the requirement of pain medications, or cannot efficiently distribute and dispense these medications once in possession of them. For example, the West African country of Burkina Faso estimated a total national requirement of 49 grams of Morphine for the entirety of 2009. Estimates for terminal cancer or end-stage AIDS patients alone in that region are 70 mg morphine over a 90-day period. Therefore, the narcotic estimate submitted by the government for an entire year was an amount that would be expected to provide pain control for a total of eight palliative patients for 3 months [10].

Failure to Enact Pain Treatment and Palliative Care Policies

Lohman et al. reported that the World Health Organization identified an inadequacy in policies addressing pain management and palliative care in public health initiatives on three separate occasions, in 1996, 2000, and 2002. A lack of distinct pain management and palliative care treatment guidelines as a component of HIV/AIDS or cancer treatment public initiatives was also identified [10].

Poor Training of Healthcare Workers

A 69-country survey performed by the Worldwide Palliative Care Alliance reported that many healthcare workers were not educated on the use of opioids in pain management during their medical training across Latin America, Asia, and Africa, (82%, 71% and 39% respectively). Furthermore, additional studies have observed that many healthcare workers in Africa report insufficient education on pain management and palliative care [10].

Restrictive Drug Control Regulations and Practices

In some countries, only oncologists may prescribe opioids and only for end-stage cancer pain management. To this point, the Worldwide Palliative Care Alliance put forth data in 2007 that showed that in Peru, Kyrgyzstan, Honduras, portions of India and Mongolia, only palliative care specialists and oncologists are legally allowed to prescribe opioids [10]. This practice restricts the number of providers as well as the diagnoses that qualify, notably patients with diseases that still carry stigma, such as AIDS.

Healthcare Workers' Fear of Legal Penalties

Criminal justice systems vary widely across the globe and there is little standardization of what constitutes legitimate medical care when it comes to use of controlled pain medication and what might be construed as illicit activity. As a result, many practitioners prefer to avoid prescribing pain medications and may go so far as to not even address pain at all. It is notable that prosecution of physicians for inappropriate opioid prescribing has increased in frequency as well as publicity, especially in the United States [10].

High Cost of Pain Treatment

Supply, transport, taxation, and distribution are common issues limiting the availability of pain medications. The most successful model to combat these barriers has been for countries to produce and manufacture their own medications. India is the clearest example of this approach and supplies many of the medications for its neighbors as well. A 2003 study describes the monthly cost of morphine for a cancer patient as roughly $10 in India and $254 in Argentina. Similar types of initiatives have been successful worldwide, such as in Uganda where the government financed an operation designed to produce a morphine solution which could be distributed cheaply around the country if needed. Vietnam has a similar system in place in which the government may commission state and other pharmaceutical entities to manufacture low-cost morphine formulations on an as-needed basis [10].

Spectrum of Providers Caring for Patients with Pain Worldwide

In the United States, pain management is a multidisciplinary specialty which draws physicians from various backgrounds. Furthermore, many specialties practice elements of pain management. This diverse knowledge-base at the medical subspecialty level allows for scientific, high-level decision making and delivery of care. In areas of deprivation, many regions struggle to provide even basic medical care to the population and as such, tasks relating to pain management are often relegated to non-physicians with varying training or knowledge-base in the field. In 2014, Song, et al. reported that nurses were often the first and only providers involved in the evaluation and treatment of pain in developing countries [11]. Downing describes three main types of models of palliative care delivery employed in sub-Saharan Africa, specifically in the nations of Kenya and Malawi. These include the specialist service model, the district hospital model, and the community model, all of which utilize a variety of caregivers. These palliative care provider roles would range from physicians, to nurses, to patient family members and religious practitioners in the local community [12]. The concept of including non-medically trained personnel to help manage pain has a long historical precedent in Africa arising from the use of community health worker (CHW) in the late apartheid South Africa [13]. These CHWs are defined as a heterogenous group of lay health workers without any formal medical or healthcare education who are chosen within a community to perform functions related to healthcare delivery. These CHWs were very popular in South Africa at around the time of the fall of apartheid and may be resurging in recent times as the utility of preventive care is being evaluated around the world. This consideration to extend medical care responsibilities beyond the role of physicians and nurses is evidenced by the 1998 study by Gilbert et al. who explored the expansion of the pharmacist's role in the delivery of medical care in South Africa [13].

Limitations of Education, Training and Knowledge of Pain and Its Treatment; Variability of Beliefs and Communication About Pain

Not only are physical resources limited in the developing world, but intangible resources such as medical and patient-care training are also lacking. Doctors in these regions often receive little training in pain management and individual nurses have been known to be responsible for wards of up to 50 patients in sub-Saharan Africa [14]. These overtaxed nurses may not be available to administer analgesic agents or may be uneducated on side effects prompting an aversion to potential harm caused by these medications. Over time, these situations may lead to non-intervention being the norm, causing patients to believe that pain should be expected from their condition and suffer quietly instead of seeking out pain relief.

In other parts of the world, legal barriers exist which preclude the distribution of opioid-based pain medications. Vranken et al. demonstrated that in 11 out of 12 Eastern European countries, including Hungary, Latvia, Lithuania, Poland, Serbia, Slovakia and Slovenia, overly restrictive legal provisions were in place that led to prohibitive requirements for dispensing. This in turn, was thought to lead to compromised pain management delivery in these countries [15].

Cost and availability of pain medication are also barriers to effective and timely pain management, as shown by De Lima et al. through their study which stratified cost as well as availability of various analgesic agents across 26 countries. They found that these medications were more readily available in nations with a higher Gross National Income (GNI). In addition, injectable and sustained release oral morphine was the most commonly available opioid medication, while methadone was found to be the most affordable [16].

It stands to reason that in nations with a lower GNI, funding for medical training is similarly diminished. This leads to less pain management advocacy which in turn leads to less legislative reform and social outreach to promote public awareness of pain management issues. Decreased awareness of the issues surrounding pain management leads to misperceptions about the legitimacy and utility of pain management as a specialty. Coupled with increased rates of terminal diagnoses that are associated with poor pain control, these areas of deprivation are caught in a downward spiral as they fall farther and farther behind in providing adequate pain control.

Research: Importance in Extending Pain Care Worldwide; Ethical and Political Issues

In their 2007 paper, Brennan, et al. describe an "inflection point" in the global field of pain management as the understanding of the multivariate nature of the specialty continues to evolve. That is to say that the field is now framed in a number of different contexts including as an ethical issue, an issue of fundamental human rights, as well as a legal issue [17]. These characterizations of pain management have brought awareness and have also served to define many of the barriers against which pain management must advance, including cultural, societal, religious and political [17].

Pain management in the developing world is sometimes overlooked in favor of prioritizing saving a patient's life; this has left a glaring gap insofar as taking into account maintaining the quality of the life saved. However, in recent years, more emphasis is being placed on pain management as a basic human right [17–19].

Societal and religious beliefs can also affect the delivery of care. Consider the resistance against the use of peripartum analgesics or nerve blocks due to the belief that pain during childbirth is biblically preordained [17]. Other societal notions of withholding pain management may be due to the impulse to prove "machismo" and that tolerating discomfort and pain is a sign of one's strength and fortitude.

According to Size et al., one of the most effective measures to take to help pain management in the developing world is to increase awareness and training. They cite as example that a majority of anesthesia providers in developing countries do not even own an anesthesia textbook [14]. As such, prior-edition publications have been circulated as a low-cost solution to impart practical information to anesthesia and pain practitioners in difficult to access places. As globalization and technology steadily march forward, the internet can provide a conduit through which these isolated practitioners may seek answers to their queries and there is anticipation that distance learning can quickly and effectively disseminate information to even the most remote corners of the globe. Face-to-face teaching is also an invaluable tool and many charities have begun to emphasize education on mission trips to further improve training in areas of pain management.

Other Clinical States; Pain Relief in Areas of Deprivation and Conflict

A newfound emphasis on pain management combined with the United States' decades-long military involvement in Iraq and Afghanistan during the global war on terror has created some interesting opportunities for research in the field. These conflicts have been noted for historically low mortality rates but high rates of non-fatal, serious injury often as a result of improvised explosive devices which leave behind particularly devastating injuries.

In these situations, appropriate, safe, and timely pain management has come to be seen as the difference between life and death, playing a crucial role in stabilizing a patient after violent and extreme injury. In looking to improving outcomes in this urgent timeframe, long-standing hospital pain management techniques such as single-shot and continuous regional anesthetics have been adapted for use on the battlefield [20].

The use of oral transmucosal fentanyl citrate in the prehospital setting on the battlefield has been shown to provide a noninvasive and safe pain management strategy [21]. Ketamine, a potent NMDA receptor antagonist, has been used successfully at the time of injury in combat and has been shown to effectively and safely reduce pain on the battlefield [22]. The increasing prevalence of the use of this medication in combination with morphine was demonstrated in a 2015 prospective multicenter observational pre-hospital combat study [23].

References

1. Saini S, Bhatnagar S. Cancer pain management in developing countries. Indian J Palliat Care. 2016;22(4):373–7.
2. McCormack VA, Schuz J. Africa's growing cancer burden: environmental and occupational contributions. Cancer Epidemiol. 2012;36(1):1–7.
3. Harding R, Powell RA, Kiyange F, Downing J, Mwangi-Powell F. Provision of pain- and symptom-relieving drugs for HIV/AIDS in sub-Saharan Africa. J Pain Symptom Manag. 2010;40(3):405–15.
4. Harding R, Stewart K, Marconi K, O'Neill JF, Higginson IJ. Current HIV/AIDS end-of-life care in sub-Saharan Africa: a survey of models, services, challenges and priorities. BMC Public Health. 2003;3:33.
5. Logie DE, Harding R. An evaluation of a morphine public health programme for cancer and AIDS pain relief in sub-Saharan Africa. BMC Public Health. 2005;5:82.
6. Harifi G, Amine M, Ait Ouazar M, Boujemaoui A, Ouilki I, Rekkab I, et al. Prevalence of chronic pain with neuropathic characteristics in the Moroccan general population: a national survey. Pain Med. 2013,14(2).287–92.
7. Cohen SP, Griffith S, Larkin TM, Villena F, Larkin R. Presentation, diagnoses, mechanisms of injury, and treatment of soldiers injured in Operation Iraqi Freedom: an epidemiological study conducted at two military pain management centers. Anesth Analg. 2005;101(4):1098–103, table of contents.
8. Carinci AJ, Mehta P, Christo PJ. Chronic pain in torture victims. Curr Pain Headache Rep. 2010;14(2):73–9.
9. Jadad AR, Browman GP. The WHO analgesic ladder for cancer pain management. Stepping up the quality of its evaluation. JAMA. 1995;274(23):1870–3.
10. Lohman D, Schleifer R, Amon JJ. Access to pain treatment as a human right. BMC Med. 2010;8:8.
11. Song W, Eaton LH, Gordon DB, Hoyle C, Doorenbos AZ. Evaluation of evidence-based nursing pain management practice. Pain Manag Nurs. 2015;16(4):456–63.
12. Downing J, Grant L, Leng M, Namukwaya E. Understanding models of palliative care delivery in sub-Saharan Africa: learning from programs in Kenya and Malawi. J Pain Symptom Manag. 2015;50(3):362–70.
13. van Ginneken N, Lewin S, Berridge V. The emergence of community health worker programmes in the late apartheid era in South Africa: an historical analysis. Soc Sci Med. 2010;71(6):1110–8.
14. Size M, Soyannwo OA, Justins DM. Pain management in developing countries. Anaesthesia. 2007;62(Suppl 1):38–43.
15. Vranken MJ, Mantel-Teeuwisse AK, Junger S, Radbruch L, Lisman J, Scholten W, et al. Legal barriers in accessing opioid medicines: results of the ATOME quick scan of national legislation of eastern European countries. J Pain Symptom Manag. 2014;48(6):1135–44.
16. De Lima L, Pastrana T, Radbruch L, Wenk R. Cross-sectional pilot study to monitor the availability, dispensed prices, and affordability of opioids around the globe. J Pain Symptom Manag. 2014;48(4):649–59 e1.
17. Brennan F, Carr DB, Cousins M. Pain management: a fundamental human right. Anesth Analg. 2007;105(1):205–21.
18. Cousins MJ, Brennan F, Carr DB. Pain relief: a universal human right. Pain. 2004;112(1–2):1–4.
19. Lohman D. Pain care as a human right. Pain Pract. 2014;14(3):199–203.
20. Buckenmaier CC 3rd, Rupprecht C, McKnight G, McMillan B, White RL, Gallagher RM, et al. Pain following battlefield injury and evacuation: a survey of 110 casualties from the wars in Iraq and Afghanistan. Pain Med. 2009;10(8):1487–96.
21. Wedmore IS, Kotwal RS, McManus JG, Pennardt A, Talbot TS, Fowler M, et al. Safety and efficacy of oral transmucosal fentanyl citrate for prehospital pain control on the battlefield. J Trauma Acute Care Surg. 2012;73(6 Suppl 5):S490–5.
22. Fisher AD, Rippee B, Shehan H, Conklin C, Mabry RL. Prehospital analgesia with ketamine for combat wounds: a case series. J Spec Oper Med. 2014;14(4):11–7.
23. Petz LN, Tyner S, Barnard E, Ervin A, Mora A, Clifford J, et al. Prehospital and en route analgesic use in the combat setting: a prospectively designed, multicenter, observational study. Mil Med. 2015;180(3 Suppl):14–8.

Correction to: Academic Pain Medicine

Yury Khelemsky, Anuj Malhotra, and Karina Gritsenko

Correction to:
Y. Khelemsky et al. (eds.), Academic Pain Medicine,
https://doi.org/10.1007/978-3-030-18005-8

The book was inadvertently published with incorrect authorships in Chapters 13, 14 and 47. It has been updated along with corresponding affiliation information as follows:

Chapter 13:
From "Karina Gritsenko" to "Ricardo Maturana, Andrew So, and Karina Gritsenko"

Ricardo Maturana
Albert Einstein College of Medicine, Montefiore Medical Center, Bronx, NY, USA

Andrew So
Albert Einstein College of Medicine, Montefiore Medical Center, Bronx, NY, USA

Karina Gritsenko
Department of Anesthesiology, Montefiore Medical Center and Albert Einstein College of Medicine, Bronx, NY, USA

Chapter 14:
From "Melinda Aquino" to "Chukwuemeka Okafor and Melinda Aquino"

Chukwuemeka Okafor
Forbes Hospital, Pittsburgh, Pennsylvania, USA

Melinda Aquino
Montefiore Medical Center, Albert Einstein College of Medicine, Bronx, NY, USA

Chapter 47:
From "Boleslav Kosharskyy" to "Guensley R. Delva, Jacquelyn K. Francis, and Demetri Koutsospyros"

Guensley R. Delva
Dartmouth Hitchcock Medical Center, Theodore Geisel School of Medicine, Lebanon, NH, USA

Jacquelyn K. Francis
Hackensack University Medical Center, Hackensack, NJ, USA

Demetri Koutsospyros
Department of Anesthesiology, Montefiore Medical Center, Bronx, NY, USA

The updated versions of the chapters can be found at
https://doi.org/10.1007/978-3-030-18005-8_13
https://doi.org/10.1007/978-3-030-18005-8_14
https://doi.org/10.1007/978-3-030-18005-8_47

Index